Handbook of
Echo-Doppler Interpretation

Dedication

Thank you . . .
Denise, for unwavering love and support
Katie, Kenny and Christian, for their love
Mom and Dad, for a nurturing disciplined childhood.
EKK

To Randall, all my love and eternal gratitude for always believing in me.
EFM

Thanks to my supportive and loving family—
Leslie, Sharon, Michael, Rachel, Danny and Matthew Alex.
GDP

Handbook of Echo-Doppler Interpretation

SECOND EDITION

Edmund Kenneth Kerut, MD FACC FASE
Director, Echocardiography Laboratory
Heart Clinic of Louisiana, Marrero, Louisiana
Clinical Associate Professor of Medicine, Division of Cardiology
Tulane University School of Medicine, New Orleans, Louisiana
Adjunct Professor of Engineering, Department of Agricultural and Biological Engineering
Mississippi State University, Mississippi State University, Mississippi
Cardiovascular Research Laboratory, Division of Cardiology, Department of Medicine
Louisiana State University Health Sciences Center, New Orleans, Louisiana

Elizabeth F. McIlwain, MHS, RDCS
Assistant Clinical Professor, Cardiopulmonary Science
School of Allied Health Professions
Louisiana State University Health Sciences Center
New Orleans, Louisiana

Gary D. Plotnick, MD, FACC
Professor of Medicine
Assistant Dean for Student Affairs
University of Maryland School of Medicine
Baltimore, Maryland

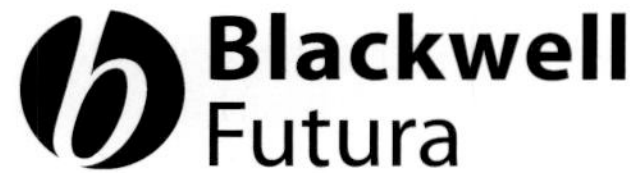

Blackwell Publishing, Inc./Futura Division, 3 West Main Street, Elmsford, New York 10523, USA
Blackwell Publishing, Inc., 350 Main Street, Malden, Massachusetts 02148-5020, USA
Blackwell Publishing Ltd, 9600 Garsington Road, Oxford OX4 2DQ, UK
Blackwell Science Asia Pty Ltd, 550 Swanston Street, Carlton, Victoria 3053, Australia

2 2007

ISBN 978-1-4051-1903-0

Library of Congress Cataloging-in-Publication Data
Kerut, Edmund Kenneth.
Handbook of echo-doppler interpretation / Edmund Kenneth Kerut, Elizabeth F. McIlwain, Gary D. Plotnick. — 2nd ed.
p. ; cm.
Includes bibliographical references and index.
ISBN 978-1-4051-1903-0
1. Doppler echocardiography.
[DNLM: 1. Echocardiography, Doppler. WG 141.5.E2 K41h 2004]
I. McIlwain, Elizabeth F. II. Plotnick, Gary D. III. Title.

RC683.5.U5K47 2004
616.1′207543—dc22 2003024704

A catalogue record for this title is available from the British Library

Acquisitions: Steve Korn
Production: Julie Elliott
Typesetter: Graphicraft Limited, Hong Kong, in 9/12pt Minion
Printed and bound in Singapore by C.O.S. Printers Pte Ltd

For further information on Blackwell Publishing, visit our website:
www.futuraco.com

The publisher's policy is to use permanent paper from mills that operate a sustainable forestry policy, and which has been manufactured from pulp processed using acid-free and elementary chlorine-free practices. Furthermore, the publisher ensures that the text paper and cover board used have met acceptable environmental accreditation standards.

Notice: The indications and dosages of all drugs in this book have been recommended in the medical literature and conform to the practices of the general community. The medications described do not necessarily have specific approval by the Food and Drug Administration for use in the diseases and dosages for which they are recommended. The package insert for each drug should be consulted for use and dosage as approved by the FDA. Because standards for usage change, it is advisable to keep abreast of revised recommendations, particularly those concerning new drugs.

Contents

Preface to the Second Edition

We wrote this second edition of the *Handbook* in an attempt to help physicians and sonographers learn practical and useful ultrasound concepts that can be applied daily in the echocardiography laboratory. Our goal is to help improve the quality of day-to-day echocardiographic studies as performed in the real world. We have broadly expanded subject content to serve as a study guide for both the physician preparing for the ASEeXAM and the sonographer studying for the RDCS or RCS examination. Addition of new subject matter and expanded discussion of all subjects covered in the first edition attempt to achieve this purpose. Over 550 photographs and illustrative drawings are included in this new edition.

The first two chapters present new subject topics, namely ultrasound physics and machine instrumentation. A section on fluid mechanics has been added within the third chapter to complement the discussion of hemodynamics. An extensive discussion of anatomy and the echo examination is then presented in Chapter 4. Chapters 5 and 6 discuss ventricular function, followed by Chapters 7 through 10 which cover various aspects of valvular disorders. Chapters 11 through 20 cover multiple topics of clinical relevance to the echocardiographer and include multiple images and drawings to illustrate points made within the text. Chapter 21 covers such divergent subjects as nonbacterial thrombotic endocarditis, drug related valvular disease, reliability of color Doppler assessment of valvular regurgitation and optimal timing of biventricular pacemakers using Doppler parameters.

We hope the reader will find the additional information and expanded discussion useful.

The Authors

List of Abbreviations

A atrial contraction causing late diastolic filling
A area
A anterior
A′ mitral annular velocity during atrial contraction
AA ascending aorta
AAA abdominal aortic aneurysm
Ac atrial contraction reversed flow in pulmonary vein
AC atrial contraction reversed flow in pulmonary vein
ACEi angiotensin converting enzyme inhibitor
ACUTE Assessment of Cardioversion Using Transesophageal Echocardiography [study]
A/D analog/digital
Adt mitral A wave deceleration time
AHA American Heart Association
AIDS acquired immunodeficiency syndrome
AIH aortic intramural hematoma
A_{jet} cross-sectional area of a color Doppler jet
AL anterior leaflet
ALPM anterolateral papillary muscle
Am TDE mitral annular motion late diastolic velocity
AML anterior mitral leaflet
Amv area of mitral valve orifice
Ao aorta
AO aorta
AQ acoustic quantification
AR aortic regurgitation
AR, Ar atrial contraction reversed flow in pulmonary veins
ARpeak peak velocity of aortic regurgitation by continuous wave Doppler
ARtvi TVI of an aortic regurgitant jet by continuous wave Doppler
ARVC arrhythmogenic right ventricular cardiomyopathy
AS aortic stenosis
ASA atrial septal aneurysm
ASD atrial septal defect
ASE American Society of Echocardiography
ASH asymmetric septal hypertrophy
AT acceleration time
AV atrioventricular
AV aortic valve
AVA aortic valve area
AVC aortic valve closure
AVD atrioventricular delay
AVco atrioventricular interval from closure to opening
AV_{long} programmed long sensed AV delay
AV_{short} programmed short sensed AV delay
AV_{opt} optimized AV programmed delay
AV_{TVI} TVI at the level of the aortic valve
$AV_{velocity}$ peak Doppler velocity at the level of the aortic valve
AVP aortic valve prolapse

BAV bicuspid aortic valve

c velocity of sound
CABG coronary artery bypass grafting
CCU coronary care unit
CHF congestive heart failure
CI cardiac index
Cm specific heat of tissue
CMP cardiomyopathy
CO cardiac output
COPD chronic obstructive pulmonary disease
CRT cathode ray tube
CS coronary sinus

CT	computerized axial tomography
CW	continuous wave Doppler
Cx	circumflex coronary artery
CXR	chest X-ray
d	distance
D	diastolic flow of pulmonary veins
2-D	two-dimensional
DA	descending aorta
dB	decibels
DGC	depth gain compensation
DI	dimensionless index
DIC	disseminated intravascular coagulation
DSC	digital scan convertor
DT	deceleration time
dyn	dyne
E	early diastolic filling
E′	mitral annular early velocity
E/A	ratio of E and A velocities
EBCT	electron beam computed tomography
ECG	electrocardiogram
EKG	electrocardiogram
EDV	end-diastolic volume
EF	ejection fraction
EI	eccentricity index
Em	TDE mitral annular motion early diastolic velocity
EOA	effective orifice area
EPSS	E-point septal separation
ER	emergency room
ERO	effective regurgitant orifice
ESV	end-systolic volume
ET	ejection time
EV	eustachian valve
EVA	effective valve area
F	force
f	frequency
FDA	Federal Drug Administration
FFT	fast Fourier transform
FR	frame rate
FS	fractional shortening
HCM	hypertrophic cardiomyopathy
HF	heart failure
HIFU	high intensity focused ultrasound
HOCM	hypertrophic obstructive cardiomyopathy
HV	hepatic vein
I	intensity
IA	innominate artery
ICE	intracardiac echocardiography
ICT	isovolumic contraction time
ICU	intensive care unit
IE	infective endocarditis
I_m	temporal average intensity of the largest half-cycle
IMH	intramural hematoma
IMI	inferior myocardial infarction
IMP	index of myocardial performance
In	innominate vein
I_{pa}	pulse average intensity
IRT	isovolumic relaxation time
I_r/I_i	reflected intensity coefficient
I_{sa}	spatial average intensity
I_{sapa}	spatial average pulse average intensity
I_{sata}	spatial average temporal average intensity
I_{satp}	spatial average temporal peak intensity
I_{sp}	spatial peak intensity
I_{sppa}	spatial peak pulse average intensity
I_{spta}	spatial peak temporal average intensity
I_{sptp}	Spatial peak temporal peak intensity
I_{ta}	temporal average intensity
I_{tp}	temporal peak intensity
IVC	inferior vena cava
IVCD	interventricular conduction delay
IVDA	intravenous drug abuse
IVRT	isovolumic relaxation time
IVS	interventricular septum
L	left
L	long axis of left ventricle
LA	left atrium
LAA	left atrial appendage
LAD	left anterior descending coronary artery
LAP	left atrial filling pressure
LAV	left atrial volume
LBBB	left bundle branch block
LC	left common carotid
LCX	left circumflex coronary artery
LM	left main coronary artery
LPA	left pulmonary artery
LS	left subclavian artery
LUPV	left upper pulmonary vein
LV	left ventricle

LVEDD left ventricular end-diastolic dimension
LVEDP left ventricular end-diastolic pressure
LVESD left ventricular end-systolic dimension
LVET left ventricular ejection time
LVFW left ventricular free wall
LVH left ventriclur hypertrophy
LVID left ventricular internal dimension
LVOT left ventricular outflow tract
$LVOT_{area}$ cross-sectional area at the level of the LVOT
$LVOT_{flow}$ flow through the LVOT (stroke volume of the LVOT)
$LVOT_{TVI}$ TVI at the level of the LVOT
$LVOT_{velocity}$ peak Doppler velocity at the level of the LVOT
LVSP left ventricular systolic pressure

MAC mitral annulus calcification
MAIVF mitral–aortic intervalvular fibrosa
MCE myocardial contrast echocardiography
MI mechanical index
MI myocardial infarction
MPA main pulmonary artery
MR mitral regurgitation
MRI magnetic resonance imaging
MS mitral stenosis
MSA mitral separation angle
MV mitral valve
MVA mitral valve area
MVG mean valve gradient
MVP mitral valve prolapse
MV_{area} area of the mitral annulus
MV_{flow} flow through the MV orifice (stroke volume of the mitral orifice)
MVG myocardial velocity gradient

N Newtons
NBTE nonbacterial thrombotic endocarditis
NSR normal sinus rhythm
NYHA New York Heart Association
Nw Womersley number

P pressure
P posterior
Pa Pascals
PA pulmonary artery
PAAU penetrating atherosclerotic aortic ulcer
PADP pulmonary artery diastolic pressure
PASP pulmonary artery systolic pressure
PAear pulmonary artery early diastolic velocity
PAED pulmonary artery end-diastolic velocity
PAMP pulmonary artery mean pressure
PAPS primary antiphospholipid syndrome
PCWP pulmonary capillary wedge pressure
PD pulse duration
PDA patent ductus arteriosus
PEP pre-ejection phase
PFO patent foramen ovale
PHT pressure half-time
P_i incident pressure amplitude
PISA proximal isovelocity surface area
PL posterior leaflet
PMBV percutaneous mitral balloon valvuloplasty
PML posterior mitral leaflet
PMPM posteromedial papillary muscle
PPH primary pulmonary hypertension
P_r reflected pressure amplitude
PR pulmonary regurgitation
PRF pulses per second
PRP pulse repetition period
PS pulmonic stenosis
PT pulmonary trunk
PTT partial thromboplastin time
PV pulmonic valve
PV pulmonary vein
PVC pulmonary valve closure
PVC premature ventricular contraction
PVR pulmonary vascular resistance
PW posterior wall (left ventricular)
PW pulsed wave Doppler
PW pulsed wave tissue Doppler

Q flow
Q quality factor
QA_{long} time from paced ventricular spike to end of a wave
QA_{opt} resultant optimized QA interval
QA_{short} time from paced ventricular spike to end of A wave
Q_P pulmonary flow
Q_S systemic flow

r radius
R right
R amplitude reflection coefficient

RA	right atrium
RAA	right atrial area
RAA	right atrial appendage
RBBB	right bundle branch block
RCA	right coronary artery
Re	Reynolds number
RF	radiofrequency
RF	regurgitant fraction
ROA	regurgitant orifice area
RPA	right pulmonary artery
RUPV	right upper pulmonary vein
RV	right ventricle
RV	regurgitant volume
RV_{aortic}	regurgitant volume of aortic regurgitation
RVFW	right ventricular free wall
RVH	right ventricular hypertrophy
RVOFT	right ventricular outflow tract
RVOT	right ventricular outflow tract
RVSP	right ventricular systolic pressure
S	systolic flow of pulmonary veins
SAM	systolic anterior motion
SATA	see I_{sata}
SAV_{long}	programmed long AV delay
SAV_{short}	programmed short AV delay
SAX_{AP}	short axis apical level
SAX_{MV}	short axis mitral valve level
SAX_{PM}	short axis papillary muscle level
SBE	subacute bacterial endocarditis
SEC	spontaneous echo contrast
SLE	systemic lupus erythematosus
SFF	systolic filling fraction
Sm	TDE mitral annular motion systolic velocity
SPAF	Stroke Prevention in Atrial Fibrillation [study]
SPPA	see I_{sppa}
SPTA	see I_{spta}
SV	stroke volume
SVC	superior vena cava
T	thickness of the shell of a 3-dimensional shape
T	transverse diameter of left ventricle
T	period
t	time
TA	transverse aorta
TCD	transcranial Doppler
TDA	traumatic disruption of the thoracic aorta
TDE	tissue Doppler echocardiography
TDI	tissue Doppler imaging
TEE	transesophageal echocardiography
TGC	time gain compensation
TI	thermal index
TIB	thermal index for bone
TIC	thermal index for the cranium
TIS	thermal index for soft tissue
TMF	transmitral inflow pattern
TOF	tetralogy of Fallot
TR	tricuspid regurgitation
TRJ	tricuspid regurgitant jet area in the right atrium
TS	tricuspid stenosis
TT	total pulmonic systolic time
TTE	transthoracic echocardiography
TV	tricuspid valve
TVI	time velocity integral, see also VTI
TVP	tricuspid valve prolapse
V_c	center velocity
V_{cf}	velocity of circumferential shortening
V_{cfc}	velocity of circumferential shortening corrected for heart rate
VEL_{pisa}	PISA aliasing velocity
V_m	mean velocity
V_p	flow propagation velocity
VS	ventricular septum
VSD	ventricular septal defect
VTI	velocity time integral, see also TVI
V_{vsd}	peak ventricular septal defect velocity
W	acoustical power
WHO	World Health Organization
WMSI	Wall motion score index
Z	impedance
ε	strain
λ	wavelength
ρ	density
μ	viscosity
σ	stress
v	velocity
ω	circular frequency of the heartbeat

CHAPTER 1

Basic Principles of Ultrasound Physics

Principles of ultrasound

Sound is mechanical energy transmitted by pressure waves through a medium. Sound carries energy (*mechanical energy*) from one location to another by causing alternate rarefactions and compressions of the traversed medium. If one could measure pressure in a medium through which sound passed, a sine wave of pressure values would be generated (Fig. 1.1). The *pressure amplitude* is the maximum pressure measured, and the *acoustic intensity* is related to the square of the pressure amplitude.

The *frequency* (f) is the number of cycles per second measured, and the *period* (T) is the inverse of frequency, the time for one cycle (oscillation) to occur:

$$f = 1/T$$

Human audible sound ranges from 20 Hz (cycles/s) to 20 000 Hz. Sound above 20 000 Hz is termed *ultrasound*. Medical equipment usually uses frequencies in the 1–20 MHz range.

Wavelength (λ) is the distance between two peaks in the sine wave. It is dependent upon the velocity of sound (c) in the medium, and is given by:

$$c = f \times \lambda$$

Wavelength is important in that image resolution is not better than one or two wavelengths, and the depth of penetration of the sound wave is less with shorter wavelengths. The *velocity of sound* is related to the stiffness and density of the medium through which it travels. Generally, as the density increases, the velocity will also (~1540 m/s in human tissue). The *range equation* is used to calculate the distance (d) an object is from an ultrasound source:

$$d = ct/2$$

where t is the time it takes for the ultrasound signal to make a roundtrip from the ultrasound emitter, bounce off the object, and be detected by the ultrasound device.

Amplitude of sound may be described in *decibels* (dB). The dB value does not represent an absolute signal level, but a ratio. The dB compares the logarithmic ratio of two amplitudes (A1 and A2) by:

$$\text{Relative amplitude level dB} = 20 \log (A2/A1)$$

If the power or intensity (I1 and I2) is given (rather than amplitude) then:

$$\text{Relative power (intensity) level dB} = 10 \log (I2/I1)$$

As a rule of thumb, with measures of amplitude, a change of 6 dB represents a doubling (halving) of

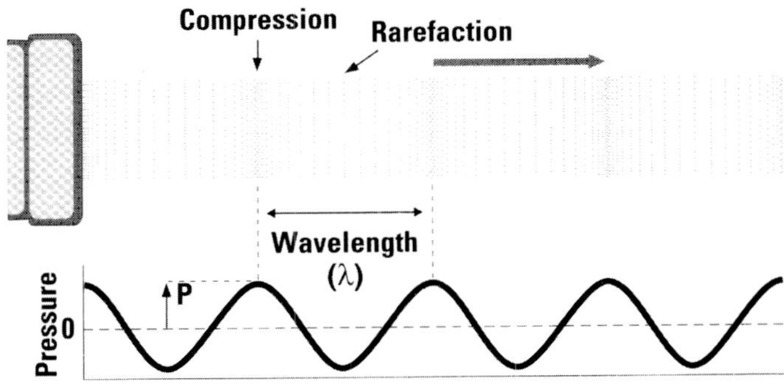

Fig. 1.1 Compressions and rarefactions noted in a medium through which a sound wave is traveling. A sine wave represents the change in pressures noted, with the *x*-axis representing distance, and the *y*-axis pressure. A pressure of 0 indicates the baseline pressure. The wavelength and pressure (*P*) are noted. (Reproduced with permission from: Zagzebski JA. Essentials of Ultrasound Physics. St Louis, MO: Mosby, 1996: p. 4, figures 1–7.)

amplitude. With measures of intensity or power, a change of 3 dB represents a doubling (halving) of intensity or power.

General properties of ultrasound waves within a medium include attenuation, reflection, refraction, and scattering. The *attenuation coefficient* for a medium quantifies the decrease over distance of an ultrasound signal amplitude. It is dependent on ultrasonic frequency, generally doubling for every doubling of frequency. It is approximately 0.5–1.0 dB/cm at 1 MHz in most tissue. Attenuation of ultrasound through tissue occurs by two mechanisms: *scattering* (described later in this chapter), and *absorption*. Absorption is the predominant cause of attenuation, and in tissues predominantly occurs from an inability of tissue molecules to completely return to their original "relaxed" position after a compression wave has passed through, and the second compression wave arrives.

The attenuation of a signal (in dB) through a given tissue is calculated by taking the attenuation coefficient for the tissue, multiplied by the distance the ultrasound signal travels:

Attenuation (dB) = attenuation coefficient (dB/cm) × distance (cm)

The depth of tissue at which generated ultrasound intensity is one-half the initial value (–3 dB drop in intensity) is the *penetration depth* (*half boundary layer*). This is clinically of the order of 0.25–1 cm depth. The penetration depth is:

Penetration depth = 3/(attenuation coefficient (dB/cm))

Reflection occurs when the ultrasound beam bounces off a boundary between two tissues with different *acoustic impedance* values. Acoustic impedance (Z), which is expressed in units of Rayls, is not a measured value, but is calculated as the product of the *tissue density* (ρ) and the *ultrasound velocity* in the tissue (c):

$$Z\ (\text{Rayls}) = \rho(\text{kg/m}^3) \times c(\text{m/s})$$

The boundary between the two differing tissues must have a lateral dimension greater than the wavelength of the ultrasound wave, and will act as a "mirror." This type of tissue interface is called a *specular reflector*. The ratio of the *reflected pressure amplitude* (P_r) to the incident pressure amplitude (P_i) (the *incident pressure amplitude* is the amplitude of the

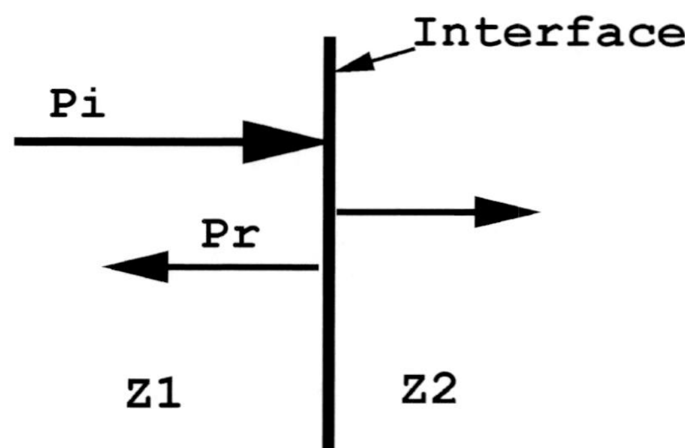

Fig. 1.2 Reflection (P_r) of an incident wave (P_i), and the continued transmission of the wave through the interface of two tissues with impedance (Z1) of the first tissue, and (Z2) of the second tissue through which the ultrasound beam passes. This is an example of a specular reflector (see text).

ultrasound wave at the moment prior to striking a boundary) is the *amplitude reflection coefficient* (R):

$$R = \frac{P_r}{P_i} = \frac{Z2 - Z1}{Z2 + Z1}$$

where Z2 is the distal tissue impedance, and Z1 is the proximal tissue impedance (Fig. 1.2). The *reflected intensity coefficient* (I_r/I_i) is R^2, since intensity is the square of ultrasound wave amplitude. If an ultrasound wave strikes a tissue boundary at an angle, the wave may or may not be reflected, as would a light beam bouncing off a mirror at an angle. As with a mirror, the reflected angle is the same as the incident angle.

Refraction is the bending of the ultrasound wave as it travels through a boundary between two tissues of different impedance, at an angle. Similarly, refraction of light occurs as it travels from water into air, distorting the perceived position of an object in the water (Fig. 1.3). *Snell's Law* states that the angle of refraction is related by:

$$(\sin \theta 1) \times V2 = (\sin \theta) \times V1$$

where V1 is the velocity of ultrasound beam through the first medium, V2 through the second medium, θ_1 is the incident angle of the ultrasound beam to the interface, and θ_2 is the angle leaving the interface (Fig. 1.4).

Diffuse scattering occurs with ultrasound interactions with tissue interfaces where the structures are usually smaller than the wavelength of the ultrasound

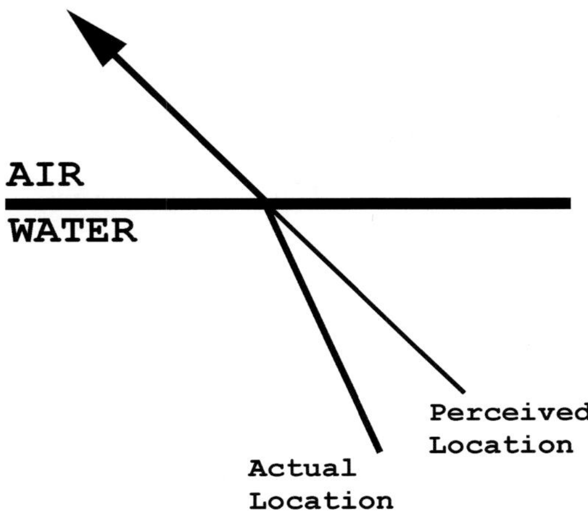

Fig. 1.3 An example of refraction (bending of light) as a light wave travels from water into air. Because the velocity of light (or any wave passing from one medium into another) is different in water and air, refraction occurs. The observer (located at the arrowhead) perceives the object position as shown. For refraction to occur, the wave (light or sound) must hit the interface at an angle other than perpendicular, and the wave must have different velocities through the two mediums.

signal. Most of the energy is directed away (scattered) from the ultrasound beam, and only a very small fraction of the original energy is reflected back towards the transducer. As opposed to specular reflectors, the property of diffuse scattering is usually independent of the ultrasound incident angle, because scattering occurs in many directions. Small changes in the acoustic impedance of these interfaces produce this diffuse scattering. *Rayleigh scattering* is a form of diffuse scattering, but from interfaces much smaller than the ultrasound wavelength. Both diffuse and Rayleigh scattering are important in tissue texture.

Interference of ultrasound waves occurs when waves emanate from more than one source. If two waves are "in phase," the amplitude of the resultant wave is the sum of both wave amplitudes. This is termed *constructive interference.* If they are "out of phase," they will tend to cancel each other out. This is termed *destructive interference.* Interference plays a role in diffuse and Rayleigh scattering, and with phased array transducer systems (see Chapter 2).

Bioeffects of ultrasound

There has been no known patient injury from diagnostic ultrasound, but very few studies have evaluated effects of low-level ultrasound on biological tissue. The biological effect of an ultrasound signal is proportional to:

- *energy* across the area of interest
- the three-dimensional *spatial pattern* of energy of the ultrasound beam
- the *time duration* of exposure to the tissue
- the ultrasound *frequency*
- the "*sensitivity*" of the tissue to ultrasound.

Acoustical power is the rate of energy transmission into the tissue (units of milliwatts). *Acoustical intensity* (milliwatts/cm^2) is the power per cross-sectional area of the beam. An ultrasound beam that is "focused" would have a higher acoustical intensity effect on the tissue within the focused area (since the cross-sectional area is smaller) than in other areas of the beam that

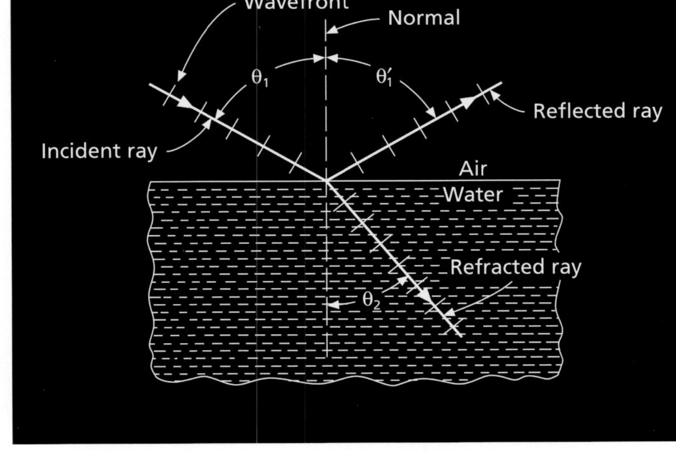

Fig. 1.4 The angle of the incident ray is related to the refracted ray angle by Snell's law. The refraction of one medium with respect to another generally varies with wavelength. The angle of a reflected ray is the same as the incident ray angle. (Reproduced with permission from: Halliday D, Resnick R. Fundamentals of Physics. New York: John Wiley, 1970: p 670, figure 36.1.)

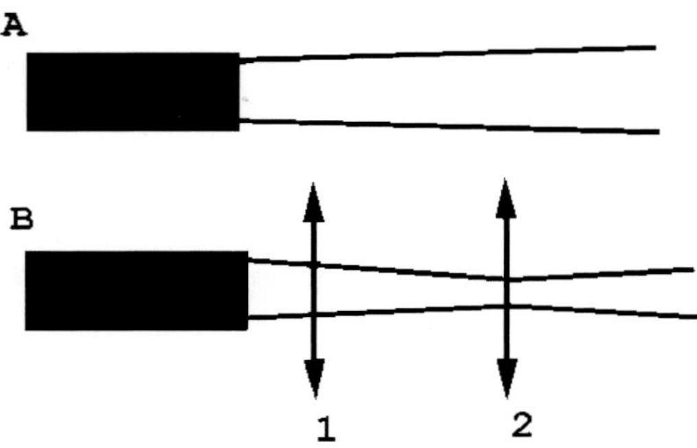

Fig. 1.5 The acoustical power transmitted by transducer A and B may be the same, but the acoustical intensity of transducer B on tissue at area 2 is higher than it is at the same distance from transducer A.

have not narrowed down (Fig. 1.5). Intensity therefore will vary according to location within the ultrasound beam (*spatial intensity*).

There are two major features of an ultrasound beam that determine its effect on tissue: (i) the *spatial distribution* of acoustic energy, and (ii) *temporal factors* (time of ultrasound exposure to tissue). The *spatial peak intensity* (I_{sp}) occurs along the beam axis at the transition point of a nonfocused transducer, and at the focal point along the beam axis of a focused transducer. The *spatial average intensity* (I_{sa}) is the I_{sp} divided by the cross-sectional area through the beam, at the area of interest, or of the cross-sectional area of the transducer face.

Since ultrasound systems operate by sending out pulsed signals, "temporal factors" are important, as energy delivered to tissues will vary through time (Fig. 1.6). "Exposure time" of tissue is determined by the *pulse duration* (PD) and the number of these pulses per second (PRF) (see Figs 2.2 & 2.3, p. 8). The *duty factor* (D) (see Chapter 2) is PD × PRF. Intensity measurements used with medical ultrasound instruments include:

- Temporal average intensity (I_{ta})—intensity averaged over one PRP.
- Spatial average temporal average intensity (I_{sata})—temporal average intensity averaged over the cross-sectional area of the beam.
- Spatial average temporal peak intensity (I_{satp})—peak intensity over a cross-sectional area (such as the transducer face) during peak emitting energy.
- Pulse average intensity (I_{pa})—intensity averaged over the pulse duration (not the PRP as with I_{ta}).
- Spatial average pulse average intensity (I_{sapa})—pulse average intensity averaged over the beam cross-sectional area.

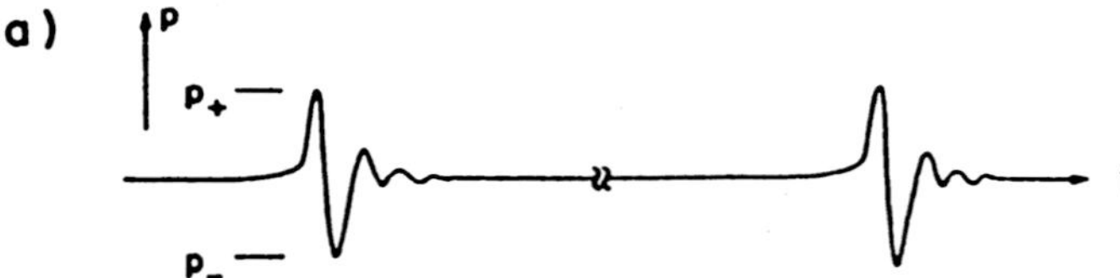

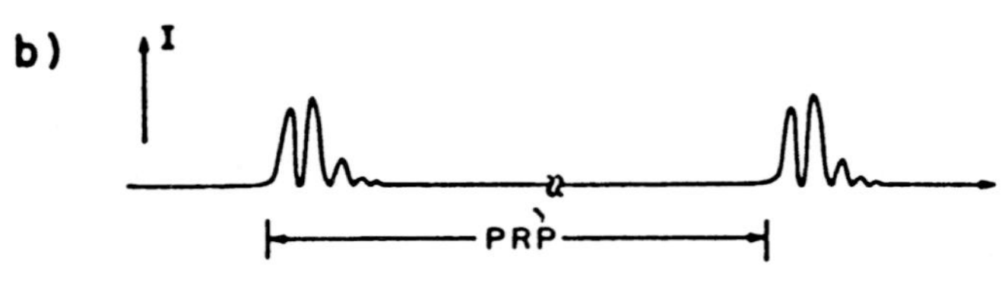

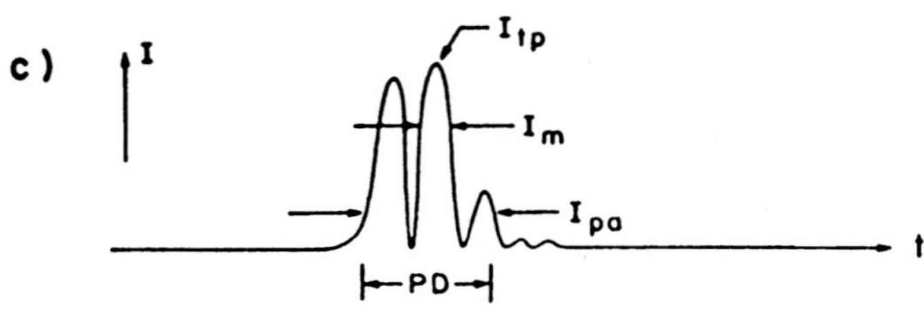

Fig. 1.6 Temporal (time-related) changes of pressure (a) and intensity (b) of an ultrasound signal at a representative single location within an ultrasound beam. Detail of an intensity impulse is shown in (c): the pulse duration (PD), temporal peak intensity (I_{tp}), the temporal average intensity of the largest half cycle (I_m), and the pulse average intensity (I_{pa}). I_{pa} is the average intensity during the time of the impulse, and the time average intensity (I_{ta}) is the average intensity over the time frame from the beginning of one impulse to the beginning of the next impulse. (Reproduced with permission from: O'Brien WD. Biological effects of ultrasound: rationale for measurement of selected ultrasonic output quantities. Echocardiography 1986; 3: 165.)

• Spatial peak pulse average intensity (I_{sppa})—pulse average intensity at the spatial location where the pulse average intensity is a maximum value.
• Spatial peak temporal average intensity (I_{spta})—temporal average intensity at the spatial location where the temporal average intensity is a maximum value.
• Spatial peak temporal peak intensity (I_{sptp})—peak intensity at the location of highest intensity during peak emitting energy (this is the highest energy value of all intensity values).
• Temporal average intensity of the largest *half-cycle* (I_m)—average intensity over the largest half-cycle of the transmitted pulse at the spatial peak location.

The I_{spta} may be the most useful of the measurements, as it describes the peak energy any tissue is exposed to over the time of ultrasound exposure. Clinical ultrasound I_{spta} (SPTA) intensity values are generally in the range of less than one to several hundred mW/cm^2 (about 10% of the average power of sunshine at Earth's surface). New "bloodless surgery" ultrasound devices (*high-intensity focused ultrasound*—HIFU) apply as much as 3000 W/cm^2 energy to a target area. Other commonly used parameters are I_{sppa} (SPPA), and I_{sata} (SATA). SATA is equal to the acoustical power (W) of the transducer divided by the cross-sectional area of the beam. For example, the SATA of transducer with 8 mW power, and a 1.5-cm-diameter surface would be:

$$\text{SATA} = W/A$$

and $A = \pi(D/2)^2$

where A = area, D = diameter of transducer face. Therefore:

$$\text{SATA} = 8/[(3.14)(1.5/2)^2] = 4.5\ \text{mW/cm}^2$$

Methods by which ultrasound may interact with tissues include: (i) *thermal effects* (local heating); (ii) *cavitation* by bubble formation or existing liquid–bubble vibration; and (iii) *mechanical effects* (radiation forces, acoustic streaming, microstreaming). Heat generated in a tissue is proportional to the intensity in the ultrasound beam. This is proportional to the attenuation coefficient and depth from the transducer. Some focused transducers will generate higher temperatures at the focal point (but overall, focused beams are less likely to have bioeffects than unfocused beams). The *rate of change of temperature* of a tissue (rate at which temperature will increase) is proportional to the tissue absorption coefficient and beam intensity at that point, and is inversely proportional to the tissue density and *specific heat of the tissue* (*Cm*—the amount heat in calories to raise 1 gram tissue by 1°C relative to water). Relatively dense tissue (muscle), because of density and specific heat, will heat slower than less dense tissue (fat). *Convection* (bloodflow through a tissue) transports heat away from tissues, and *conduction* decreases local heating by direct diffusion through the surrounding tissue. Thermal effects are most likely to occur clinically, and would occur closest to the surface of the transducer.

Cavitation (bubble formation) occurs with oxygen and carbon dioxide dissolved within tissues. Rarefactions (Fig. 1.1) of the ultrasound beam result in a decreased pressure locally within tissue, and the dissolved gas will then "boil" out of suspension. Formed bubbles (*stable cavitation*) will resonant (vibrate) under the influence of ultrasound and will absorb energy, converting that energy to heat. At very high local ultrasound intensity, cavitation will occur during a rarefaction, and collapse of the bubble will occur during compression (*transient cavitation*). Tremendous energy is generated with a marked local increase in pressure. This effect does not occur at power levels used by diagnostic ultrasound equipment. Bubble formation is hindered in tissue (compared to water) because of tissue viscosity. Mechanical effects may include *microstreaming*, where an oscillating bubble could shear molecules, but how relevant this is to clinical diagnostic ultrasound is questionable.

Cavitation and mechanical effects are thought not to be significant in clinical diagnostic ultrasound, but thermal effects may be relevant clinically:
• Possible *thermal effects on the fetus* are in question (bone absorbs greater acoustic energy than soft tissues), and for this reason some suggest that studies on the fetus should be as short as possible, with minimal power levels used. Doppler is associated with higher energy, and for this reason Doppler is recommended only when information to be obtained is necessary. Also, an ultrasound beam traveling through amniotic fluid will result in higher temperatures to the fetus than would be expected.
• Most transesophageal echocardiography (TEE) probes have an automatic "shut-off switch" if the temperature at the face of the probe rises above a certain temperature. This may actually cause a problem for patients with a febrile illness at the time of the TEE study.

Methods used to measure the power generated by ultrasound equipment include a *radiation force balance device*, and methods to measure pressure include a *hydrophone*. The radiation force balance is a sensitive device that measures the force exerted on it by the transducer, which is proportional to the total emitted power. A hydrophone is a small probe with a piezoelectric element that will convert pressure energy to an electrical voltage, which is proportional to the pressure amplitude. A *calorimeter* is an instrument that will convert the acoustic power generated by an ultrasound transducer into heat. The rate of rise of the temperature is proportional to the power of the ultrasound transducer.

Whereas ultrasound machines have been labeled as having transmit power in terms of percentage, dB, or low/med/high (all subjective descriptions), they are now quantified with the *thermal index* (TI), and the *mechanical index* (MI). The TI is the ratio of the acoustical power produced by the transducer to the power needed to raise the temperature of tissue by 1°C. TIS is the TI for soft tissue, TIB for bone (relevant for fetal bone), and TIC for cranial bone. The MI reflects the probability of cavitation at a power level. TI values and exposure times, for which no biologic effect in mammals has been reported, are: 1 min (TI = 6), 10 min (TI = 4.3), and 100 min (TI = 2.7). The MI for an instrument and transducer is calculated from the generated peak rarefaction pressure and the ultrasound frequency (MI is proportional to peak rarefaction pressure, and inversely proportional to the square root of frequency), and comparing this to cavitation threshold values found in the laboratory. No injury has been reported in mammals for a MI approximately less than 0.3. Diagnostic ultrasound machines may produce minor hemorrhage in the presence of a gas-filled cavity, and has been noted in mammals with direct ultrasound beams on the lung. *It seems prudent to keep the TI and MI as low as possible* while still obtaining a useful study (the *power* (energy transmitted into the tissue) should be as low as possible, and *gain* (amplification of the signal after returning back to the transducer) increased as needed).

CHAPTER 2

Principles of Instrumentation and Echo-Doppler Modalities

Transducer types and echo imaging

The cardiac ultrasound machine is basically made up of three components: (i) the transducer; (ii) the echocardiography unit and circuitry; and (iii) display and recording systems. The function of the ultrasound *transducer* (a transducer is a device which is capable of converting one form of energy into another) is based on the *piezoelectric* (pressure-electric) *effect* in which certain materials have the property that the application of an electric voltage to that material causes a mechanical deformation (vibration). The magnitude of the mechanical deformation is proportional to the applied voltage within the elastic limits of the material. Similarly, the application of a mechanical stress (vibration) to a piezoelectric material will cause a voltage to be produced across the material, in proportion to the magnitude of the applied deformation. The simplest transducer is based on a single piezoelectric crystal (Fig. 2.1).

The characteristic frequency of a transducer is a wavelength such that the piezoelectric element has a thickness one-half of that wavelength. At this wavelength is the *fundamental resonant frequency* of the transducer (velocity of ultrasound signal through the element divided by two times the thickness). The *bandwidth* of the transducer is the range of frequencies around the resonant frequency, and the *quality factor* (Q) is defined as the number of oscillations in the pulse (which is proportional to the fundamental resonant frequency divided by the bandwidth).

Matching layers of one-quarter wavelength thickness between the piezoelectric element and the body surface help to markedly reduce reflective losses from *impedence mismatch* (see Chapter 1) between the piezoelectric element and the body surface.

A transducer spends most of the time "listening" for returning echoes bouncing back from the tissue studied. The fraction of time that the transducer transmits an ultrasound signal is the *duty factor* (see also Chapter 1), and in clinical ultrasound machines is usually less than 1%. The *pulse duration* is the length of the pulse from its beginning to the end of the same pulse. Usually the higher the frequency of the transducer, the shorter the pulse duration. The *pulse repetition period* is the time from the beginning of a pulse to the beginning of the next pulse (Fig. 2.2). The time between each pulse is spent listening for returning echoes. By use of the range equation (see Chapter 1), the total distance traveled by the pulse, and therefore its depth before reflecting back, are known (Fig. 2.3). The *pulse repetition frequency (PRF)* is defined as the rate at which ultrasound pulses are generated by the transducer.

The pulse transmitter delivers to the transducer a short burst of electricity and the piezoelectric element

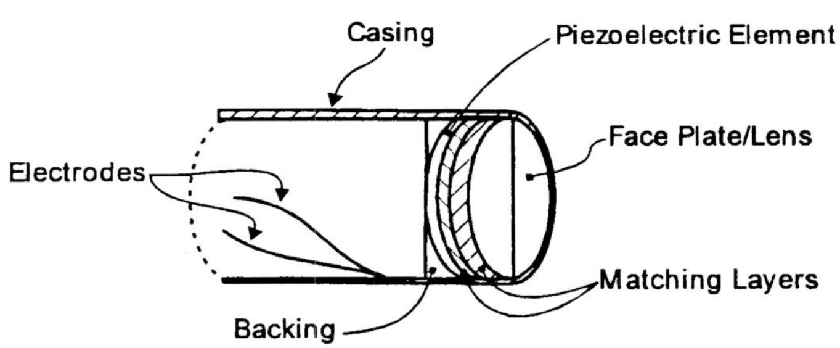

Fig. 2.1 A single piezoelectric element ultrasound transducer. The piezoelectric element produces an ultrasound signal when a voltage is passed through the element. The same piezoelectric element also receives ultrasound signals, and they are converted to a voltage, which is then transmitted through the electrodes to the ultrasound machine.

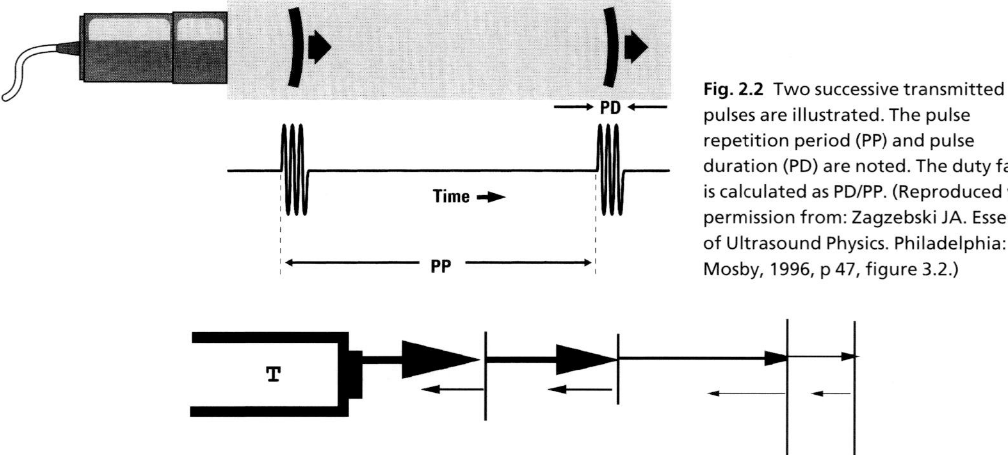

Fig. 2.2 Two successive transmitted pulses are illustrated. The pulse repetition period (PP) and pulse duration (PD) are noted. The duty factor is calculated as PD/PP. (Reproduced with permission from: Zagzebski JA. Essentials of Ultrasound Physics. Philadelphia: Mosby, 1996, p 47, figure 3.2.)

Fig. 2.3 An impulse is transmitted from the transducer (T), and is reflected back along its path. The transducer then "listens" for returning echoes. By application of the range equation, the distance traveled by each returning echo is known. The "collection" of returned signals from one transmitted pulse, reflected from progressive depths, is known as a **vector**.

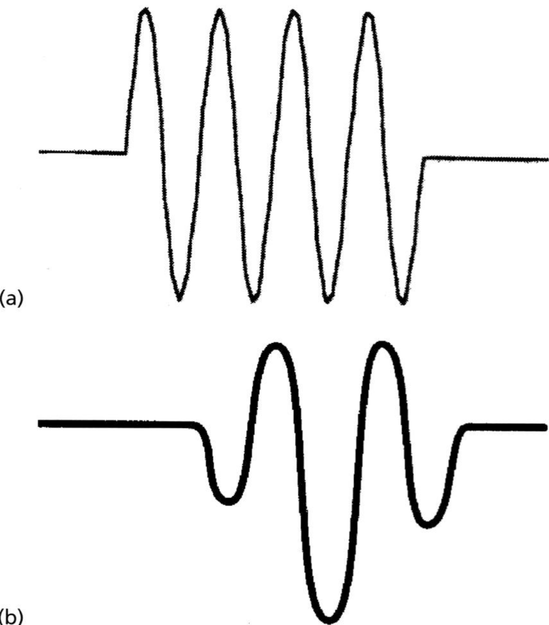

Fig. 2.4 Ultrasound pulse waveforms. (a) A short pulse duration with rapid onset and termination results in a wide range of frequencies (broad bandwidth) transmitted around the fundamental resonant frequency of the transducer. This results in improved images with "multifrequency blending" and less speckle along B-scan lines. (b) The waveform is short with a "gradual" onset and end, resulting in a narrow frequency bandwidth. This is important with second harmonic imaging (discussed later in this chapter), where it is desirable not to transmit energy at the desired harmonic frequency.

vibrates. The element sends out an ultrasound signal. The element would continue to vibrate for some time were it not for damping from *backing material* adjacent to the element. Most transducers emit a short pulse for best axial resolution. This results in transmission of a fairly wide spectrum of frequencies, other than the fundamental frequency. In certain applications (*second harmonic imaging*) this wide spectrum of frequencies is undesirable and a waveform with a "tight" frequency transmission at the fundamental frequency is desirable (Fig. 2.4).

The ultrasound signal that returns to the transducer causes the piezoelectric element to vibrate, and an electrical signal is generated. This electrical pulse is called a *RF (radiofrequency) signal* (Fig. 2.5). It is then amplified by the *RF amplifier*. As signals return to the receiver they are generally progressively weaker, because of attenuation from the increasing distance traveled. Compensation for this is accomplished by continuously increasing amplification. The returning RF signals then undergo *rectification* (display all values of the signal whether positive or negative as positive values). After rectification the "envelope" of the signal (termed *video signal*) is produced, and many times the first derivative of the "envelope" signal is obtained. If only the positive values of the derivative are used, this will help in locating the leading edge of the RF signal better, and in better identifying an accurate depth of the reflector from which the RF signal returned, since the leading edge of the signal is the best indicator of

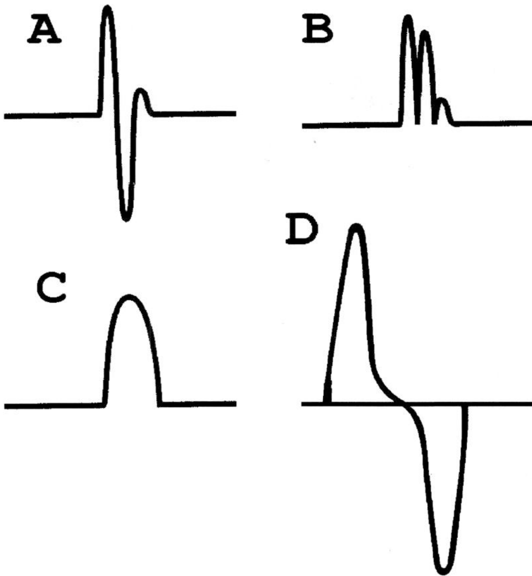

Fig. 2.5 Sequence of events for demodulation of the returning RF signal. In (A) the original signal has been amplified, and then it is (B) rectified, by taking the absolute value of the signal. In (C) the video signal is obtained by taking the "envelope" of the rectified signal. If the first derivative (D) of the envelope signal is obtained, better depth localization (see text) is possible. This differentiated signal is also less sensitive to alterations upon changing the amplification of the RF signal.

the distance traveled. This process of changing the RF signal is called *demodulation* and allows for a suitable waveform for display purposes. The magnitude of the signal is proportional to the "strength" of the reflector from which it returned, and correlates with the intensity of the corresponding location on a display. Because there will be a wide range of values for magnitude from returning signals, *log compression* of the magnitude values is performed, so that they may all be displayed on a monitor. *"Digital ultrasound"* machines will change the RF signal early in the processing procedure from an "analog" signal to a "digital" signal, which can then be manipulated by computer processing (see Chapter 1).

Several modes of image presentation have been used. Basically they are the *A-mode* (amplitude mode) and the *B-mode* (brightness mode) with its variations (*M-mode* (motion mode) and *two-dimensional imaging*) (Fig. 2.6). With A-mode, distance is represented along the vertical axis and the length of a "spike" depicts the reflected image intensity. The A-mode modality is no longer used in routine studies. With B-mode, distance is again represented along the vertical axis, but image intensity is indicated by brightness of the "dots." If the B-mode is "swept" across the cathode ray tube (CRT) screen, an M-mode image will result.

There are three basic types of transducers used for imaging: phased-array, mechanical (rotating and oscillating), and linear-array (Fig. 2.7). Each of these transducers will produce a two-dimensional image (other terms sometimes used include "cross-sectional" or "real-time" imaging). A transducer will "build" an image by rapidly displaying many B-mode lines to form the two-dimensional image, and hence is sometimes called B-mode imaging. There are three main ways to present two-dimensional images using multiple B-mode "lines." They are the *sector scan, linear scan*, and *arc scan* (Fig. 2.8). The sector scan is the most popular method for cardiac imaging, as it is best used with narrow ultrasound "acoustic windows" found when imaging the heart.

Mechanical transducers use crystals that mechanically move in a fluid-filled housing. Older transducers

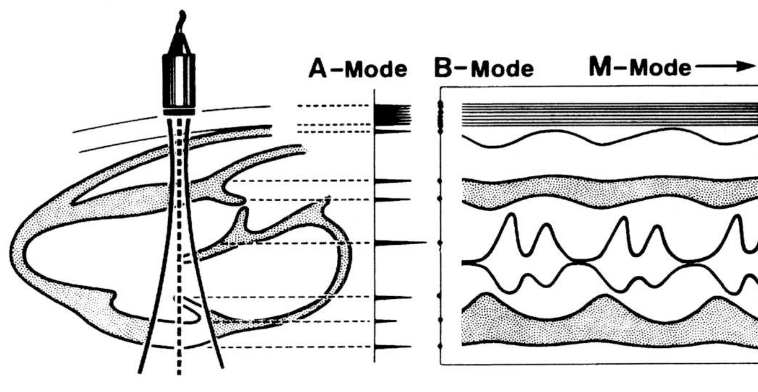

Fig. 2.6 Types of pulse-echo imaging displays. By A-mode, the distance of the interfaces from the transducer is noted by horizontally directed "spikes" along the vertical axis, with the amplitude of the reflection indicated by the length of these spikes. By B-mode the spikes are replaced by "dots," where the intensity of the dots corresponds to the length of A-mode spikes. M-mode is basically the B-mode format swept across a screen. (Reproduced with permission from: Weyman AE. Principles and Practice of Echocardiography, 2nd edn. Philadelphia: Lea & Febiger, 1994).

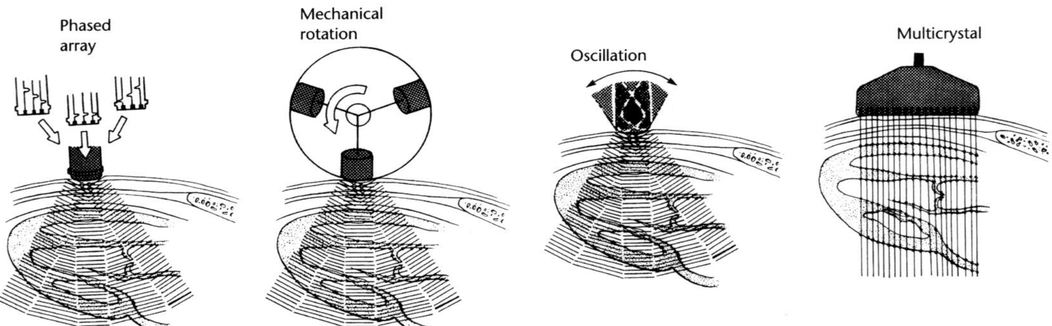

Fig. 2.7 The three general types of transducers include phased-array, mechanical (of which there are rotary and oscillating), and linear-array (see text). (Reproduced with permission from: Snider AR, Serwer GA, Ritter SB. Echocardiography in Pediatric Heart Disease, 2nd edn. St Louis: Mosby, 1997.)

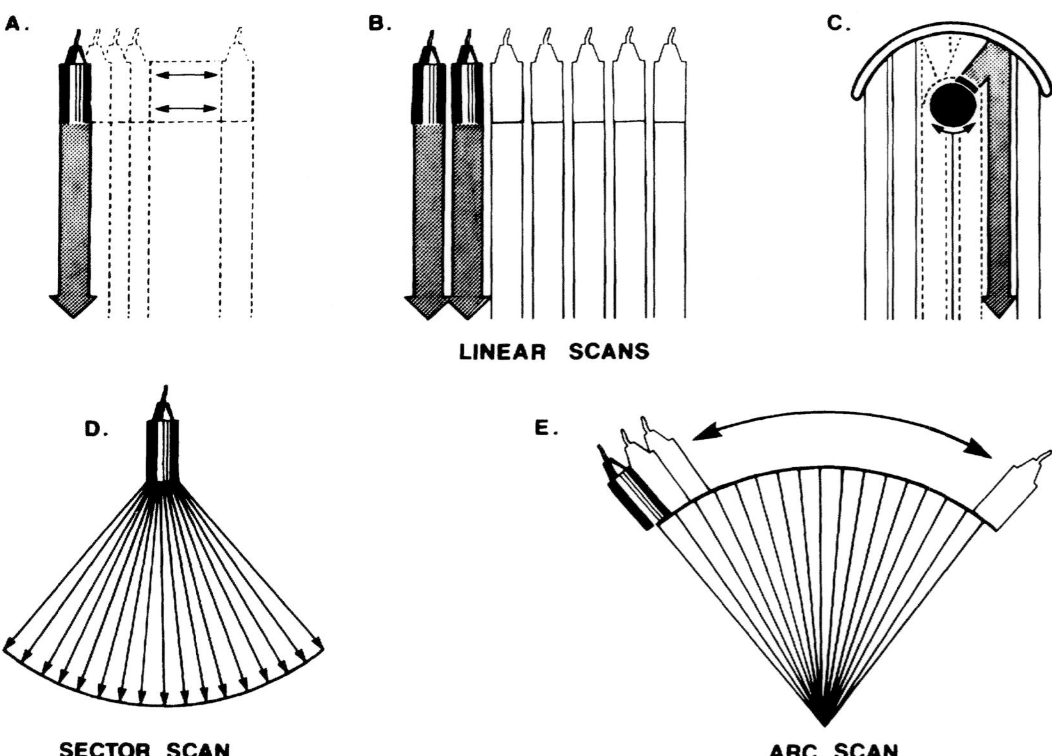

Fig. 2.8 The three main two-dimensional scan formats include the following: (A,B,C) linear scan; B represents the popular linear-array transducer used in vascular studies (see text); the sector scan (D), where the transducer remains in a fixed position while the ultrasound signals are sequentially swept across an arc; and (E) the arc scan where the transducer is moved in an arc, and the ultrasound beam is continuously pointing at a fixed distant point. (Reproduced with permission from: Weyman AE. Principles and Practice of Echocardiography, 2nd edn. Philadelphia: Lea & Febiger, 1994.)

(*oscillatory transducers*) used a single crystal that oscillated back and forth to form many B-scan lines and subsequently build a two-dimensional image. These transducers significantly vibrate and have a problem of uneven B-line distribution because the transducer must slow down, stop and change directions at each edge of the two-dimensional image formed. Mechanical transducers subsequently were built that house three or four crystals around a central hub. The *rotary transducers* rotate with each crystal used sequentially, building a sector image from the multiple B-scans. The *annular-array* transducers are a form of array transducers with a set of piezoelectric elements arranged concentrically as rings around a central disk-shaped element. These transducers must be mechanically moved by a motor, with rapid starts and stops, corresponding to each B-scan line. During ultrasound emission and "listening" for each B-scan line, the transducers are motionless. The advantage of this design over the phased-array system in cardiac imaging is improved focusing with narrow focusing in all three directions (spherical focusing ability), whereas the phased-array system has resolutions that are different in the three directions (axial, lateral, elevational). The disadvantage is that the number of rings in the transducer makes its size large, and limits the acoustic windows for cardiac imaging.

Array transducers consist of a single row of closely spaced elements, each of which has its own electrical wire connections to the ultrasound machine. Each element is in effect a "mini-transducer." Each element transmits an individual ultrasound pulse, and RF signals are received by each element. They are then individually amplified before combination with other RF signals from other elements.

On transmit, *phased-array transducers* electronically sweep through an arc to form a sector (Fig. 2.9a). On receive, the sequential elements must "listen" for returning signals at sequential delays in timing since the elements are at different distances from the target.

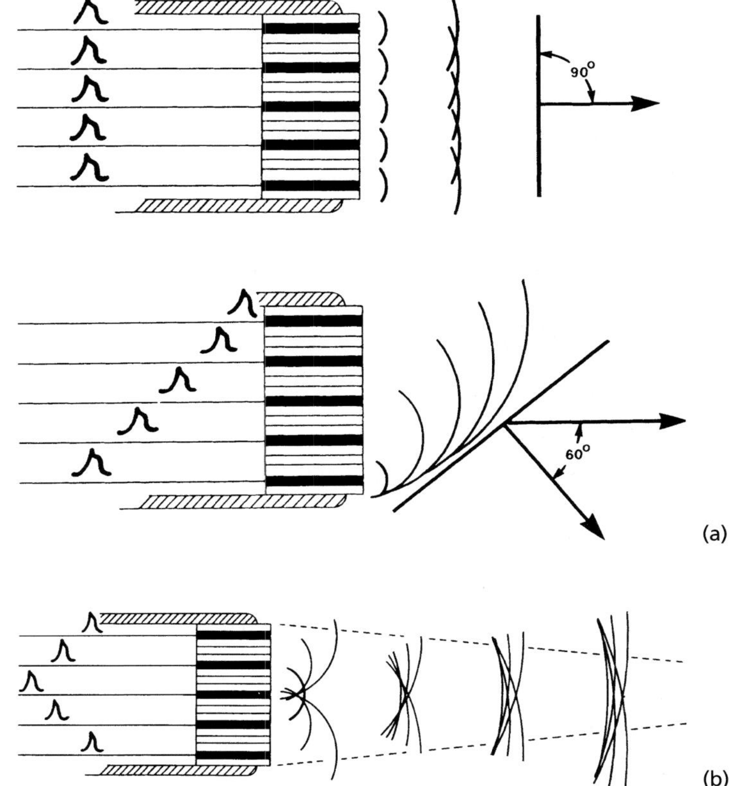

Fig. 2.9 Electronic steering and focusing of a phased-array transducer. In the upper panel of (a) simultaneous pulses summate (constructive interference—Chapter 1) to form an ultrasound beam (Huygen's principle) with most of the signal along a central beam that gradually narrows and then diverges (see also Fig. 2.10a). The lower panel of (a) illustrates sequential activation of elements, with a resultant ultrasound beam directed out toward the tissue at an angle. By varying timing of sequential activation of elements, a continuous "fan" of ultrasound pulses is produced, to yield a sector image. (b) The lower panel demonstrates that by varying timing of element activation electronic focusing of the phased-array transducer system will result by both constructive and destructive interface. (Reproduced with permission from Weyman AE. Principles and Practice of Echocardiography, 2nd edn. Philadelphia: Lea & Febiger, 1994.)

The timing of the sequential delays of the elements will vary according to the target distance away from the transducer (*dynamic receive focusing*). Focusing on receive is not sonographer selected and is automatic within the ultrasound machine electronics. Echoes that are received from other directions will have a tendency to be out of phase (destructive interference) and will be negligible. Focusing electronically is achieved in delaying timing of element activation (Fig. 2.9b). The focal distance of an array transducer is varied electronically by changing the timing of activation of the elements (the *transmit focal distance* is selected by the sonographer). If *multiple transmit focal zones* are used, multiple ultrasound pulses, with each focused at a different depth along the B-scan line, is performed. This will slow down the image frame rate. The transmit focal distance is usually indicated on the ultrasound machine video screen as the "focus." If an array transducer transmits signals through all its elements simultaneously it behaves as an *unfocused transducer* (Fig. 2.10a), as opposed to changing the timing of sequential activation of the elements for a focused array transducer. The focus is more complex for an electronically focused array transducer (Fig. 2.10b).

Dynamic aperture is a process where the transducer attempts to make the ultrasound beam width the same with depth, and maintain lateral resolution (see below). As ultrasound impulses return to the transducer from deeper within the tissues, the number of elements activated to sense returning signals continuously increases from a small number of elements for close structures to a large number of elements for distant structures.

Axial resolution (minimum distance between two reflectors along a pulse that can be detected) of a transducer system is proportional to the pulse duration and to the frequency and bandwidth. Practically, the axial resolution is about twice the ultrasound wavelength, therefore higher frequency transducers have better axial resolution. With a wider bandwidth (shorter pulse duration) resolution is also better. *Lateral resolution* (the ability to detect two reflectors side-by-side and perpendicular to the ultrasound) is related to the beam width (which is related to system gain), and transducer size, frequency, side and grating lobe artifact (discussed later in this chapter), and focusing properties. The narrower the ultrasound beam width at a particular depth, the better the lateral resolution. Because the beam diverges in the far field, lateral resolution deteriorates with distance. *Elevational resolution* is the "slice thickness" of tissue that contributes to the signal. It is the resolution perpendicular to the signal. Elevational resolution is very dependent on transducer focusing properties (Fig. 2.10b) and side lobe artifact. Of these three resolution directions, the axial direction is most precise, with the most

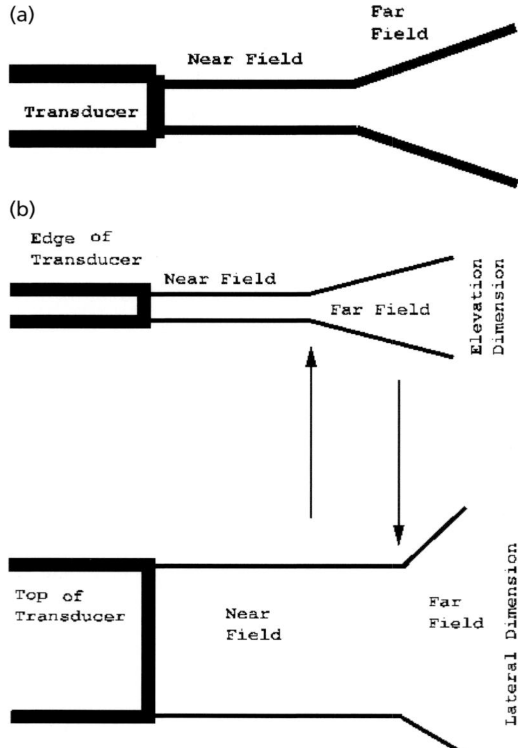

Fig. 2.10 Focusing of a transducer. (a) An unfocused transducer. The near field (*Fresnel zone*) is the zone from the transducer to the focus, and the far zone (*Fraunhofer zone*) is after the focus. The *focus* is the location where the diameter of the ultrasound beam is narrowest, and the *focal zone* (also termed *transition zone*) is the region surrounding the focus. The *focal length* is the distance from the transducer to the focus, and is proportional to both the crystal diameter and ultrasound frequency (for a wider diameter crystal and higher frequency the longer the focal length therefore the longer the Fresnel zone). The length of the Fresnel zone is the radius of the ultrasound-generating surface squared then divided by the wavelength. (b) A focused phased-array transducer. Because the width of the transducer is greater than its height, the focal length in the horizontal (along the transducer width) direction is longer than in the vertical (along the transducer height) direction (arrows).

accurate measurements made in this axial direction. An advantage of an annular array transducer over that of a phased-array system is that the resolution of the annular system in the "elevational" direction is the same as the lateral direction at all depths, whereas elevational resolution significantly deteriorates in a phased-array system with distance (Fig. 2.10b). For imaging small objects, the annular system may have some advantage.

Linear array transducers originally transmitted a pulse simultaneously from each element, and then received each pulse to generate each B-mode line to form a rectangular image (*simple switched array*). Later linear array transducers were developed (*grouped switched array*) for an increase in the number of B-lines per imaged area with improved resolution. By using phased-array technology, a grouped switched linear array transducer may use the first four elements to send out an impulse and form the first B-line signal from those. The second B-line would then be formed by combining the second through fifth elements, and the third B-line would be formed by combining the third through sixth element, and so forth.

Side lobe artifacts, found in all types of transducers, result from returning signals from the far field or focal region that are not part of the main ultrasound beam. Side lobes are caused by laterally directed waves from the edges of the transducer and will occur when the distance to the edge of the transducer face traveled by the returning ultrasound beam is one wavelength different from the main beam. Because ultrasound pulses tend to have a wide bandwidth (wide range of wavelengths around the center frequency), side lobes will many times "smear" out and not be much of a problem. To further reduce side lobes, however, the transducer may transmit progressively weaker signals from the center of the element outward to the edge (*apodization*). The larger the number and smaller the size of the elements, the smaller the side lobes.

Grating lobe artifact is the result of the transducer being divided into small individual elements that are regularly spaced. This artifact appears more problematic for linear array transducers. The angle of the artifact from the center of the sector image is dependent on the spacing between elements and the wavelength of the ultrasound beam. By reducing the spacing of the elements to one half wavelength or less, this artifact is reduced in amplitude and is also further displaced from the midline of the image.

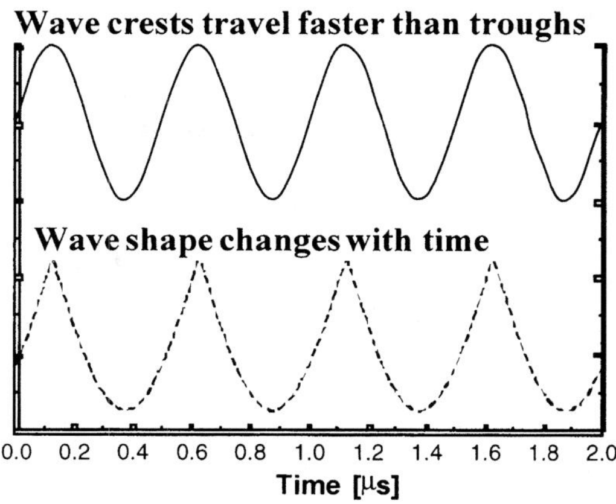

Fig. 2.11 As the fundamental frequency travels through tissue (a compressible medium—see text), the shape of the propagation wave will change, due to slight changes in the velocity of the ultrasound with compression compared to rarefaction. The "sharp" peaks are the developing harmonic frequencies. (Reproduced with permission from: Thomas JD, Rubin DN. Tissue harmonic imaging: why does it work? Journal of the American Society of Echocardiography 11(8): 804.)

Principles of harmonic imaging (tissue and contrast)

The term *harmonic imaging* refers to a form of B-mode scanning where a transducer will transmit at its fundamental frequency but "listen" at twice this frequency. As the fundamental frequency propagates through tissue, progressively small amounts of new *harmonic frequencies* are generated. (Harmonic frequencies are frequencies that are integer multiples of the fundamental frequency. If the fundamental frequency is 2 MHz, then the second harmonic is 4 MHz.) Harmonic frequencies are generated because tissue is slightly compressible. Since the velocity of sound is proportional to tissue density, as a wave travels through tissue (see Fig. 1.1), the velocity of the peak (compression) is slightly faster than when at a trough (rarefaction). This will result in a progressive slight change in the appearance of the propagated sine wave to more of a "peaked" sine wave containing not just the fundamental transmitted frequencies, but also small energies at harmonic frequencies (Fig. 2.11). The amount of harmonic frequency energy will slowly increase with distance traveled. Also, the magnitude of energy at the second harmonic is exponentially related to the fundamental frequency power (example: for a doubling of input fundamental power,

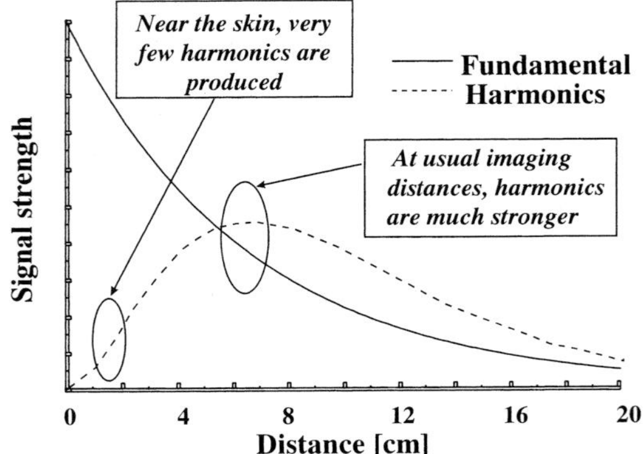

Fig. 2.12 As the distance traveled by the fundamental frequency increases, harmonic frequency amplitude will increase (see text). The amplitude of the harmonic signal is exaggerated in this image. The actual amplitude compared to the fundamental signal amplitude is much weaker. (Reproduced with permission from Thomas JD, Rubin DN. Tissue harmonic imaging: why does it work? Journal of the American Society of Echocardiography 11(8): 805.)

there will be a quadrupling of the second harmonic energy).

Harmonic imaging without contrast agents is termed *tissue harmonic imaging*, and is associated with improved B-mode images for several reasons. With routine fundamental imaging much artifact results from nearfield scatter near the chest wall. Because harmonic energies are progressively generated with increasing distance, very little harmonic frequency energy has been generated when the transmit impulse has just left the transducer (near the chest wall), and these artifacts are not yet present at the higher harmonic frequency (Fig. 2.12). Also, side lobe artifact is essentially nonexistent at harmonic frequencies, since the generation of side lobe artifact is exponentially proportional to the energy of the applied pressure (Fig. 2.13). Lateral resolution is improved because low energy ultrasound waves are processed (as the energy is increased, the resolution decreases as discussed earlier in this chapter). Lastly, because the returning frequencies are higher, the resolution is inherently improved.

As discussed earlier, the transmit impulse for harmonic imaging is preferably a smooth onset-offset short narrowband impulse (Fig. 2.4). A wideband transmit impulse will have some energy at the desired "listening" frequency, but a narrowband impulse will have essentially no energy at the "listening" frequency, which improves the returning signal clarity (Fig. 2.14). For routine "fundamental" B-mode imaging, a wideband impulse is preferred, as the broad range of transmitted frequencies have improved axial resolution and somewhat less side band artifacts (see discussion earlier in this chapter). The transducer used for harmonic imaging must have a wide *dynamic range* (a measure of the range of signal intensities that can be evaluated in decibel units), since the second harmonic energy is at least 10–20 dB less than the returning fundamental frequency energy.

Harmonic imaging with microbubble contrast is a second way to use the harmonic frequency. It is thought that when microbubbles in the circulation come in contact with ultrasound, they will oscillate at predominately twice the fundamental frequency. By having the transducer "listen" at the harmonic frequency, mostly contrast and little tissue/structures will be visualized. When performing harmonic imaging with contrast, the power should be lower than normally used (as opposed to relatively high output power when using tissue harmonic imaging), as increasing ultrasound acoustic pressure will dramatically destroy contrast bubbles. At a "low" range of acoustic pressures, there is a linear response of contrast similar to that of tissue. At a desirable "medium" range of acoustic pressures, the bubbles resonate at

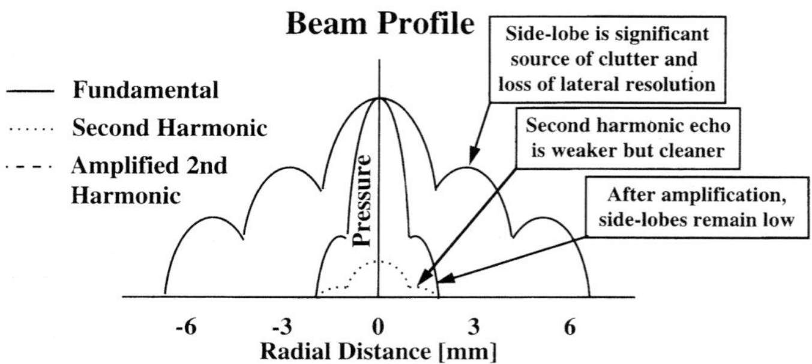

Fig. 2.13 The fundamental frequency has significant side lobe strength, whereas side lobe strength remains relatively low, even after the harmonic signal has been amplified (see text). (Reproduced with permission from: Thomas JD, Rubin DN. Tissue harmonic imaging: why does it work? Journal of the American Society of Echocardiography 11(8): 805.)

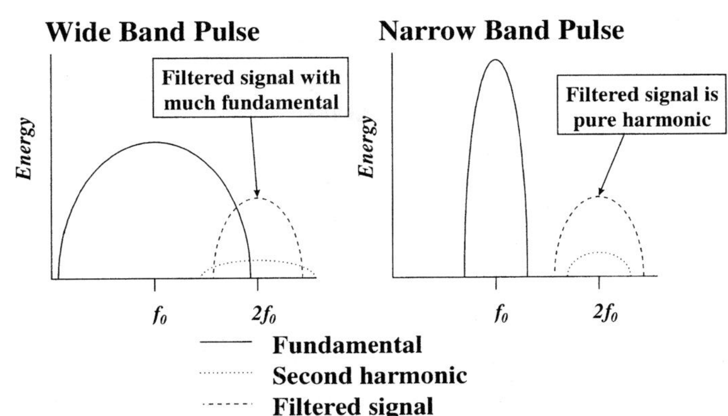

Fig. 2.14 With a wideband transmit signal, energy is present all the way up to the second harmonic frequency, but with a narrowband transmit signal, there is essentially no energy transmitted at the second harmonic frequency. A narrowband transmit signal will result in "sharp" returning signals having energy at the fundamental and harmonic frequency, but very little energy between these frequencies. (Reproduced with permission from: Thomas JD, Rubin DN. Tissue harmonic imaging: why does it work? Journal of the American Society of Echocardiography 11(8): 805.)

the harmonic frequencies allowing higher signal intensities. At higher acoustic pressures, the bubbles emit a final high energy broad-spectrum signal, before collapsing.

To further prolong microbubble "life" *transient response imaging* (*intermittent imaging, triggered response imaging*) may be used, in which exposure of the microbubbles to ultrasound energy occurs during selected phases of the cardiac cycle. Ultrasound transmission is decreased by triggering frame rates to once every cardiac cycle instead of continuously (normally 30 or more frames/s standard B-mode frame rates). Another way to prolong bubble life is to design and produce bubbles that are more resistant to acoustic pressure.

Harmonic power Doppler imaging (see also section on Doppler principles and instrumentation, p. 19), or *angiomode*, displays the intensity of a Doppler signal reflected from the contrast agent by using a color on the B-mode image. Tissue artifact is reduced, with an improved signal-to-noise ratio. This modality yields the highest returning signal intensity from microbubbles compared to contrast fundamental or second harmonic imaging.

An echo-pulse method called the *pulse inversion technique* has shown promise for imaging of microbubbles. Microbubbles are "nonlinear scatterers" and myocardium is a "linear scatterer." The transducer will emit pairs of pulses, with the second pulse inverted (Fig. 2.15). These two sequential pulses are processed together to form a single B-line. The returning signals will cancel each other out if reflected from a linear scatterer (myocardium), and summate from nonlinear scatterers (microbubbles). This method should provide the advantage of greater image resolution, better contrast detection, and improved contrast visualization even at a low acoustic power.

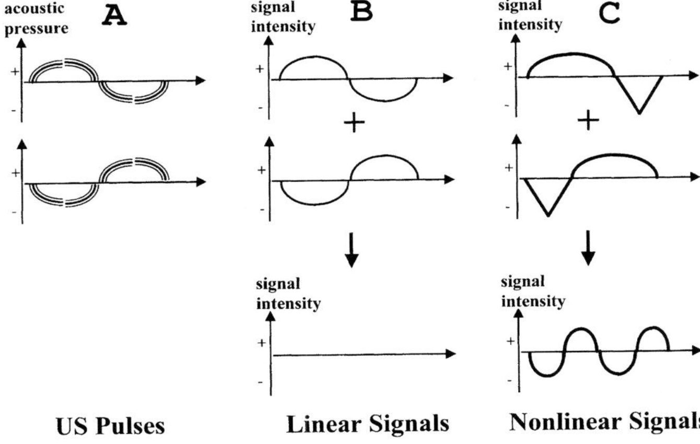

Fig. 2.15 The pulse inversion technique. (A) The transducer emits two sequential echo-pulses for each B-line. (B) The two returning signals will "cancel out" if reflected from tissue "linear scattering." (C) If scattered from microbubbles, the returning signals again are summated, but this time will not cancel out, and will be detected and then processed by the transducer. (Modified with permission from Bibra HV, Voigt JU, Froman M, *et al*. Interaction of microbubbles with ultrasound. Echocardiography 1999; 16(7 part 2): 740.)

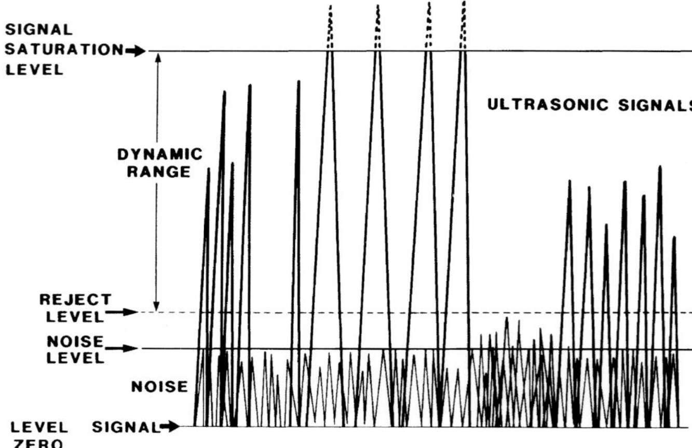

Fig. 2.16 The dynamic range of ultrasonic signals. Ultrasound machines have a *reject level*, which removes noise and low intensity echoes just above noise level. Signals increase in amplitude until the signal *saturation level* is achieved, which is the brightest possibly attained. The *dynamic range* is that between the system reject and signal saturation level, and is representative of signals that appear on the display. (Reproduced with permission from: Weyman AE. Principles and Practice of Echocardiography, 2nd edn. Philadelphia: Lea & Febiger, 1994.)

B-mode processing and display

The strength of the ultrasound signal generated by the transducer is termed the *acoustic power* (*output gain, energy output*). The maximum power the transducer can generate is 0 dB (–3 dB would be one half the maximum and –6 dB one quarter the maximum power output) (see Chapter 1).

As discussed earlier in the chapter, the returning RF signals from a single transmitted pulse are progressively amplified because of progressive attenuation from returning signals from further depths (Fig. 2.3). This is termed *time gain compensation* (TGC) or *depth gain compensation* (DGC). Echo signals returning from more distant reflectors are amplified more than signals from close to the transducer. Ultrasound machines will also have an operator-adjusted set of TGC knobs to adjust the *gain curve* for returning signals. A higher frequency transducer requires a steeper gain curve (quickly increasing gain for increasing depth) because of increased attenuation. *Compensation* will make echo signals arising from similar reflectors appear the same intensity, despite the depth (and henceforth increased attenuation) of the different reflectors.

After the RF signal has been modified to obtain the magnitude envelope (demodulation described earlier in the chapter), logarithmic signal *compression* (mentioned earlier in the chapter) is performed on the data to reduce the *dynamic range*. The dynamic range is the range of signals measured in decibels that are utilized by the ultrasound system. The dynamic range is the ratio of the largest signal amplitude that can be utilized (before saturation of the signal) to the smallest signal amplitude that can be detected (above the reject level) The sampled range (around 12 bits) is then reduced to that of an output display (8 bits) (Fig. 2.16). The range of data is nonlinearly compressed to map the dynamic range to enhance the darker gray levels at the expense of brighter gray levels. *Reject* is a filter that will remove low amplitude noise and echoes from the returning signals in order to allow the desirable higher amplitude signals to be displayed "crisper" and allow increased contrast of these signals on the display.

It should be noted that many newer generation ultrasound units are described as having "digital architecture," implying that the analog voltage is digitized (the process of analog-to-digital conversion through an A/D converter) after the RF signal has been amplified. An *analog* signal is a function that is defined over a continuous range of time and in which the amplitude may assume a continuous range of values (the voltage generated by the piezoelectric crystals of the transducer). A *digital* signal is a function in which both time and amplitude are quantified. A digital signal may always be represented by a sequence of numbers in which each number has a finite number of digits. An *A/D converter* takes the transducer-generated analog voltage and transforms it into a digital format (binary number). The *resolution* of the A/D converter is the precision with which the digital signal is generated, expressed in bits (for example 8 bits is 2 raised to the 8th power, which is 256). The *sampling rate* of the A/D converter is the number of digital points sampled per second (Hertz). The sampling rate of the A/D

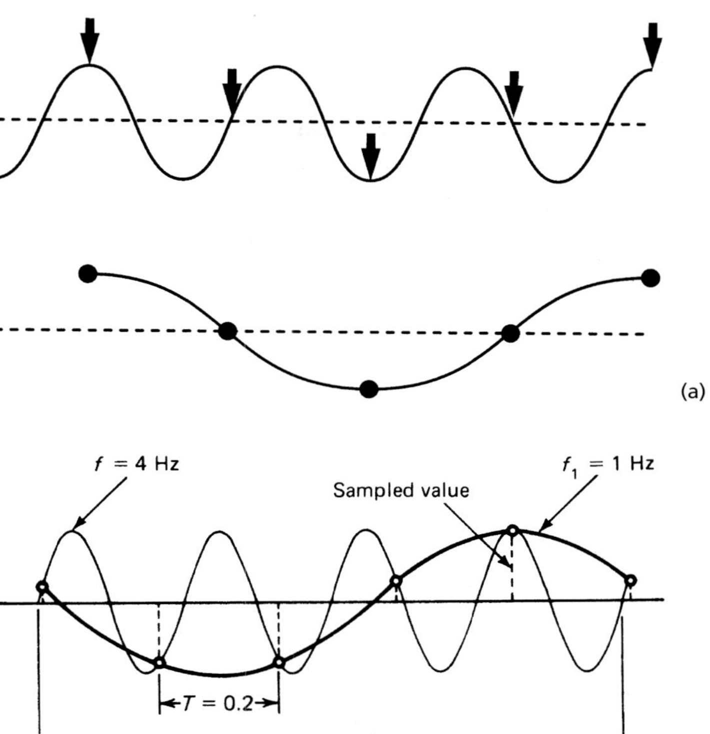

Fig. 2.17 Aliasing of a signal occurs when an analog signal is digitally sampled at less than twice the maximum frequency within that signal. (a) Sampling below the Nyquist rate produces a digital frequency (lower panel) that is less than the original analog frequency (upper panel). (b) The original analog frequency (*f*) is 4 Hz. Sampling occurs at 5 Hz (the Nyquist rate in this example is 8 Hz), and the resultant digital frequency (f_1) is only 1 Hz. For the digital frequency to accurately reflect the analog frequency, digital sampling must occur at a minimum of 8 Hz. ((a) Reproduced with permission from: Zagzebski JA, Essentials of Ultrasound Physics. Philadelphia: Mosby, 1996: p 103, figure 5.30. (b) Reproduced with permission from: Ahmed N, Natarajan T. Discrete-Time Signals and Systems. Reston Publishing, 1983: p 124, figure 4.31.)

converter must be at least twice the frequency of the highest transducer frequency used, according to *the Nyquist theorem* (also called the *sampling theorem* described by Shannon in 1948). The highest frequency in a signal (e.g. the generated RF signal) is called the *Nyquist frequency*, and the minimum sampling rate at which the signal could theoretically be recovered is called the *Nyquist rate* (twice the Nyquist frequency). If the sampling rate of the A/D converter is below the Nyquist rate, *aliasing* of the signal will occur (Fig. 2.17). If above the Nyquist rate, the signal can be theoretically uniquely determined by its sampled values. Aliasing results if a signal is not sampled at a sufficiently high rate. An analog frequency will be mistakenly represented as a lower frequency when digitized. Higher digitization sample rates are needed for A/D converters located at the transducer, as opposed to A/D converters located after the RF signal has been demodulated, since demodulated signals have lower frequencies than preprocessed "raw" RF signals. A typical sampling rate of a "raw" RF signal for a transducer with a 7.5-MHz center frequency is on the order of 36 MHz. Basically the higher the number of bits of an A/D converter, the higher the resolution; and the higher the sampling rate, the better the temporal resolution of the digitized signal.

After the signal has been digitized (in newer generation ultrasound machines) and processed (demodulation, amplification, compensation, compression, reject) it enters the *digital scan converter* (DSC). B-mode lines (and color flow Doppler) are in polar coordinates, and must be converted to a Cartesian raster output format for the display screen (Fig. 2.18). Each number represents a shade of gray (B-mode) or a color (color flow Doppler), and is called a pixel. (A digital image can be considered a matrix whose row and column indices identify a point in the image and the corresponding matrix element value identifies the gray level at that point. The elements of this digital array are termed *image elements, picture elements, pixels*, or *pels*.)

To be presented on a video screen, the digital output of the DSC must undergo digital-to-analog conversion (through a *D/A converter*). A typical size of a DSC matrix comparable in quality to a monochrome television image is a 512 × 512 size array with 128

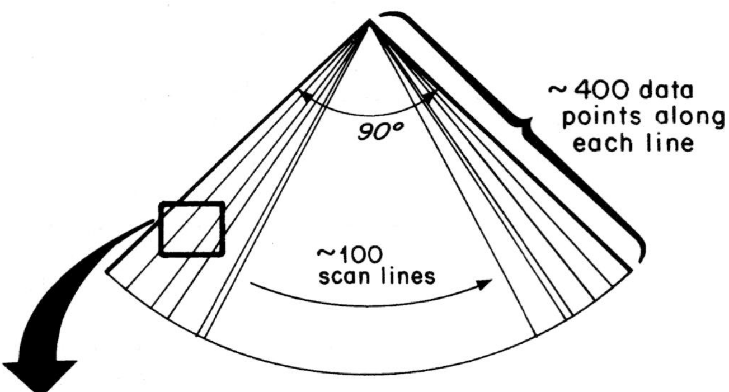

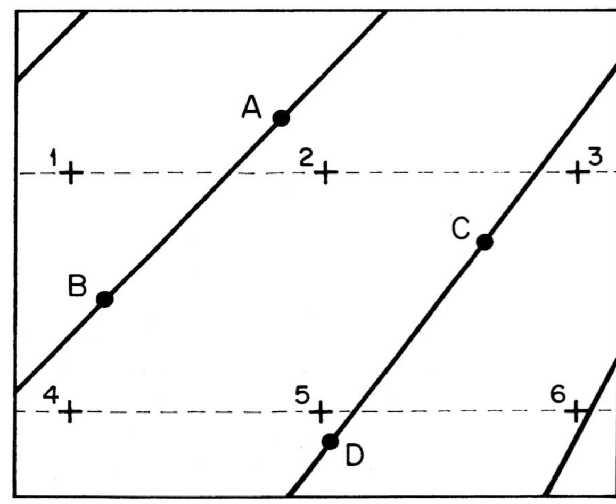

Fig. 2.18 The digital scan converter will take polar coordinate data (A, B, C, D in lower panel) and convert that data to rectangular coordinates (1, 2, 3, 4, 5, 6 in lower panel). Because the generated rectangular coordinate data may not exactly correlate to a value from the polar coordinate system, data must be interpolated. For example, to obtain the value at position 2, the values from points A and C might be averaged. This process is termed *interpolation.* (Reproduced with permission from: Weyman AE. Principles and Practice of Echocardiography, 2nd edn. Philadelphia: Lea & Febiger, 1994.)

gray levels (7 bits). Analog signals are generated corresponding to raster lines (there are 525 horizontal raster lines that make up a television image) of the monitor. First, odd lines (1,3,5 . . . , 525), then even lines (2,4,6 . . . , 524) are generated and displayed. Since the number of raster lines is different than the number of digital lines (rows) in the DSC, interpolation of the digital lines occurs to generate the analog signals. The first *field* (odd raster television lines) is displayed in 1/60 second, and the second field (even raster television lines) is displayed in 1/60 second. It therefore takes 1/30 second for all the information to be displayed, but by displaying odd lines first, and even lines next, the human eye will not perceive television screen flicker. It becomes evident that the B-mode ultrasound transducer (and color flow Doppler) sweep rate is usually different from the display rate of the television monitor.

The *frame rate* of a B-mode sector scan is basically limited by the travel time of ultrasound pulses within tissue. Given that the velocity of sound in tissue is 1540 m/s, one can calculate the time required to travel a known depth (and back) in tissue as:

$$T_{line} = (2 \times D)/(1540 \text{ m/s})$$

$$T_{line} \times (0.0012987 \text{ s/m}) \times D$$

$$T_{line} = 0.13 \times D(\text{cm})$$

where T_{line} is the time for a signal to travel down and back one scan line, and D is the distance from the transducer to the reflector. The time required to form a single frame (T_{frame}) from a single sweep is calculated as:

$$T_{frame} = (N) \times (T_{line})$$

$$T_{frame} = (N) \times (0.13 \times D) \text{ cm}$$

where N is the number of B scan lines. The frame rate (FR) that is maximally allowable (due to the velocity of sound in tissue) is:

$$FR = 1/T_{frame}$$

Substituting yields the following useful equation:

$$FR = 77\ 000/(N \times D)$$

FR is then the number of frames that may be maximally generated in 1 s, and D is in units of centimeters.

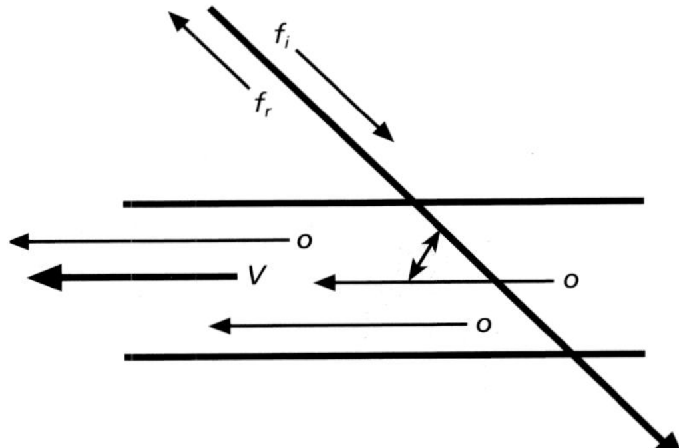

Fig. 2.19 An example of the Doppler shift. An incident soundwave (light or any other wave) with frequency (f_i) will reflect off a moving target (o) with a velocity V. There results a change in the reflected soundwave frequency to f_r. The angle between the incident soundwave and the moving target (double-headed arrow) is the angle θ (see text).

Doppler principles and instrumentation

The principle of the *Doppler* effect states that the frequency of a soundwave (lightwave or any other wave) is altered when the source of the soundwave is moving relative to the observer (or receiver device). If the object is moving toward the source, the reflected frequency will be higher than the original frequency, and if the object is moving away from the source, then the reflected frequency will be lower. This change in frequency is called the *Doppler shift* or *Doppler frequency* (Fig. 2.19). The Doppler equation calculates this change in frequency (f_d) as:

$$f_d = f_i - f_r = (2)(f_i)(V)(\cos\theta)/c$$

where f_i is the transmit initial frequency, f_r the reflected frequency, V the velocity of the moving object, c the velocity of the soundwave, and θ the angle between the soundwave and the direction of the moving target. In clinical Doppler studies of blood flow, the shifted frequency (f_d), is usually within the audible range of frequencies. The Doppler angle θ is important in clinical ultrasound, since the calculated f_d is dependent on its cosine. For an angle of 0°, the cos is 1 and will not affect the Doppler equation, but for increasing angles of θ properly measuring the correct angle becomes important. From the above equation, it is apparent that the Doppler shift frequency (f_d) is proportional to the transmit initial frequency (f_i) and the moving object velocity (V), and inversely proportional to the velocity of the soundwave (c) through the medium.

The frequency of the returning reflected ultrasound signal is calculated by the ultrasound machine using a *spectrum analyzer* (the "frequency spectrum" is calculated, thus the name); hence, the Doppler shift frequency is then calculated as ($f_i - f_r$), and the moving object velocity (V) is then known. Two basic methods have been used to calculate the frequency content of a Doppler signal returning from a moving reflector. The first is the method of *zero crossings*. Since a sine wave crosses the zero line twice for each cycle, the frequency of that sine wave is the number of zero crossings divided by 2. Unfortunately, the signal returning to the ultrasound transducer is not a "pure" sinusoidal wave, but is made up of many returning signals forming a complex signal. This method therefore falls short in analysis of the returning signal, and has not been used in ultrasound equipment since the early 1980s. The second method used to analyze a Doppler signal returning from a moving reflector is *Fourier analysis* (using a computer algorithm called a *fast Fourier transform—FFT*) for determination of the frequency content of a signal (*frequency domain analysis*). Fourier analysis provides a mathematical tool to extract frequency information from a signal and identify the frequencies that make up that signal. This is the method of spectrum analysis used by most

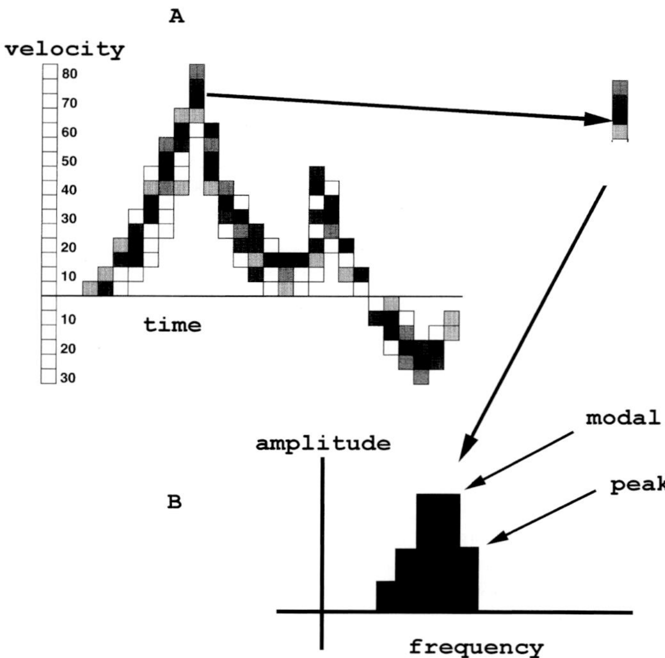

Fig. 2.20 (A) Each vertical set of pixels of a Doppler spectral display, representative of a small increment of time, is generated by a single FFT calculation of the ultrasound signal returning to the transducer. (B) A frequency plot (power spectral plot) is first generated. The Doppler shift frequency (f_i–f_r) is then converted to velocity by use of the Doppler equation to obtain the Doppler spectral display. The *modal* frequency (frequency at which the amplitude of the frequency plot is greatest, which presumably correlates with the greatest number of reflectors moving at that corresponding velocity) will correlate with the modal velocity; likewise the *peak* frequency of the frequency plot will correlate with the peak velocity of the Doppler spectral display. The *spectral width* is the range of frequencies generated by an FFT calculation at a particular time.

ultrasound manufacturers. To generate and display a Doppler signal, many sequential FFTs are performed with one FFT calculation representing a specific unit of time. Each FFT output will result in a set of spectral data for that unit of time (Fig. 2.20).

Doppler transducers require more power for "weak" reflectors (blood) than sector scanning transducers. Gain settings should be increased until background noise is just noticeable. Lower frequency transducers are required for adequate tissue penetration. A dynamic range of 25–30 dB should be adequate, but decreasing the dynamic range further may help diminish excessive background noise. In addition to the desired signal returning from flowing blood, the returning signal contains clutter from surrounding tissue and slowly moving vessel walls. The *clutter signal* may be very strong (about 40 dB stronger than blood signal) and of low frequency. A *wall filter* (a *high-pass filter* which only allows high frequency signals to "pass through") will remove these low frequency strong signals (these strong low frequency signals are used for *tissue Doppler imaging*). The wall filter should be set at as low a frequency as possible without removing desired velocity information. The *focal zone* of a Doppler probe (on phased-array systems) should be adjusted to the depth of interest.

Pulsed wave Doppler

A Doppler transducer will transmit an ultrasound signal and listen for the returning signal using a *depth-gated receiver*. The receiver only analyzes returning signals during a preselected time frame that corresponds to the distance of a particular area of interest.

A *pulsed wave Doppler* (PW) transducer will emit a series of individual pulses at a rate limited by the PRF (a pulse takes a certain amount of time to be emitted and return to the transducer). *Range ambiguity* (uncertainty in determining the distance of the reflector—distance traveled by a returning ultrasound signal) will result if a pulse is transmitted before the previous pulse returns. The returning ultrasound signals will each have a shifted phase in relation to each other (Fig. 2.21), and from this information the Doppler-shift frequency due to the moving reflectors is generated. The PRF of the pulsed Doppler system must be at least twice the cycle of the Doppler-shifted frequency, otherwise *aliasing* will occur (Fig. 2.17).

To eliminate aliasing from a pulsed wave signal, increasing the velocity on the ultrasound unit display will increase the PRF automatically on many machines. Since the highest frequency that can be detected is PRF/2 (the *Nyquist limit* or *Nyquist frequency*), by increasing the PRF the detected frequency

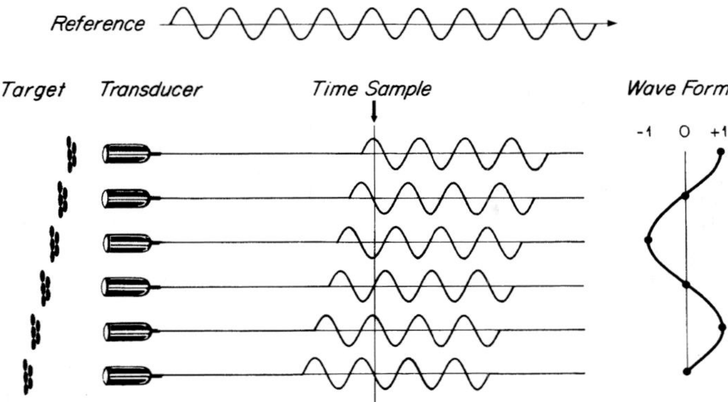

Fig. 2.21 A series of ultrasound pulses are transmitted at a maximum rate determined by the PRF. Each returning ultrasound pulse will change its "*phase*" relative to each other. This noted phase shift contains the Doppler shift information. The received pulses are compared to a sine wave "*reference*", and by a process called *coherent demodulation*, the resultant signal "*wave form*" is the Doppler shift frequency. Gated Doppler spectral estimation will track Doppler frequencies at a single spatial location over time by collecting a significant number of pulses—of the order of 256 pulses in clinical instruments, and then perform an FFT on this "*wave form*" to obtain the spectral plot for a single moment of time. (Reproduced with permission from: Weyman AE. Principles and Practice of Echocardiography, 2nd edn. Philadelphia: Lea & Febiger, 1994.)

(and hence velocity) will then be increased. Shifting the axis of the Doppler scale will also help to eliminate aliasing (Fig. 2.22). The advantage of pulsed wave Doppler is *range resolution* (known position of the ultrasound reflector), and the significant disadvantage is an inability to record high velocities.

High pulse repetition frequency Doppler

When a higher velocity is to be determined than that possible with pulsed wave Doppler, some instruments have a *high PRF* mode. Instead of considering only one pulse to be "within the body" at a time as with pulsed Doppler, high PRF will transmit pulses at an interval too short to allow reflections to return to the transducer from deep structures. This will lead to range ambiguity, but higher velocities will be detected because of the higher PRF (Fig. 2.23).

Continuous wave Doppler

Continuous wave Doppler (CW) will continuously and rapidly transmit ultrasound signals. Signals will also continuously return to the transducer. Because the signal is a continuous single frequency the returning frequency has the narrowest frequency and the best frequency resolution. As opposed to PW, there is essentially no velocity that will alias with CW, but CW cannot determine the depth from which the reflected signal originated.

Color flow Doppler

Color flow Doppler is only possible with phased or annular array technology. It is in many respects similar to pulse-echo gray scale (B-mode) imaging. Whereas reflector amplitude is measured with B-mode gray scale imaging, color Doppler measures reflector velocity. For color flow Doppler imaging, a B-mode sector scan is displayed, with a second color sector scan "superimposed" on the B-mode sector scan.

Ultrasound impulses are transmitted in a similar fashion as a B-mode sector scan, but the ultrasound pulse duration (PD) is longer, and therefore has a narrower frequency bandwidth than the PD of a gray scale impulse. Not only is the returning signal amplitude noted, but also its *phase*. Whereas PW Doppler obtains velocity information by a method as illustrated in Fig. 2.21, color Doppler technology will emit a group of ultrasound pulses (maximum emitted rate is the PRF) for each pixel in the color scan. Pairs of returning pulses are compared for a shift in phase compared to each other (Fig. 2.24). This shift is indicative of motion of a reflector (blood cells) from one ultrasound pulse to the next. The amount of shift

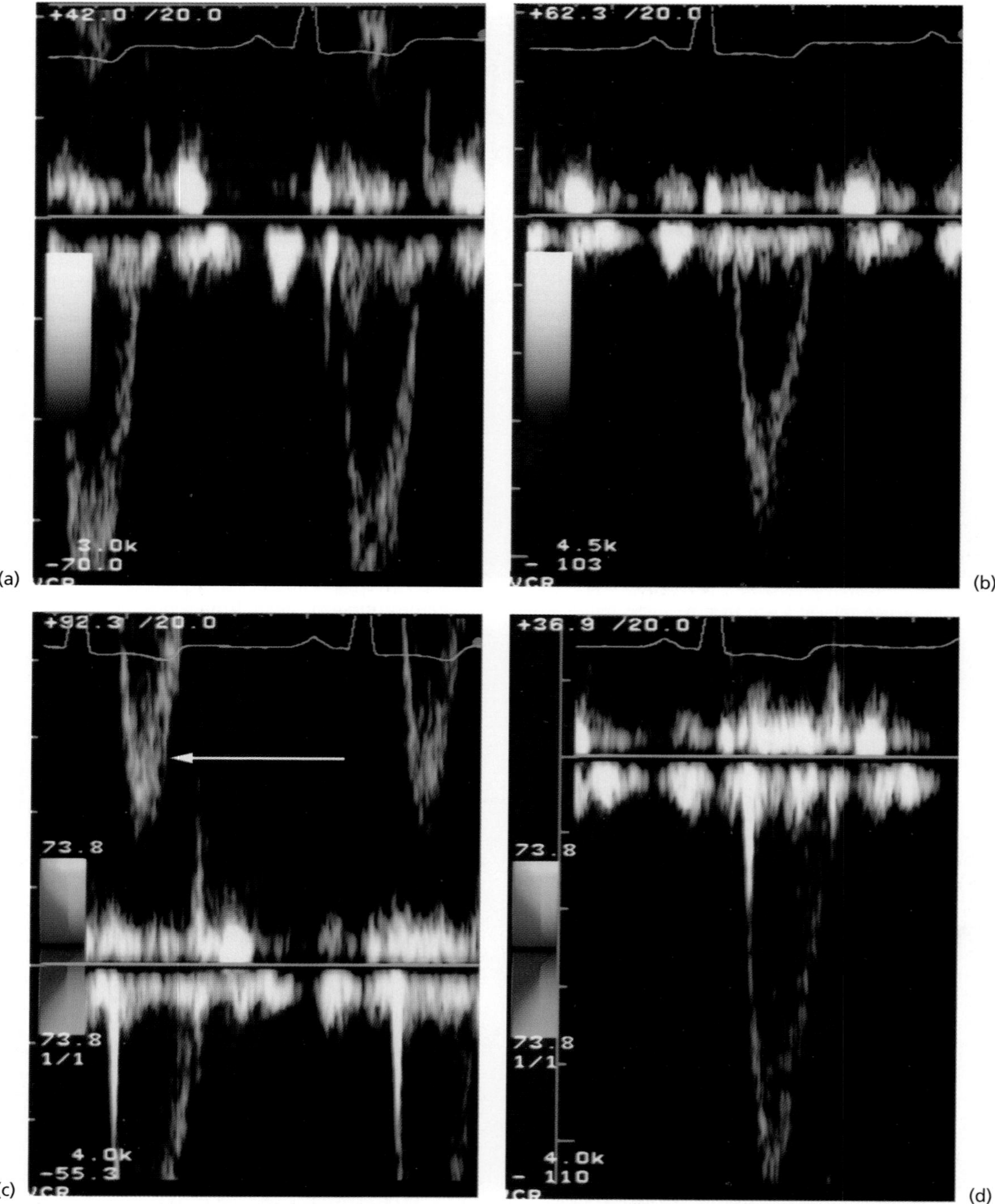

Fig. 2.22 Two ways to increase the velocity with PW Doppler is: (i) to increase the PRF and (ii) shift the baseline. In (a) the PW Doppler recording aliases, but in (b) the PRF has been increased to record the entire Doppler envelope. In (c) the signal again aliases, with "wraparound" noted (arrow), but (d) by shifting the baseline, the entire Doppler recording is noted.

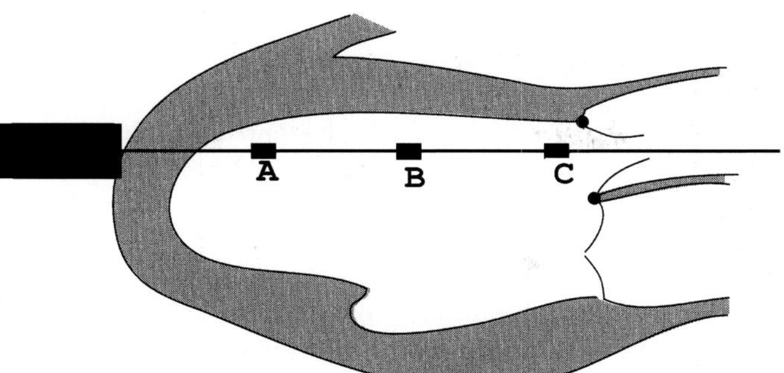

Fig. 2.23 Multiple Doppler sample volumes are evident in high PRF mode. If the velocity of flow at gate C is desired, the maximum possible velocity measured will be higher because the PRF has been increased. However, range ambiguity is introduced into the system, with velocities at gates A and B simultaneously measured. Multiple pulses are within the body at once; it is not possible to determine whether a given reflected signal resulted from one pulse or another, and therefore the resultant range ambiguity (unknown duration of time that a signal has been traveling within the body, and therefore unknown distance traveled).

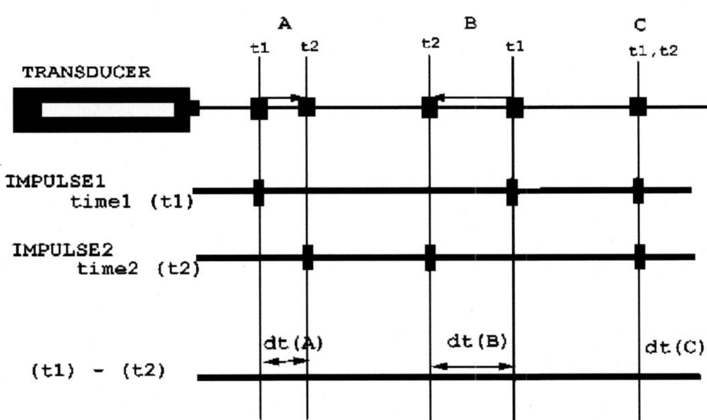

Fig. 2.24 The method of color flow Doppler. Reflector A is moving away, B toward, and C is stationary relative to the transducer. Time of return from the first impulse (IMPULSE1) is recorded and stored for three representative positions (A, B, C) in this example. A second impulse (IMPULSE2) is then transmitted, and the return times measured. For reflector A, the second impulse "round-trip" will be longer than the first impulse, because the reflector has moved a distance dt (A) away from the transducer. The time value dt (A) is proportional to the distance the reflector has moved; therefore the reflector velocity, relative to the transducer, is then calculated. Similarly, for reflector B the "round-trip" time for IMPULSE2 is less than IMPULSE1, and the velocity toward the transducer is calculated. Reflector C is stationary, therefore there will be no "phase shift" between IMPULSE1 and IMPULSE2, and the impulses will "cancel out". IMPULSE1 and IMPULSE2 are pulse-pairs. Multiple pulse-pairs are transmitted along a single ultrasound scan line to obtain an average velocity, velocity variance, and magnitude.

in phase between the two pulses is proportional to reflector velocity. A group of pulse "pairs" will be analyzed at each pixel, with the total number of impulses referred to as the *packet size* (*color packets* or *pulse packets*, or also sometimes termed *ensemble length*). The final velocity at the pixel being evaluated is the average of the calculated velocities from these pulse pairs. Because there are many reflectors (blood cells) within the pixel region, it is more accurate to have a relatively large packet size. Three quantities are obtained: *mean phase shift* (indicative of mean velocity), *variance* of the mean value (indicative of either turbulence of acceleration), and *amplitude* information (suggestive of the number of reflectors at that velocity).

Importantly, before calculating color Doppler velocity information a *clutter filter* (*clutter rejection filter*) must be employed (a wall filter is an electronic high-pass filter used to filter out low frequency signals) to remove stationary reflectors (reflector C in Fig. 2.24). Stationary reflectors are predominantly tissue and muscle, and are usually high amplitude (and very low velocity) signals. These signals must first be removed in order to obtain the very low amplitude signals from moving reflectors (blood flow). Once these high amplitude/low velocity signals are removed, the low amplitude/relatively high velocity signals (representative of blood flow) are amplified. These signals are then processed to obtain velocities by one of two methods. The most common method to detect velocity is a *phase-shift* velocity estimate using an *autocorrelation* computer algorithm. Basically, the algorithm mathematically compares both signals of a pulse pair to see how "similar" they are to each other. The other method used to detect velocity is a *time-shift* velocity estimate. This method tracks movement of a group of reflectors (red blood cells) by evaluating the reflected amplitude. A computer *cross-correlation* technique compares consecutively transmitted pulses along a beam line. Using the infrequently used time-shift method theoretically will remove aliasing with color Doppler and is generally thought to be more accurate, but increased velocity estimates require a large pulse-packet, and computing capability will limit this computer mathematical technique's ability.

Color flow Doppler maximal frame rate calculation is somewhat more detailed than that for frame rate calculations for B-mode sector scans. One must take into account the pulse-packet size and also time spent sending ultrasound pulses for the underlying B-mode sector scan. *Color Doppler frame rate* (FR_c) maximally obtainable may be expressed as:

$$FR_c = (PRF)/(n \times N)$$

where PRF is the pulse repetition frequency, n the size of the pulse-packet, and N the number of lines per frame. Note that for an increasing number of pulse packets or number of color lines, the color Doppler frame rate necessarily decreases.

Properties of color are described by *hue* (what color by the wavelength of light), *saturation* (how much white is blended into the hue . . . a totally saturated color is a pure hue and one light wavelength), and *intensity* (brightness). By convention, red is indicative of flow toward and blue away from the transducer. In some color maps less saturation (more white blended into the hue) indicates higher velocities. Intensity may also be indicative of velocity. *Variance* (flow disturbance) is expressed as another color . . . usually yellow or green.

Generally, the transmit power is set at a maximum unless scanning at close range or during fetal echocardiography. Gain is increased until background "color clutter" is evident, then slowly dialed down to optimize the blood-flow envelope. A color pixel represents the flow within that area it covers. By increasing the pixel size the signal-to-noise ratio is reduced, the signal strength is increased, and color frame rates are increased, but at the cost of a decreased color resolution. *Color versus echo write priority* (available on some machines) allows the sonographer to decide if color or B-mode information predominates on the screen.

Tissue Doppler principles

Tissue Doppler echocardiography (TDE) analyzes motion from relatively slow moving "strong" reflectors, such as LV myocardium, valves, and other masses. Whereas traditional color flow Doppler of bloodflow evaluates relatively high velocity signals (range on the order up to 2 m/s) and "weak" ultrasound reflectors (red blood corpuscles), tissue velocity is approximately an order of magnitude lower (in the range of approximately 1–20 cm/s) and a strong echo reflector. TDE may be represented as two different "types": *tissue Doppler imaging* (TDI) and *pulsed wave tissue Doppler* (PWTD).

The principles of a TDI system are similar to that of color flow Doppler except that the signal is not passed through a high-pass filter (clutter filter described earlier), and all low amplitude returning signals are rejected (Fig. 2.25).

PWTD echocardiography will quantify velocity information about myocardial motion. As with TDI, the high-pass filter is not used and low amplitude signals are disregarded. This method provides a better temporal resolution and velocity range than TDI, but TDI provides better spatial information as compared to PWTD. This method represents motion at the PW Doppler cursor. This velocity profile may not only represent true tissue motion, but also motion caused

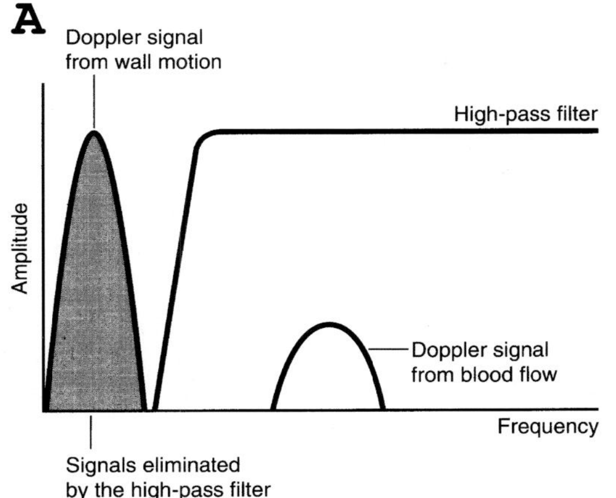

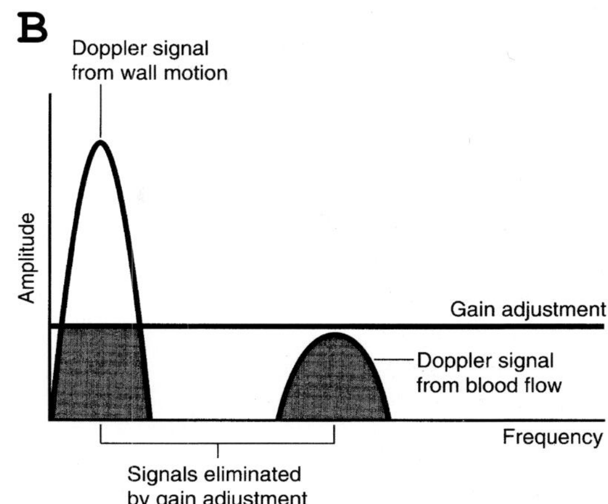

Fig. 2.25 Doppler signals returning to the transducer are either relatively high amplitude/low velocity (tissue) or relatively low amplitude/high velocity (blood). (A) For traditional color flow Doppler of blood, the returning impulses are high-pass filtered (clutter filter) to only obtain bloodflow signals. (B) Tissue Doppler imaging will reject relatively low amplitude signals, thus only the high amplitude signals are retained. (Reproduced with permission from: Yamazaki N. Principle of Doppler tissue velocity measurements. In: Erbel R, Nesser HJ, Drozdz J, eds. Atlas of Tissue Doppler Echocardiography TDE. New York: Springer, 1995.)

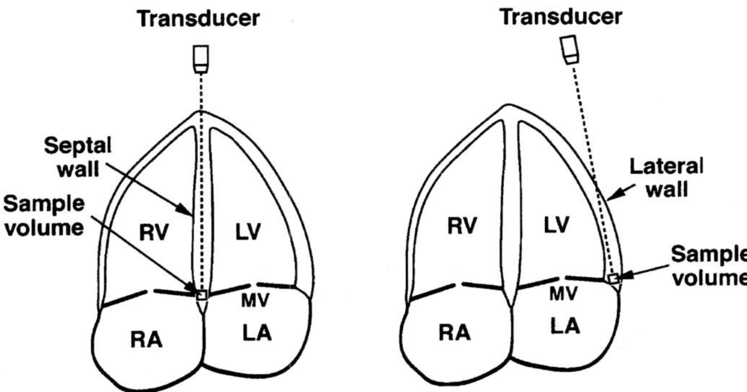

Fig. 2.26 PWTD of mitral annular motion for assessment of LV diastolic function and preload (see Chapter 6). (Reproduced with permission from: Sohn DW, Chai IH, Lea DJ, *et al.* Assessment of mitral annulus velocity by Doppler tissue imaging in the evaluation of left ventricular diastolic function. J Am Coll Cardiol 1997; 30: 474–480.)

by myocardial translation and rotation relative to the transducer. PWTD of myocardial segments may be performed to evaluate global and regional cardiac function. PWTD may assess diastolic function independent of LV preload (Fig. 2.26). The sample volume may be set to 3–7 mm, gain reduced significantly, power often to the lowest setting, and wall filters minimized so that low velocities may be recorded.

3

CHAPTER 3

Basics of Fluid Mechanics and Hemodynamic Equations

Introduction to fluid mechanics

A *fluid* cannot resist a stress (*stress* may be thought of as the opposite of compression . . . if a bar is pulled from both ends stress is exerted on the material within that bar) without moving, as can a solid. Fluids may be classified as a liquid or gas. A *liquid* has intermolecular forces that keep it together so that it has volume but no definite shape. In describing a fluid system, if we follow not any individual fluid molecule as it travels (*Lagrangian description*), but watch a particular point in space as fluid flows through that point; the velocity, acceleration and other properties at that point as a function of time may be measured (*Eulerian description*).

Stress is defined as the force exerted on an object divided by its cross-sectional area (Fig. 3.1, and see Chapter 5). *Pressure* in a nonmoving fluid is defined as the normal compressive force per unit area (normal stress) acting on a surface immersed in that fluid. This pressure is termed *hydrostatic pressure. Viscosity* (μ) is a measure of a fluid's resistance to shear when that fluid is in motion (Fig. 3.2).

Fluid flow may be considered to be *ideal* (flow has no internal friction and is laminar—no fluid is truly ideal, but many bloodflow conditions are considered such for analysis), *viscous*, or *turbulent*. *Laminar flow* (purely viscous flow) is fluid flow in layers (laminas), as opposed to turbulent flow in which random velocity fluctuations are imposed upon the mean velocity. An example of a transition from laminar to turbulent fluid flow is that of smoke rising from a candle . . . initially it is a smooth laminar flow, but then widens and becomes turbulent. In turbulent flow shear stresses predominate over viscous forces. To predict if a flow will be laminar or turbulent one can calculate the *Reynolds number* (Re) for the fluid system. The Reynolds number (a dimensionless number) is defined as:

$$\text{Re} = \text{Inertial forces/Viscous forces} = [(\rho)(V_m)(d)]/\mu$$

where ρ is fluid density, V_m is the average fluid velocity across the cross-sectional area, d is the tube diameter, and μ is viscosity. If Re is less than 1200 the flow will be laminar, at 1200–2300 flow is described as transitional, and at greater than 2300 turbulent.

As fluid enters a pipe the *average* velocity throughout the pipe will remain constant (see "Continuity equation" below). Because of fluid viscosity, layers that are adjacent to the stationary layer at the vessel wall boundary will slow down, but in order to maintain a constant average velocity profile, the center fluid columns will accelerate (Fig. 3.3). Flow will finally assume a parabolic profile with the velocity of the fluid at the vessel wall remaining as zero. Depending to a

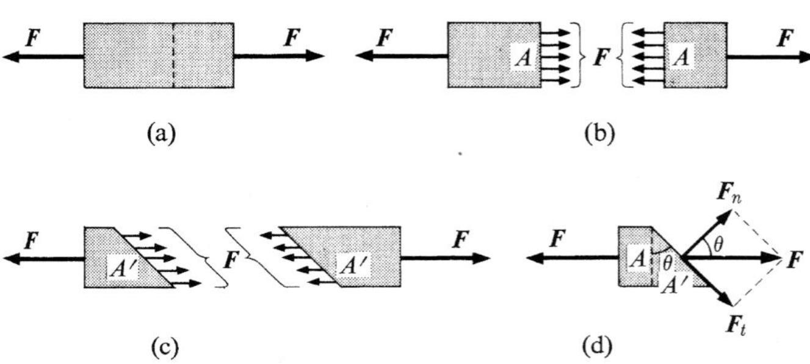

Fig. 3.1 (a) A bar in tension. (b) The stress on the bar in the perpendicular direction (*normal stress*) equals *F/A*. If one looks at a section (c) of the bar at an angle the stress may be resolved into a normal component (F_n/A') and a tangential (*shear stress*) component (F_t/A'). (Reproduced with permission from: Sears FW, Zemansky MW. University Physics, 4th edn. Reading, MA: Addison-Wesley Publishing, 1970.)

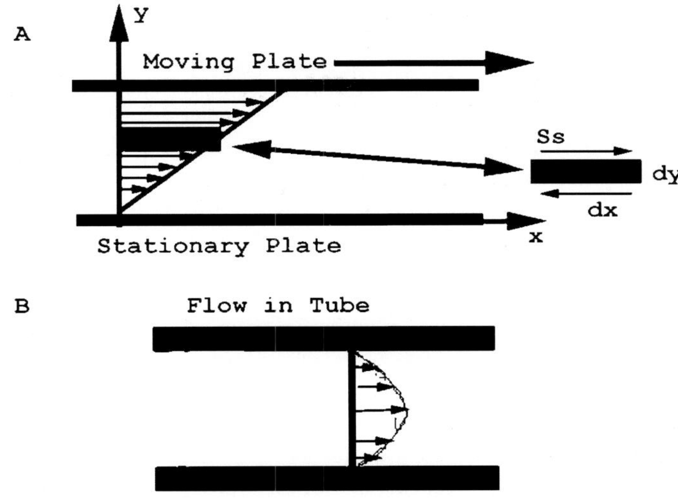

Fig. 3.2 (A) Flow demonstrating shear stress (Ss) of a fluid between two plates at a representative small element within the moving fluid. The top plate is moving toward the right, and the bottom plate is stationary. The shear stress is the viscosity (μ) multiplied by the small change in velocity in the *y* direction (d*v*) divided by the small distance (d*y*) . . . Ss = μ[d*v*/d*y*]. This simple relationship between shear stress and velocity gradient is known as a Newtonian relationship (*Newton's Law of Viscosity*), and fluids that obey such a relationship are termed *Newtonian fluids*. (B) Laminar flow velocity is a parabolic shape in a tube. Note that at the wall of the tube the fluid velocity is zero, and the maximum fluid velocity is in the center of the tube.

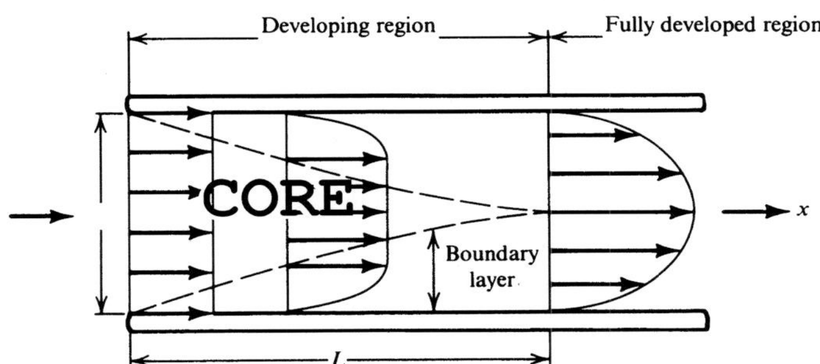

Fig. 3.3 As fluid enters a pipe it progresses along and will assume a parabolic shape. The length *L* is the *developing region* (*unestablished flow*), and when flow then becomes parabolic it is the *developed region* (*established flow*). The developing region will become dominated by the growth of the *boundary layer*, and a diminishing *core* of fluid at the center of the pipe. Established flow will result from the merging of the boundary layers. The velocity of the core flow will increase progressively as it approaches the fully developed region, but the *average* velocity along each cross-section remains constant along the entire length of pipe. (Modified with permission from Granger RA. Fluid Mechanics. New York: Dover Publications, 1995.)

large extent on the Reynolds number, the boundary layer and established flow may be turbulent, instead of laminar. The average velocity, however, will remain constant, as is the case with laminar flow. Core flow may be thought of as frictionless, and the drop in pressure along the pipe may be calculated (from known core velocities along the pipe) from the Bernoulli equation. The equation to describe the profile of the parabola (for laminar flow only) is (Hagen–Poiseuille flow profile):

$$V/V_c = (1 - (r^2/R^2))$$

where V is velocity at a radial location r, V_c is the center velocity, and R is the radius of the pipe. The mean velocity of flow (V_m) is described as the *Hagen-Poiseuille equation*:

$$V_m = (R^2/8\mu)(dp/dx)$$

where dp/dx is the pressure drop per unit distance x, and μ is the viscosity. *Poiseuille's law* describes flow through a tube:

$$Q = \pi(R^4)[P_1 - P_2]/(8\,\mu L)$$

where Q is flow, R is the radius of the tube, P_1 the pressure at the beginning of the tube, P_2 the pressure at the end of the tube and L the length of the tube. The pressure drop along L is the energy needed for the movement of the fluid.

Turbulence occurring with pulsatile flow may be transient. Transition of flow from laminar to turbulent requires a certain amount of time to develop, therefore if flow is pulsatile, turbulence may not develop. In a similar fashion, if flow is turbulent, but the status now favors laminar flow, the transition may be delayed. Acceleration of flow tends to favor laminar flow, whereas deceleration of flow tends to favor turbulent flow (e.g. many times pulsed wave Doppler recordings show spectral broadening on the "downslope" of recordings). The Reynolds number required for turbulence to develop in pulsatile flow is necessarily higher than for nonpulsatile flow, and is described as a function of the *Womersley number* (Nw):

$$Nw = (R)\sqrt{[\rho\omega/\mu]}$$

where ω is the circular frequency of the heartbeat. As the calculated Nw for a system increases, the required value of Re for turbulence to occur also increases.

Time velocity integral/stroke volume, shunt and regurgitant fraction calculations

The *time velocity integral* (*TVI*), also called *velocity time integral* (*VTI*), is the area measured under the Doppler velocity envelope for one heartbeat. The Doppler sample (pulsed wave) is placed at the level of the annulus of the valve, and parallel to blood flow direction (using color Doppler helps "line up" flow parallel to the Doppler probe direction). Many times the *modal velocity* (darkest part of the signal indicative of the greatest number of reflectors—red blood cells—at that particular velocity) is used for *TVI* measurement (Fig. 3.4).

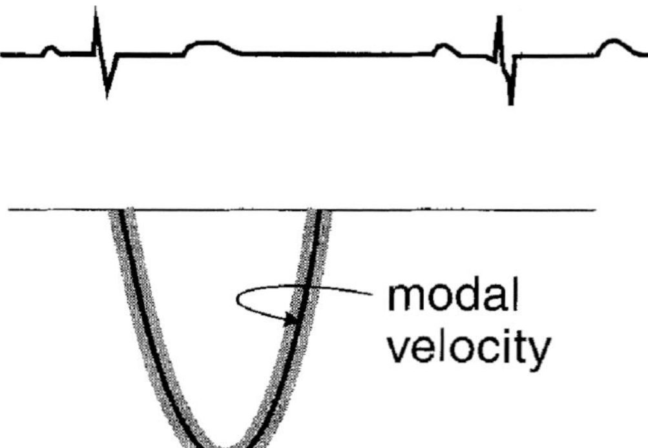

Fig. 3.4 The time velocity integral (*TVI*) is obtained by tracing the area of the PW envelope of flow. The modal velocity (darkest part of the waveform) is used, as this represents the predominant velocity of the majority of red blood cells. Units are in length (m or cm). The Doppler horizontal axis is in units of seconds (s), and vertical axis often as m/s, therefore [m/s × s] will be meters for the units of the *TVI*.

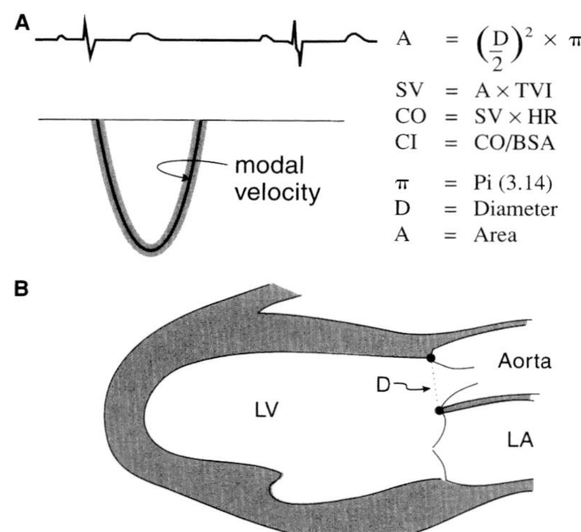

Fig. 3.5 Determination of the *TVI*, *SV* (stroke volume), *CO* (cardiac output), and *CI* (cardiac index). In (A) the *TVI* is obtained from the apical five-chamber view, by planimetering the area of flow, and in (B) the diameter is obtained in early mid systole, from the parasternal long axis, using the inner-edge-to-inner-edge method. Both measurements are made from the same level. Importantly, significant error may be introduced in *SV* calculations by slightly inaccurate diameter (*D*) measurements, since this term is squared when obtaining the area (*A*).

From the *TVI* the *stroke volume* (*SV*), and hence *cardiac output* (*CO*) and *cardiac index* (*CI*) may be calculated (Fig. 3.5) (SV may be also calculated as the planimetered end-diastolic volume minus the end-systolic volume discussed in Chapter 5). The *area* (*A*) is obtained at the same level as the *TVI* measurement was made. Left ventricular *SV* may by calculated as follows:

$$SV = TVI_{ot} \times A_{ot}$$

$$SV = TVI_{ot} \times [D/2]^2 \times \pi$$

$$SV = TVI_{ot} \times D^2 \times 0.785$$

where D is the LVOT diameter in centimeters, TVI_{ot} is the *TVI* of the LVOT in centimeters, and A_{ot} is the calculated area of the LVOT.

TVI and area measurements can be made at many sites including the ascending aorta, aortic annulus, mitral inflow, tricuspid inflow, and pulmonary valve levels. Generally, the diameter measurement is made from a stop-frame in the mid-portion of the cycle corresponding to flow (early mid systole for aortic and pulmonic measurements and early mid diastole for tricuspid and mitral measurements). *The inner-edge-to-inner-edge method* for diameter measurements should be used. The general equation for calculating area uses *D*/2, but when using the mitral annulus, since it is not circular, one should measure the diameter in the apical 4 (D_1), and also apical 2 chamber (D_2) views. The area equation at the mitral valve orifice (A_{mv}) is then:

$$A_{mv} = [(D_{1/2}) \times (D_{2/2})]^2 \times \pi$$

The aortic annulus is the most accurate of all the valves for *SV* measurements. The aortic diameter is measured in the parasternal long axis in early mid systole, and the pulsed wave Doppler (PW) aortic *TVI* is obtained from the apical five-chamber view. The PW sample is placed at the same level as where the diameter measurement was made. *SV* measurements at the level of the tricuspid valve (TV) are generally not very accurate.

This method of *SV* determination makes the assumption that:

- The velocity profile is flat.
- The area of the orifice is constant during the time obtaining the *TVI*.
- Flow is laminar (not turbulent).

Other potential *clinical pitfalls* in calculation of the *SV* include:

- Best beam alignment is not obtained.
- The best LVOT velocity profile is not obtained (one should obtain the maximum velocity profile for *SV* measurements . . . for a proper LVOT profile during aortic valve area (AVA) measurements, "inch" up toward the stenotic valve from the apical five-chamber view, until the LVOT signal begins to show spectral broadening, then obtain the waveform just proximal to that).
- Failure to obtain the modal velocity.
- Failure to measure the diameter early in the cardiac cycle, and failure to use diameter measurements from the mitral valve using two orthogonal measurements.
- Failure to accurately measure the inner-edge-to-inner-edge.

TVI measurements and subsequently *SV* calculations allow for shunt calculations and also measurement of valvular regurgitant fraction. *Shunt ratios* (Q_P/Q_S) may be calculated knowing that *SV* can be calculated at multiple levels. Q_P is pulmonic flow (right-sided stroke volume) and Q_S is systemic flow (left-sided stroke volume). The following table shows which valve levels may be measured to obtain shunt ratios for a particular defect:

Defect	Q_P	Q_S
ASD	TV, PV	MV, AV
VSD	MV, PV	TV, AV
PDA	MV, AV	TV, PV

See List of Abbreviations, p. vii for definitions.

Generally, use of the aortic and pulmonary valves is preferred to that of mitral or tricuspid valves for *SV* measurements. The most accurate is the AV level, followed by PV (measured from a high parasternal short axis for both *TVI* and diameter measurements), MV (apical 4 and 2), and the TV level.

Example: Calculate an ASD shunt ratio using (Q_P/Q_S) given the following:

$LVOT_d$	aortic annulus diameter	2.0 cm
$LVOT_a$	aortic annulus area	
TVI_{ot}	LVOT TVI	24 cm
PUL_d	pulmonic annulus diameter	2.2 cm
PUL_a	pulmonic annulus area	
TVI_{pul}	pulmonic TVI	28 cm

$$Q_P = TVI_{pul} \times PUL_a$$

$$PUL_a = \pi(PUL_d/2)^2$$

$$Q_P = (TVI_{pul})[\pi(PUL_d/2)^2]$$

$$Q_P = 28 \times 3.14 \times (2.2/2)^2$$

$$Q_P = 106.4$$

$$Q_S = TVI_{ot} \times LVOT_a$$

$$LVOT_a = \pi(LVOT_d/2)^2$$

$$Q_S = (TVI_{ot})[\pi(LVOT_d/2)^2]$$

$$Q_S = 24 \times 3.14 \times (2.0/2)^2$$

$$Q_S = 75.4$$

$$Q_P/Q_S = 106.4/75.4$$

$Q_P/Q_S = 1.4$ the shunt ratio is 1.4 : 1

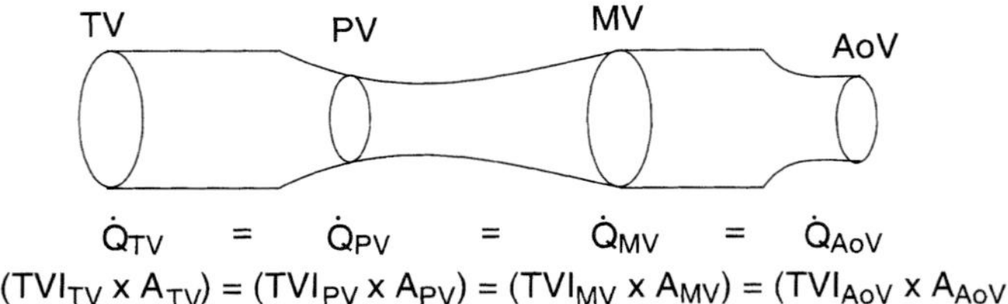

Fig. 3.6 The continuity equation, which is valid only in the absence of significant valvular regurgitation or an intracardiac shunt.

The regurgitant jet area (seen on color flow Doppler imaging) depends not only on the regurgitant volume, but also jet velocity, receiving chamber compliance, and ventricular function. Using color Doppler imaging may at times be difficult to interpret. The *regurgitant fraction* (*RF*) is the amount of blood flowing retrograde (regurgitant volume) divided by the total amount of blood ejected by the LV (total *LV SV*). It is the percentage of regurgitant volume compared to the total flow across the valve that is regurgitant. This method truly quantitates regurgitation.

RF = (Regurg. volume)/Total *LVSV* = (Total *LVSV* – Systemic flow)/Total *LVSV*

The following parameters can be fit into the above equation for mitral regurgitation (MR) or aortic regurgitation (AR):

	Total *LVSV*	Systemic flow
MR	2DSV or *MVSV*	*AVSV*
AR	2DSV or *AVSV*	*MVSV* or *PVSV*

2DSV = *SV* by 2D echo measurement (*EDV* – *ESV*) (see description of method of discs in Chapter 5).
MVSV = *TVI* × *A* at mitral orifice.
AVSV = *TVI* × *A* at LVOT.
PVSV = *TVI* × *A* at pulmonic valve level.

Generally, regurgitant fraction (*RF*) measurements >0.20 are considered hemodynamically significant:

RF	Severity
<0.20	Mild
0.20–0.40	Moderate
0.40–0.60	Moderate to severe
>0.60	Severe

Practically, measurement of the RF is prone to several possible errors, and for that reason is not usually done in routine day-to-day clinical situations.

Continuity equation

The *continuity equation* states that the amount of blood flow through one cardiac chamber (or valve orifice) is the same as the blood flow through the other chambers and orifices (Fig. 3.6). It is based on the principle of conservation of mass. The continuity equation most commonly is applied to calculation of the aortic valve area (*AVA*) in aortic stenosis. Flow at the level of the valvular stenosis (obtained with continuous wave (CW) Doppler) and that of the LVOT, just below the valve orifice are generally used (Fig. 3.7). The three variables on the right side of the equation in Fig. 3.7 are measured, allowing us calculate the *AVA*. When using the LVOT, the continuity equation is still valid in the presence of aortic regurgitation, because the same amount of blood is still going through both "orifices" being measured (see Chapter 7).

Potential clinical pitfalls found with the continuity equation when calculating the *AVA* include (see Chapter 7):

- Inaccurate measurement of the LVOT diameter.
- CW underestimation of the peak stenotic jet.
- Inaccurate positioning of the LVOT PW Doppler signal . . . if too far back into the LV the peak velocity is too low, if too close to the stenotic valve, then spectral broadening is noted, and the peak velocity is too high.
- Measurement with arrhythmia . . . for example, with atrial fibrillation the stroke volume varies beat by beat.
- With coexistent subaortic stenosis the LVOT measurement is inaccurate.

Bernoulli equation

Bernoulli described the conversion of energy in a fluid from one form to another, as occurs when fluid flows in a tube that suddenly either increases or decreases its diameter. *Bernoulli's law* states that total energy at all points along a tube is the same—conservation of

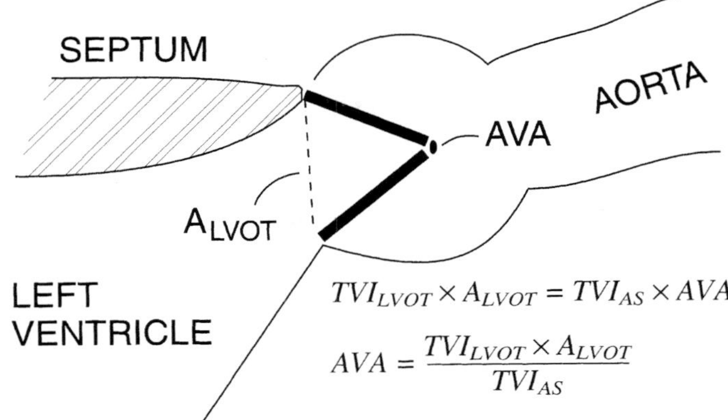

Fig. 3.7 Application of the continuity equation for calculation of the *AVA* (aortic valve area). The *TVI* of the left ventricular outflow tract (LVOT) is obtained from the apical five-chamber, the *TVI* of the stenotic AV from the best obtainable view (see Chapter 7), and the area of the LVOT from the parasternal long axis.

energy. *Energy* (the ability to do work) is composed of *pressure energy* (pressure × the volume of fluid), *kinetic energy* (fluid in motion has kinetic energy . . . which is proportional to the mass and the velocity squared; *mass* is density × volume), and *gravitational energy* (the product of density, volume, height above a surface, and the gravitational constant). Gravitational energy is not significant when describing bloodflow, but pressure energy and kinetic energy are important; therefore, according to Bernoulli's law, the sum of pressure energy and kinetic energy is the same at all points in the path of a tube. Since kinetic energy is proportional to the fluid velocity squared, if fluid enters a narrowed section of a pipe (e.g. a stenotic aortic valve), the velocity will increase (termed *convective acceleration*), and the kinetic energy at that point will increase. In order that total (hydraulic) energy remains constant, the pressure energy must decrease (pressure at the constriction will decrease) (Fig. 3.8). Summarizing, pressure in a fluid stream is less in constrictions, where the fluid will travel faster than in other portions of a tube. If there was no decrease in pressure at the narrowing, there would be no pressure gradient to produce the acceleration needed to push the fluid through it!

The *Bernoulli equation* relates pressure gradients and velocities within a fluid system. It is derived as follows (refer to Fig. 3.8)—since total energy is preserved, according to Bernoulli's law the sum of the kinetic and pressure energies at each point is the same (omitting the gravitational energy component):

(Pressure at 1) + (Kinetic energy at 1)
= (Pressure at 2) + (Kinetic energy at 2)

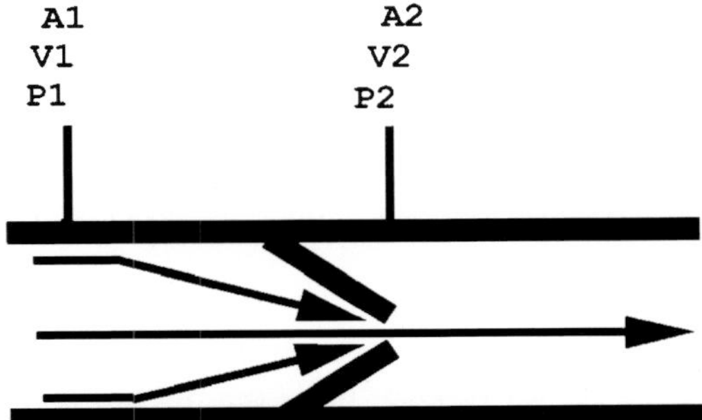

Fig. 3.8 As fluid approaches a narrowing within a pipe it will accelerate ($V_1 < V_2$). According to Bernoulli's law, in order that hydraulic energy remain constant at every point in the pipe, the pressure will necessarily decrease ($P_1 > P_2$). A_1 and A_2 are cross-sectional areas at the respective locations along the pipe (see text).

$$P_1 + (1/2)\rho(V_1)^2 = P_2 + (1/2)\rho(V_2)^2$$

The velocity terms (V_1 and V_2) are average velocity at locations 1 and 2. Rearranging terms yields:

$$P_2 - P_1 = (1/2)\rho[(V_1)^2 - (V_2)^2]$$

The value $(1/2)\rho$ in bloodflow analysis is about 4, so the equation becomes:

$$P_2 - P_1 = 4[(V_1)^2 - (V_2)^2]$$

By multiplying both sides by the value −1, the equation becomes:

$$P_1 - P_2 = 4[(V_2)^2 - (V_1)^2]$$

If V_1 is ≤1 m/s (or $V_1 << V_2$), then clinically this term may be ignored, and the equation becomes the *simplified Bernoulli equation*:

$P_1 - P_2 = 4V^2$

This derived equation does not take into account fluid *viscous friction* and energy needed to overcome *inertial force* that are caused by a changing flow rate (as found in a pulsatile system as with the circulation). Taking these two effects into account, the Bernoulli equation becomes:

$$\underset{\text{Kinetic + pressure}}{(P_1 - P_2) = (1/2)\rho[(V_2)^2 - (V_1)^2]} + \underset{\text{Inertial}}{\rho\int[dV/dt]ds} + \underset{\text{Viscous}}{R(V)}$$

where dV/dt is the change in velocity with respect to time, ds is the change in distance, and $R(V)$ are the viscous frictional forces with respect to velocity. The inertial term (dV/dt is acceleration) only is important at the onset or termination of a pulsatile flow cycle (it is zero at the peak of a velocity profile where velocity peak gradients are measured . . . the first derivative at the peak velocity is zero).

Clinical examples of use of the Bernoulli equation are provided in respective chapters. *Potential pitfalls* with clinical use of the Bernoulli equation include the following:

- The Doppler beam is not parallel to the bloodflow jet.
- The maximum velocity jet is not obtained.
- Long, tubular stenoses—the viscous friction component $R(V)$ is significant.
- Blood viscosity is altered—polycythemia.
- The V_1 term is significant (proximal velocity jet) and must be included (cannot use the *simplified* Bernoulli equation).

Pressure half-time and deceleration time

The *pressure half-time* (*PHT*) is defined as the time (in milliseconds) required for the peak initial pressure (P_1) to drop by one half (P_2). Keeping in mind that the Doppler signal measures *velocity*, one must apply the modified Bernoulli equation to convert velocity to pressure (Fig. 3.9). It may be seen that the *PHT* is the time (in milliseconds) for the velocity to drop to ~0.707 of the maximum velocity . . . $V_2 = (0.707) \times V_1$. The *PHT* is clinically used most frequently in evaluating mitral stenosis and aortic regurgitation (see Chapters 7 & 8).

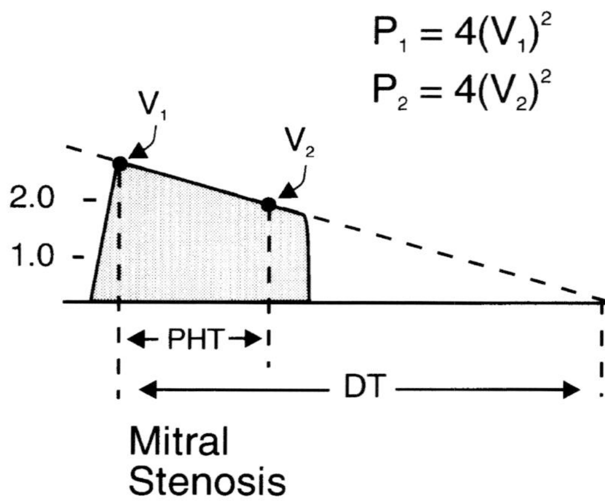

Fig. 3.10 The DT is the time required for the velocity, beginning with the peak value, when extrapolated, to cross the zero baseline.

The *deceleration time* (*DT*) is defined as the time from the peak velocity of the Doppler jet, when extrapolated, to cross the zero baseline (Fig. 3.10). *PHT* and *DT* are always related by the following equation:

$PHT = 0.29 \times DT$

Proximal isovelocity surface area

The *proximal isovelocity surface area* (PISA) method is based on the fact that as a fluid approaches a narrow orifice (e.g. regurgitant valvular lesion, stenotic valvular

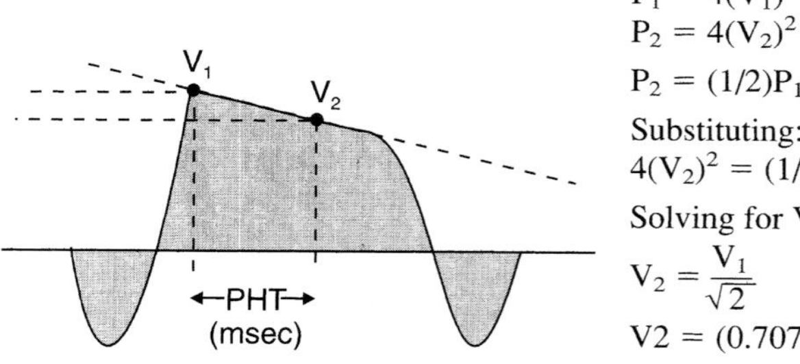

$P_1 = 4(V_1)^2$
$P_2 = 4(V_2)^2$
$P_2 = (1/2)P_1$
Substituting:
$4(V_2)^2 = (1/2)4(V_1)^2$
Solving for V2:
$V_2 = \frac{V_1}{\sqrt{2}}$
$V2 = (0.707)V1$

Fig. 3.9 Diagram demonstrating calculation of the pressure half-time (PHT) from a CW Doppler aortic regurgitant jet (see text).

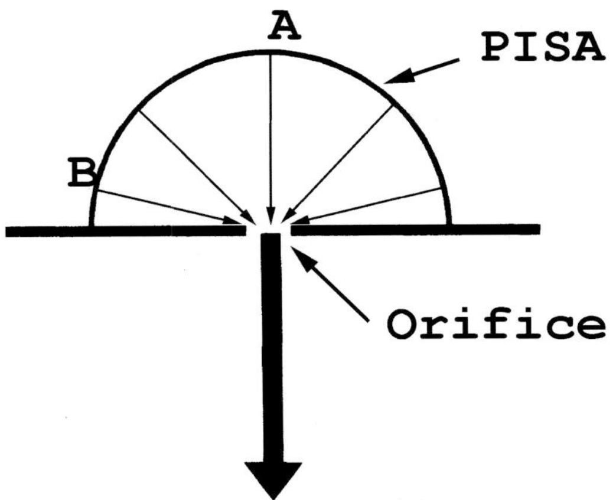

Fig. 3.11 Principle of the proximal isovelocity surface area (PISA). As a bloodflow approaches an orifice it will increase in velocity. Color flow Doppler will register the increase in flow, and aliasing will then occur at a known velocity noted on the color map of the echo machine monitor. According to the continuity equation the flow (area × velocity) at the PISA will be the same as through the narrowed orifice. The area of the "shell" at the PISA is $2\pi r^2$, and the flow through the PISA will be this area × the noted aliasing velocity. One should measure the radius of the shell at point A (parallel and "in line" with the ultrasound transducer) and not where flow is at an angle to the transducer beam . . . point B (see text).

lesion, prosthetic valve regurgitation, and narrow orifice intracardiac shunts) the velocity of the fluid will increase (and pressure drop to conserve energy—Bernoulli's law). According to the conservation of mass (continuity equation), the flow through any and each hemispheric surface proximal to that lesion will be the same as through the narrowed orifice (Fig. 3.11). By using color flow Doppler, the aliasing velocity, as flow accelerates toward the orifice, will be known, by the color map on the echo machine monitor. By shifting the baseline of the color map (away from the transducer direction for blood flowing away from the transducer, and toward the transducer direction for blood flowing toward the transducer) aliasing will occur at a lower velocity, and therefore a larger hemisphere will be generated, leaving less room for measurement error. An aliasing velocity of 20–40 cm/s is probably ideal. One should note to measure the radius of the hemisphere "in line" and parallel to the ultrasound transducer (point A in Fig. 3.11). As blood approaches the orifice at an angle to the transducer (point B in Fig. 3.11), velocity will be "seen" by the transducer as lower than it is, by the cosine of the angle of the transducer beam and true blood flow direction (see Chapter 2). Using a higher frequency transducer, a relatively low color velocity scale, and shifting the color baseline all may help reduce potential error. In high flow states with a relatively small orifice, setting the aliasing velocity "too low" may result in overestimation of the flow through the PISA hemisphere. Likewise, in low flow states and a large orifice, setting the aliasing velocity relatively high will result in underestimation of flow through the hemisphere.

Theoretically, the PISA method should work well as accelerating fluid will not become turbulent despite a very high Reynolds number, and viscosity is essentially nonexistent. However, PISA measurements may be affected by the fact that the orifice may be an odd shape (a hemi-ellipsoid model for calculating the PISA volume is possibly better than the hemispheric model, but it is practically difficult to obtain two orthogonal radius measurements), or the two valves on either side of the orifice may not be parallel (e.g. mitral stenosis with flow within the LA approaching the "domed" leaflets—see example of mitral stenosis below).

In order to calculate the *effective regurgitant orifice area* (*EROA*) of mitral regurgitation for example, we start knowing (continuity equation) that the flow through the PISA hemisphere (Q_{pisa}) equals the flow through the regurgitant orifice (Q_{mr}):

$$Q_{pisa} = Q_{mr}$$

$$2\pi r^2 \times V_{pisa} = EROA \times V_{mr}$$

where r is the radius of the PISA jet, V_{pisa} is the aliasing velocity of the PISA jet, and V_{mr} is the maximum velocity obtained, using CW Doppler, of the MR jet. Solving for *EROA* yields:

$$EROA = [(2\pi r^2 \times V_{pisa})/V_{mr}]$$

The *regurgitant volume* (*RV*) is calculated as the *EROA* multiplied by the *TVI* of the MR jet (TVI_{mr}):

$$RV = EROA \times TVI_{mr}$$

This equation assumes that the orifice size is constant throughout the time of regurgitation, which may not necessarily be true. A calculated mitral *EROA* of less than 0.1 cm^2 suggests mild MR, and a value greater than 0.5 cm^2 severe MR.

To calculate the valve area of mitral stenosis (applies equally for tricuspid stenosis), for example, one again applies the continuity equation as follows:

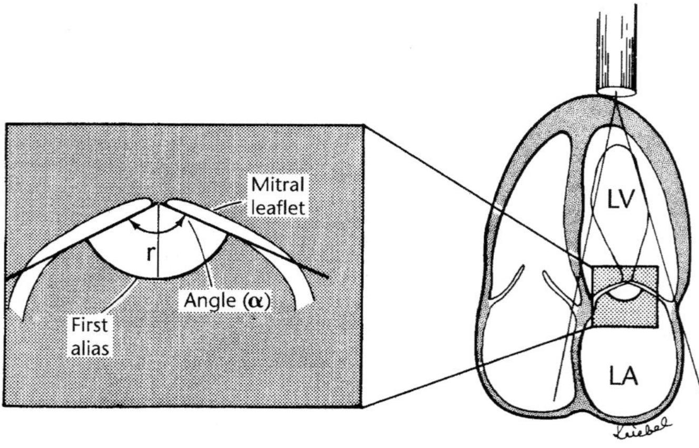

Fig. 3.12 Example of calculation of the mitral valve area (*MVA*) using the PISA method. The radius of the aliasing velocity is *r*, and α is the angle formed by the valve leaflets to form a "funnel" as flow approaches the orifice. (Reproduced with permission from: Rodriquez L, *et al*. Validation of the proximal flow convergence method: calculation of orifice area in patients with mitral stenosis. Circulation 1993; 88: 1160.)

$$Q_{pisa} = Q_{ms}$$

where Q_{pisa} is flow through the color aliasing "hemisphere," and Q_{ms} is flow through the stenotic mitral valve (Fig. 3.12). In this situation Q_{pisa} is:

$$Q_{pisa} = (2\pi r^2) \times (\alpha/180) \times (V_{pisa})$$

where α is the angle formed by the valve leaflets. Mitral valve area (*MVA*) can then be calculated:

$$MVA = Q_{pisa}/V_{ms}$$

where V_{ms} is the peak mitral stenosis inflow velocity.

The vena contracta and pressure recovery phenomenon

The *vena contracta* ("the contracted vein") is the minimal cross-sectional area of fluid flowing through a narrowed orifice. This minimal area is distal to the actual orifice, and is smaller in diameter than the anatomic orifice; hence the highest fluid velocity is at the vena contracta (and not the anatomic orifice), and the lowest pressure is also at the vena contracta. The continuity equation actually measures an effective valve area (the area at the vena contracta) and not the true anatomic orifice area (Fig. 3.13). The relationship of the true anatomic area and the vena contracta area is complex, but depends to some extent on the shape of the orifice and the Reynolds number.

The *pressure recovery* phenomenon is illustrated (Fig. 3.14). Distal to the vena contracta, the "pipe" will widen and therefore average velocity will decrease. To preserve total energy (Bernoulli's law) pressure must increase as the velocity decreases. Because of viscous and turbulent effects within the system, however, pressure will not return to what it was proximal to the orifice. The pressure recovery phenomenon has been noted in patients with tight native aortic stenosis, prosthetic aortic valve stenosis, hypertrophic cardiomyopathy, tunnel-like ventricular septal defects, and subpulmonary stenosis. In this situation, the Doppler valve gradient will be higher than that measured by catheterization, as the gradient measured by CW Doppler is $(P_1 - P_3)$, and that by catheterization

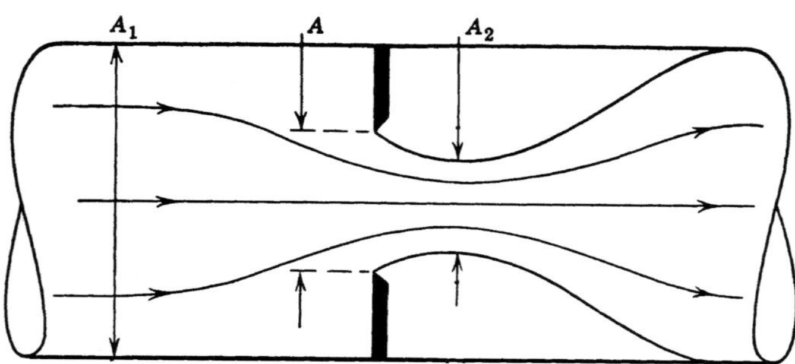

Fig. 3.13 Fluid flowing through a tube of diameter A_1 approaches an orifice of diameter *A*. The fluid will continue to narrow to a minimal diameter at A_2 somewhat distal to the orifice. It is this "effective valve area" at A_2 and not the true anatomic area at the orifice, that is calculated using the continuity equation. The system's lowest pressure is also at A_2 and not at the anatomic orifice.

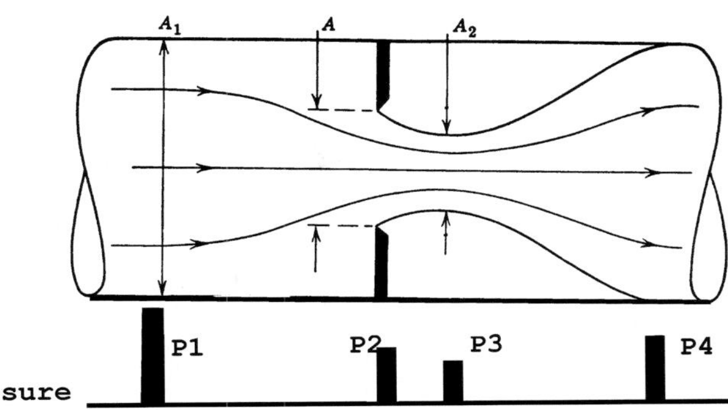

Fig. 3.14 The pressure will drop from its original value (P_1) as fluid enters an orifice (P_2). The minimum pressure is at the vena contracta (P_3). As the velocity then diminishes past the vena contracta, through a wider pipe "downstream," the pressure must increase (P_4), but will not fully recover to the value of P_1 (see text).

using standard catheters ($P_1 - P_4$), unless the catheter tip is located within the vena contracta.

Jet momentum

Newton's First Law of Motion states "a body at rest or in motion will remain at rest or in motion unless some external force is applied to it." *Newton's Second Law of Motion* tells us how the motion of a body changes under the action of a given force. *Newton's Third Law of Motion* states that "to every action force there is always an equal and opposite reaction force."

The *Momentum Equation* is based on the principle of *conservation of momentum*. Force (F) acting on a particle or system of particles is described by *Newton's Second Law of Motion:*

$$F = dM/dt$$

where dM is the change in momentum (M), and dt is the change in time (t). Momentum (M) is defined as:

$$M = \text{mass} \times \text{velocity}$$

and

$$F = \text{mass} \times \text{acceleration}$$

When discussing liquid flow, momentum is described in terms of that through a fixed region per unit time. With regards to fluids, conservation of momentum states that the momentum across a jet is constant throughout the extent of that jet (Fig. 3.15). The momentum across any plane that is perpendicular to the jet direction must be constant throughout the length of the jet. In Fig. 3.15, the momentum of "plane a" is the same as that of "plane b". Momentum (M) is defined as density (ρ) × flow (Q) × velocity (v):

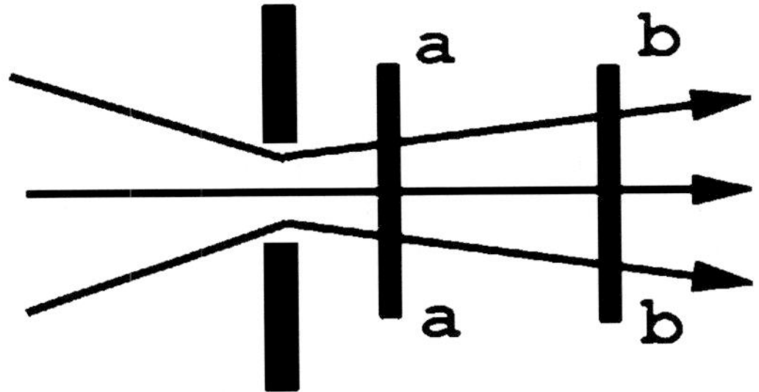

Fig. 3.15 Momentum of a fluid jet is the same through plane "a" as through plane "b," as momentum through any perpendicular plane is equal to that of any other perpendicular plane. The momentum is also equal at the jet orifice. To calculate regurgitant orifice area (*ROA*) of a regurgitant valve, theoretically one could make use of this. Momentum of the orifice (M_o) is *ROA* × v^2 (using CW Doppler), and momentum through a plane (M_p) is jet area ($AREA_{jet}$) × velocity of the plane (V_p^2). Since $M_o = M_p$, one may theoretically solve for *ROA*, as $ROA = [AREA_{jet} \times V_p^2]/v^2$. As the velocity through $AREA_{jet}$ is not uniform, but decreases from the center outward, the term V_p changes, and an integral equation must be applied to obtain V_p (see also Fig. 3.16). Although theoretically promising, this method for calculating a regurgitant orifice area has not been clinically used as of yet.

$$M = \rho Q v$$

Since flow (Q) is orifice area (A) × velocity (v), the above equation may be written as:

$$M = \rho A v^2$$

Since momentum (M) is proportional to area (A) × the square of the velocity (v^2), and momentum is unchanged through the length of the jet, as the regurgitant area distal to an orifice increases, velocity must decrease. The simplified Bernoulli equation states:

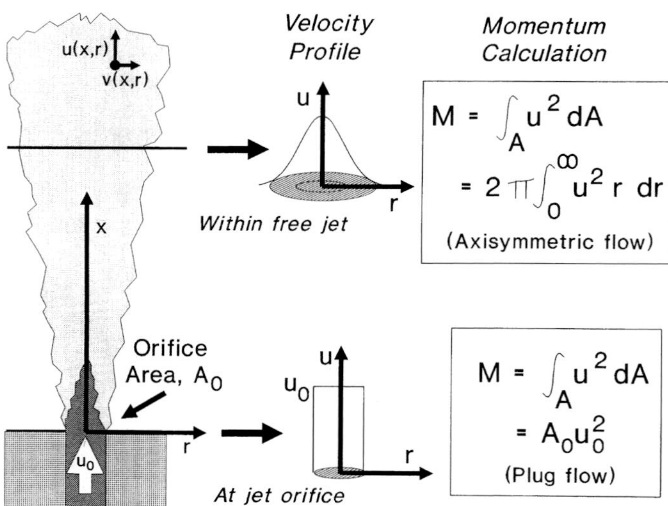

Fig. 3.16 Turbulent flow through an orifice. The *x*-axis lies along the jet direction, and *r* represents the radial distance away from the centerline. At the orifice the velocity profile across the orifice is essentially the same (Plug flow), but within the free jet the velocity diminishes as one travels further from the centreline (see also Fig. 3.15). The velocity across a representative plane may be represented mathematically by an integral equation (Axisymmetric flow). (Reproduced with permission from: Thomas JD, Liu CM, Flachskampf FA, *et al.* Quantification of jet flow by momentum analysis: an in vitro color Doppler flow study. Circulation 1990; 81: 247–259.)

$$\Delta P = \tfrac{1}{2}\rho v^2$$

where ΔP is the change in pressure. From this the momentum equation may be rewritten as:

$$M = 2A\Delta P$$

Since momentum is equal at different locations downstream in a regurgitant jet (Fig. 3.16), theoretically one may calculate momentum at a point downstream in the receiving chamber (the LA for mitral regurgitation—use color Doppler to obtain velocity at the aliasing velocity). Knowing the velocity at the valve orifice (from the continuous wave Doppler velocity) calculate ΔP (from the modified Bernoulli equation). One then knows momentum and ΔP, and therefore can solve for A (effective valve orifice area).

4

CHAPTER 4

Echo Examination and Echo Anatomy

Preparation for the echo examination

Transthoracic echocardiography

Simultaneous electrocardiographic (ECG) monitoring is usually conducted while performing an echo study. The rhythm is then displayed with the M-mode or two-dimensional (2-D) scan on the cathode ray tube (CRT) screen. On occasion it is helpful to also record respirations with a respirometer, for example, to evaluate potential pericardial constriction or tamponade.

Both patient and sonographer should be in a comfortable position, with the patient in a left lateral decubitis position with some degree of head elevation to begin a study. Commercially available "echo tables" are advantageous and will provide a section on the side of the bed that may be removed to facilitate scanning of the cardiac apex when the patient is in a left lateral decubitis position. The left lateral decubitis position facilitates gravity pulling the heart (LV apex) closer to the transducer. Some views (subcostal, suprasternal) will require the patient to lie flat, or to assume the right lateral decubitis position (right upper parasternal for continuous wave (CW) Doppler of aortic stenosis).

A gown that opens in the front allows access to all the acoustic windows with the least problems. Routinely, studies are performed in quiet dimly illuminated rooms to allow the sonographer to best see the video screen.

Holding the transducer with the right or left hand is the choice of the sonographer but using the right hand usually requires the sonographer to reach over the patient to scan the heart.

Transthoracic echocardiography (TTE) in the critically ill patient (ICU, CCU, ER) may be suboptimal (due to patient immobility, ventilator, surgical incisions, multiple lines and tubes). Because of this, TEE may be necessary in these environments.

Transesophageal echocardiography

Transesophageal echocardiography (TEE) is "semi-invasive" and is associated with a small but real probability of complications. The procedure should be performed only by specially trained physicians. *Informed consent* should be obtained before the procedure is performed. Elective cases (in the endoscopy lab or a special room in the echo lab) and cases performed in the critical care setting should preferably be performed by the physician with a nurse in attendance. The patient should be fasting for at least 4 h prior to the procedure. An intravenous line should be placed to use for sedation medications and agitated saline contrast injections. Preferably a 20 or even 18 gauge intravenous catheter should be placed in the right antecubital vein. For saline contrast studies, a three-way stopcock should be placed close to the intravenous catheter for sonication of saline for contrast studies. Dentures should be removed and the patient should be monitored. The echo procedure room should have the following available:

- blood pressure monitoring (automatic cuff)
- oxygen per nasal cannula (unless contraindicated, such as patients with severe CO_2 retention)
- continuous pulse oximetry
- topical anesthesia (lidocaine spray, benzocaine spray, viscous xylocaine)
- intravenous sedation
- suction and resuscitation equipment/"crash" cart.

Topical anesthesia is given to reduce gagging and the potential for laryngospasm, but there is a risk of aspiration. For this reason, the patient should not receive anything by mouth for at least 2 h after the procedure.

Medications used for an elective (awake) patient for TEE include:

• topical anesthesia: lidocaine spray, benzocaine spray, viscous xylocaine.
• intravenous sedation: diazepam (Valium), midazolam (Versed), meperidine (Demerol).
• drying agents: subcutaneous atropine, glycopyrrolate (Robinul).

Glycopyrrolate (Robinul, 0.2 mg), used to dry secretions and reduce the likelihood of aspiration, has only been rarely used by us over the past several years, as we have found these agents not very helpful, and they have a tendency to increase heart rate (especially with atrial fibrillation) and may cause blurry vision. We also have subjectively found a higher incidence of postprocedure transient "sore-throat" and hoarseness.

Intravenous sedation is provided to help the patient remain calm and cooperative. It is important, however, not to "oversedate" the patient, in that a cooperative patient will make swallowing and passage of the probe easier and oversedation may lead to respiratory depression. In critically ill, hemodynamically unstable patients we use rapid-acting, short half-life sedation. Midazolam should be used carefully in elderly patients as respiratory depression may be a problem. In our experience, meperidine has been especially beneficial in younger adults as it also tends to suppress the gag reflex.

A nasogastric tube usually will not interfere with the TEE insertion or with imaging. An endotracheal tube in place is usually not a problem. On occasion the "balloon" needs to be temporarily deflated to allow the tip of the TEE probe to be advanced past that same level within the esophagus. The balloon is then reinflated as soon as the probe tip is advanced past it. If a patient is being "weaned" from the ventilator and a TEE procedure is anticipated, usually it is safer (and easier) to perform the procedure prior to extubation. In ventilated patients, the patient is usually supine. Having the echo machine on the left side of the patient's bed and passing the probe and examining from the right side has been found by our group to be easiest. A TEE in the critical care situation is generally a "goal-directed" study. That is, one should evaluate the patient quickly, initially, trying to answer the specific question asked and then complete the remainder of the study, if possible. Many times a study must be curtailed before a complete exam is performed.

A bite block is used, many times even in patients that are orally intubated. The probe tip is introduced with the transducer "face" towards the tongue, with slight angulation (flexion) of the probe as it is guided into the posterior pharynx. As the probe is introduced, the left index finger may help press on the tongue, and guide the probe through the posterior pharynx. At that point the patient is asked to swallow (usually at around 18 cm from the incisors), and while swallowing, the probe advanced into the esophagus.

Endocarditis prophylaxis is somewhat controversial, but over the past several years *subacute bacterial endocarditis* (SBE) resulting from a TEE study, even in patients with prosthetic heart valves, has not been problematic. It seems prudent, however, at the present time to use SBE prophylaxis in patients at "high risk" for development of SBE, using American Heart Association (AHA) guidelines.

Complications of the transesophageal echocardiography procedure

For the physician, sonographer, and nurse involved, it is important to be aware of the potential *complications of TEE*, and to know how to respond to these. Patients with *severe esophageal* or *gastric disease* should generally not have the TEE procedure performed. These problems include *esophageal diverticuli* (Fig. 4.1), *stricture*, *perforation*, *varices*, *esophageal tumors*, *postradiation* esophageal complications, and *scleroderma*. If there is a question as to the safety of an anticipated esophageal intubation, on occasion we have had the patient evaluated first by a gastroenterologist. Patients with *severe cervical disk disease* and *chest radiation* are also at increased risk of complications. Usually a patient on intravenous heparin will not have a problem with the TEE procedure, but a *severe coagulopathy* is associated with increased risk. The authors are aware of a case of an elderly female with degenerative cervical spine disease on aspirin and intravenous heparin with a PTT > 190, who developed a retropharyngeal hematoma 30 h after the procedure without a pharyngeal or esophageal tear, and who required emergent tracheostomy for airway obstruction. This is similar to a reported case of delayed upper airway obstruction in a patient on aspirin and intravenous heparin. In this patient heparin at subtherapeutic levels was used during the study, but the dosage was increased afterwards to therapeutic levels (Saphir *et al.* 1997).

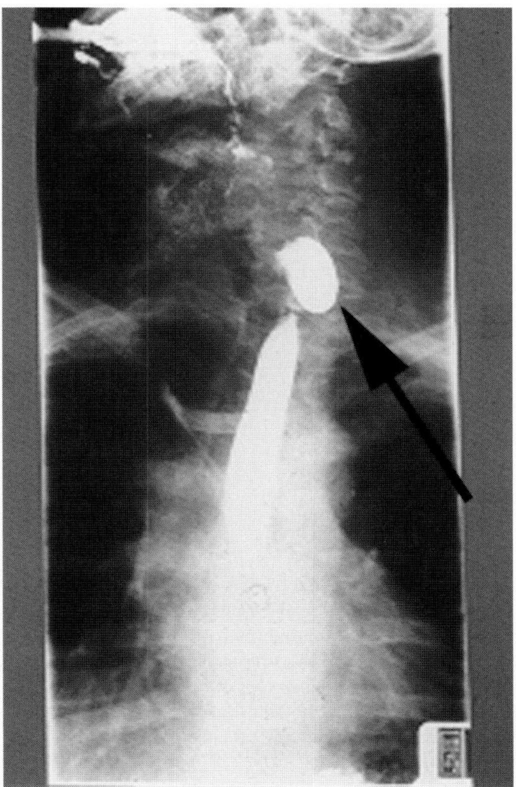

Fig. 4.1 Esophageal intubation was attempted in a middle-aged male, but at approximately 16–18 cm from the incisors the probe met resistance. A barium swallow was performed, revealing a Zenker's diverticulum. The patient's history was unremarkable for any swallowing difficulties.

Most *complications of TEE* are relatively benign (*transient hypotension* or *desaturation*, *supraventricular tachycardia*, *hypertension*, *parotid swelling*, *transient hoarseness*, or *sore throat*). Severe complications may occur, however, and include *sustained ventricular tachycardia*, *laryngospasm*, *aspiration*, *reaction to sedation*, *esophageal perforation*, and even *death*. When introducing the probe, it is important not to "force" the probe when significant resistance is met (Fig. 4.1).

"*Buckling*" of the tip of the TEE probe may occur if the steering cables become stretched and elongated (Fig. 4.2). When attempting to remove the probe from the esophagus, resistance may be encountered. This may also occur if the control knob for flexion is "fixed." By advancing the probe into the stomach and straightening the tip, it can subsequently be removed.

Complications of topical and intravenous anesthetics may occur. Excessive sedation may be caused by *midazolam* (*Versed*), similar to that found with other benzodiazepines. This side-effect may be reversed with *flumazenil* (*Romazicon*). (In adults this may by initiated with 0.2 mg intravenously over 15 s. If a satisfactory level of consciousness is not obtained after another 45 s, a further dose of 0.2 mg can be injected and repeated at 60-s intervals up to a maximum of four additional times. The maximum dose is 1.0 mg—*see package insert.*) Respirations, pulse, and blood pressure should be monitored and supportive measures given, with particular attention to maintenance of a patent airway and oxygen. Fluid and vasopressors may be required.

Meperidine (*Demerol*) is a narcotic analgesic with actions qualitatively similar to morphine, most prominently central nervous system and smooth muscle effects, with therapeutic effects of analgesia and sedation (*see package insert*). Meperidine is contraindicated in patients who are on or who have recently received monoamine oxidase (MAO) inhibitors. Overdosage is characterized by respiratory depression, extreme somnolence progressing to stupor or coma, and sometimes bradycardia and hypotension. Treatment includes attention to respirations and the airway, oxygen, intravenous fluids, and vasopressors as clinically indicated. *Naloxone* (*Narcan*), an opioid antagonist, is a specific antidote against respiratory

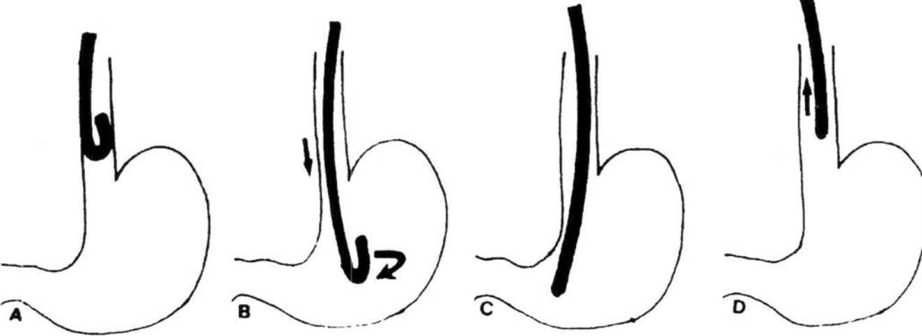

Fig. 4.2 "Buckling" of the tip of the transesophageal echocardiography (TEE) probe. (Reproduced with permission from: Kronzon I, *et al*. Buckling of the tip of the transesophageal echocardiography probe: a potentially dangerous technical malfunction. Journal of the American Society of Echocardiography 1992; 5: 176.)

depression. Naloxane is not recommended in the absence of clinically significant respiratory or cardiovascular depression. (Naloxane may be diluted for intravenous use in normal saline or 5% dextrose; in adults an initial dose of 0.4–2 mg may be used and if improvement in respirations is not obtained, it may be repeated at 2- to 3-min intervals. If no response is observed after a total of 10 mg, the diagnosis should be questioned—*see package insert*).

Toxic methemoglobinemia has been reported to occur rarely (0.115% reported incidence from the Cleveland Clinics) with *topical benzocaine spray*. Treatment is with intravenous *methylene blue*, 1–2 mg/kg as a 1% solution over 5 min. For persistently elevated levels (>30%) with symptoms, repeat administration of methylene blue may be needed, but should not exceed 7 mg/kg body weight. Exchange transfusion or dialysis may be needed in cases of a poor response to methylene blue therapy. This may occur in patients with glucose-6-phosphate deficiency or in severe methemoglobinemia (levels >70 mg percentage). For less severe cases, ascorbic acid (vitamin C) may be used. One reported mild case was treated successfully with vitamin C, 600 mg qid, for 1 day.

This is a rare consequence of exposure of normal red blood cells to oxidizing drugs such as benzocaine, dapsone, nitrates, acetaminophen, amyl nitrite, aniline dyes, nitroglycerin, nitroprusside, metoclopramide, nitric oxide, and sulfonamides. Within minutes of receiving these drugs the patient may develop dyspnea, tachypnea, cyanosis, and a significant drop in oxygen saturation. This may progress to lethargy, dizziness, stupor, arrhythmias, seizures, and circulatory failure. Using 100% oxygen facemask the partial pressure of oxygen may increase, but the oxygen saturation not rise substantially. If a cardiac or pulmonary etiology of the decrease in oxygen saturation is not found, an arterial blood gas with methemoglobin level should be obtained. The blood sample will have a distinctive chocolate-brown color. A methemoglobin level will be elevated, and the oxyhemoglobin level of the order of up to 50%. It is important to quickly recognize and treat this potentially life-threatening problem (Fig. 4.3). Factors thought to predispose to toxic methemoglobinemia include elderly age, excessive administered doses, hypoxia, enzyme deficiency, malnutrition, mucosal erosions or recent oropharyngeal instrumentation, sepsis, and tracheobronchial exposure to benzocaine.

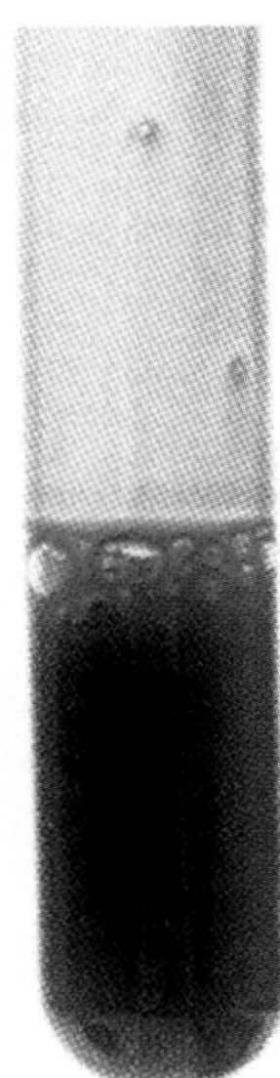

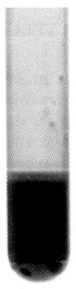

Fig. 4.3 The test tube on the left is an EDTA-treated (to prevent clotting) tube of venous blood, which demonstrates the chocolate-brown color which is characteristic of methemogloginemia. The test tube on the right is from a normal subject for comparison. (Reproduced with permission from: Donnelly GB, Randlett D. Images in clinical medicine: methemoglobinemia. New England Journal of Medicine 2000; 343: 337.)

The transthoracic echocardiography examination

By convention an *index mark* on the transducer indicates the edge of the imaging plane and indicates the part of the image plane that will appear on the right side of the display screen. The index mark is positioned either toward the patient's head or to the left side of the body.

The primary anterior acoustic windows for imaging are illustrated (Fig. 4.4). These windows represent the most common imaging positions, but imaging should be performed from any location in which useful information can be obtained. Some of the other views include the right and left *supraclavicular* and *right parasternal* windows. The left posterior thorax is occasionally used to image cardiac structures through a left pleural effusion (see Chapter 12).

When performing the examination, regions of interest should intersect the *central ray* of the transducer. The central ray is the B-scan line directly extending outward from the long axis of the scanning

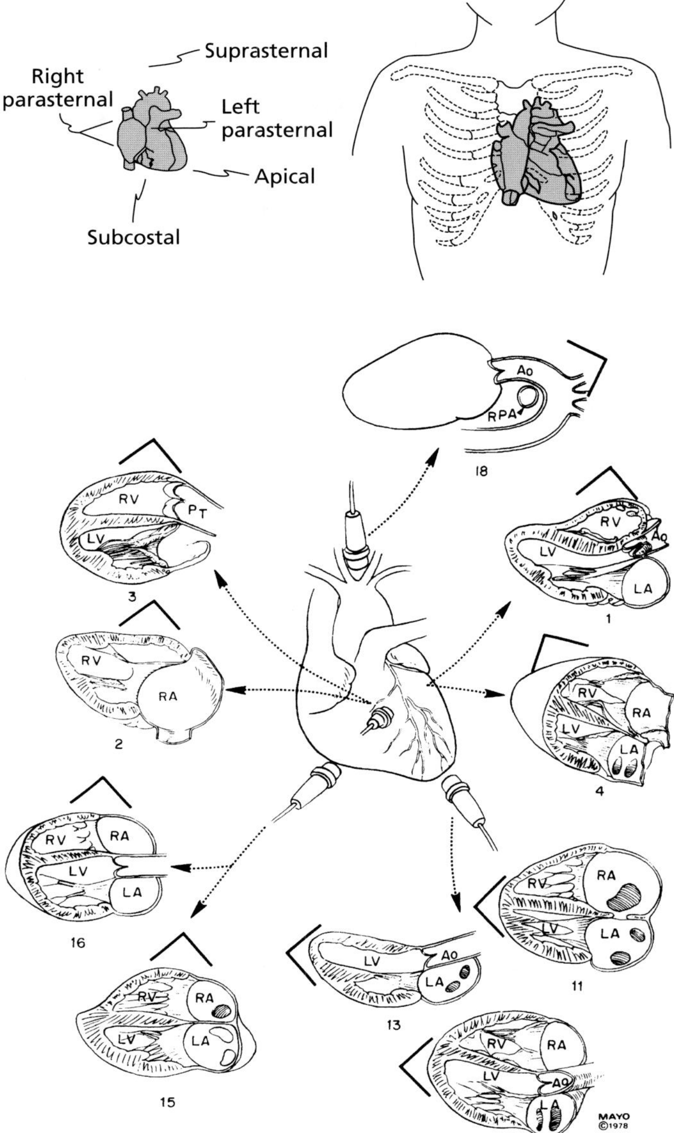

Fig. 4.4 Anterior acoustic window and the relation to the bony thorax. The right parasternal window is frequently used with the patient in the *right* supine position, and the suprasternal and subcostal views from a flat supine position. In the suprasternal window frequently the neck is slightly extended, and with the subcostal window, the knees are "pulled up" to improve imaging.

Fig. 4.5 Long axis images of cardiac structures from the primary acoustic windows: (1) parasternal long axis; (4) parasternal RV inflow; (11) apical four-chamber; (12) apical five-chamber; (13) apical three-chamber; (15) subcostal four-chamber; (16) subcostal long axis (five-chamber); (18) suprasternal long axis. (Reproduced with permission from: Tajik AJ, *et al.* Two-dimensional real-time ultrasonic imaging of the heart and great vessels. Mayo Clinic Proceedings 1978; 53: 271.)

transducer. The examination is usually begun from a *left parasternal* imaging plane including the third, fourth, and fifth intercostal spaces adjacent and to the left of the sternum (Figs 4.5(1) & 4.6(5–9)). When the term "parasternal view" is used here, it implies the left parasternal view. The patient is usually best imaged in a left lateral decubitis position with the left arm positioned under the head.

The *parasternal long axis* view should be obtained by positioning the transducer beam generally from the patient's left hip to the right shoulder. Proper positioning of the transducer from the left parasternal area usually requires a slight leftward tilt of the transducer (toward left shoulder). If properly obtained, *the ventricular septum and anterior aortic root will be aligned "straight across the sector beam,"* and the anterior MV leaflet and posterior aortic root will appear to be continuous (Fig. 4.7). The LV apex will appear foreshortened as the ultrasound plane is medial to the apex. The plane of the left ventricular outflow tract (LVOT)

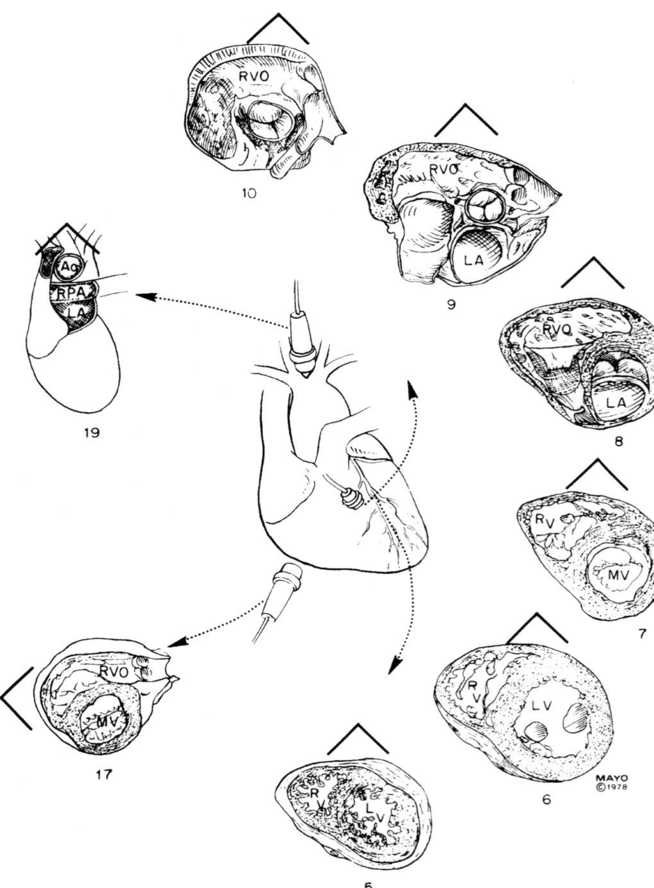

Fig. 4.6 Short axis images of cardiac structures from the primary acoustic windows. Parasternal short axis views (5–10): (10) aortic valve view with cranial angulation to show bifurcation of the main pulmonary artery (PA); (9) aortic valve and LA; (8) RV outflow tract (7); mitral valve (MV) level; (6) papillary muscle level; (5) apical short axis (imaged from a position just above the palpated LV apex); (17) subcostal short axis; (19) suprasternal short axis. (Reproduced with permission from: Tajik AJ, *et al.* Two-dimensional real-time ultrasonic imaging of the heart and great vessels. Mayo Clinic Proceedings 1978; 53: 271.)

and aortic annulus with proximal aortic root is not in the same plane as the LV extending to the apex. For quantitative M-mode measurements (see Chapter 5) the right and left septal surfaces and the endocardium of the posterior wall should be lined up perpendicular to the transducer. The *left ventricular internal dimension (LVID)* is measured at the chordal level between the tips of the MV and papillary muscle tips (see section on M-mode measurements). Other structures that may be visualized include the *left inferior pulmonary vein* emptying into the LA posteriorly. The *coronary sinus (CS)* appears in the posterior atrioventricular groove, and appears to "move with the heart," as opposed to the descending aorta behind the LA, which "does not move."

One can also use the parasternal long axis position to obtain other views, including the *tricuspid inflow (right ventricular inflow)* view (Figs 4.5(4) & 4.8). This is a good view for evaluating tricuspid regurgitation velocities with CW Doppler. The anterior and posterior TV leaflets will be seen, as will the coronary sinus, the inferior vena cava orifices, and the *Eustachian valve (EV)*.

The *parasternal short axis* views are obtained by then rotating the transducer clockwise by about 90°, so that the transducer "pointer" is directed toward the right supraclavicular area, and the beam is along a line from the left shoulder to the right side of the abdomen. By then angulating the transducer in a superior to inferior direction, the heart is "breadloafed" into different imaging planes (Fig. 4.6(6–10)).

The *aortic valve level* of the parasternal short axis (Figs 4.6(9) & 4.9) demonstrates all three aortic valve leaflets. Often, the origin of the left main coronary artery (3–4 o'clock position) above the left coronary cusp, and right coronary artery (10–11 o'clock

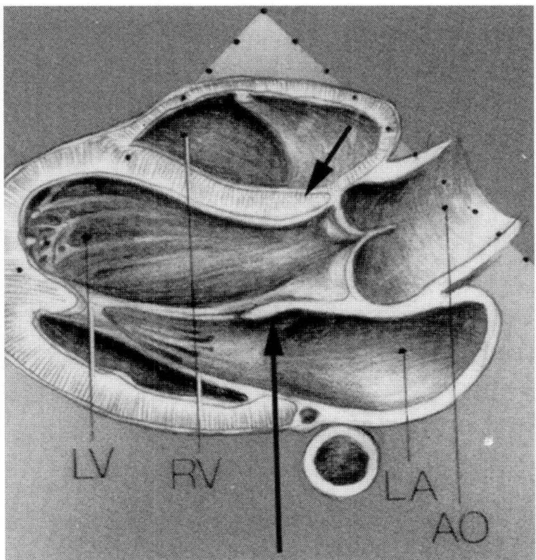

Fig. 4.7 Parasternal long axis view. The interventricular septum (IVS) and anterior aortic root should be aligned (short arrow), as should the anterior MV leaflet and posterior aortic root (vertical arrow). (Reproduced with permission from: Snider AR, Serwer GA, Ritter SB. Echocardiography in Pediatric Heart Disease, 2nd edn. St Louis, MO: Mosby, 1997.)

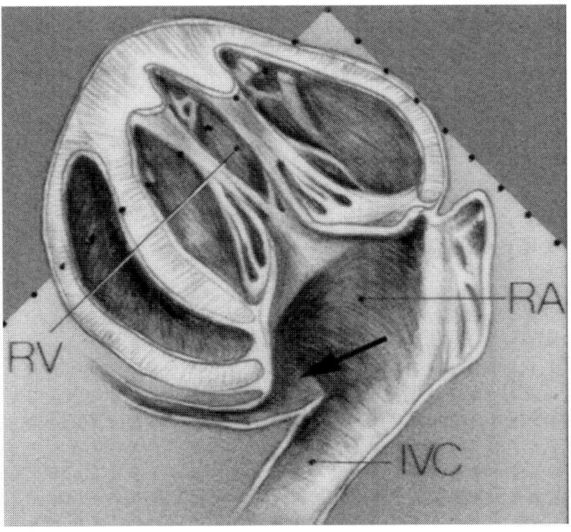

Fig. 4.8 RV inflow view (parasternal RV long axis) demonstrates posterior and anterior tricuspid valve (TV) leaflets, the coronary sinus (CS; arrow) and IVC orifices, and Eustachian valve. (Reproduced with permission from: Snider AR, Serwer GA, Ritter SB. Echocardiography in Pediatric Heart Disease, 2nd edn. St Louis, MO: Mosby, 1997.)

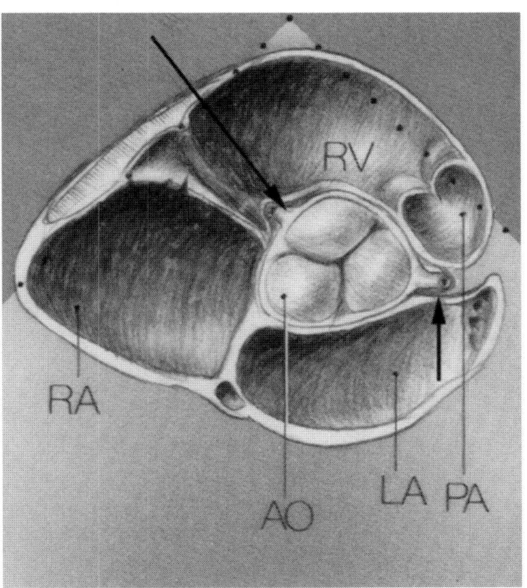

Fig. 4.9 Parasternal short axis aortic valve level demonstrating all three aortic leaflets (right, left, noncoronary). The right coronary artery origin (long arrow) originates above the right aortic valve leaflet and the left coronary artery (short vertical arrow) above the left aortic valve leaflet. Sometimes the proximal left anterior descending coronary artery (LAD; branches toward the transducer) and proximal circumflex artery (branches away from the transducer) may be seen. The noncoronary cusp is also shown (AO). The anterior wall of the RV and part of the right ventricular outflow tract (RVOT) are noted. The pulmonic valve (excellent view for Doppler across the pulmonic valve) and proximal PA are also noted. (Reproduced with permission from: Snider AR, Serwer GA, Ritter SB. Echocardiography in Pediatric Heart Disease, 2nd edn. St Louis, MO: Mosby, 1997.)

position) above the right coronary cusp, will be noted. The atrial septum may be visualized, and the LA size should be measured in both the anteroposterior and medial-lateral dimensions. Angling the transducer superiorly and leftward may reveal the bifurcation of the main PA into the proximal left and right pulmonary arteries (Fig. 4.6(10)). The left atrial appendage (LAA), especially if enlarged, may be seen inferior to the main PA. Visualizing the *tricuspid valve* (septal and anterior leaflets) requires moving the transducer to optimally visualize this structure. This view is good for obtaining continuous wave (CW) Doppler of tricuspid regurgitation (TR) and evaluating diastolic tricuspid inflow.

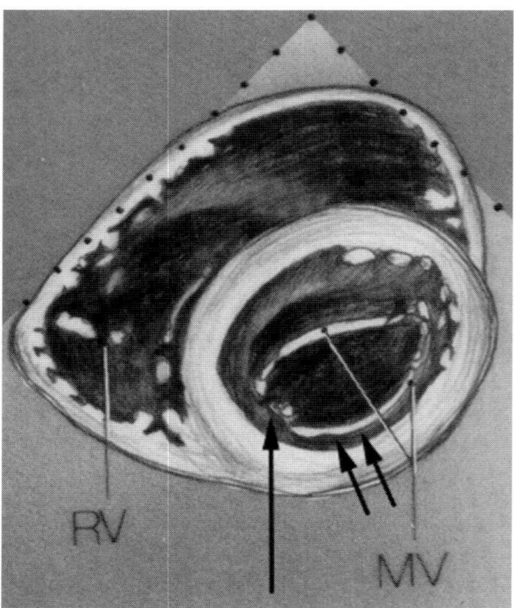

Fig. 4.10 Parasternal short axis MV level view demonstrates both anterior and posterior (two small parallel arrows) MV leaflets, and the posteromedial commissure (vertical arrow), and anterolateral commissure. (Reproduced with permission from: Snider AR, Serwer GA, Ritter SB. Echocardiography in Pediatric Heart Disease, 2nd edn. St. Louis, MO: Mosby, 1997.)

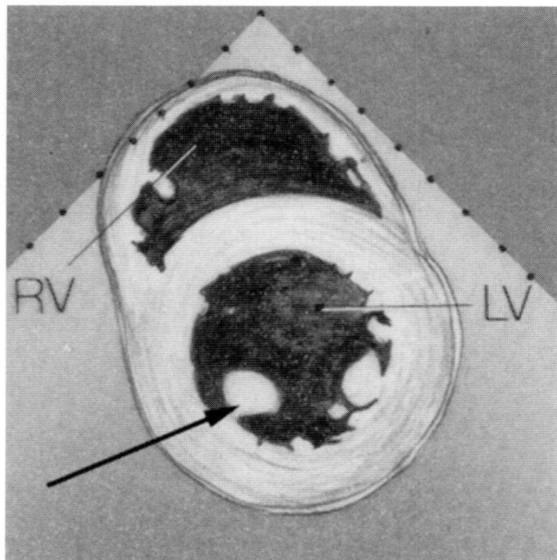

Fig. 4.11 Parasternal short axis at the papillary level. The posteromedial (arrow) and anterolateral papillary muscles are noted. (Reproduced with permission from: Snider AR, Serwer GA, Ritter SB. Echocardiography in Pediatric Heart Disease, 2nd edn. St Louis, MO: Mosby, 1997.)

The *mitral valve level* of the parasternal short axis (Figs 4.6(7) & 4.10) reveals both anterior and posterior MV leaflets (so-called *fishmouth* view of the MV in diastole). Both commissures should also be noted. A short axis image plane just below the MV plane is good to visualize small posterobasal LV aneurysms, which may be missed if not careful.

The *papillary muscle level* of the parasternal short axis (Figs 4.6(6) & 4.11) in the 4th or 5th left intercostal space should reveal the posteromedial and anterolateral papillary muscles. The interventricular septum and apical portion of the RV may be noted.

A short axis view of the *cardiac apex* area, below the papillary muscle level, should be recorded from a position just above the apical impulse and below that when recording the papillary muscles. This (*bread-loaf of the apex*) view has proven useful in patients when looking for apical thrombi.

The next area usually imaged is the *apical acoustic window*. This is also performed in the left lateral decubitis position. One can palpate the cardiac apex, and place the transducer just lateral to this. By *inching* the transducer laterally, the left ventricular cavity will less likely be foreshortened. The *LV four-chamber*, *five-chamber*, *two-chamber*, and *three-chamber* views are usually obtained from this position (Figs 4.5(11–13) & 4.12).

In the *apical four-chamber* view the inferior aspect of the ventricular septum is in the imaging plane. If the transducer is not located at the true apex, the LV will be foreshortened. The tricuspid annulus plane is slightly *closer to the apex* than the mitral annulus plane, with the tricuspid valve (TV) septal and anterior leaflets recorded. The RV apex does not extend as far away from the base of the heart as does the LV apex. The RV also usually has more *trabeculations and muscle bundles* than the LV. The RA includes the Eustachian valve which covers the ostium of the IVC. The flap of the foramen ovale is located on the LA side (usually not able to differentiate by TTE). The pulmonary veins may be difficult to visualize entering the LA from this view, and the descending aorta may be noted lateral to the LA.

The *apical five-chamber* view should be obtained by angling the transducer anteriorly. The LVOT and aortic valve will also be seen. This view is good for obtaining flow measurements from the LVOT (for stroke volume calculations and application of the

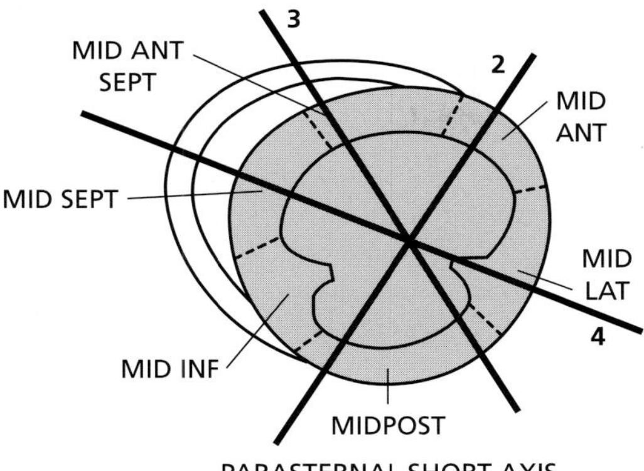

Fig. 4.12 Parasternal short axis view at the papillary level demonstrates the relationship of the two-, three-, and four-chamber apical views. These apical views "slice through" the LV as shown. The apical five-chamber view is obtained by angulating the transducer *anteriorly* (the left ventricular outflow tract (LVOT) and aortic valve are anterior structures) from the four-chamber position. By angulating the transducer posteriorly from the apical four-chamber view, the CS in the atrioventricular groove may be seen.

continuity equation for aortic valve area (AVA) measurements) and imaging LVOT abnormalities.

Rotating the transducer counterclockwise (around 60°) from the four-chamber view yields the *apical two-chamber* view. This will image the LA and LV. The RV in particular is *not* seen in this view. This plane is approximately orthogonal to the four-chamber view, and is used with the four-chamber view in LV volume measurements. This view images the anterior and posterior LV walls.

The *apical three-chamber* view (*apical long axis*) may be obtained by rotating the transducer another ~60° counterclockwise. The LV, LA, LVOT and aortic valve (AV) will be seen. The anteroseptum (right side of display screen) and posterior wall (left side) of the LV should be recorded. This view is equivalent to the parasternal long axis. The apex is well recorded, however, but the MV and AV are further from the transducer. LVOT and AV Doppler may be obtained from this view.

The *subcostal window* should be visualized by first having the patient lie supine on the scanning table and lowering any head tilt to 0°. The knees may be flexed with the feet kept on the table to help maintain a soft and relaxed abdomen. The transducer should be then positioned in the epigastric region and depressed until it is under the level of the ribs. The probe is then tilted superiorly and toward the left clavicular area to initiate an optimal scanning plane. The subcostal view is especially helpful in patients with lung disease and also in neonates and infants. The *subcostal long axis* view images the LV free wall and the RV posterolateral free wall, along with both atrial and ventricular septa. The *subcostal right ventricular outflow tract (RVOT) long axis (LV short axis) view* (Fig. 4.6(17)) visualizes the MV and also the entire RVOT. Doming of the pulmonary valve leaflets in pulmonary stenosis is well seen. An important structure to visualize is the abdominal aorta, in that an abdominal aortic aneurysm (AAA) may be detected (a screening study found an AAA in 6.5% of patients ≥50 years with hypertension).

The *suprasternal notch* is usually best imaged from the supine position. By having the patient slightly hyperextend the neck, sometimes aided by a small "rolled-up" towel under the shoulders, an improved access to this window may be achieved. The head may be tilted to either the right or left side at about 45° to facilitate transducer positioning. The *suprasternal aortic long axis* (Figs 4.5(18) & 4.13)) can be imaged

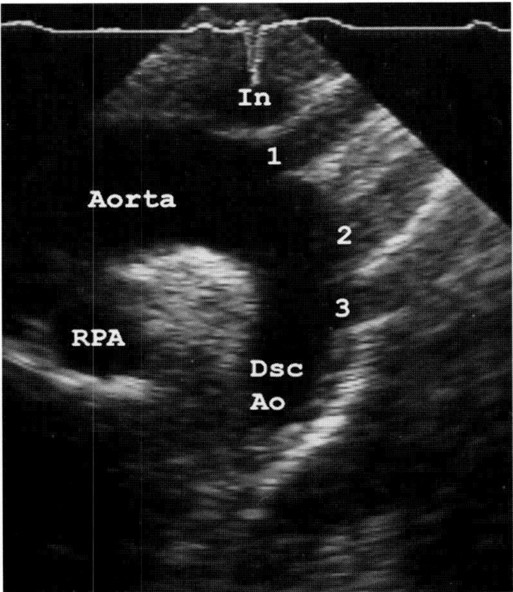

Fig. 4.13 Suprasternal long axis image of the aorta, in which the upper ascending (Aorta), transverse, and descending (Dsc Ao) aorta are visualized. The innominate artery (1), left common carotid artery (2), and left subclavian artery (3) are seen. The left innominate vein (In) is also visualized in this view as it courses from the left to right in subsequently joining the SVC.

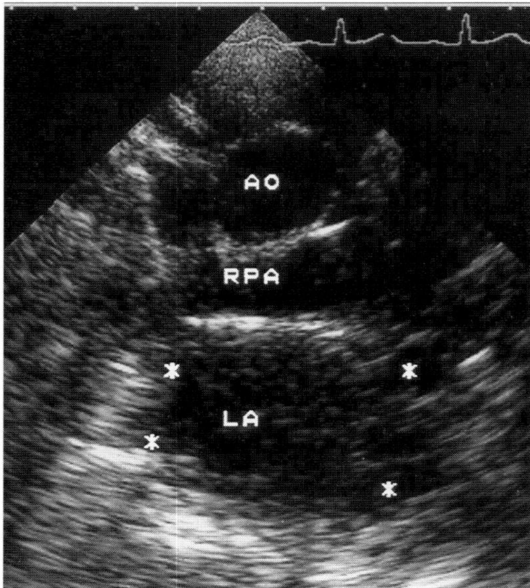

Fig. 4.14 Suprasternal short axis of the aorta (AO) with the right pulmonary artery (RPA) below it, in a longitudinal view. Below the RPA is the LA, and on occasion all four pulmonary veins (*) will be noted to enter the LA, yielding the so-called "crab" view.

with the transducer "marker" facing the right supraclavicular fossa, and the *suprasternal aortic short axis* (Fig. 4.6(19)) with the "marker" rotated posteriorly. In the suprasternal aortic long axis view the transverse aorta is seen longitudinally and the right pulmonary artery (RPA) in cross-section. The upper ascending aorta, occasionally even the aortic valve itself, the brachiocephalic vessel origins, and the proximal descending aorta are imaged. With the suprasternal aortic short axis view, the upper ascending aorta is in cross-section, and the RPA will be longitudinally seen. Inferior to the RPA is the LA. Sometimes all four pulmonary veins will be noted to enter the LA, yielding the "crab" view (Fig. 4.14), usually only seen in pediatric echocardiograms.

The *right parasternal* imaging windows lie in the intercostal spaces adjacent to the right sternal border. Improved imaging is usually obtained by having the patient lie in a *right* lateral decubitis position. This position is sometimes helpful in obtaining a maximum Doppler velocity with aortic stenosis (especially congenital) and in imaging the proximal ascending aorta.

M-mode recordings

As reviewed earlier, the M-mode (motion mode) recording uses a continuous B-mode line that is "scrolled" across the display screen. A "marker line" is projected onto a 2-D image to obtain the M-mode recording. Modern ultrasound transducers use 2-D images for "M-mode guidance" (Fig. 4.15). Standard M-mode studies are performed from the parasternal window. Using "2-D guidance" to obtain the M-mode slice through the LV cavity insures that *the cursor is at 90° to the muscle border*, to insure proper measurements of chamber dimension and LV wall thickness. When performing LV measurements, the method frequently used is the American Society of Echocardiography (ASE) standard, the *leading-edge to leading-edge* method (Fig. 4.16). This method is reproducible and least dependent on instrument gain or machine processing. Other measurement methods have been used also (Fig. 4.17). In the past, several

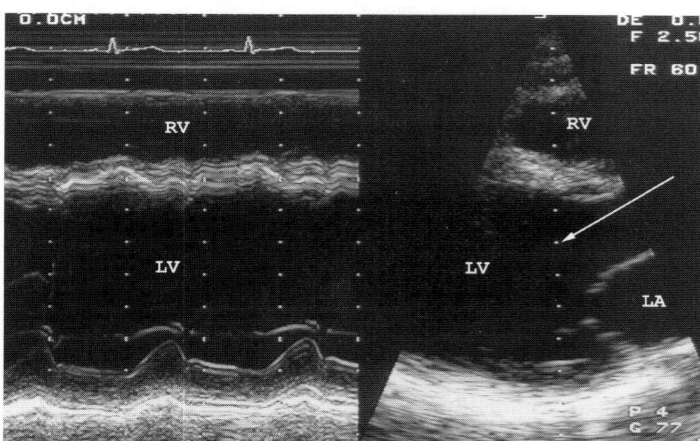

Fig. 4.15 M-mode and two-dimensional (2-D) recordings in a patient with an old anterior wall myocardial infarction. The "M-mode cursor" (arrow) is shown on the 2-D image. Most modern transducers perform M-mode recordings with 2-D scanners, allowing 2-D "guidance" of the M-mode beam.

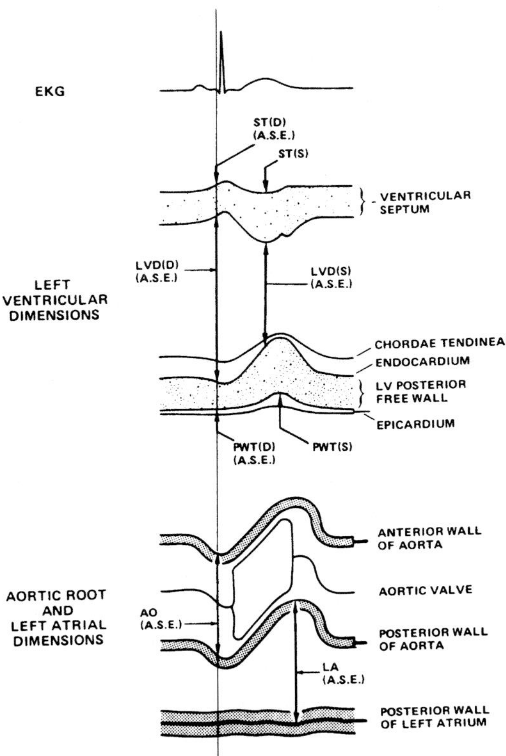

Fig. 4.16 M-mode measurements according to ASE standards. (Upper panel) End-diastolic measurements are made with the onset of the QRS. End-systolic measurements are defined by ASE guidelines at the peak posterior motion of the ventricular septum. Some laboratories define end-systole as the peak anterior motion of the LV posterior wall. LVD(D), LV end-diastolic dimension; LVD(S), LV end-systolic dimension; ST(D), septal end-diastolic dimension; ST(S), septal end-systolic dimension; PWT(D), LV posterior wall end-diastolic dimension; PWT(S), LV posterior wall end-systolic dimension. (Lower panel) Aortic valve and LA size measurements are illustrated. The aortic root dimension is measured at end-diastole as leading-edge to leading-edge, and the LA dimension is measured at end-systole as the leading edge of the posterior aortic wall to the *dominant line* representative of the posterior wall of the LA. (Reproduced with permission from: Feigenbaum H. Echocardiography, 5th edn. Philadelphia: Lea & Febiger, 1994: p. 660.)

studies published "normal" M-mode parameter tables using the inner-edge to inner-edge method, which yields slightly different results from the ASE standard.

M-mode recording at the aortic valve level (Fig. 4.16) demonstrates the LA posterior to the aortic root and valve. Aortic valve closure is noted as a thin line in the aortic root in diastole, and the right (anterior leaflet) and noncoronary cusp (posterior leaflet) form a *box* in systole.

At the level of the mitral valve, the M-mode recording (see Chapter 8) demonstrates both anterior (AML) and posterior (PML) mitral leaflets (Fig. 4.18). The distance between the maximum AML excursion (E) and the ventricular septum is the *E-point to septal separation* (*EPSS*). This is normally 6 mm or less and will be larger with LV dilatation, unless mitral stenosis is present or aortic regurgitation is present with the regurgitant jet "deforming" the MV leaflet in diastole.

General approach to the Doppler examination

The goal of a Doppler examination is to identify and confirm normal flow patterns and detect and evaluate abnormal flow. The color flow Doppler exam along with pulsed wave (PW) and continuous (CW) Doppler allow the sonographer to obtain valuable information within a reasonable period of time.

From a *parasternal window* color flow interrogation should be started from the *parasternal long axis*, observing flow patterns across the MV and AV, looking for evidence of mitral (MR) or aortic (AR) regurgitation. The right side of the interventricular septum can be evaluated for jets of left-to-right flow. PW Doppler helps differentiate timing of abnormal flow from the normal diastolic inflow of the TV. From the 2-D *RV inflow* view TV flow can be recorded and TR can be searched for. Often, prominent flow from the IVC can be seen entering the RA. Coronary sinus flow may also be detected. CW Doppler of TR flow velocity (to be used for RV pressure calculation) is performed from this view. From the *parasternal long axis of the pulmonary artery*, systolic flow patterns of the RVOT and proximal pulmonary artery are recorded. Pulmonary regurgitation (PR) should be recorded also. The *high parasternal short axis* plane allows pulmonary artery flow to be further examined. Color flow patterns should be assessed for the diastolic retrograde flow characteristic of a patent ductus arteriosus (PDA) (see Chapter 16) and for flow of PR.

Begin sampling at the *apical window* with the transducer positioned in the *four-chamber view*. Flow patterns across the mitral and tricuspid valves can be recorded to assess diastolic function. MR and TR can be initially noted with color flow Doppler. CW

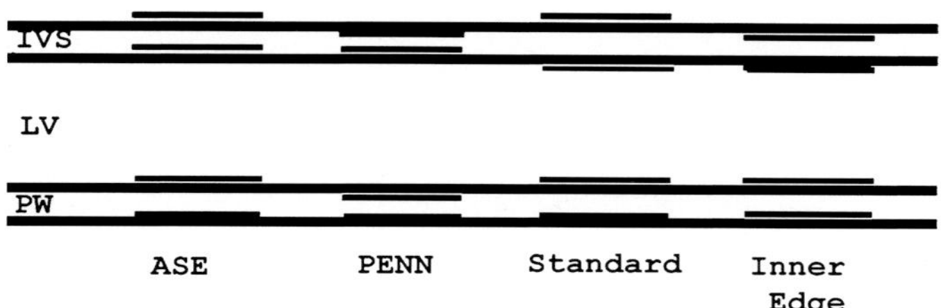

Fig. 4.17 The various methodologies used for M-mode LV measurements. The interventricular septum (IVS) is represented by the upper pair of parallel lines, the posterior LV wall (PW) by the lower pair of parallel lines, and the LV cavity (LV) between the IVS and PW. The American Society of Echocardiography (ASE) convention uses the leading-edge to leading-edge method. The PENN convention has been used in LV mass calculations by M-mode measurements. The Standard convention (first M-mode method of measurement introduced in the late 1960s) used leading-edge to trailing-edge for the LV septum, and leading-edge to leading-edge for the LV posterior wall. The inner-edge to inner-edge method is also used by several laboratories.

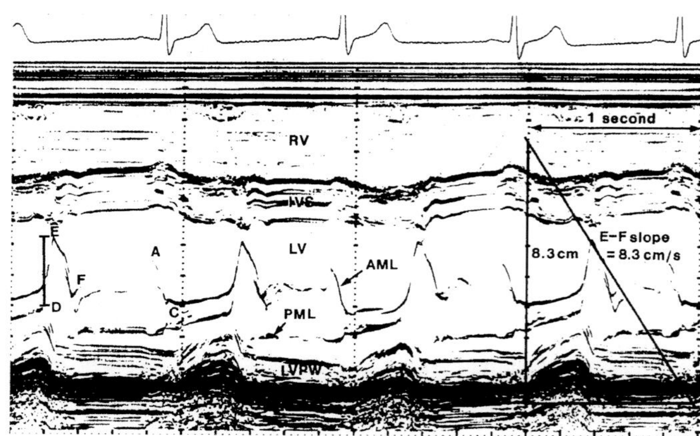

Fig. 4.18 M-mode recording at the level of the mitral valve. The E-point to septal separation (EPSS) is the distance from the maximum excursion of the anterior leaflet of the MV to the interventricular septum (see text), and the E–F slope is the distance of the EF line over 1 s (see also Chapter 8).

Doppler is used to obtain the maximum velocity of TR in pressure calculations.

The apical *five-chamber view* (and also the *three-chamber view*) is used to access LVOT flow by PW Doppler in stroke volume calculations, and in the use of the continuity equation in calculation of aortic valve area in aortic stenosis. Aortic regurgitation (AR) is well noted from these views (as well as the parasternal long axis view).

The *suprasternal notch* allows sampling of flow in the ascending aorta and in the descending aorta for evaluation for coarctation of the aorta (see Chapter 16). Reversed diastolic flow in the descending thoracic aorta may be noted in patients with a PDA, AR, and left-to-right shunting (such as a large upper extremity dialysis arteriovenous shunt). The suprasternal short axis view may reveal the SVC as it turns toward the RA, and color and PW Doppler flow may be recorded. SVC flow helps in differentiating the etiology of respiratory variation in venous return (see Chapter 12).

With the patient in the *right lateral decubitis* position, color flow guided CW of the aortic valve and proximal ascending aorta should be performed from the *right upper parasternal position* in patients with aortic stenosis. The maximal velocity may be obtained from this view, in particular in patients with congenital valvular stenosis. On occasion, the *right lower parasternal* position may be of benefit, as for example in evaluating the IVC–RA junction in patients with giant left atrium.

The transesophageal echocardiography exam

Monoplane TEE probes were the first commercially available transducers. The imaging plane (termed

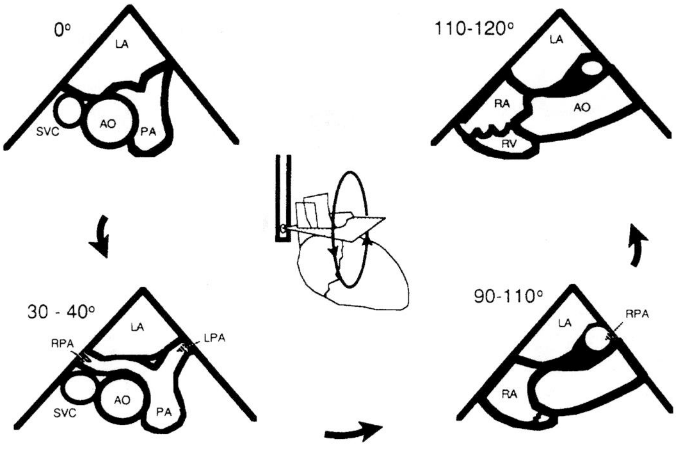

Fig. 4.19 Sections of the aorta and pulmonary artery that may be obtained from the *upper esophagus* by multiplane TEE imaging. AO, ascending aorta; LPA, left pulmonary artery; RPA, right pulmonary artery. (Reproduced with permission from: Pandian NG, *et al.* Multiplane transesophageal echocardiography: imaging planes, echocardiographic anatomy, and clinical experience with a prototype phased array omniplane probe. Echocardiography 1992; 9: 649.)

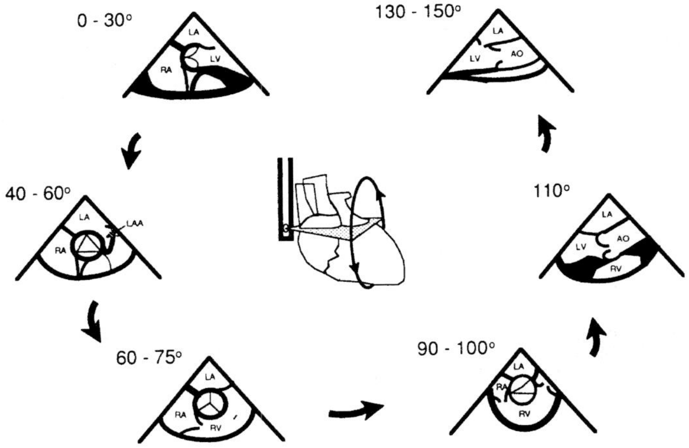

Fig. 4.20 Sections of the aortic valve and right ventricular outflow region from the *mid-upper esophagus*. LAA, left atrial appendage; LV, left ventricle. (Reproduced with permission from: Pandian NG, *et al.* Multiplane transesophageal echocardiography: imaging planes, echocardiographic anatomy, and clinical experience with a prototype phased array omniplane probe. Echocardiography 1992; 9: 649.)

horizontal plane or at an angle of 0°) is perpendicular to the plane of the probe. Imaging of structures are obtained by advancing or withdrawing the probe, rotation about the long axis of the probe shaft, medial and lateral probe tip angulation (not available on monoplane probes), and anterior and posterior (flexion and anteflexion) probe tip angulation. Subsequently *biplane TEE probes* were introduced. This probe has another *vertical plane* (angle of 90°) transducer located proximal to the horizontal plane transducer on the end of the probe. The vertical plane is parallel to the axis of the shaft of the probe. Because the biplane probe contains two separate transducers, imaging in the horizontal and longitudinal planes is not exactly at the same level. The transducer must be advanced or withdrawn slightly when switching from one plane to another in order to image structures at the same level.

Multiplane TEE probes have been made available by all of the major ultrasound companies. These probes have both imaging (M-mode and 2-D) and Doppler (PW, CW, color) ability. The transducer rotates around a central axis on the probe to allow essentially an infinite number of planes at any esophageal depth. Probes with variable transducer frequencies are available, allowing for adjustment between approximately 3.75 and 6 MHz as a study is being performed. Higher frequencies can be used for imaging structures relatively close to the transducer, whereas lower frequencies are necessary for structures relatively distant.

Multiplane imaging views from the esophagus and stomach are illustrated (Figs 4.19–4.25). The ASE/SCA Guidelines for Intraoperative Multiplane Transesophageal Echocardiography recommends 20

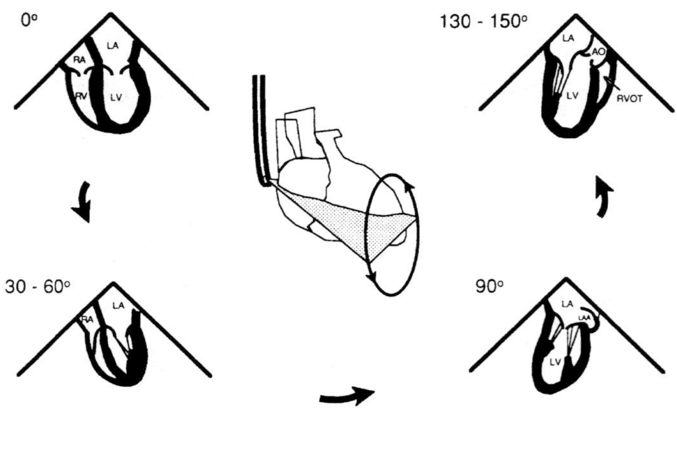

Fig. 4.21 Representative sections of the *mid esophagus* level. (Reproduced with permission from: Pandian NG, *et al.* Multiplane transesophageal echocardiography: imaging planes, echocardiographic anatomy, and clinical experience with a prototype phased array omniplane probe. Echocardiography 1992; 9: 649.)

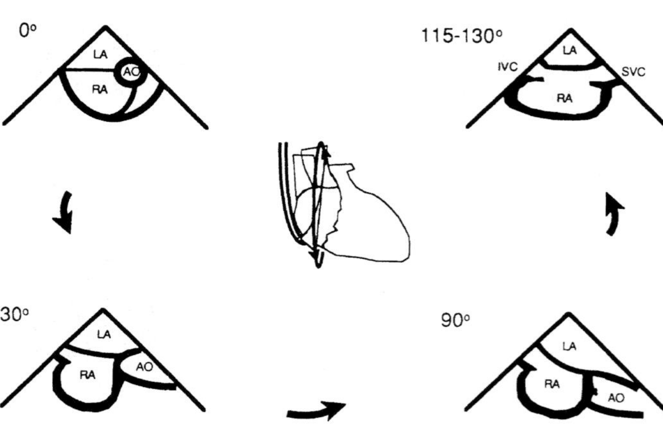

Fig. 4.22 Representative sections of the *mid-lower esophagus* level. (Reproduced with permission from: Pandian NG, *et al.* Multiplane transesophageal echocardiography: imaging planes, echocardiographic anatomy, and clinical experience with a prototype phased array omniplane probe. Echocardiography 1992; 9: 649.)

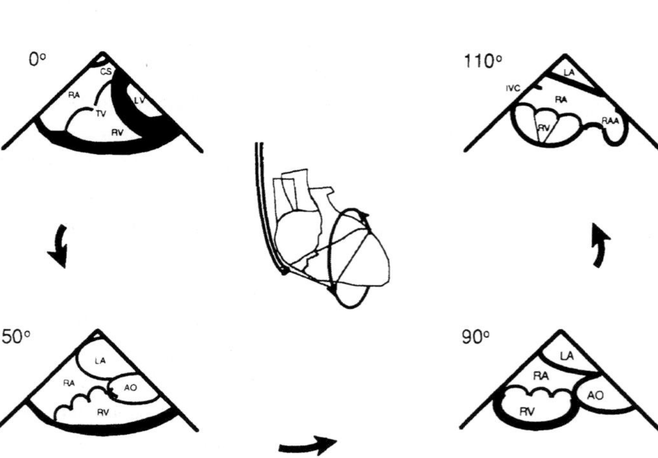

Fig. 4.23 Representative sections of *lower esophagus* level. (Reproduced with permission from: Pandian NG, *et al.* Multiplane transesophageal echocardiography: imaging planes, echocardiographic anatomy, and clinical experience with a prototype phased array omniplane probe. Echocardiography 1992; 9: 649.)

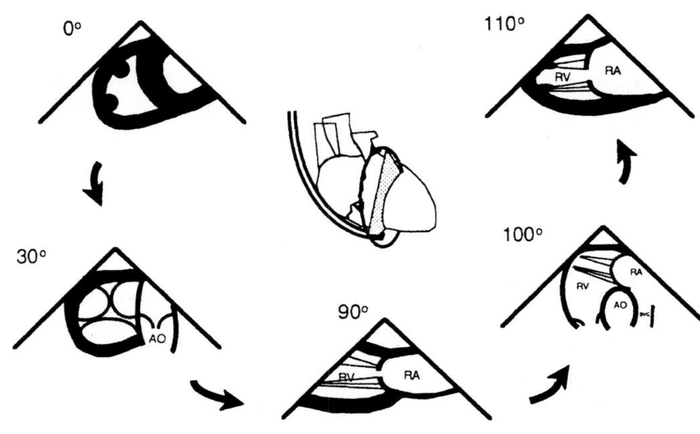

Fig. 4.24 Representative sections of the right heart obtained in the transgastric level. (Reproduced with permission from: Pandian NG, *et al.* Multiplane transesophageal echocardiography: imaging planes, echocardiographic anatomy, and clinical experience with a prototype phased array omniplane probe. Echocardiography 1992; 9: 649.)

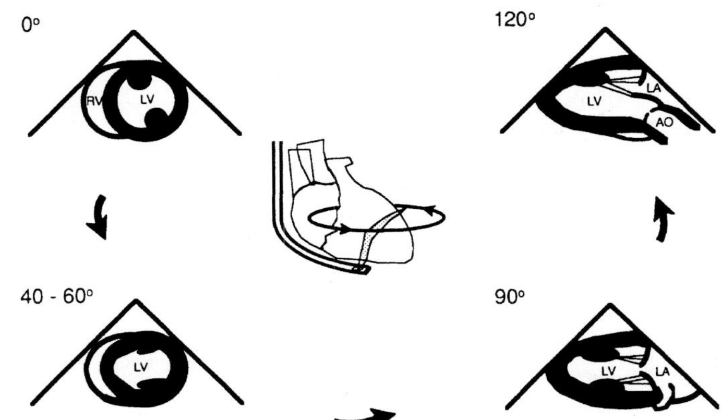

Fig. 4.25 Representative sections of the left heart obtained in the transgastric level. (Reproduced with permission from: Pandian NG, *et al.* Multiplane transesophageal echocardiography: imaging planes, echocardiographic anatomy, and clinical experience with a prototype phased array omniplane probe. Echocardiography 1992; 9: 649.)

basic cross-sectional views of the heart and great vessels (Fig. 4.26, Chapter 15).

Visualization of the great vessels may be performed by TTE as described earlier, and by TEE imaging (see Chapter 19). Anatomy of the great vessels may vary on occasion (Fig. 4.27). For imaging normal great vessel anatomy, TEE has been helpful. By withdrawing the probe from the descending aorta (horizontal plane) toward the transverse aorta and switching to the longitudinal plane, these vessels will be seen. Rotation of the transducer shaft clockwise will image the innominate artery (most anterior takeoff from the aorta) and counterclockwise rotation will image the left common carotid and left subclavian vessels (more posterior takeoff from the aorta). Normally, the innominate and left subclavian PW Doppler waveforms will have only systolic flow (high resistance), and the left common carotid will have both systolic and diastolic forward flow velocities (low resistance).

General Indications for transesophageal echocardiography

As a general rule, TEE should be performed only if the results obtained *will potentially significantly affect patient management*. TEE is used both within and outside of the operating room. Within the operating room, TEE is used during cardiac and noncardiac surgery for the evaluation of cardiac structure and for monitoring of LV function and hemodynamics. Outside the operating room, both hospitalized and outpatients are studied in the endoscopy lab (or a specially prepared room in the echo lab). Critically

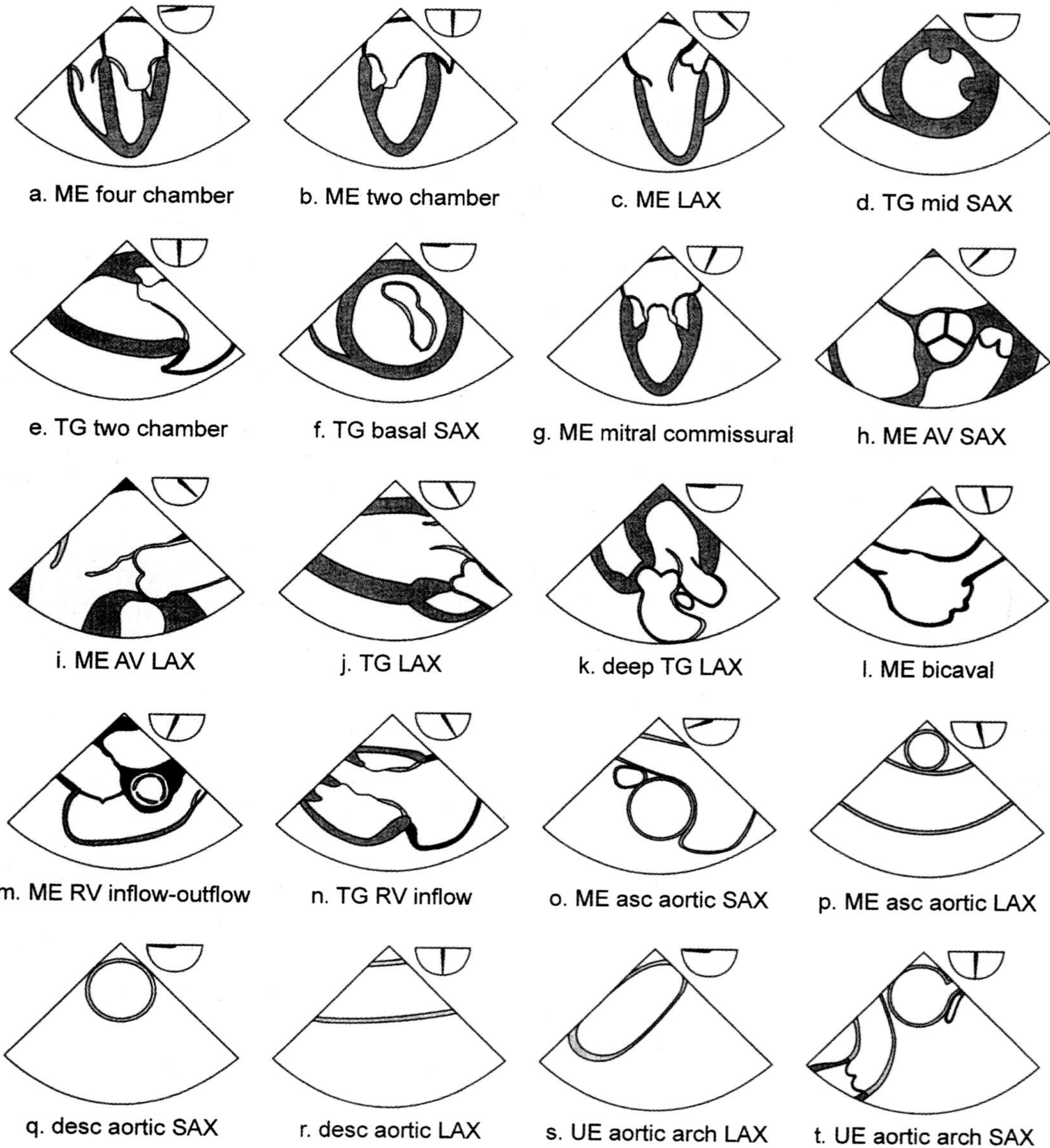

Fig. 4.26 The 20 views for a comprehensive TEE examination, as recommended by the ASE/SCA Guidelines. ME, mid esophagus; LAX, long axis; TG, transgastric; SAX, short axis; AV, aortic valve; asc, ascending; desc, descending; UE, upper esophagus. (Reproduced with permission from: ASE/SCA Guidelines for Performing a Comprehensive Intraoperative Multiplane Transesophageal Echocardiography Examination. Recommendations of the American Society of Echocardiography Council for Intraoperative Echocardiography and the Society of Cardiovascular Anesthesiologists Task Force for Certification in Perioperative Transesophageal Echocardiography. Journal of the American Society of Echocardiography 1999; 12: 884–900.)

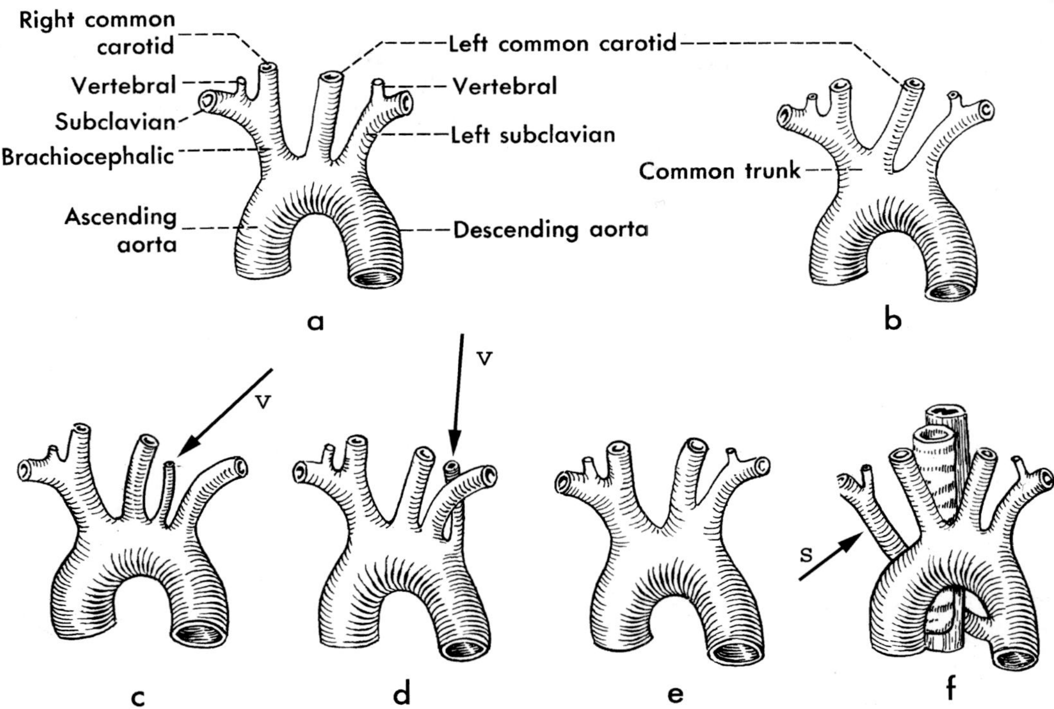

Fig. 4.27 "Normal" (a) anatomy of the great vessels and several variants. In (c) and (d) the *left vertebral artery* arises from the aortic arch (arrows labeled "V"). In (f) a relatively common variant is noted in which the *right subclavian* (arrow labeled "S") arises anomalously and passes behind the trachea and the esophagus. (Reproduced with permission from: Hollinshead WH. Textbook of Anatomy, 3rd edn. New York: Harper & Row, 1974: p. 522.)

ill and emergency room patients are studied at the bedside. Please see the specific chapters for application of TEE to specific areas.

Specific indications for the use of TEE include:

- *Outside the operating room*—technically difficult TTE study, native valve dysfunction, prosthetic valve dysfunction, embolic events, endocarditis, aortic pathology, masses/tumors, congenital diseases, critical care/emergency room, coronary arteries, interventional procedures.
- *Within the operating room*—monitoring structure and hemodynamics during cardiac surgery and noncardiac surgery.

CHAPTER 5

Ventricular Measurements and Systolic Function

Factors affecting contractility

Cardiac systolic function may be assessed by multiple modalities (Fig. 5.1), including echocardiography. Echo methods of assessment of systolic performance include M-mode, two-dimensional (2-D) and Doppler methods (see Chapter 3). "Systolic function" is affected by *ventricular preload, ventricular afterload, intrinsic ventricular contractility*, and *heart rate. Asynchronous ventricular contraction* secondary to coronary artery disease or a ventricular pacemaker may also affect systolic function.

The influence of *preload* on contractility is described by the *Frank–Starling relationship*, which states that increasing initial muscle length will result in an increased force and velocity of subsequent contraction. This continues to a point where eventually a further increase in initial fiber length will result in no change or a reduction in the force of contraction (Fig. 5.2). As preload increases (increased diastolic filling pressure) the LV fibers will lengthen in diastole, and subsequently the force of systolic contraction will increase. Preload is commonly estimated as the ventricular end-diastolic pressure (or end-diastolic diameter or volume).

Whereas preload affects the ventricle during diastole, *afterload* is the force the ventricle faces when it is contracting in systole. Afterload (*systolic wall stress*, see Fig. 3.1, p. 26 and below) is directly related to ventricular systolic pressure and ventricular radius and is inversely related to ventricular wall thickness. (Afterload will vary throughout systole, and may be calculated at various times in systole, such as at AV opening or at end-systole.) From this, one can see that although *ventricular systolic pressure* and *systemic vascular resistance* affect afterload, they are not the same as afterload. An increasing afterload will result in a reduced ventricular force and velocity of contraction (reduced myocardial fiber shortening) (Fig. 5.3) and lead to an increase in end-systolic volume.

Intrinsic contractile function is a basic attribute of the myocardium, which is reflective of the *intensity* of its active state. It is reflective of calcium availability and the actin–myosin interactions within the muscle cells. Several drugs and hormones, and the sympathetic nervous system, will increase myocardial intrinsic contractility. *Heart rate* will affect the heart by first increasing cardiac output as the heart rate increases. With higher heart rates, calcium levels may be higher within the muscle cells, and therefore the force of contraction will increase.

Stress and strain

Stress (see also Fig. 3.1) is defined as the force exerted on an object divided by its cross-sectional area, as:

$$\sigma = F/A$$

where σ is stress (often described as Newtons per square meter, N/m^2, which is *Pascal*, Pa), F is force (often in Newtons—a force of 1 *Newton* can accelerate a body of mass 1 kg to 1 cm/s^2, and a force of 1 *dyne* (dyn) can accelerate a body of mass 1 g to 1 cm/s^2), and A is cross-sectional area. *Normal stress* is that stress vector acting perpendicular to the surface of an object, and *shear stress* is that stress parallel to a surface (see Fig. 3.1, p. 26). Stress is described in units of Newtons/m^2, or dynes/cm^2.

For a *sphere*, stress is described as:

$$\sigma = [(P) \cdot (r)]/2(T)$$

where P is pressure, r the radius, and T the thickness of the shell of the sphere. Left ventricular shape is more complex than that of a sphere, therefore one may describe *meridional stress* (in the direction along the axis from the apex to the base) and *circumferential*

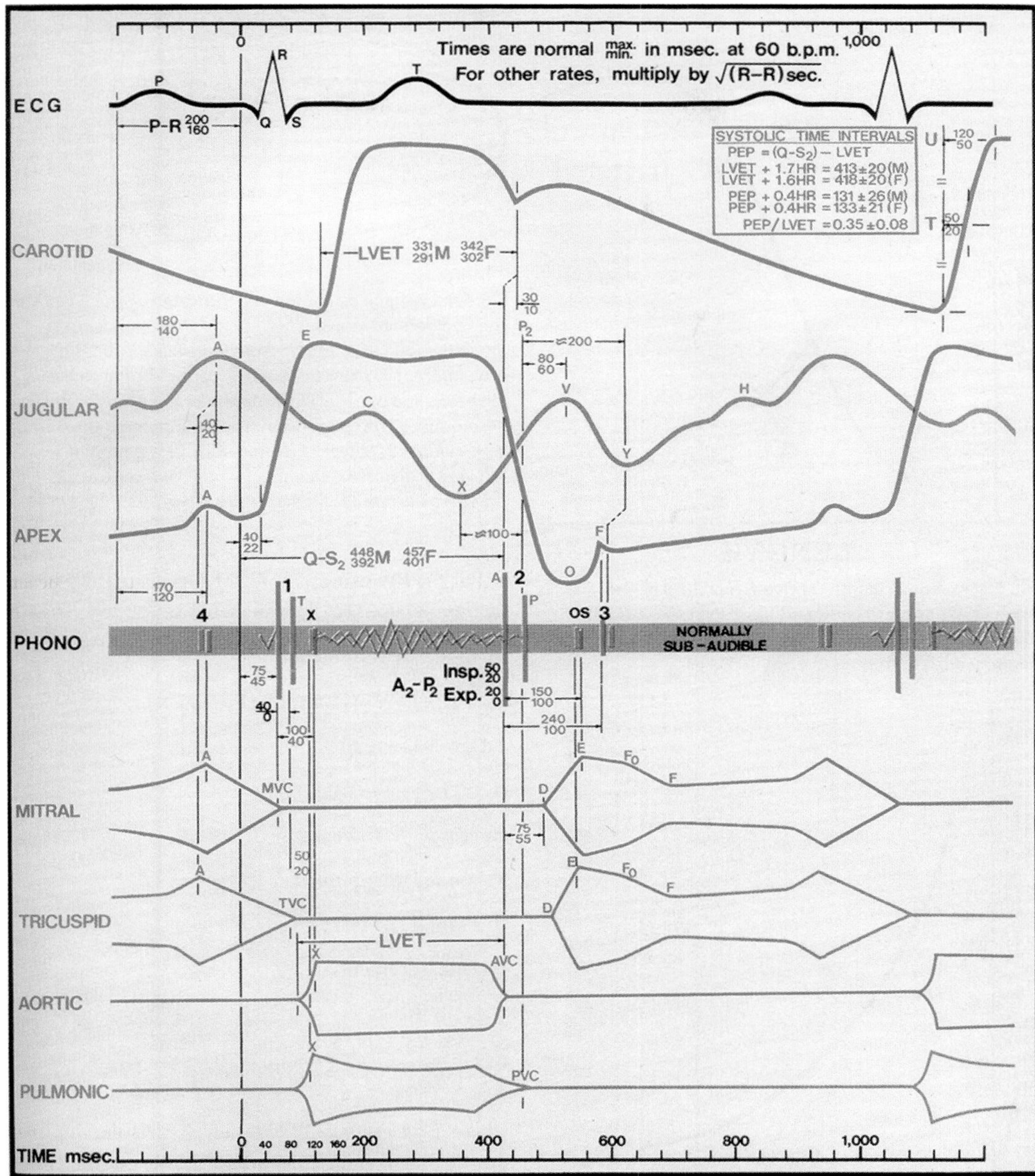

Fig. 5.1 Measurement of time intervals, reflective of cardiac function. The EKG is used for "timing." *Carotid pulse tracing, jugular pulse tracing, apexcardiogram, phonocardiogram,* and M-mode tracings of the four cardiac valves for measurement of time intervals are included. LVET, left ventricular ejection time; PEP, pre-ejection phase; AVC, aortic valve closure; PVC, pulmonic valve closure. (Reproduced with permission from: Tavel ME. Clinical Phonocardiography and External Pulse Recording, 4th edn. Chicago: Year Book Medical Publishers, 1985.)

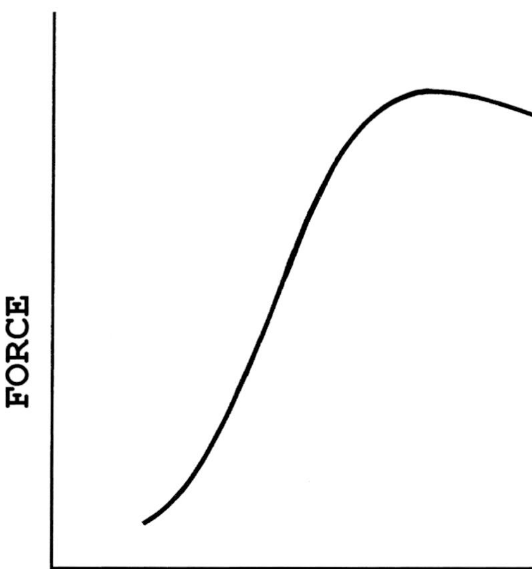

Fig. 5.2 As muscle length (*preload*) increases at end-diastole, the force of contraction will increase, but when muscle is stretched to a point, the force of contraction will begin to decrease.

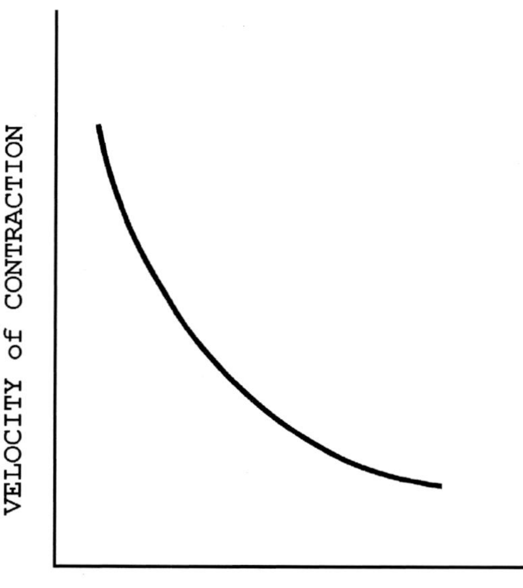

Fig. 5.3 As *afterload* increases, the force of contraction will decrease.

stress (otherwise termed *hoop stress*), which is perpendicular to the long axis (Fig. 5.4). The predominate strength and volume of LV ejection is produced by circumferential muscle bundles, with meridionally directed shortening less effective in ejection.

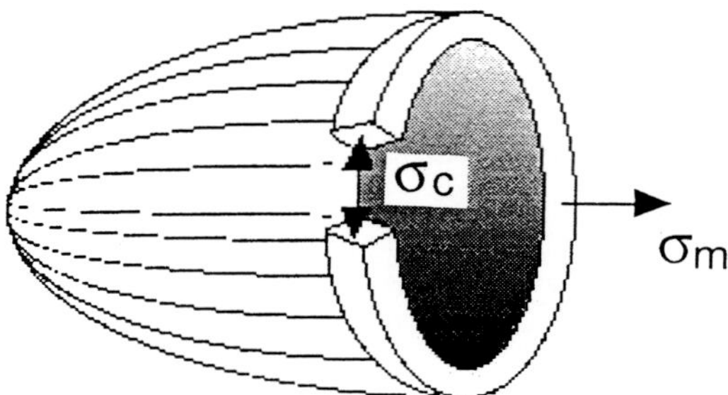

Fig. 5.4 LV shape estimated as a *truncated ellipse* illustrates the two defined stresses. *Meridional stress* (σ_m) is stress along the long axis, and opposes long axis shortening. *Circumferential stress* (σ_c) is stress perpendicular to the long axis, and opposes circumferential fiber shortening. (Reproduced with permission from: Aurigemma GP, Gaasch WH, Villegas B, Meyer TE. Noninvasive assessment of left ventricular mass, chamber volume, and contractile function. Current Problems in Cardiology 1995; 20: 375.)

For the LV, using a model of a *truncated ellipse*, the *meridional stress* (σ_m) is calculated as:

M-mode measurement

$$\sigma_m = (P)(LVID)/[4(T)(1 + (LVID/T))]$$

2-D measurement

$$\sigma_m = (1.33)(P) \cdot (A_m/A_c)$$

and *circumferential stress* (σ_c) as:

M-mode measurement

$$\sigma_c = P(a^2)[1 + (b^2/r^2)]/(b^2 - a^2)$$

2-D measurement

$$\sigma_c = \left(\frac{1.33P\sqrt{A_c}}{\sqrt{A_m + A_c} - \sqrt{A_c}}\right)\left(\frac{\frac{4(A_c)^{3/2}}{\pi L^2}}{\sqrt{A_m + A_c} - \sqrt{A_c}}\right)$$

where P is pressure, $LVID$ left ventricular internal dimension, T ventricular wall thickness, a the endocardial radius, b the epicardial radius, and r is the midwall radius. A_t is the 2-D area surrounded by epicardium and right side of the ventricular septum, A_c is the area surrounded by endocardium, and A_m is $A_t - A_c$. Stress measurements using M-mode and 2-D methods yield different results, with M-mode measurements higher than 2-D. *Afterload* is obtained as the stress calculation performed at end-systole, using end-systolic echo measurements. For pressure (P), the systolic blood pressure is often substituted for end-systolic pressure, but a more accurate method is to use the systolic pressure at the dicrotic notch of an arterial pulse recording (Fig. 5.1). *Preload* is obtained as the end-diastolic wall stress, using the end-diastolic pressure for *P*, and end-diastolic echo measurements.

A force applied to a solid object causes a *deformation*, whereas a force applied to a liquid causes *flow*. *Strain* is a measure of deformation, defined as:

$\varepsilon = (L - Li)/Li$

or has also been defined as:

$\varepsilon = (L - Li)/L$

where ε is strain (it is dimensionless), L is the final length to which an object has been stretched (or compressed), and Li is the original length. It is important to know which definition of strain is being used.

Stress and strain for many materials are linearly related for comparatively small values of strain. This linear relation between elongation and the force causing it is called *Hooke's law*, and is denoted as:

$E = \sigma/\varepsilon$

where E is the *modulus of elasticity* (*Young's modulus*). E has the same units as the stress, since strain is dimensionless.

Measures of regional strain within myocardial segments are reflective of regional function and attempts to measure strain of the myocardium have been made with techniques such as magnetic resonance imaging. With echocardiography, the *rate of deformation* of muscle (*strain rate*) has been evaluated. This measurement has been performed using *tissue Doppler imaging* (TDI), where shortening velocity has been obtained between two points within a segment of myocardium. The *myocardial velocity gradient* (MVG) between the two points of interest identifies the strain rate for the tissue segment (Fig. 5.5). Ventricular myocardium is often considered *incompressible*. That is a deformation in one direction is associated with expansion in the perpendicular direction. Therefore, measures of strain rate are thought to be equivalent, whether measured from the LV apex (longitudinally directed LV thickening) or the parasternal window (meridional thickening).

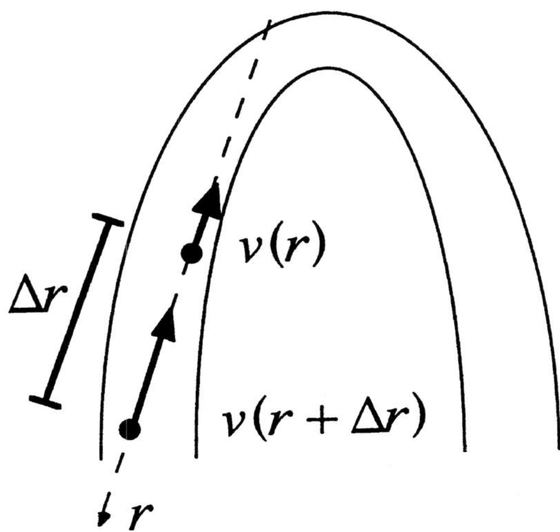

Fig. 5.5 Calculation of the strain rate of a tissue segment of length Δr. Each arrow at both points is a vector representing the velocity at that point. The *strain rate* is the difference in velocities between the two points. (Reproduced with permission from: Heimdal A, Stoylen A, Torp H, Skjaerpe T. Real-time strain rate imaging of the left ventricle by ultrasound. Journal of the American Society of Echocardiography 1998; 11: 1013–1019.)

Patient position and image acquisition

When performing studies for mass and volume measurements one should try to reduce variablility in measurements as much as possible (see also Fig. 5.6). Factors to consider include: *patient positioning, respirations, examination table position and angle, EKG waveform, image processing*, and *transducer position.*

To preserve uniformity, the *lateral left recumbency* position should be used for patient positioning. A wedge pillow against the patient's back may be helpful. Different *echo table tilt* angles may result in different measurement results. Ideally an attempt should be made to keep the echo table angle unchanged. Recording during *suspended* end-expiration (or mid-expiration) helps preserve uniformity and reduces translational motion. To perform quantitative measurements comparable to established data, R-wave gating to the EKG signal is performed. Many laboratories use end-systole as the frame preceding initial diastolic MV opening, or if the MV is not seen, then the frame with the smallest LV cavity is used. The first frame in which the QRS complex is apparent may be used as end-diastole.

During attempts to image the apical 2-D view (for volume and mass calculations), the transducer is usually impeded by the echo bed. A removable wedge from the mattress will facilitate transducer positioning. The patient remains in the lateral decubitis

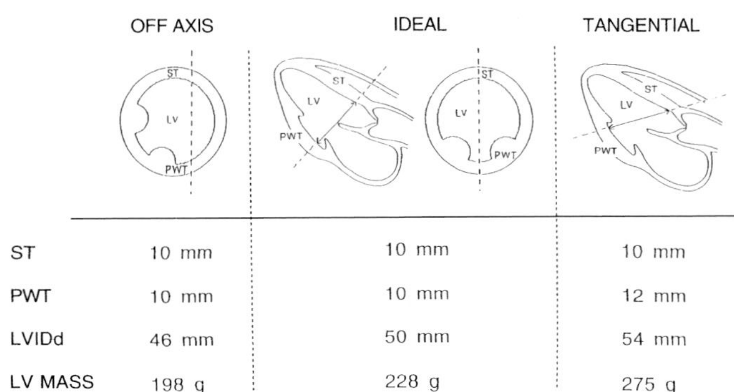

OFF AXIS
IDEAL
TANGENTIAL
ST
LV
PWT
ST 10 mm 10 mm 10 mm
PWT 10 mm 10 mm 12 mm
LVIDd 46 mm 50 mm 54 mm
LV MASS 198 g 228 g 275 g

Fig. 5.6 M-mode LV measurements from short and long axis views. Calculation of LV mass from off-angle measurements will result in large errors in mass calculations. ST, diastolic septal thickness; PWT, diastolic posterior wall thickness; LVIDd, end-diastolic LV internal dimension. (Reproduced with permission from: Aurigemma GP, Gaasch WH, Villegas B, Meyer TE. Noninvasive assessment of left ventricular mass, chamber volume, and contractile function. Current Problems in Cardiology 1995; 20: 386.)

position, and the transducer is initially positioned along the posterior axillary line, posterior to the palpable LV apex location. The transducer should be slowly moved anteriorly until the maximum size of the LV is noted. With enlarged ventricles in particular, not starting laterally may result in under-measurement of LV size. If in the two-chamber view the apex "curves out" of the image, the tracing of the LV outline should end at the limits of the sector and not be "fabricated".

Ventricular volume, mass, and shape

M-mode

M-mode echo has been used for LV mass and volume calculations. Parasternal long and short axis *2-D-guided* M-mode measurements are made *between the tip of the MV in diastole and the tips of the papillary muscles*. In systole, the ventricles exhibit motion of *rotation* (rotation of the LV about the long and short axes), *translation* (motion of the LV in space), and *longitudinal axis shortening*. Rotation may affect the short axis image, whereas the spherical end-diastolic image will become more elliptical in end-systole. Translation will have little effect on short axis 2-D measurements, but M-mode measures may change with respiration, as the LV shifts medially as the diaphragm flattens with inspiration. The M-mode cursor will be subsequently more laterally placed through the LV chamber. Measurements acquired in suspended respiration will help reduce this error. Longitudinal axis shortening in systole will result in a more basal part of the LV transected by the M-mode and 2-D scans towards end-systole. This will result in what appears to be a larger end-systolic cavity and diminished excursion of the myocardium with systole. Relatively small errors in M-mode measurements result in relatively large mass calculation errors (Fig. 5.6); therefore it is important for the M-mode beam to be perpendicular to the ventricular septal and posterior wall surface.

LV mass quantification using M-mode is based on the assumption that the LV is a prolate ellipsoid with a 2 : 1 long/short axis ratio. This assumption is fairly accurate for normal shaped ventricles, but for patients with LV segmental wall motion abnormalities or valvular regurgitation with altered LV geometry, this may not be accurate.

The well-validated *cube formula* for *LV mass calculations using M-mode echo* is:

$$\text{LV mass} = 0.8\{1.04[(IVS + LVID + PWT)^3 - LVID^3]\} + 0.6\ \text{g}$$

where (*ASE guidelines* for measurements) *IVS* is diastolic interventricular septal thickness, *LVID* is diastolic LV internal dimension and *PWT* is diastolic posterior LV wall thickness. The *Penn convention* has also well described LV mass by another form of the cube formula:

$$\text{LV mass} = 1.04[(IVS + LVID + PWT)^3 - (LVID)^3] - 13.6\ \text{g}$$

Using this formula, normal mass values included for males are 93 ± 22 g/m^2 body surface area, and for females 76 ± 18 g/m^2.

LV volumes using M-mode, may be made using a cube formula ($V = LVID^3$), but dilated (spherical) ventricles will have an overestimated volume. The

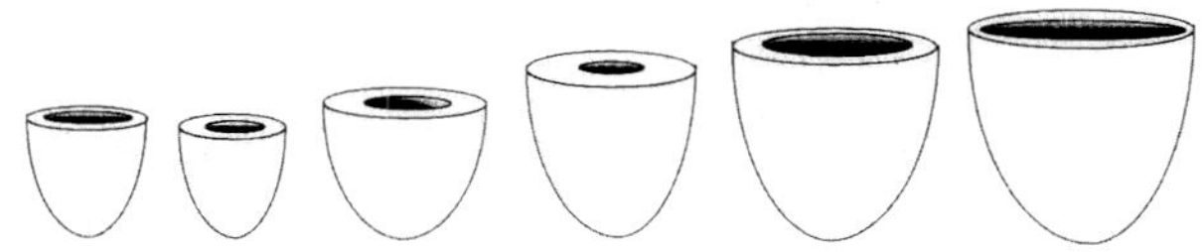

	NORMAL	CONCENTRIC REMODELING	CONCENTRIC HYPERTROPHY	HYPERTROPHIC CARDIOMYOPATHY	ECCENTRIC HYPERTROPHY	DILATED CARDIOMYOPATHY
MASS	N	N	↑	↑	↑↑	↑↑
VOLUME	N	N-↓	N	N-↓	↑↑	↑↑↑
RWT	N	↑	↑	↑↑	N-↓	↓
V/M	N	↓	↓	↓↓	N-↑	↑

Fig. 5.7 Various changes of the LV as classified by LV mass, volume, relative wall thickness (*RWT*), and volume/mass (*V/M*) ratio. (Reproduced with permission from: Aurigemma GP, Gaasch WH, Villegas B, Meyer TE. Noninvasive assessment of left ventricular mass, chamber volume, and contractile function. Current Problems in Cardiology 1995; 20: 385.)

Teichholz equation gives the *best M-mode formula for estimating LV volume*:

$$V_{diastole} = [7/(2.4 + LVID)] \cdot [LVID^3]$$

The *relative wall thickness* (*RWT*) is defined as the following:

$$RWT = 2(PWT/LVID)$$

As systolic pressure increases, the RWT will increase in both normal and compensated hypertensive ventricles. The RWT normally is (0.0027) × (peak systolic pressure). An elevated RWT (compared to what it should be based on the patient's systolic blood pressure) may be found in the so-called *hypertensive hypertrophic cardiomyopathy of the elderly*, in *hypertrophic cardiomyopathy*, occasionally in *aortic stenosis*, and rarely in *hypertension*. A relatively low RWT in patients with a dilated cardiomyopathy predicts that the patient will not respond to dobutamine with an increase in ejection fraction, as would be expected (Fig. 5.7).

For patients with untreated hypertension, LV mass and RWT measurements categorize patients into one of the following four groups: (i) *concentric hypertrophy* (↑ LV mass and ↑ RWT); (ii) *eccentric hypertrophy* (↑ LV mass and normal RWT); (iii) *concentric remodeling* (normal mass and abnormally ↑ RWT); and (iv) normal LV mass and RWT. Among patients with untreated hypertension, the group with normal LV mass and RWT was *most commonly* found, and concentric hypertrophy *least* often found. Concentric hypertrophy was associated with a higher incidence of adverse events than those with eccentric hypertrophy. Concentric remodeling is also associated with an increased incidence of adverse events.

Two-dimensional

Two-dimensional methods are used most often for measurement of *LV volumes*, and from these ejection fraction and LV mass measurements. The *area-length method* (which assumes the LV is a *cylinder-hemiellipsoid*) is the most practical method for calculating *LV mass*. This method calculates volume (V) as:

$$V = (5/6)(A)(L)$$

where A is the planimetered short axis area at a high papillary muscle level, and L is the LV length obtained from the apical four-chamber view. The volume of the "inner" shell (endocardium) is subtracted from the volume of the "outer" shell (epicardium), and multiplied by 1.05 to obtain LV mass. The *truncated ellipsoid method* has also been used to calculate LV mass (Fig. 5.8). Normal LV mass values (truncated ellipsoid method) are on the order of: males 148 ± 26 g, 76 ± 13 g/m^2 (body surface area), and females 108 ± 21 g, 66 ± 11 g/m^2. At autopsy, left ventricular hypertrophy (LVH) has been defined as a LV mass of 220 g or greater, and by echo as a LV mass of 215 or 225 g.

LV volume (most commonly for ejection fraction measurements—see "Systolic function—global" below) is calculated with either the biplane *method of disks* (*modified Simpson's rule* or otherwise termed *disk summation method*), or if only a single plane is

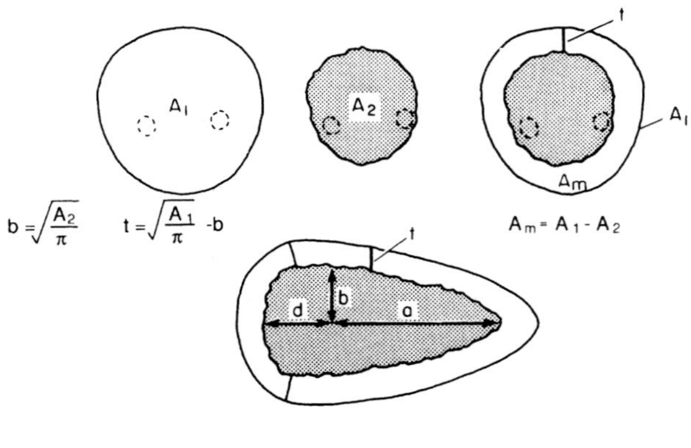

$$\text{LV Mass (AL)} = 1.05 \left\{ \left[5/6\, A_1 \; (a + d + t) \right] - \left[5/6\, A_2 \; (a + d) \right] \right\}$$

$$\text{LV Mass (TE)} = 1.05\, \pi \left\{ (b + t)^2 \left[2/3\, (a + t) + d - \frac{d^3}{3\,(a + t)^2} \right] - b^2 \left[2/3\, a + d - \frac{d^3}{3a^2} \right] \right\}$$

Fig. 5.8 Calculation of LV mass using the *area–length (AL)* and *truncated ellipsoid (TE)* methods. The short axis view of the LV is at the level of papillary muscle tips. Epicardial and endocardial perimeters are traced to calculate thickness (*t*), short axis radius (*b*), and the areas (A1 and A2). The papillary muscles are not included in the planimetry. In the figure, the parameter (*a*) is the long (semi-major) axis from the widest minor axis radius to the apex, and (*d*) is the truncated semi-major axis from the widest short axis diameter to the mitral annulus plane. As shown by the equations above that calculate *b* and *t*, these two values are "back calculated" from the traced areas. The area–length method is probably less difficult to implement. (Reproduced with permission from: Schiller NB, Shah PM, Crawford M, *et al*. Recommendations for quantification of the left ventricle by two-dimensional echocardiography. Journal of the American Society of Echocardiography 1989; 2(5): 364.)

obtained, the *single plane area length method* (Fig. 5.9). For LV volume using the method of disks, two nearly orthogonal apical views (four- and two-chamber) are obtained.

Systolic function—global

M-mode *fractional shortening* (FS) is defined as:

$$FS\% = 100 \times [(LVEDD) - (LVESD)]/(LVEDD)$$

where *LVEDD* is the LV end-diastolic dimension and *LVESD* is LV end-systolic dimension. It is a commonly used M-mode index of systolic performance. If there are no segmental LV wall motion abnormalities, the *FS* and ejection fraction (*EF*) correlate well. Normal values are greater than 30%.

The *velocity of circumferential shortening* (V_{cf}), in circumferences per second (c/s), indicates the mean velocity of LV shortening through the LV minor axis:

$$V_{cf} = FS/ET$$

where *ET* is *ejection time*. The ejection time is obtained from either the M-mode measure of aortic valve opening to aortic valve closure, aortic flow by Doppler, or by an external pulse recording of the carotid artery (Fig. 5.1). Normal values for V_{cf} are 1.1 c/s or greater. The V_{cf} may be heart rate corrected (V_{cfc}) to the preceding electrocardiographic RR interval as:

$$V_{cfc} = V_{cf}/\sqrt{(RR)}$$

M-mode tracings of *mitral annular excursion* toward the LV apex (recorded from the apex) in systole correlate with systolic function. The magnitude of systolic motion is proportional to the shortening of the LV longitudinally. Normal annular systolic motion is 8 mm or greater, with the average 12 ± 2 mm from both four- and two-chamber views. If annular systolic motion is less than 8 mm, the *EF* is likely to be less than 50%.

The E-point to septal separation (EPSS) describes the distance from the maximum MV early diastolic excursion (E-point) to the LV septum (see Chapter 4). It is normally 6 mm or less. With reduced LV systolic function, the EPSS may be increased (Fig. 5.10). The *mitral separation angle* (MSA) is the 2-D counterpart of the EPSS. The MSA is the angle between the

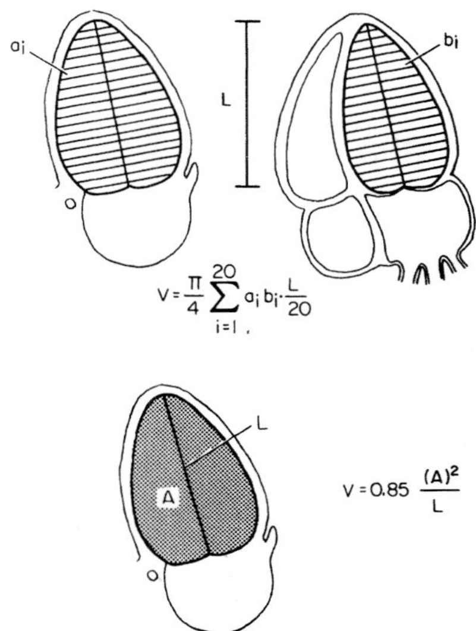

Fig. 5.9 Calculation of LV volume (usually for ejection fraction calculations) is performed by either the biplane method of disks (upper panel), or the single plane area length method. To calculate LV volume by the *method of disks*, two nearly orthogonal apical views are obtained, and the endocardium is planimetered (diastolic volume in end-diastole and systolic volume in end-systole). The volume of the LV is generated by summing up multiple disks that are generated (at least 20 disks, and many times more). If the length of the ventricle is different in the two planes, usually the longest length is assumed correct. If the difference in length between the two views is over 20%, then the method of disks should probably not be used. The *area–length method* (equation is shown for volume calculation) is used if only one plane is obtained. (Reproduced with permission from: Schiller NB, Shah PM, Crawford M, *et al.* Recommendations for quantification of the left ventricle by two-dimensional echocardiography. Journal of the American Society of Echocardiography 1989; 2(5): 362.)

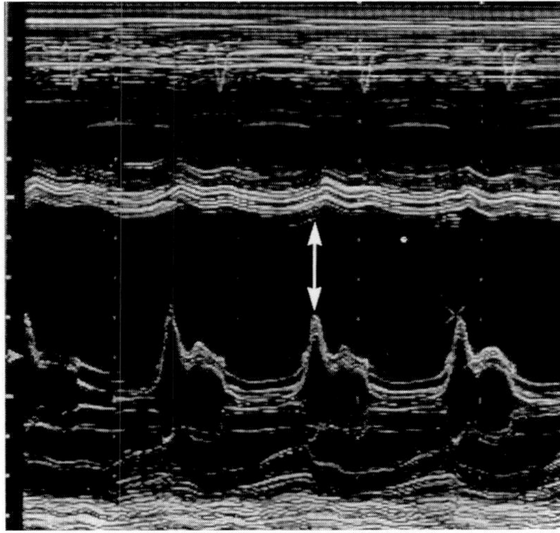

Fig. 5.10 M-mode of mitral valve in a parasternal view demonstrating an increased E-point to septal separation (EPSS) (arrow).

anterior MV leaflet and the LV side of the interventricular septum during maximal leaflet excursion. It is best seen in the apical four-chamber view, with normal values being 5–30°. The EPSS and MSA may be diminished not only with depressed LV systolic function, but also with significant aortic regurgitation also.

Ejection fraction (*EF*) is the stroke volume (*SV*) divided by the end-diastolic volume (*EDV*):

$$EF = (SV/EDV) \times 100\%$$

and since

$$SV = (EDV - ESV)$$

therefore

$$EF = [(EDV - ESV)/EDV] \times 100\%$$

where *ESV* is end-systolic volume (Chapter 3 for *Doppler derived calculations of stroke volume*). *EF* is a global index of systolic function and one of the most commonly used markers of systolic function. *Qualitative estimation* (eyeball estimation) of *EF* may be reasonably accurate with experienced interpreters, and is usually reported as a value in intervals of 5–10%, or commonly within a range of within approximately 10%. Errors in *EF* estimation may result from:

- Underestimation of *EF* because of endocardial echo dropout and the eyeball seeing mostly epicardial motion.
- Underestimation of *EF* when the LV cavity is significantly enlarged. A large LV can eject a larger volume with less endocardial motion.
- Overestimation of *EF* in a normal or small LV (opposite of the above).
- Significant LV regional wall motion abnormalities. The LV cavity area will change differently in different echo views, so the reader must "integrate" these views to arrive at an accurate estimate.

Quantitative methods to calculate *EF* are usually preferable. LV volumes are obtained (see "Ventricular volume, mass, and shape" above), and from this the

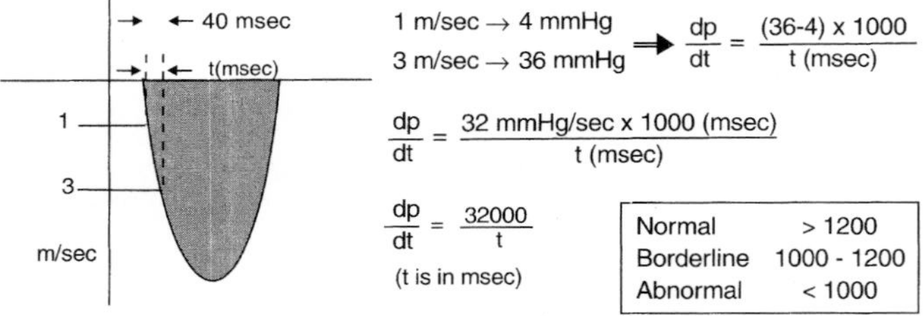

Fig. 5.11 Calculation of dp/dt. In this example $t = 40$ m/s. Therefore $dp/dt = (32 \times 1000)/40$, which is 800 mmHg/s, indicative of abnormal LV systolic function.

EF calculated. For an accurate *EF* calculation, one must be able to obtain proper positioned images along with good endocardial visualization. If the modified Simpson's method (method of disks) is not possible (difficult endocardial definition or foreshortened image from the apex), then a method described by Dr M.A. Quinones' laboratory measuring several LV diameters (*LV diameter method*) may be used. An LV diameter at the upper, mid and lower third of the LV cavity in at least one, but preferably three, apical long axis views, and two diameter measurements in the parasternal long axis (since the apex is not usually seen in this view) are obtained. From the apex, the first measure (D1) is about 1 cm below the MV leaflet tip, D2 is about halfway between the MV and apex, and D3 at the lower third of the LV (about the same distance from D2 as D2 is from D1). Measurements are perpendicular to a line drawn from the mid MV plane to the LV apex. All of these diameters are averaged for end-diastole (D_d) and end-systole (D_s).

$$EF = [(D_d^2 - D_s^2)/D_d^2] + [(D_s^2/D_d^2) \times ((L_d - L_s)/L_d)]$$

where L_d and L_s are the apical long axis measurements at end-diastole and end-systole. This method of *EF* calculation is particularly suited for acoustically difficult cases.

A simpler method uses only parasternal long axis guided M-mode derived end-diastolic diameter (*EDD*) and end-systolic diameter (*ESD*):

$$EF = \{[(EDD^2 - ESD^2)/EDD^2] \times 100\%\} + K$$

where *K* is a correction factor for the LV apex, and is 10% for a normal apex, 5% for hypokinesis, 0% for akinesis, and –5% for dyskinesis. This method is useful in patients with "symmetric" ventricles, who do not have major wall motion abnormalities.

Using continuous wave (CW) Doppler (see Chapter 8) the "rate of rise" of the mitral regurgitation (MR) jet is correlated with LV systolic function. A slow "rate of rise" (dp/dt) of the MR signal (from 1 m/s to 3 m/s) indicates poor systolic function, and correlates with a slow rise of intracavitary LV systolic pressure (Fig. 5.11). In order to calculate dp/dt by this method one must first have MR present, and record the maximal Doppler spectra, which may be difficult with eccentric jets.

The *eccentricity index* (*EI*) is defined as left ventricular length (*L*) divided by the transverse diameter (*T*):

$$EI = L/T$$

where *L* is the longest distance from the mitral annulus plane to the apex of the left ventricle, and *T* is the distance at the mid-point of *L*. In patients with more

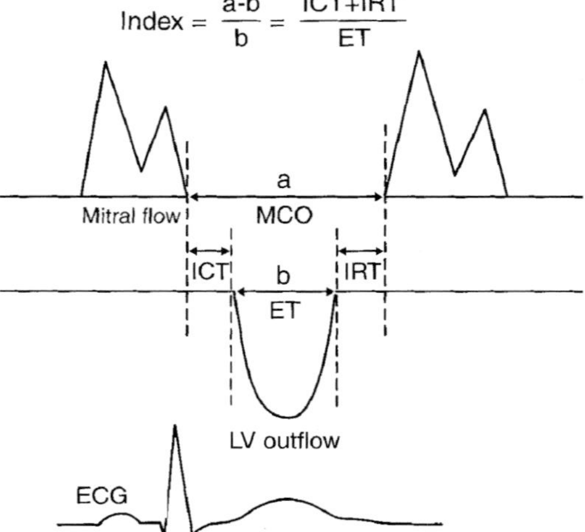

Fig. 5.12 Measurement of the index of myocardial performance (IMP). In this illustration (a) is the interval between atrioventricular valve closure and opening (MCO) (AV_{co}—see text), and (b) is the ejection time (ET). (Reproduced with permission from: Oh JK, Seward JB, Tajik AJ. The Echo Manual, 2nd edn. Philadelphia: Lippincott Williams & Wilkins, 1999.)

spherical ventricles, *EI* is lower. *EI* is a quantitative measure of left ventricular remodeling (see Chapter 11).

The *index of myocardial performance* (IMP), introduced by the Mayo Clinics, incorporates both systolic and diastolic time intervals for evaluation of global ventricular performance. Whereas systolic dysfunction will result in a prolonged *isovolumic contraction time* (*ICT*) and a shortened *ejection time* (*ET*), both systolic and diastolic dysfunction results in a prolonged *isovolumic relaxation time* (*IRT*).

$$IMP = (ICT + IRT)/ET$$

Tei *et al.* (1995: see Further reading, p. 358) found the following range of values:
LV, normal—0.39 ± 0.05
LV, dilated CMP—0.59 ± 0.10
RV, normal—0.28 ± 0.04
Primary pulmonary hypertention—0.93 ± 0.34.

In order to obtain the *IMP* (Fig. 5.12), one should obtain either a pulsed wave (PW) Doppler of the atrioventricular inflow signal, or use continuous wave (CW) to obtain the atrioventricular regurgitant signal. Then one should measure the interval between atrioventricular valve closure and opening (AV_{co}). Next, one should obtain the semilunar outflow signal using either PW or CW and measure the ejection time (*ET*). From this, the *IMP* may be calculated.

$$IMP = (AV_{co} - ET)/ET$$

In summary, there are multiple methods available to determine LV systolic function. When endocardium is well defined, from a clinical standpoint most echocardiography laboratories today employ either subjective or objective estimates of ejection fraction. Other methods may be used as complementary to or as a substitute, particularly if the endocardium is not well seen on 2-D imaging.

6

CHAPTER 6

Diastolic Function

Background—determinants of LV filling, mitral and pulmonary vein flow

Diastolic dysfunction may be a significant factor in myocardial disorders including hypertension, coronary artery disease, pericardial disease, and various forms of cardiomyopathy. Diastolic dysfunction *is nearly always* present in patients with LV systolic dysfunction and usually *precedes* systolic dysfunction in most disease processes. It appears that diastolic function may be important in patients with systolic dysfunction in determining symptom class. For example, some patients with poor systolic function have New York Heart Association Class III or IV congestive heart failure (CHF) symptoms, whereas other patients with similar systolic dysfunction have only mild Class I or II symptoms. The difference in the symptomatic state is the diastolic parameters. Whereas one third of patients diagnosed with heart failure have *normal* systolic function (this percentage increases with increasing age), therapy that improves systolic function may not be appropriate for "pure" diastolic dysfunction. Diastole has been defined as beginning with aortic valve closure, and ending with mitral valve closure (see Fig. 5.1, p. 55).

Four phases of diastole have been described (Fig. 6.1). Briefly, *isovolumic relaxation* begins with aortic valve closure and lasts until mitral valve opening. The ventricle is a "closed" chamber during this period of ventricular relaxation (both aortic and mitral valves are closed), hence LV volume is unchanged as ventricular pressure is decreasing. The rate of decline of pressure during isovolumic relaxation may affect LV filling after the MV opens.

The *rapid filling phase* begins as the MV opens. The rate of filling is related to the pressure gradient between the LA and LV. This pressure gradient is mostly determined by the *LA pressure* at MV opening, and the *rate of active decline* of the LV pressure. The ventricle continues to *actively* relax, and the LV volume continues to *increase*, despite a *decreasing* LV pressure (evidence of diastolic suction).

The third phase of diastole is *diastasis*, which consists of *passive* LV filling in which LA and LV pressures are nearly equal. LV filling is mostly the result of pulmonary venous flow (the LA is a "passive conduit" allowing flow from the pulmonary veins directly into the LV).

The fourth phase is *atrial systole* (atrial contraction) in which about 15% of LV filling occurs in normal patients, and probably more in several myocardial disorders. Atrial systole ends with MV closure, and is affected by *myocardial stiffness*, *pericardial restraint* on LV volume "expansion," *atrial resistance* to contraction (and lack of atrial contraction with arrhythmias such as atrial fibrillation), and so-called *LV-LA synchrony* (the PR interval on the ECG recording). The three phases of diastole during which the MV is open (rapid filling, diastasis, atrial systole) are termed *auxotonic relaxation*, in that the LV volume continues to increase, but pressure change varies.

Normal diastolic function is manifested by adequate ventricular filling at rest and with exercise without an abnormal increase in diastolic filling pressures. Abnormal diastolic function is manifested by an increased ventricular diastolic pressure due to an increased diastolic volume, delayed relaxation or increased stiffness of the ventricle.

LV filling is determined by active and passive forces. During *early* diastole, both *active relaxation* (requires active expenditure of energy within myocardial cells) and recoil from elastic energy, which may have been stored in the myocardium from the previous systole (termed "*diastolic suction*"), mostly determine LV filling. This active process is usually completed, or nearly so, by mid-diastole. During *late* diastole, the *passive* properties of the myocardium (*myocardial*

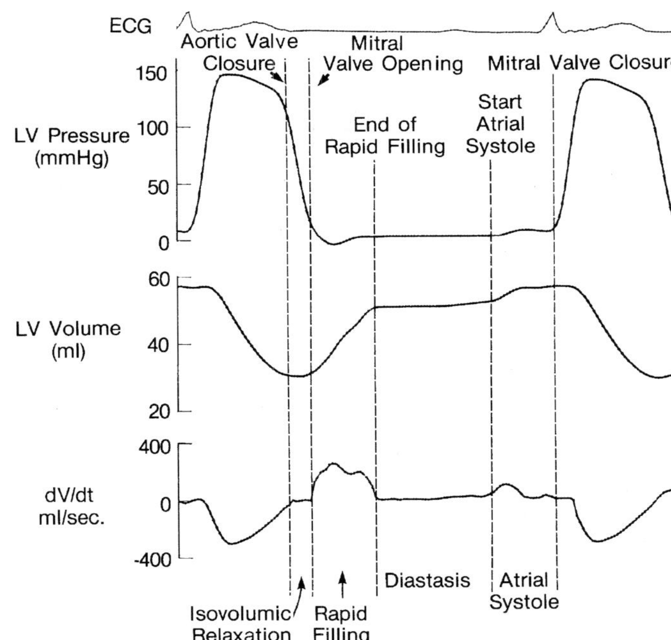

Fig. 6.1 Recording of LV pressure, volume, and the change in volume as a function of time (d*V*/d*t*). The four phases of diastole are illustrated (see text). (Reproduced with permission from: Little WC, Downes TR. Clinical evaluation of left ventricular diastolic performance. Progress in Cardiovascular Diseases 1990; 17(4): Jan/Feb 274.)

compliance—the "inverse" of stiffness) predominate. Late in diastole, interactions between the LV and RV, and also the pericardium, become important.

Several indices describe early active relaxation. These include peak $-dp/dt$, *tau* (τ), and *isovolumic relaxation time* (IVRT). The peak $-dp/dt$ is the fastest rate of pressure decline occurring during early relaxation after aortic valve closure. It may be measured using the pressure decay of a mitral regurgitant (MR) jet with continuous wave Doppler (see Fig. 5.11, p. 62 where dp/dt of MR upstroke is measured). The time interval in milliseconds is measured between 3 m/s and 1 m/s on the Doppler velocity deceleration. A normal calculated value is -2000 ± 400 mmHg/ s, with a less negative value noted with impaired active relaxation due to ischemia. This value will vary dependent on sym-pathetic tone and aortic pressure, and is not often used in clinical practice. τ describes pressure drop during isovolumic relaxation. It assumes mono-exponential decay in LV pressure from the point of aortic valve closure to a point 5 mmHg above the left ventricular end-diastolic pressure (LVEDP) (approximation of MV opening). Values are converted to logarithmic scale and fitted to a straight line. The negative reciprocal of the slope of the line represents τ in milliseconds. Normal values range from 25 to 40 ms, with higher values noted with impaired active relaxation. This measurement is impractical in most clinical situations and is not easily reproducible. IVRT measurement is used more frequently and will be described later in this chapter.

Assessment of diastolic function and loading conditions

M-mode/two-dimensional imaging

Left Ventricle

One of the most common causes of LV diastolic abnormality is reduced systolic dysfunction. Therefore, *in a patient with systolic dysfunction noted by echo, diastolic dysfunction will also be present* and will be the predominant cause of the patient's congestive symptoms. In addition, diastolic dysfunction most often *precedes* development of systolic dysfunction in most disease processes. LV *wall motion abnormalities*, suggestive of coronary artery disease/infarction are also clues to the presence of ventricular diastolic dysfunction. Diastolic dysfunction is associated with *left ventricular hypertrophy* (LVH) of any etiology.

Left Atrium

An enlarged LA with reduced LA contractility suggests elevated LV filling pressures and diastolic dysfunction either presently or in the past. The LA should be

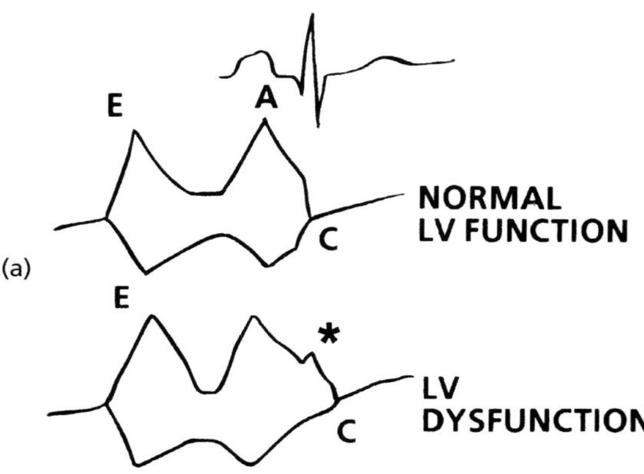

*** SYNONYMS: B - bump; Beta - inflection; interruption of AC slope by plateau or notch**

(b)

Fig. 6.2 Normal M-mode mitral AC slope (a) and prolonged AC slope (b). A B-bump is evident (*). (Reproduced with permission from: D'Cruz IA, Kleinman D, Aboulatta H, Orander P, Hand RC. A reappraisal of the mitral B-bump (B-inflection): its relationship to left ventricular dysfunction. Echocardiography 1990; 7(1): 70.)

evaluated using 2-D imaging and not just M-mode measurement, as the latter shows only one dimension of the LA size.

Left atrial volume (LAV), normalized to body surface area (BSA), as an index of atrial size is better reflective of cardiovascular disease than M-mode left atrial dimension (LAD). LAV may be calculated, using an ellipse formula, as:

$$\mathrm{LAV} = \frac{\pi}{6}(\mathrm{D}_1)(\mathrm{D}_2)(\mathrm{LAD})$$

Where D_1 is the LA dimension in a long-axis measurement from the mitral coaptation point to the LA posterior wall, and D_2 is the transverse LA dimension. LAD is measured using ASE guidelines. All are measured as end-systole. Median normal values using this method for women is 21 ml/m^2, and for men 22 ml/m^2. If one calculates LA volume using the biplane method of discs (Simpson's method), normal volumes are similar. As Simpson's method requires one to trace the LA endocardium, this ellipse formula method appears somewhat easier.

IVRT and B-bump

Although usually obtained by Doppler techniques (see section below), the IVRT may be determined by M-mode measurement of the time between aortic valve closure and MV opening.

On M-mode tracings of MV motion, a *B-bump* may suggest an elevated LV end-diastolic pressure (also seen with tricuspid valve (TV) M-mode tracings with an elevated RV end-diastolic pressure). Normally the AC segment of the MV M-mode tracings is a rapid slope (see Fig. 6.2a), from the A peak to the C point (complete closure). The point of abrupt closure is the B point. The B-bump is a delay in MV leaflet closure (Fig. 6.2), and usually represents an LVEDP of at least 20 mmHg.

Doppler

Figure 6.3 is a diagram of mitral and pulmonary vein flow. Pulmonary systolic flow may be biphasic with an S1 (early) and S2 (late) wave (Fig. 6.3b). IVRT recorded with MV Doppler inflow is the first phase of diastole. Rapid filling occurs with the Doppler E wave, and the A wave represents filling from atrial contraction. S1 of pulmonary venous flow represents atrial relaxation. There is a drop in atrial pressure with atrial relaxation, leading to an increase in the pulmonary vein–LA pressure gradient and a resultant increased pulmonary vein (PV) forward flow. S2 occurs after RV contraction, which results in increased PV forward flow. The PV D wave occurs after MV opening with the decrease in LA pressure due to blood emptying into the LV. The AC wave (Fig. 6.3b) is reversed flow back into the pulmonary veins, secondary to atrial contraction.

Clinically useful measured diastolic parameters include isovolumic relaxation time (IVRT), deceleration time (DT), E and A velocities, E/A ratio, pulmonary vein S, D and AC velocities, and the duration of A seen on the transmitral flow pattern compared to the duration of AC on the pulmonary vein flow pattern (Fig. 6.3). There are basically four mitral inflow patterns by PW Doppler (Fig. 6.4), with a general range of measured parameters (Table 6.1). In normal young patients, atrial contraction contributes little to LV filling but with *increasing age*, active relaxation will decrease with an associated increase in the passive-filling component and the active atrial contraction contribution to filling (Fig. 6.5). By age 65 years, the E velocity approaches A velocity, and by 70 years, the E is usually less than A. PV flow patterns demonstrate a progressive decrease in D velocity, and an increase in S velocity.

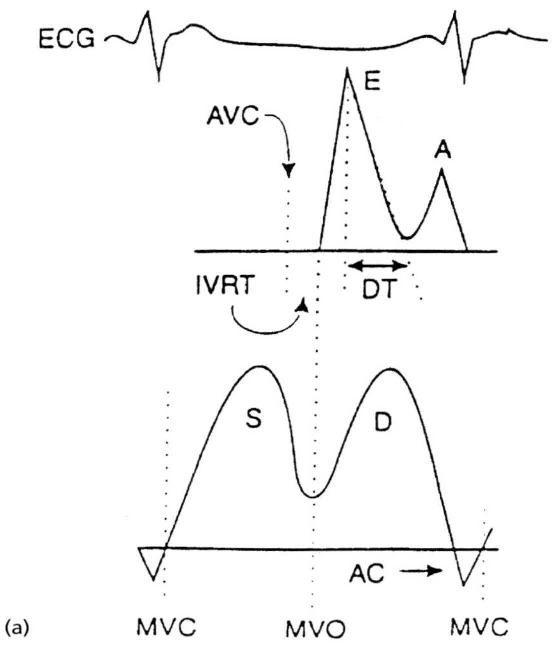

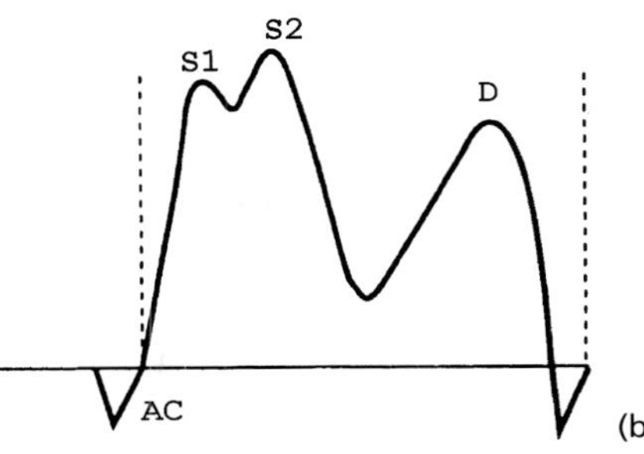

Fig. 6.3 Pulsed wave (PW) Doppler mitral inflow and pulmonary vein flow patterns. In (a) isovolumic relaxation time (IVRT) is the time from aortic valve closure (AVC) to mitral valve opening (MVO). Pulmonary vein systolic (S) and diastolic (D) flow, atrial contraction (AC), and mitral valve closure (MVC) are illustrated. Deceleration time (DT) is the time for the peak E velocity to decline to the zero baseline. In (b) the pulmonary vein systolic flow is biphasic with an early (S1) and late (S2) systolic wave.

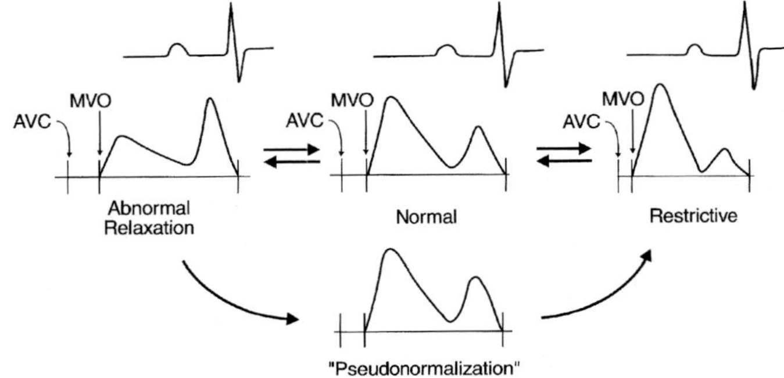

Fig. 6.4 Patterns of mitral inflow by PW Doppler, recorded at the "tips" of the mitral valve, recorded in an apical four-chamber view (see text).

Table 6.1 Parameters of diastolic filling: obtained from the MV inflow using PW Doppler for normal/pseudonormal, abnormal relaxation, and restriction to filling.

	Abnormal relaxation	Normal	Restriction
DT	>240 ms	160–240 ms	<160 ms
E	↓	0.8–1.5 m/s	↔↑
A	↑	0.75 m/s	↓
E/A	E < A	E < A(>1.0)	E >> A
IVRT	↑	55–90 ms	<70 ms

DT, deceleration time; E, E wave; A, A wave; E/A, E wave/A wave ratio; IVRT, isovolumic relaxation time.

Patients with impaired myocardial relaxation will have a pattern of *abnormal relaxation* (Figs 6.4 & 6.5). Reduced active relaxation as seen with myocardial disorders (hypertrophy of any type, ischemia/infarction, and early stages of infiltrative disorders) will result in a prolonged IVRT and DT, and a reduced E velocity and E/A ratio (Fig. 6.6). A pattern of "abnormal relaxation" (E < A with ↑ IVRT and ↑ DT) may also be seen in patients with normal intrinsic diastolic function who have a markedly reduced preload. This may occur

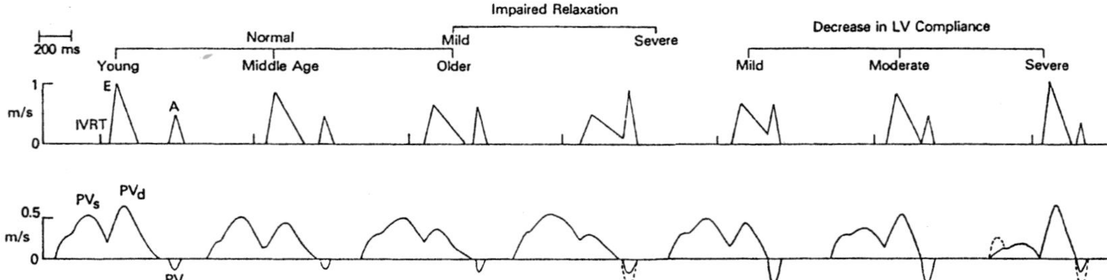

Fig. 6.5 The three MV inflow patterns on the left of the diagram represent changes in flow patterns with *normal aging*. Associated normal pulmonary vein (PV) flow patterns are drawn below each mitral valve (MV) pattern. Note the age-related trend toward an abnormal relaxation pattern, with a PV decrease in D velocity and increase in S velocity (see text). The four inflow patterns on the right of the diagram demonstrate an *abnormal relaxation* pattern evident in various cardiac disorders, indicative of reduced active relaxation. The atrial reversed flow component (PV flow of middle drawing) may be normal, indicative of a normal end-diastolic pressure, or it may be increased (dashed line in middle PV drawing), indicative of an elevated end-diastolic pressure (increase in atrial pressure with atrial contraction). With a progressive increase in preload (increased atrial pressure) the IVRT and DT begin to shorten, and E velocity and E/A ratio increase. The MV inflow may appear normal (termed "*pseudonormal*"), but the PV flow pattern will demonstrate a reduced S/D ratio, and prominent atrial reversed flow (second panel from right), in distinction from a PV "normal pattern" (left three panels). With a progressive increase in preload, the E velocity and E/A ratio continue to increase, with a further shortening of the IVRT and DT. PV flow demonstrates an increased D velocity with an associated rapid D wave deceleration time ("*restriction to filling*"). The S velocity is markedly blunted, and atrial reversal (and S1) may also be blunted because of depression of atrial systolic function (see text). (Reproduced with permission from: Appleton CP, Hatle LK. The natural history of left ventricular filling abnormalities: assessment by two-dimensional and Doppler echocardiography. Echocardiography 1992; 9(4): 453.)

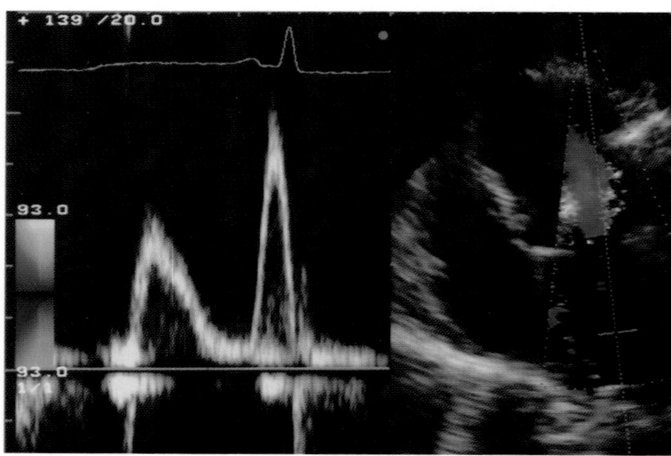

Fig. 6.6 Mitral inflow pattern in a 74-year-old male with a history of hypertension and left ventriclur hypertrophy (LVH) by two-dimensional (2-D) imaging. The E/A ratio is less than 1, and DT is prolonged.

in patients with severe acute volume loss secondary to severe bleeding, or dehydration. An abnormal relaxation pattern usually is indicative of a normal *mean* LV diastolic filling pressure. The exception to this is in patients in whom there is markedly prolonged active relaxation due to severe LVH. In that situation, an abnormal relaxation pattern may be present despite a high mean LV diastolic filling pressure.

As a rule of thumb, pulmonary vein flow D velocity and its DT always parallels the MV flow E wave and its DT. Therefore, with abnormal relaxation, pulmonary vein D velocity and its DT are reduced and pulmonary vein S velocity is relatively increased. The atrial reversal wave (Ar or AC) in the PV is reflective of end-diastolic pressure. If it is prominent (Ar usually equal to or greater than 0.4 m/s, and Ar duration is

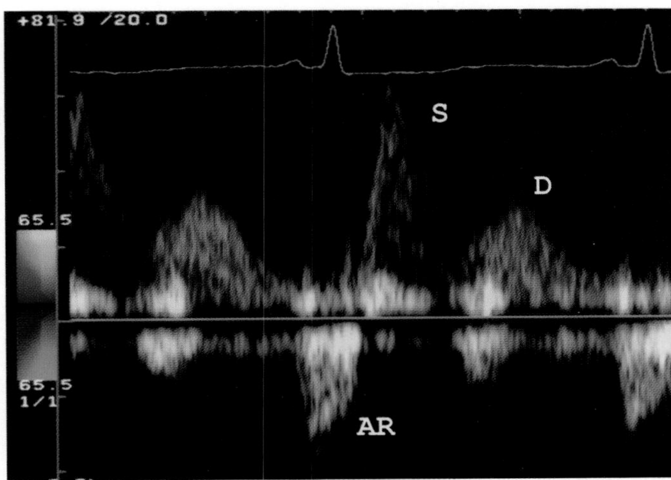

Fig. 6.7 Pulmonary vein flow pattern in the patient shown in Fig. 6.6. The S/D ratio is less than 1, consistent with abnormal relaxation (either low or normal *mean* left ventricular diastolic pressure), but a prominent atrial reversal wave (AR) suggests an elevated LV end-diastolic pressure.

30 ms greater than the duration of the mitral A wave), end-diastolic pressure is probably elevated (Fig. 6.7).

There is a correlation between the mitral A wave deceleration time (Adt) and LVEDP. Because there is an abrupt cessation of the A wave with an elevated LVEDP, the Adt will be shortened also. A previous study demonstrated a correlation between an Adt of 65 ms or less and a LVEDP greater than 18 mmHg. This measurement was not valid in patients with mitral stenosis, atrial fibrillation, or other arrhythmias. With tachycardia and EA fusion, the Adt may be the only reliable measurement of LVEDP.

When a pattern of abnormal relaxation is present in the presence of an increased preload, the mitral filling pattern approaches a normal pattern, termed *pseudonormalization* (Fig. 6.4). The PV pattern, however, will help differentiate this from a normal pattern (Fig. 6.5). The S velocity will be blunted, and the Ar wave will be prominent. Other clues when performing an echo examination to help differentiate normal from pseudonormal MV inflow may include:

- Patients with LV systolic dysfunction, hypertrophy, or LA enlargement would be expected to have diastolic abnormality, and therefore a MV inflow pattern of abnormal relaxation. A "normal" pattern in these patients would then be suggestive of pseudonormalization (diastolic dysfunction with an elevated preload).
- Preload may be reduced during the strain phase of a *Valsalva maneuver* or by *nitroglycerin*. In a patient with a transmitral pseudonormalized pattern, these maneuvers may cause a transient reduction in preload and allow the pattern to revert transiently to an abnormal relaxation pattern. In distinction to this, a normal transmitral pattern will demonstrate reduced E and A velocities in proportion, so that the E/A ratio will not change.
- Evaluation of *right-sided diastolic parameters* may help in that if the LV demonstrates diastolic abnormality, usually the RV will also; therefore if a pseudonormal pattern is present across the MV, a pattern of abnormal relaxation may be noted across the TV.

If a patient with pseudonormalization continues with a progressive increase in preload, the MV inflow pattern will develop a pattern of *restriction to filling* (Figs 6.4 & 6.5). With a progressive increase in LA pressure, the MV will open earlier. Therefore, the IVRT will be shorter and the E velocity will be higher (a higher gradient from the LA to LV across the MV). The DT and A wave duration will be both shortened (Fig. 6.8). With a marked increase in LA pressure (as with severe acute aortic regurgitation), diastolic MR may be noted between the E and A wave (Figs 6.9 and 7.28).

Occasionally low velocity flow will be noted to occur during diastasis (Fig. 6.10). Termed an *L wave*, it is felt to represent abnormal relaxation with marked delayed active relaxation and elevated filling pressures. Typically, the L wave may be seen in an elderly patient who has LVH with excellent systolic function and coexistent moderate mitral regurgitation.

The E wave peak velocity is predictive of mortality in patients with *dilated cardiomyopathy* and heart failure. Patients with dilated cardiomyopathy and a

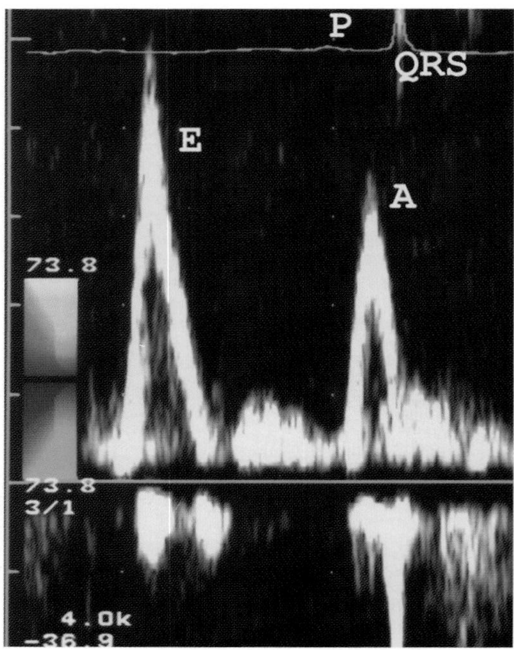

Fig. 6.8 Pulsed wave MV inflow pattern in a 74-year-old male with an ischemic cardiomyopathy and symptoms of heart failure. The patient would "normally" be expected to have an abnormal relaxation pattern based on age and reduced LV systolic function. The E/A ratio is greater than 1 and DT is reduced. The A wave is shortened at the onset of the QRS, consistent with high LV filling pressures. P, P wave; QRS, QRS on the ECG rhythm strip.

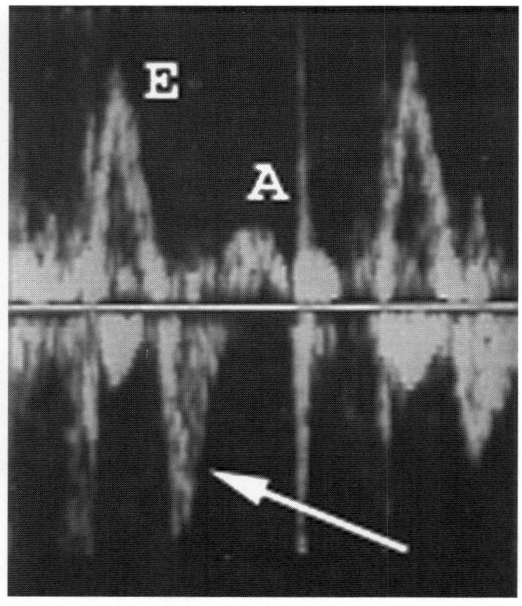

(a)

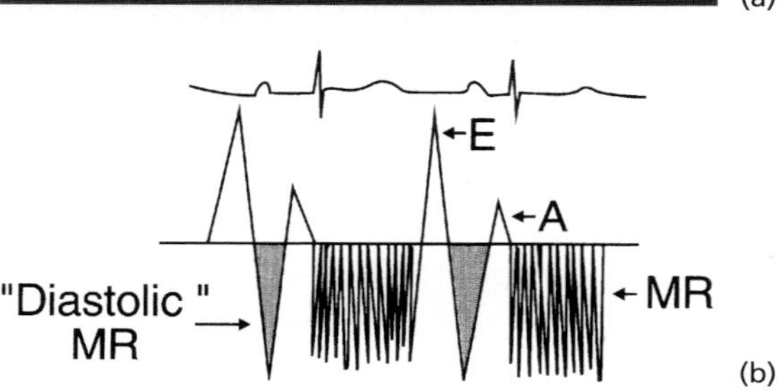

(b)

Fig. 6.9 (a) Pulsed wave MV inflow pattern in a young adult drug addict with acute bacterial endocarditis involving the aortic valve. The patient developed sudden severe aortic regurgitation. The MV inflow pattern reveals diastolic mitral regurgitation (MR; arrow), consistent with a markedly elevated LV diastolic filling pressure. (b) The PW Doppler pattern illustrated (see also Chapters 7 & 18).

restrictive pattern appear at greater risk than those with an abnormal relaxation pattern, and these patients are at particularly high risk if the restrictive pattern can not be reverted to the abnormal relaxation pattern with maneuvers that reduce preload. For example, if an adequate Valsalva is performed in a patient with systolic dysfunction and a restrictive pattern does not appear pseudonormalized (and DT remains short), prognosis is poor (Fig. 6.11). As a corollary, if a patient with systolic dysfunction and an abnormal relaxation pattern has preload increased (e.g. by a leg-raising maneuver) and a "restrictive" pattern results, the prognosis is also poor.

Physiologic influences on diastolic parameters

A mitral inflow pattern of abnormal relaxation may be seen with *RV pressure overload* (acute pulmonary embolus, primary pulmonary hypertension) or acute RV infarction. Pulmonary abnormalities with *labored respirations* secondary to severe *obesity* or *chronic obstructive pulmonary disease (COPD)* cause a mitral restrictive pattern. Respiratory variation similar to that seen with constrictive pericarditis may be recorded (see Chapter 12).

An *increase in preload* increases the E wave velocity and shortens the DT and IVRT. An *increase in afterload* has the same effect on MV and PV flow patterns as a decrease in preload. With an increase in heart rate, the A wave increases relative to the E wave. The IVRT will shorten, but DT is unaffected. Eventually, the E

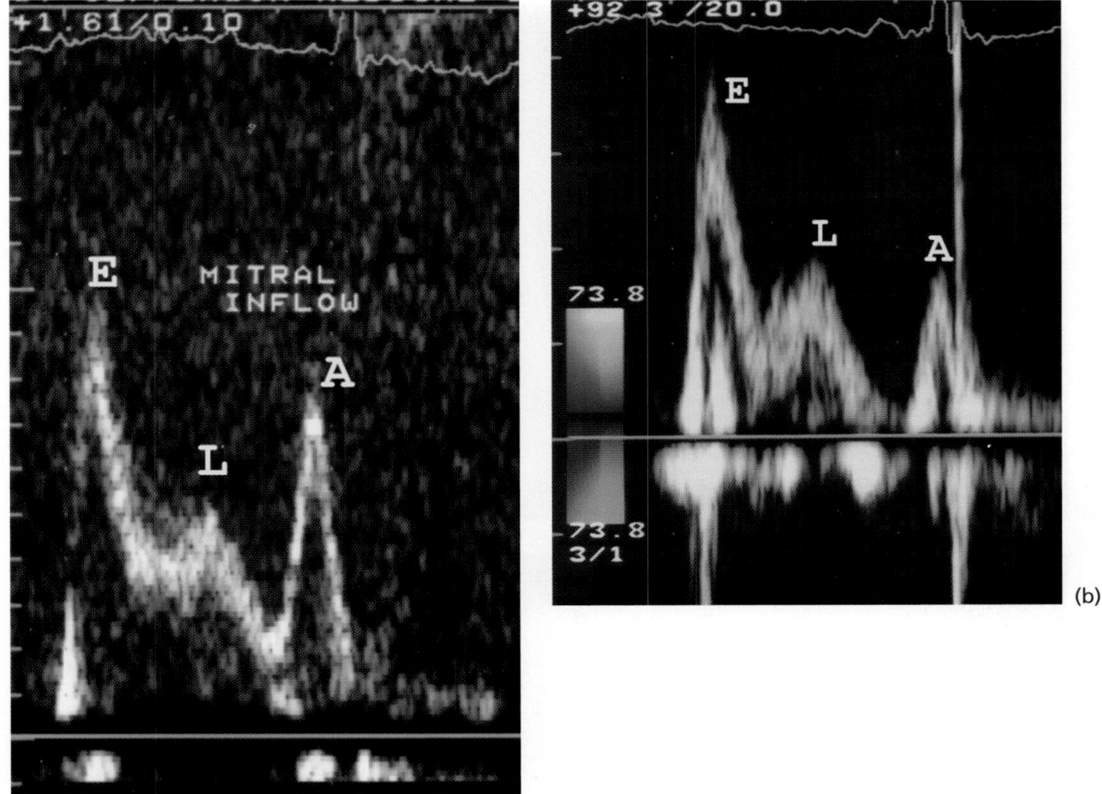

Fig. 6.10 (a,b) MV inflow patterns in two different patients with longstanding hypertension and moderate mitral regurgitation. A prominent low velocity L wave is noted during diastasis (see text).

Fig. 6.11 Patterns of MV inflow at (Baseline) and with the Valsalva maneuver (Maximum), causing a reduction of LV preload. Valsalva patterns are after 10 s of strain. Note the difference between Normal and Pseudonormal. (Reproduced with permission from: Appleton CP, Firstenberg MS, Garcia MJ, Thomas JD. The echo-Doppler evaluation of left ventricular diastolic function: a current perspective (Kovacs SJ, guest ed). Cardiology Clinics 2000; 18(3): 525, figure 12.)

Pattern	Baseline	Maximum	Interpretation
Normal			Normal
Impaired Relaxation			Normal Pressures
Impaired Relaxation			↑LV A Wave, ↑EDP
Pseudonormal			Pseudonormal
Restrictive			Preload Sensitive Partially Reversible
Restrictive			Fixed Restrictive

(a)

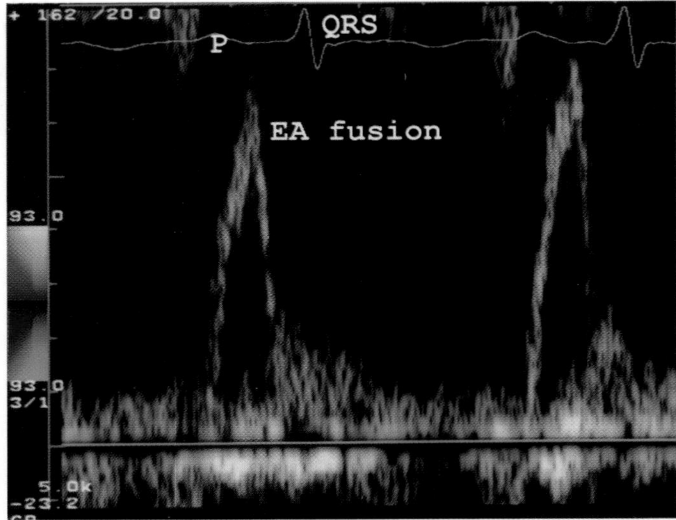

(b)

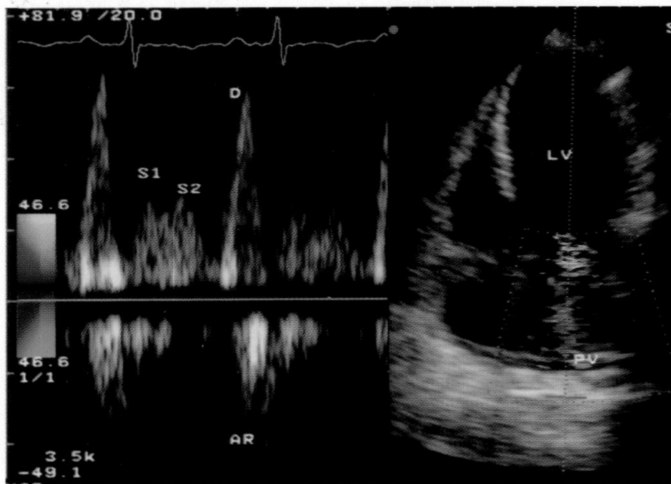

Fig. 6.12 A 35-year-old female with an idiopathic dilated cardiomyopathy presented with congestive heart failure. She was noted to have a heart rate of 137 bpm. In (a) the mitral inflow pattern reveals a fused E and A wave, and therefore measurement of diastolic parameters are not possible. In (b) pulmonary vein flow measurements reveal a blunted S1 and S2, with a prominent D wave, suggesting an elevated mean LV diastolic filling pressure. A prominent atrial reversal wave (AR) suggests an elevated left ventricular end-diastolic pressure (LVEDP).

and A wave will merge, and MV inflow patterns are not helpful. In this situation, the PV flow patterns may still be helpful (Fig. 6.12).

In *atrial fibrillation*, the MV and PV A waves will not be present, as an organized atrial contraction is not present. The IVRT and E wave velocities are somewhat useful for estimation of filling pressures. Systolic flow in the pulmonary veins is blunted.

A *long PR interval* causes an augmented A wave. In *heart block*, the E and A velocities vary, depending on the relation between the P and QRS complexes (Figs 6.13 & 6.14). The EA fusion velocity will generally be higher than an E wave alone. *Abnormal left ventricular depolarization* due to left bundle branch block (LBBB) or a *post-premature ventricular contraction (PVC)* may cause a diastolic pattern of abnormal relaxation (dyssynchronous contraction and subsequent dyssynchronous relaxation).

Mitral regurgitation (MR; see Chapter 8) affects both mitral inflow and pulmonary vein flow according to the severity of the regurgitation. As MR severity increases, the LA pressure will increase, and MV inflow pattern will progress toward a restrictive filling pattern. PV flow develops a diminished forward systolic flow with prominent atrial contraction (2+ to 3+ MR), and progresses to reversed PV systolic flow with 4+ MR (Fig. 6.15). It is important to obtain PV flow recordings in both right and left PVs, as MR

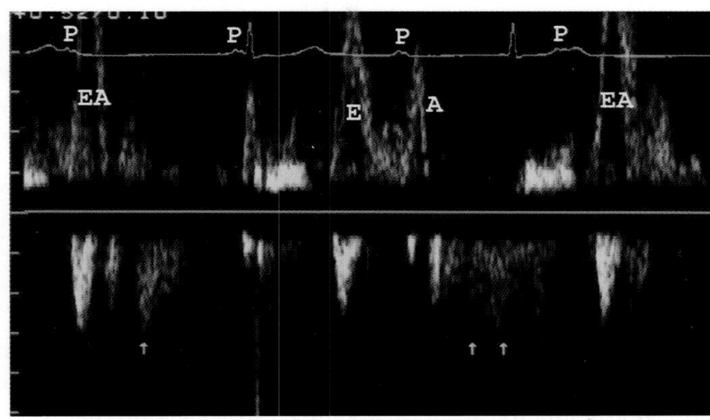

Fig. 6.13 Pulsed wave MV inflow pattern in a young adult patient with congenital third degree AV block. Following each P wave is a mitral A wave. Depending on its relation to the QRS, the A wave may be fused (EA) with the E wave. Arrows point out low velocity *diastolic MR* secondary to the prolonged P-QRS intervals noted.

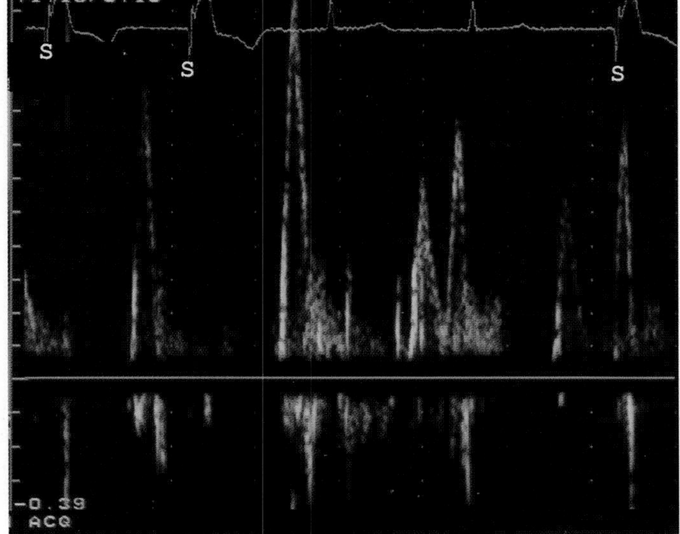

Fig. 6.14 A patient with an electronic ventricular pacemaker in the demand mode, and an underlying sinus rhythm. Electronic spikes (S) and the patient's own intrinsic rhythm compete, causing varying mitral inflow patterns.

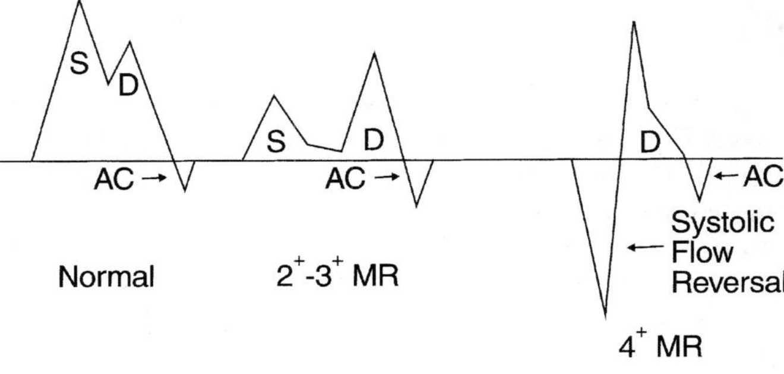

Fig. 6.15 Diagram of pulmonary vein flow with MR. Note a decreased systolic/diastolic flow ratio with 2+ to 3+ MR, and *pulmonary vein (PV) systolic flow reversal* usually indicative of 4+ MR. It is important to obtain PV flow recordings from both right and left pulmonary veins, as an MR jet may be directed toward one PV causing systolic flow reversal in one PV and not the other (see text and Chapter 8).

is often directed toward one or the other PV, with systolic flow reversal noted in PVs only on one side of the LA. If systolic flow reversal is noted within a PV, it usually indicates 4+ MR, but a jet of lesser magnitude may "spray" directly into one PV.

Significant *aortic regurgitation* is associated with a restrictive mitral filling pattern. When severe, LV diastolic pressures rise quickly, and *diastolic mitral regurgitation* develops (Fig. 6.9). In normal hearts and patients with prolonged PR intervals (Fig. 6.13; see

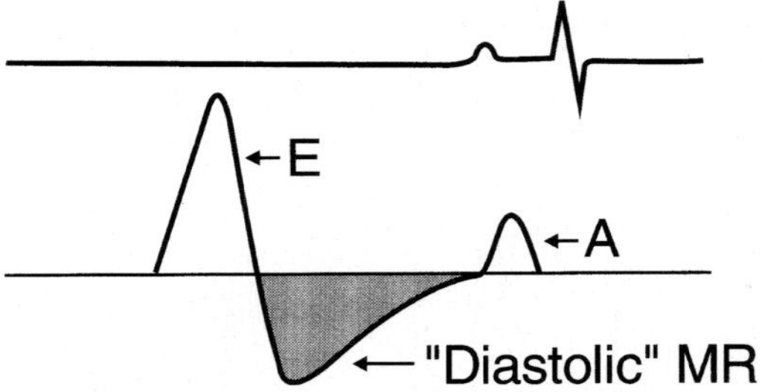

Fig. 6.16 Normal mitral inflow with low velocity diastolic MR in a normal heart.

Chapter 8), however, diastolic MR may occasionally be seen, and does not indicate an abnormality (Fig. 6.16).

Isovolumic relaxation time flow

Patients with hypertrophic cardiomyopathy or vigorous LV function with some degree of *cavity obliteration* may have an apically directed flow during the IVRT (while the LV is a "closed chamber" with both mitral and aortic valves closed). This flow may result from asynchronous LV relaxation and/or elastic recoil of LV wall segments around the obliterated cavity, and then development of intraventricular pressure gradients, as the apex relaxes prior to the base (Fig. 6.17). Patients with *apical hypertrophy* or *midventricular hypertrophy* may demonstrate IVRT flow directed toward the LV base (Fig. 6.18). This flow may extend briefly into the rapid filling stage.

Practical evaluation of mitral, pulmonary vein, tricuspid, hepatic–inferior vena cava, and superior vena cava flow

Doppler frequency for both PW and CW should be as low as possible (~2 MHz). The lowest possible machine gain setting improves velocity resolution. PW wall filters should be as low as possible (200 Hz), but with CW higher filters (800–1200 Hz) improve high frequency signals. Initially a recording chart speed of 50 mm/s is used to look for respiratory effects on the signal, but flow duration measurements should be made at the fastest possible recording speed. The ECG signal should be on the recording also. A respirometer recording is helpful when respiratory variation is evaluated during diastolic measurements.

After obtaining M-mode and 2-D recordings, diastolic evaluation begins with measurement of *mitral inflow* from the apical four-chamber view, using PW Doppler. Color Doppler is used as a guide to help with placement of the sample box within maximum flow and parallel to the flow profile. The sample box should be narrowed to 1–2 mm and the wall filter to ~200 Hz, with recording chart speed preferably 100 mm/s. A small sample box will result in sharper velocity profiles. Mitral flow is recorded at the level of the *leaflet tips*, with the sample box in the center of flow or slightly closer toward the posterior MV leaflet. MV flow should be directed toward the transducer,

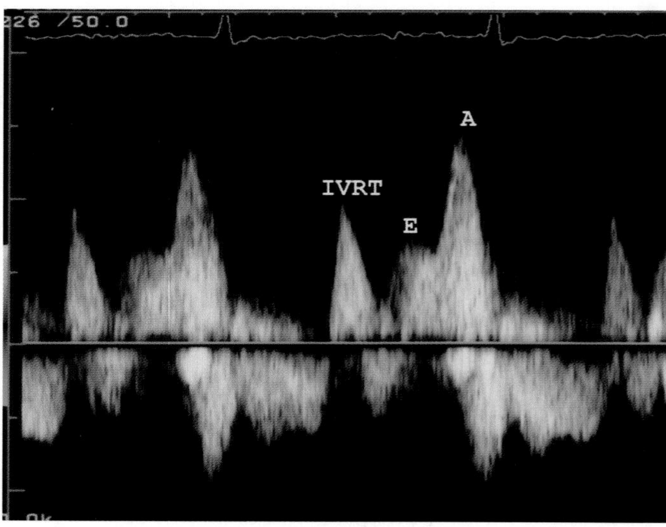

Fig. 6.17 Continuous wave Doppler of LV flow demonstrating IVRT flow toward the LV apex in a patient with LVH and systolic cavity obliteration.

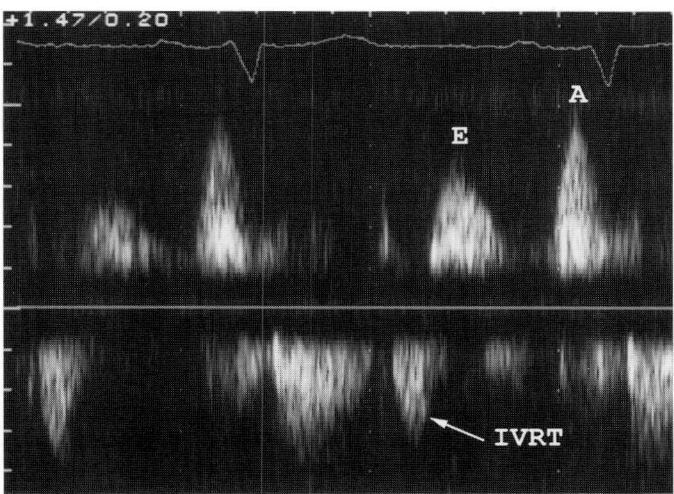

Fig. 6.18 Continuous wave Doppler LV flow demonstrating IVRT flow toward the LV base in a patient with abnormal relaxation.

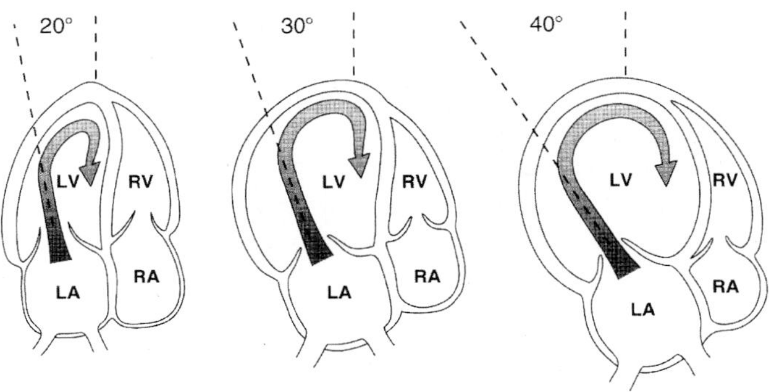

Fig. 6.19 MV inflow as recorded in the 2-D apical four-chamber view. Normally MV inflow is ~20° laterally directed, but increases as the LV enlarges. The transducer should be laterally placed with respect to the LV apex, so that MV inflow is directed straight toward the transducer. Color flow Doppler superimposed on the 2-D image helps transducer and PW cursor positioning. (Reproduced with permission from: Appleton CP, Jensen JL, Hatle LK, Oh JK. Doppler evaluation of left and right ventricular diastolic function: a technical guide for obtaining optimal flow velocity recordings. Journal of the American Society of Echocardiography 1997; 10(3): 272.)

therefore the transducer should be placed lateral to the apex (more lateral than usual for recording an apical four-chamber image) (Fig. 6.19). *Maximal* (not modal) velocities should be measured for E and A peak velocities. DT measurement begins at the E peak with a line drawn along the outer envelope of the spectral display to the baseline (Fig. 6.20). Measurement variability is potentially greatest with DT. It is important to pay attention to details, such as making certain the transducer is parallel to MV flow and using suggested settings. The *A wave duration* may be obtained by recording as described above, but at the level of the MV annulus.

IVRT recording should be on the fastest possible chart speed. Either PW or CW may be used in the apical five-chamber view (we use CW almost exclusively for IVRT measurements). With PW, the sample box should be opened to 3–4 mm and placed between MV and AV flows to capture the aortic valve closing click and the onset of MV flow. With CW, the cursor should be placed between the MV and AV from the apical five-chamber view. The initiation of IVRT is the AV closing click and not the cessation of recorded aortic flow. The end of the IVRT is the initiation of recorded MV flow. Doppler IVRT measurement is about 10–25 ms longer than that obtained using

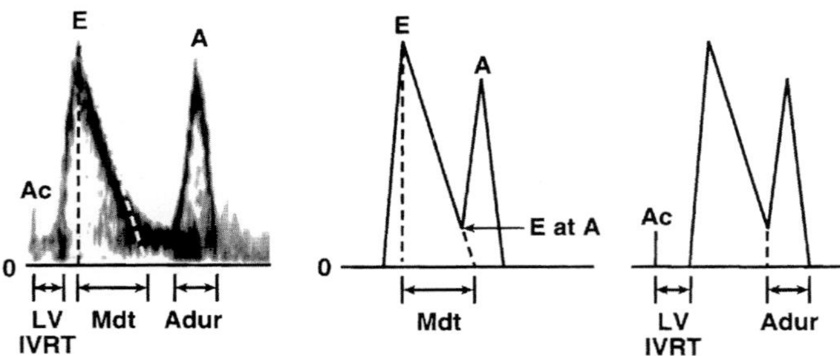

Fig. 6.20 Measurement of the E and A peak, mitral deceleration time (Mdt), IVRT, and A wave duration (Adur). The *E-at-A* point is shown. When present, Adur is measured beginning at the E-at-A (far right panel). When the E-at-A is greater than 20 cm/s (seen with tachycardia, delayed MV opening, ↑PR interval, variable heart block), partial fusion of the E and A will cause an increased A velocity and Adur, making interpretation of the MV inflow patterns problematic. (Reproduced with permission from: Appleton CP, Firstenberg MS, Garcia MJ, Thomas JD. The echo-Doppler evaluation of left ventricular diastolic function: a current perspective (Kovacs SJ, guest ed). Cardiology Clinics 2000; 18(3): 519, figure 5.)

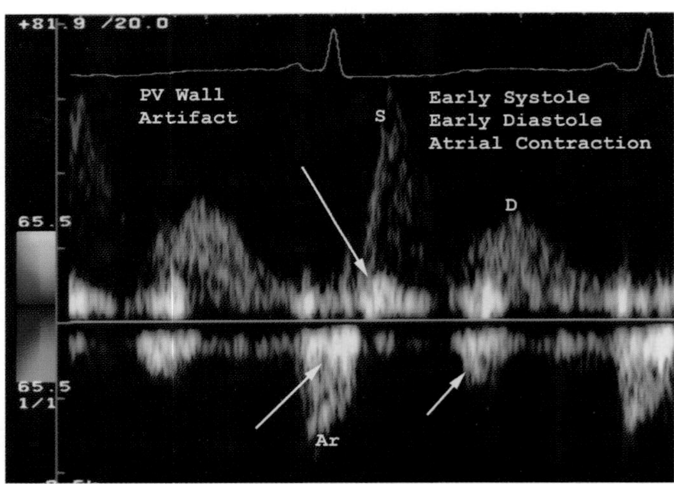

Fig. 6.21 Arrows point to recording artifact from the PV wall. An early systolic artifact is seen above the baseline, and two artifacts below the baseline are seen in diastole (early and late diastole). The late diastolic artifact may be confused with the atrial reversal wave.

M-mode recordings because MV flow is slightly delayed from initiation of MV opening. The MV opening click by phonocardiography correlates roughly with the peak E wave velocity on the Doppler tracing.

Pulmonary vein flow is measured with PW, using color flow Doppler to help guide sample box positioning. By transthoracic echocardiography (TTE), recording is from the apical four-chamber view, with slight anterior transducer angulation so that part of the aortic valve may be seen. The right upper PV, which enters the LA near the interatrial septum, is most often sampled. With a sample box of 3–4 mm, sampling should be performed within the PV 1–2 cm from its orifice. A low wall filter (200 Hz) and rapid chart speed should be used. Recording should be made for several beats, as some changes may be noted with respiration. On occasion, the left upper pulmonary vein may be recorded, or recording of PV flow may be obtained from the parasternal short axis or even the suprasternal notch (so-called "crab" view—see Fig. 4.14). A small PW Doppler sample box results in a weak Doppler signal and too large a sample box will result in unclear signals. Wall motion artifact from the PV wall is a common problem (Fig. 6.21).

With settings similar to that for MV inflow recordings, diastolic *tricuspid inflow* should be performed from an apical four-chamber view with PW Doppler, again using color Doppler to properly align the PW Doppler sample box parallel to flow. The transducer

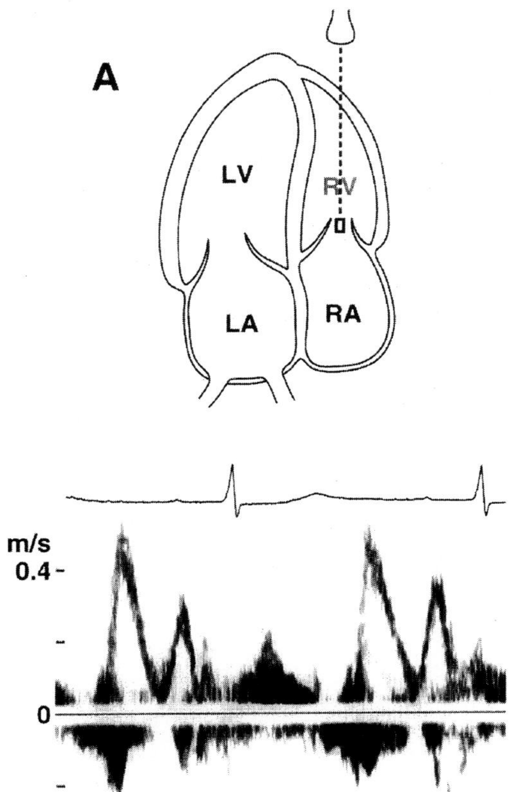

Fig. 6.22 PW recordings of tricuspid inflow. The sample box is kept 1–2 mm, velocity wall filters ~200 Hz, and chart recording speed set preferably at 100 mm/s. E and A peak velocity, and E wave DT are most often measured. (A) The PW Doppler probe is parallel to tricuspid valve (TV) inflow, resulting in a preferred narrow spectral signal. (B) PW recording is misaligned from TV inflow, with resultant velocities that are lower, with some broadening of the Doppler signal. (Reproduced with permission from: Appleton CP, Jensen JL, Hatle LK, Oh JK. Doppler evaluation of left and right ventricular diastolic function: a technical guide for obtaining optimal flow velocity recordings. Journal of the American Society of Echocardiography 1997; 10(3): 287.)

should be located medially from the LV apex. The sample box is placed at the level of the TV tips (Fig. 6.22).

For *hepatic vein* (HV) flow measurements, the short axis subcostal view is used. Flow should be parallel to the PW Doppler signal, using color Doppler to help guide positioning. The sample box will usually be 1–3 mm in size, and placed 1–3 cm in the HV (right superior HV) from its junction with the inferior vena cava (IVC). If flow is lost because of respiratory motion, using a slightly larger sample box may help. Filling can be assessed during normal respiration and suspended respiration. *IVC dynamics* are also assessed from the subcostal short axis view. M-mode through the IVC (perpendicular to the IVC) during normal respiration, and then with a cough or "sniff," helps to evaluate for IVC collapse.

Superior vena cava flow is obtained with the patient flat (no pillow) and the head turned toward the left. The transducer should then be placed in the right supraclavicular fossa. Color Doppler guidance helps with PW Doppler probe placement. The depth for recording is about 5–8 cm. One should use a PW sample box of 1–3 mm, 200 Hz wall filter, a rapid recording chart speed, and lowest possible gain settings.

Tissue Doppler echocardiography

Tissue Doppler echocardiography (TDE) allows for quantitative measurement of myocardial motion (see

Pearls of diastolic function analysis

1 The MV inflow and pulmonary vein S and D waves are generally indicative of mean LV diastolic filling pressure, whereas the pulmonary vein Ar wave is reflective of LV end-diastolic pressure (LVEDP). The LV mean diastolic filling pressure correlates with the pulmonary capillary wedge pressure (PCWP) obtained by right heart catheterization, and LVEDP with that obtained by measuring the LVEDP with a catheter in the LV during cardiac catheterization.

2 The mitral E wave and PV D wave "follow" each other.

3 Based on the patient history (and importantly age) and M-mode/2-D echo findings, think about what should be expected for the appearance of the mitral and PV flow patterns (should diastolic abnormality be present?). If a different pattern is found, do altered loading conditions explain it?

4 If needed, consider altering preload with the leg lift or Valsalva maneuver.

5 Consider obtaining tricuspid inflow patterns when trying to decide if the MV inflow patterns are normal or "pseudonormal" (if there is left-sided diastolic abnormality, then right-sided diastolic abnormality usually also exists).

6 Patients with hypertrophic cardiomyopathy probably have less correlation of diastolic filling patterns with LV filling pressures, probably due to more significant abnormal active relaxation (MV inflow may continue to show an $E/A < 1$ despite elevated filling pressures).

7 A normal mitral inflow pattern in a patient without cardiac history or symptoms probably has normal diastolic function.

8 Any patient with an $E/A < 1$ (without hypovolemia) probably has abnormal active relaxation.

9 A patient with heart failure symptoms or heart disease with an $E/A > 2$ probably has restriction to filling.

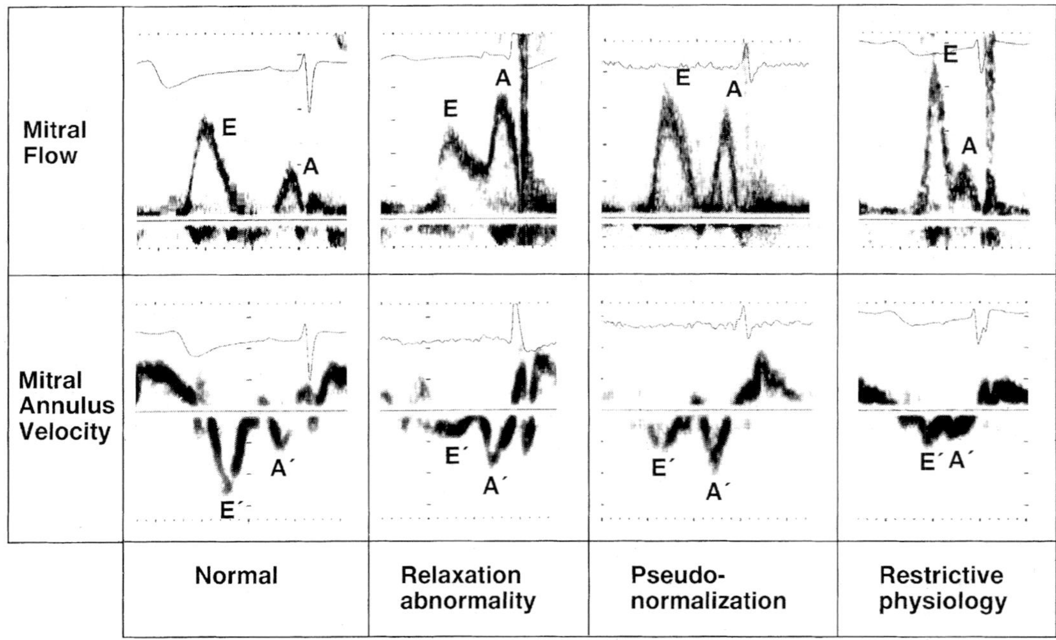

Fig. 6.23 Mitral annulus velocity profiles and associated mitral inflow patterns. Note that with pseudonormalization, the early to late diastolic flow ratio is less than 1. (Reproduced with permission from: Sohn DW, Chai IH, Lea DJ, *et al.* Assessment of mitral annulus velocity by Doppler tissue imaging in the evaluation of left ventricular diastolic function. Journal of the American College of Cardiology 1997; 30: 474–480.)

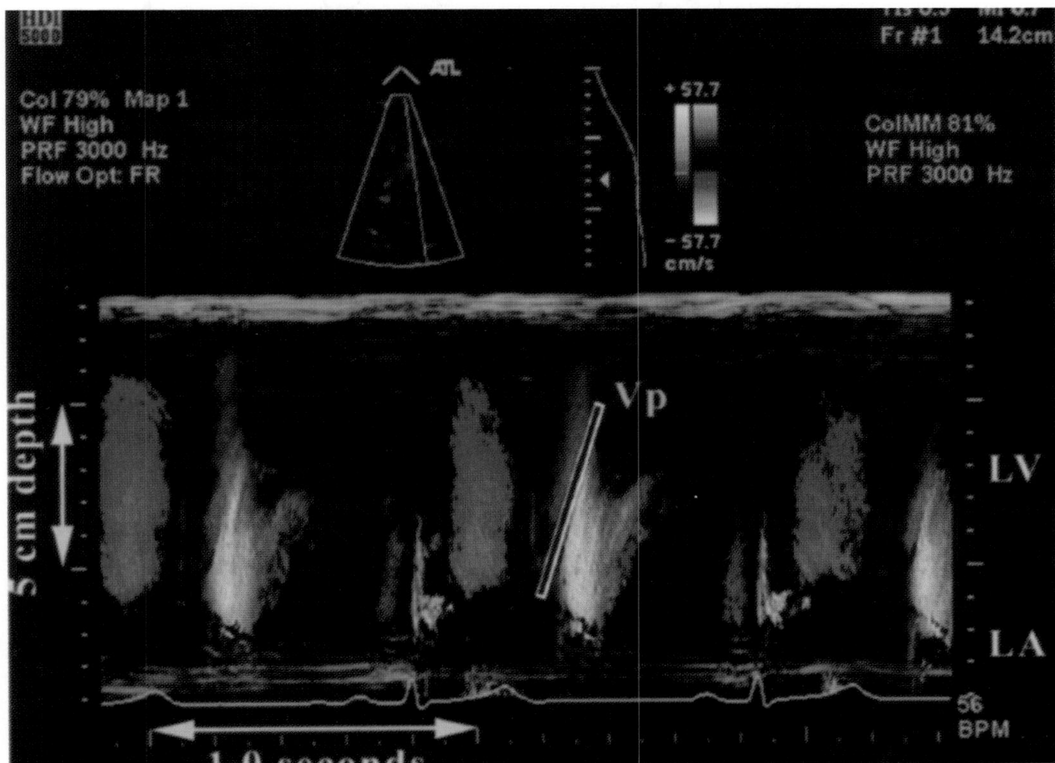

Fig. 6.24 M-mode color image demonstrating measurement of flow propagation velocity (V_p). In this example the aliasing velocity was set as 57.7 cm/s. (Reproduced with permission from: Firstenberg MS, Levine BD, Garcia MJ, *et al*. Relationship of echocardiographic indices to pulmonary capillary wedge pressures in healthy volunteers. Journal of the American College of Cardiology 2000; 36: 1666.)

Chapter 2). Mitral annulus velocity in diastole is reflective of changes in velocity for the LV long axis. In normal hearts, the long axis and circumferential motion is approximately the same. By recording mitral annulus motion from the apex, the effect of myocardial translation is minimized. A typical spectral pattern will demonstrate a single systolic velocity toward the LV centroid (Sm), and two signals away from the centroid during early (Em) and late (Am) diastole. This method appears to be relatively insensitive to preload, therefore it may help differentiate normal from pseudonormal filling (Fig. 6.23). With abnormal active relaxation, mitral annulus motion during late diastole (atrial systole) is increased. Mitral annulus velocity is markedly reduced with restrictive cardiomyopathy, but with constrictive pericarditis, the velocities are preserved (see Chapter 12). With aging, the Em : Am ratio decreases.

For mitral annulus spectral recordings the PW sample box should be 3–7 mm, the TDI function activated, Doppler gain reduced (often 0% power), and wall filters minimized. At the mitral annulus the sample box may be placed in the septum, lateral, anterior or inferior aspects (usually the septum or lateral) to help differentiate pseudonormal from normal filling. For the young, normal Em is greater than 10 cm/s, and for the adult, normal Em is greater than 8 cm/s. For abnormal relaxation, pseudonormal and restriction to filling Em should be less than 8 cm/s.

Color M-mode flow velocity propagation

Color M-mode Doppler allows for assessment of velocities both temporally and spatially over a line. From the apical four-chamber view, color Doppler

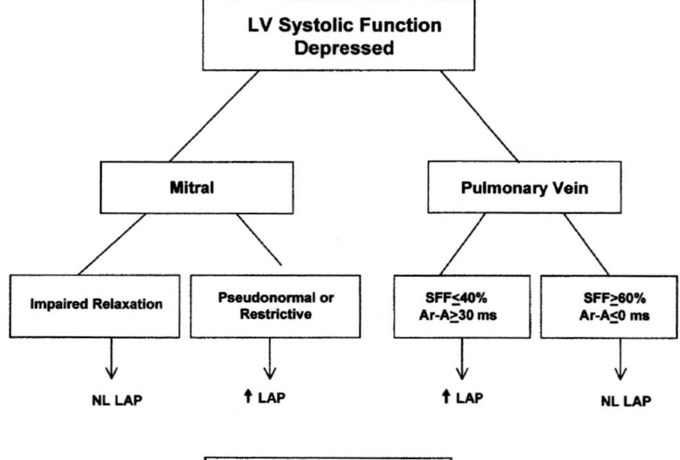

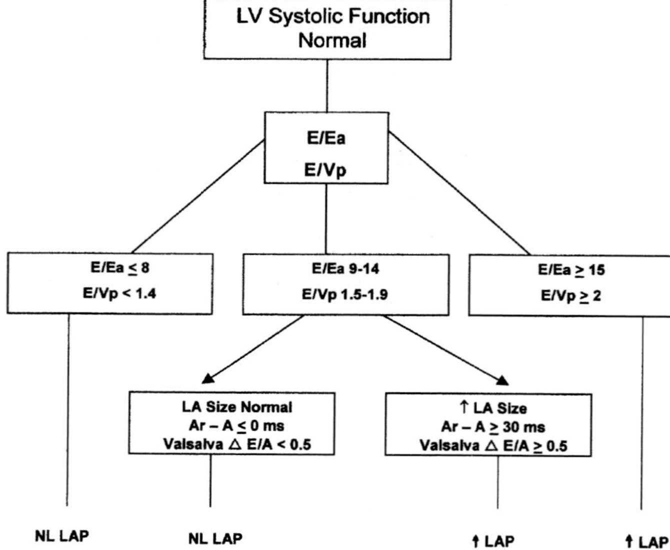

Fig. 6.25 Algorithms to assess LV preload in patients with depressed (A) and normal (B) LV systolic function. The *systolic filling fraction* (SFF) is the time velocity integral of the pulmonary vein systolic wave divided by the total pulmonary vein flow time velocity integral. Tissue Doppler and color flow propagation are more important in patients with normal LV systolic function. Ar–A, the difference in duration of the PV atrial reversal wave and the mitral inflow atrial wave; NL LAP, normal LA pressure; E, mitral E velocity; Ea, early diastolic velocity at the mitral annulus; V_p, flow propagation velocity. (Reproduced with permission from: Nagueh SF, Zohgbi WA. Clinical assessment of LV diastolic filling by Doppler echocardiography. ACC Current Journal Review 2001; Jul/Aug: 49.)

should be activated. The M-mode cursor includes the mitral valve and LV with part of the LA. Color aliasing should be initially set to 55–60 cm/s and sweep speed set at 100–200 mm/s. The first diastolic flow is E wave flow and the second A wave flow. The *flow propagation velocity* (V_p) is the early diastolic flow pattern, and the measurement most often made. Recording should be made at suspended end-expiration with the V_p measured from a still frame. It is the slope connecting any isovelocity line (aliasing line) from the MV tips to the LV apical region (Fig. 6.24). One should be careful not to measure intracavitary flow during the IVRT. With heart block or a prolonged first degree AV block it may be difficult to separate early from late diastolic filling. In young normal individuals V_p should be greater than 55 cm/s, and in adult normals V_p should be greater than 45 cm/s. For abnormal relaxation, pseudonormal patterns and restriction to filling V_p should be less than 45 cm/s.

A proposed set of algorithms (S. Nagueh, W. Zoghbi, M. Quinones, Baylor College of Medicine, Houston, Texas) use Doppler measurements to estimate LV preload. TDI and V_p appear most helpful in patients with normal LV systolic function, and help to confirm findings in patients with LV systolic dysfunction (Fig. 6.25).

CHAPTER 7

Aortic Valve

Fine systolic fluttering of normal aortic valve leaflets by M-mode imaging is often noted (Fig. 7.1). Stenotic valves generally will not demonstrate *systolic fluttering* (Fig. 7.2). A flail aortic valve leaflet will demonstrate coarse fluttering in systole and/or diastole. *Diastolic fluttering is abnormal* (Fig. 7.3). In patients with acquired aortic stenosis (not congenital) the amount of leaflet separation may give clues to the severity of the stenosis. Stenosis is probably severe if leaflet separation is less than 8 mm whereas if separation is greater than 15 mm, it is probably mild.

Aortic stenosis

In addition to valvular aortic stenosis (AS), causes of LV outflow obstruction include *dynamic subaortic obstruction* (see Chapter 11), *fixed subaortic obstruction* (see Chapter 16), and *supravalvular aortic stenosis*. The most common etiologies of valvular aortic stenosis are *calcific, rheumatic* (Fig. 7.4), and *bicuspid*.

Calcific AS involves calcification on the aortic side of the leaflets with resultant leaflet immobility. The commissures are not involved. Significant AS increases with age but is most prevalent in patients of 70 years old or older.

Rheumatic aortic stenosis is characterized by fusion of aortic valve commissures (Fig. 7.5) (as occurs with rheumatic mitral disease) and often systolic doming will be noted. Rheumatic disease almost always involves the mitral valve; therefore, when rheumatic AS is present, the mitral valve will also be affected. *Valve doming* (Fig. 7.6) is an important 2-D sign for

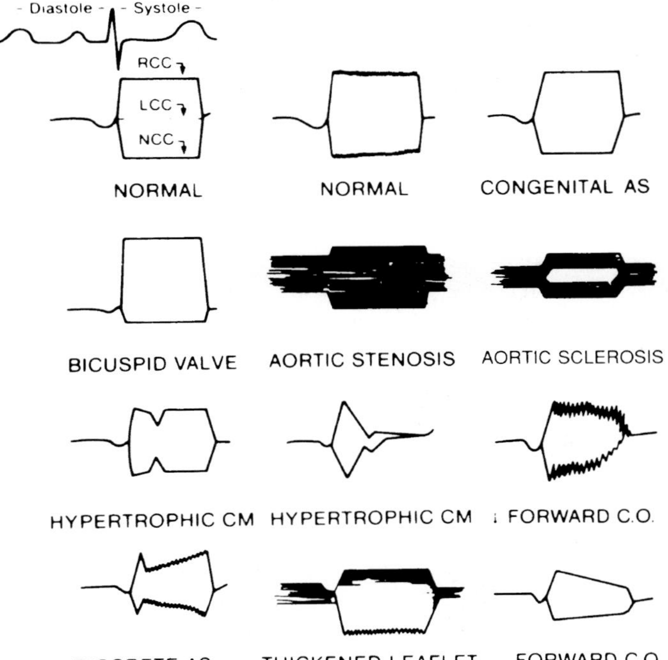

Fig. 7.1 Various M-mode patterns of the aortic valve. The left coronary cusp (LCC) is usually not seen. RCC, right coronary cusp; NCC, noncoronary cusp. (Reproduced with permission from: Felner JM, Martin RP. The echocardiogram. In: Schlant RC, Alexander RW, eds. The Heart, 8th edn. New York: McGraw-Hill, 1994: p. 401.) (*Continued on p. 82.*)

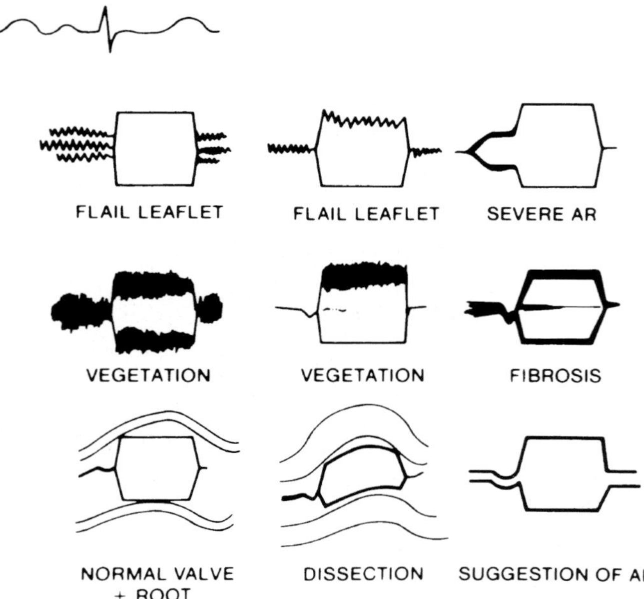

Fig. 7.1 *(cont'd)*

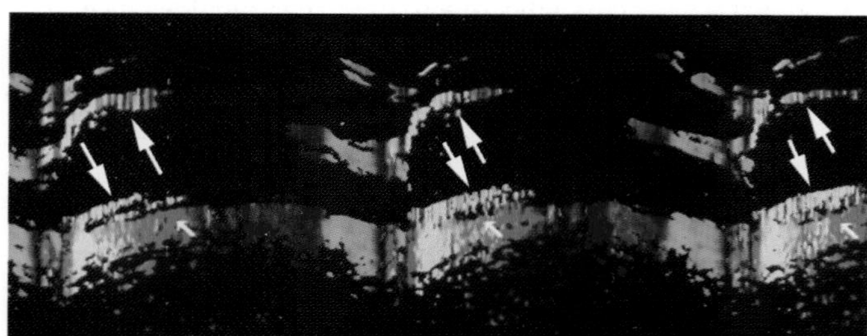

Fig. 7.2 M-mode tissue Doppler imaging (TDI) of fine fluttering (arrows) of a nonstenotic aortic valve. TDI color codes motion, therefore the fine fluttering is highlighted.

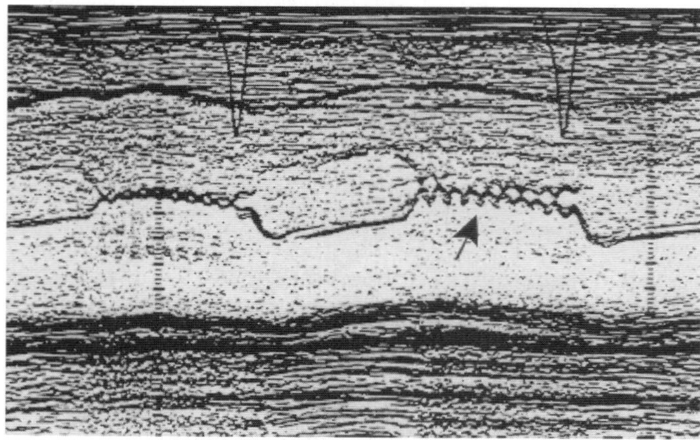

Fig. 7.3 Coarse diastolic fluttering noted on an M-mode of a flail aortic valve leaflet.

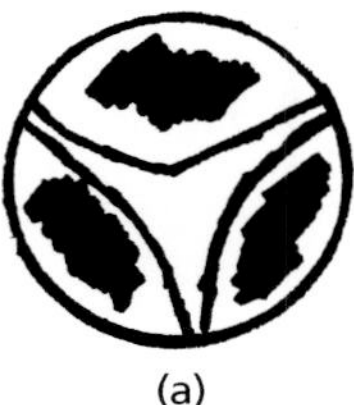
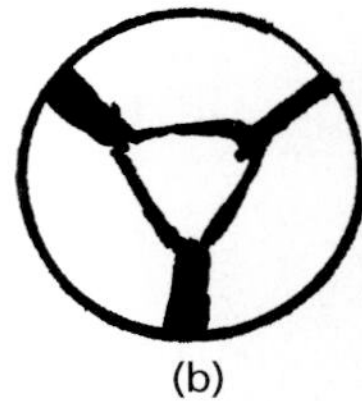

(a) (b)

Fig. 7.4 *Calcific aortic stenosis* (a) and *rheumatic aortic stenosis* (b). Calcification of the aortic side of valve leaflets is noted with calcific aortic stenosis (AS), sparing the commissures. With rheumatic AS, the commissures fuse, and almost always the mitral valve will evidence rheumatic involvement.

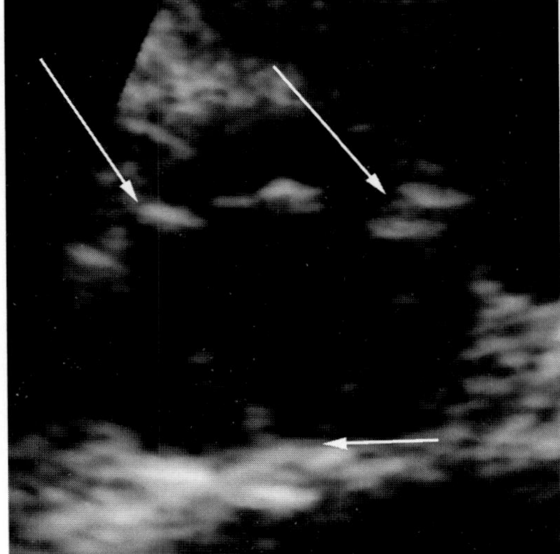

Fig. 7.5 Parasternal short axis systolic image of mild rheumatic involvement of the aortic valve. Note evident commissural fusion (arrows). This patient had evident rheumatic mitral valve involvement and aortic valve systolic doming.

any form of valvular (congenital or acquired) stenosis (tricuspid, pulmonic, mitral, and aortic).

A *bicuspid aortic valve* (BAV) is present in ~2% of the adult population. There appears to be some clustering of BAV in families, with a male : female ratio of 4 : 1. Echocardiographic screening of first-degree family members is prudent. A bicuspid valve is the most common congenital defect and has been associated with aortic aneurysm, aortic dissection, and coarctation of the aorta. Identification of a BAV is important as the patient should receive endocarditis prophylaxis for medical and dental procedures. A bicuspid valve may demonstrate a *right* and *left cusp*

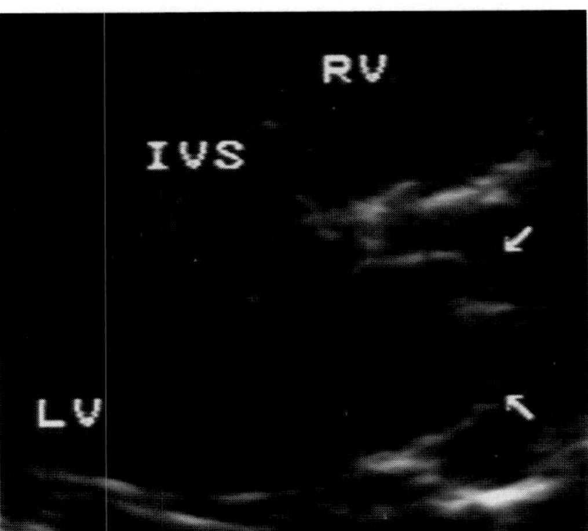

Fig. 7.6 Parasternal long axis image of an aortic valve demonstrating systolic doming (arrows). IVS, interventricular septum.

(the origin of the right coronary artery is in the right cusp, and the left coronary artery in the left cusp), or an *anterior* and *posterior cusp* (both right and left coronary arteries originate in the anterior cusp).

M-mode of a BAV may demonstrate an *eccentric line of closure* (Fig. 7.7), but an eccentric line of closure may also be seen in patients with a tricuspid leaflet aortic valve and a "normal" line of closure may be seen in patients with a BAV. In the parasternal and transesophageal short axis (Figs 7.8 and 7.9) the valve anatomy may appear normal in diastole as a raphe may simulate three commissural lines. However, in systole the valve will have a "fish-mouth" appearance. In the parasternal long axis, the valve may appear domed in systole (Fig. 7.6) and appear prolapsed in diastole (Table 7.1). When performing a color Doppler "screening," if even trivial aortic regurgitation is noted, one should look closely for a BAV.

A *unicuspid aortic valve* is very rare (Fig. 7.10), and can easily be misidentified as bicuspid. The *acommissural* type has a single membrane-like leaflet with a central orifice. There is no lateral attachment to the

Table 7.1 Features to look at for in parasternal views of a bicuspid valve.

	Long axis	Short axis
Systole	Doming	"Fish-mouth"
Diastole	Prolapse	Raphe—normal appearance

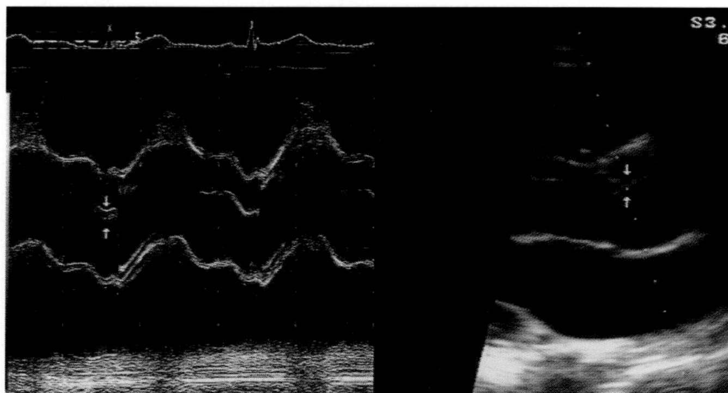

Fig. 7.7 M-mode and two-dimensional (2-D) image (diastolic long axis) of a bicuspid aortic valve with eccentric closure (arrows).

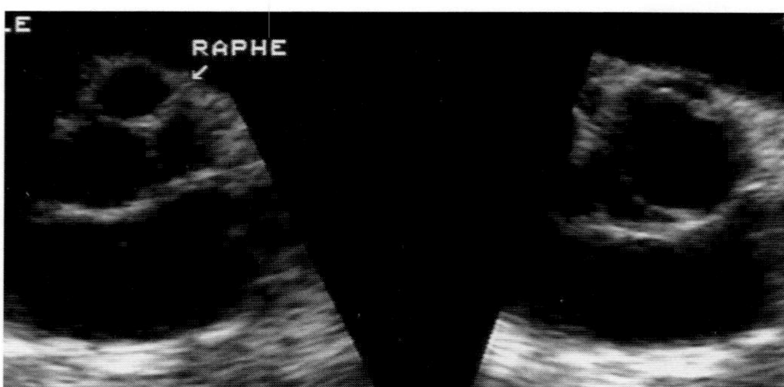

Fig. 7.8 Two-dimensional short axis image of a bicuspid aortic valve. The diastolic image (left panel) appears normal as the raphe may appear as a commissure, but the systolic image (right panel) has a typical "fish-mouth" appearance.

(a)

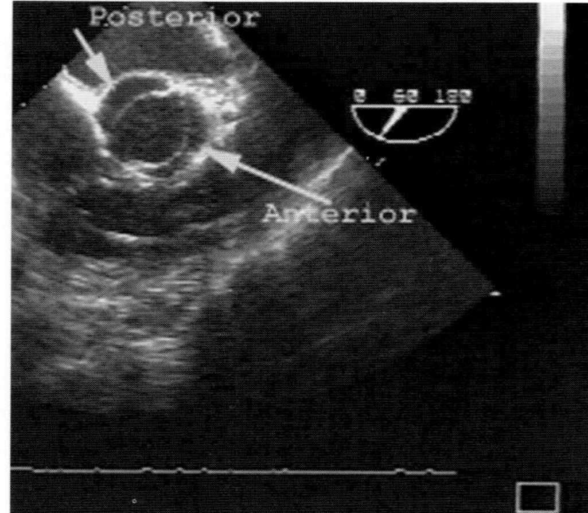

(b)

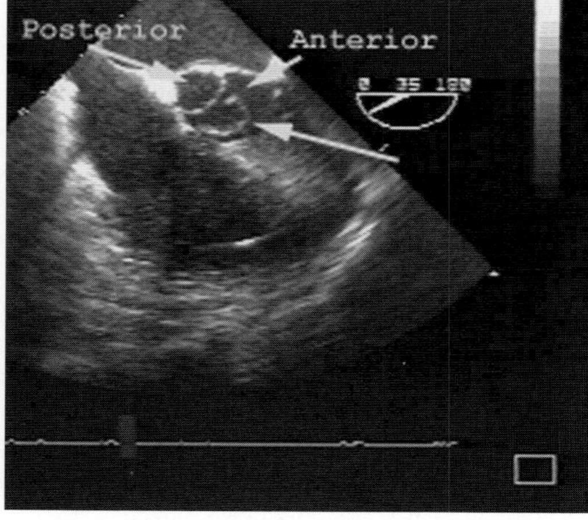

Fig. 7.9 Transesophageal echocardiography (TEE) performed preoperatively for aortic valve repair. In systole (a), a short axis image (60°) reveals the typical fish-mouth appearance, and in diastole (35°) (b), the anterior leaflet prolapses. (Courtesy Dr Nabil A. Munfakh, Department of Cardiothoracic Surgery, Washington University, School of Medicine, St Louis, MO.)

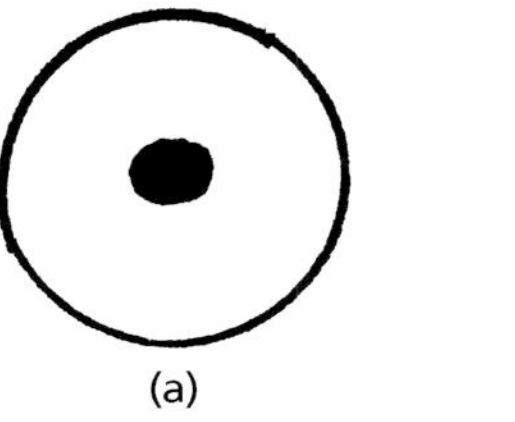
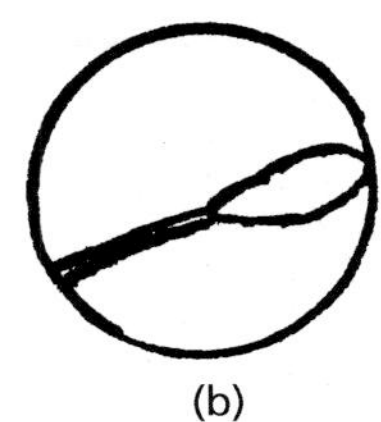

Fig. 7.10 *Acommissural* (a) and (b) *unicommissural unicuspid aortic* valves. On very rare occasion a unicuspid aortic valve will present in adulthood.

aorta. The *unicommissural type* is the most common form, and has one commissure attached to the aorta (two commissures attach to the aorta with a BAV). Usually unicuspid valves present in infancy but they may present in adulthood. A *quadricuspid aortic valve* is very rare and may be associated with normal function. Up to half of the patients with a quadricuspid aortic valve have been reported to have aortic regurgitation and rarely AS (Fig. 7.11). A quadricuspid valve (or more leaflets) has been associated with truncus arteriosus.

Quantification of aortic stenosis

(see also Chapter 3)

A time delay exists between the LV and aortic peak pressures. The *instantaneous peak pressure gradient* obtained by Doppler is greater than the *peak-to-peak pressure gradient* obtained in the catheterization laboratory (Fig. 7.12). Doppler and catheterization

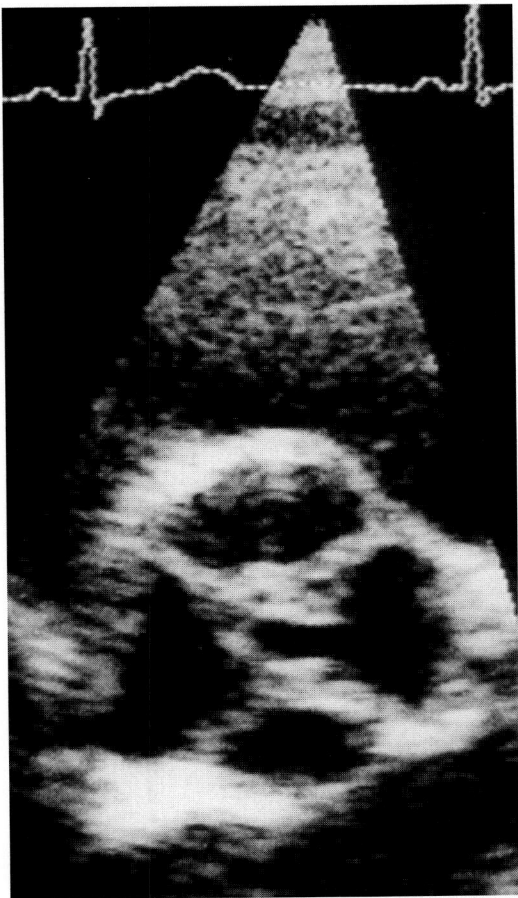

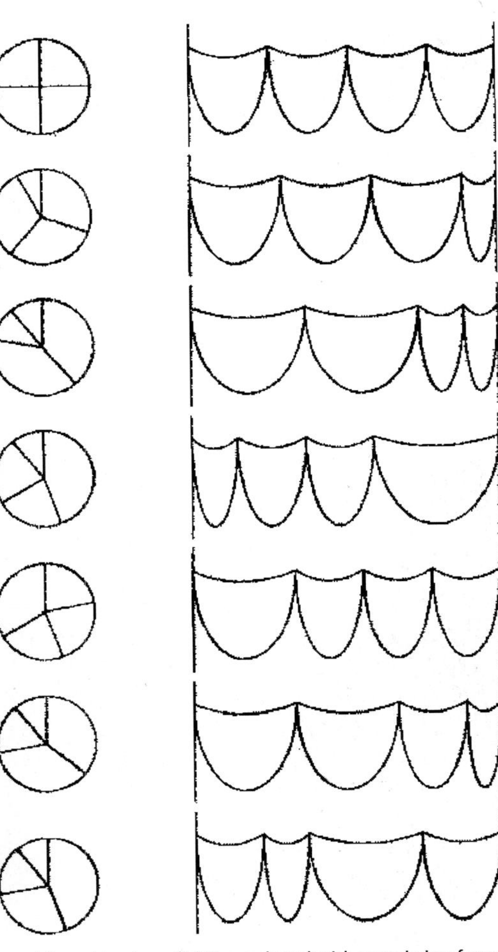

Fig. 7.11 (a) A normally functioning quadricuspid aortic valve visualized in a systolic parasternal short axis view in an asymptomatic adult male. (b) Anatomic variations of quadricuspid valves. ((b) Reproduced with permission from: Hurwitz LE, Roberts WC. Quadricuspid semilunar valve. American Journal of Cardiology 1973; 31: 623–626.)

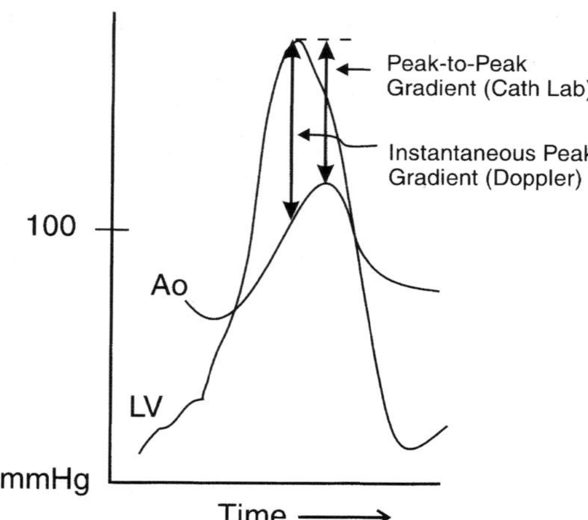

Fig. 7.12 Hemodynamic profile of the LV and ascending aorta (Ao) demonstrate *the peak-to-peak pressure gradient* (obtained in the catheterization laboratory) and *instantaneous peak pressure gradient* (obtained by Doppler).

laboratory derived *mean pressure gradient* measure the same physiologic parameter and should coincide if done at similar times.

Color flow Doppler helps guide the continuous wave (CW) transducer position. It is important to use all Doppler windows to find the highest velocity. A "good" Doppler signal may be found in one window, and the sonographer tempted to stop and use that as the maximum velocity. If one continues, an even greater velocity may be found from another window. A "good" Doppler envelope may be obtained despite a poor two-dimensional (2-D) image and a poor Doppler signal may be seen despite a good 2-D image.

Eighty per cent of the time, an *apical five-chamber* window will be the best window to obtain the maximum velocity in calcific aortic stenosis (Fig. 7.13). The *suprasternal window* may provide the highest velocity in younger patients. Velocity from the *right upper parasternal window* can be best visualized with the patient in the right lateral decubitis position (Fig. 7.14). This latter view may be best for congenital bicuspid aortic stenosis. Other windows include the *left parasternal, subcostal,* and *apical right-sided.* With the apical right-sided window, the CW transducer "cuts" through the right heart chambers and can also scan the aortic valve and proximal aorta.

The aortic valve *time velocity integral* (TVI) and left ventricular outflow tract (LVOT) TVI are obtained by planimetry of the Doppler signal. The aortic TVI is obtained with CW and the LVOT TVI is obtained with PW Doppler. The *peak (instantaneous) valve gradient* is determined by applying the modified Bernoulli equation to the peak velocity (Fig. 7.15). The *mean valve gradient* is obtained by applying the modified Bernoulli equation to multiple velocity measurements over the CW pressure waveform (Figs 7.15 & 7.16). It is important to remember that the mean pressure gradient *cannot* be obtained from the mean (or average) aortic velocity, but must be calculated by making multiple instantaneous gradient (and hence pressure calculations) measurements, and then averaging those instantaneous pressures.

The aortic valve area (Fig. 7.17) is calculated using the continuity equation (see Chapter 3). Flow through the LVOT is the same as flow through the aortic valve (*this holds true in the presence of coexistent aortic regurgitation, therefore the continuity equation remains valid*

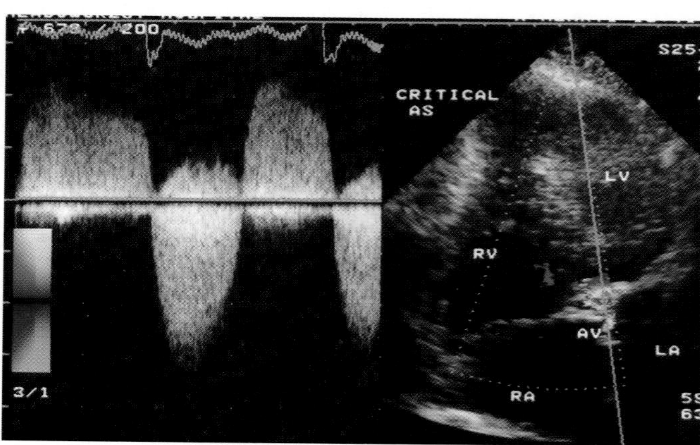

Fig. 7.13 Apical five-chamber view with color flow Doppler used to "line-up" the colour wave (CW) Doppler to measure the aortic valve gradient in an elderly female with severe dyspnea and a murmur of aortic stenosis. The measured peak velocity across the severely stenotic valve was over 6 m/s. Mild aortic regurgitation was also noted by CW Doppler.

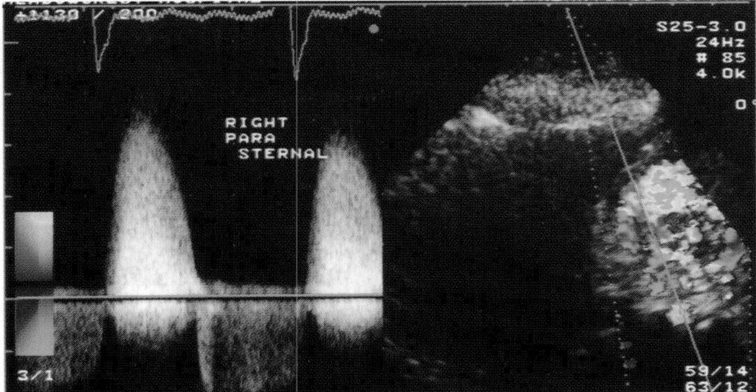

Fig. 7.14 CW Doppler profile obtained from the same patient as in the previous figure from the right upper parasternal window. The patient assumed a right lateral decubitis position. Color flow Doppler will help "line-up" the CW Doppler probe.

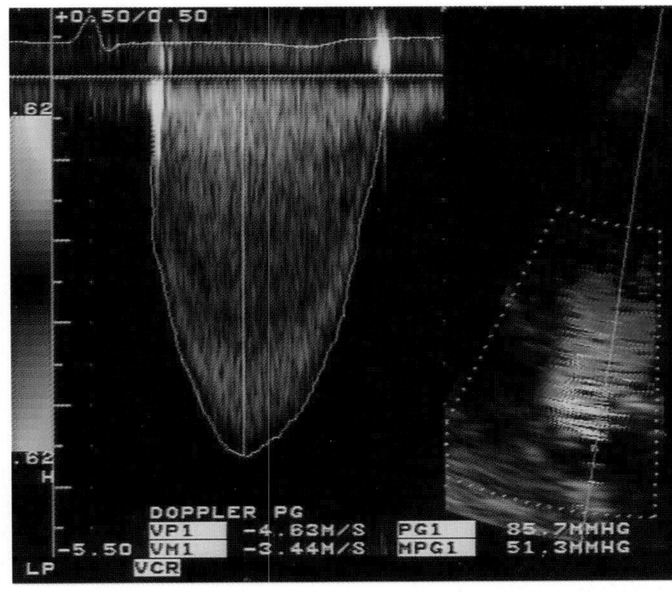

Fig. 7.15 Apical five-chamber view with CW Doppler across a patient with aortic stenosis. The peak valve gradient is obtained by applying the modified Bernoulli equation to the maximum velocity (4.63 m/s yields 85.7 mmHg). The mean valve gradient (see also Fig. 7.16) is obtained by planimetry of the CW Doppler waveform. The ultrasound machine will apply the modified Bernoulli equation to multiple velocity measurements and use the average as the mean pressure gradient (3.44 m/s yields 51.3 mmHg).

when using the LVOT to calculate the aortic valve area (AVA)). The only "unknown" is the AVA; therefore one may solve the equation for this.

Since LVOT flow is stroke volume $[(LVOT_{tvi}) \times (LVOT_{area})]$, this measurement may also be made from volume measurements of the LV at end-diastole (*EDV*) and end-systole (*ESV*):

$$[(LVOT_{tvi}) \times (LVOT_{area})] = EDV - ESV$$

therefore:

$$EDV - ESV = (AV_{tvi}) \times AVA$$

rearranging yields:

$$AVA = (EDV - ESV)/(AV_{tvi})$$

where $LVOT_{tvi}$ is the TVI of the LVOT, $LVOT_{area}$ is the cross-sectional area at the level of the LVOT, and AV_{tvi} is the TVI of the stenotic aortic valve.

If the LVOT cannot be used as part of the continuity equation (inability to measure an accurate LVOT diameter, hypertrophic obstructive cardiomyopathy (HOCM)), use another flow site (pulmonary, mitral). One must keep in mind, however, that the continuity equation requires the same flow through both orifices. Hence, significant valvular insufficiency of either valve, or a shunt, would not allow the continuity equation to be applied.

A "short cut" method for AVA measurement substitutes peak Doppler velocities for TVI planimetered waveforms:

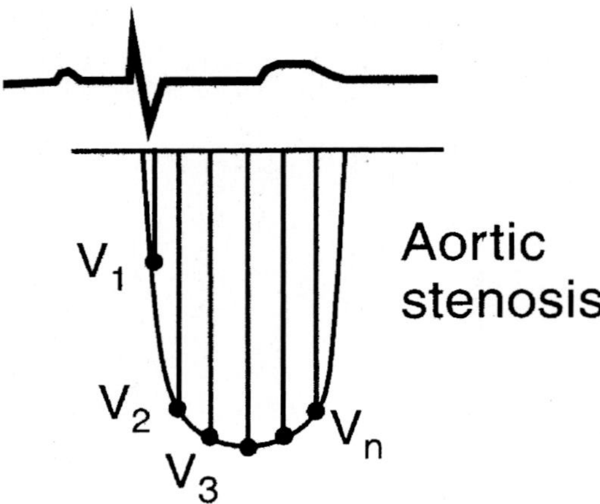

Fig. 7.16 The mean valve gradient is obtained by applying the modified Bernoulli equation to multiple velocities, adding up the pressures and dividing by the number of measurements made to obtain the average value. This procedure is automatically performed in modern ultrasound machines.

$$AVA = [(LVOT_{area}) \times (LVOT_{velocity})]/(AV_{velocity})$$

where $LVOT_{velocity}$ is the peak Doppler velocity at the level of the LVOT and $AV_{velocity}$ is the peak velocity of the stenotic aortic valve. Generally, an AS peak Doppler velocity of 3 m/s or less is not critical (unless there is markedly diminished forward cardiac output), and an AS jet greater than 4.5 m/s indicates severe AS (unless there is an elevated cardiac output).

The ratio of LVOT to aortic valve TVI or peak velocities is termed the *dimensionless index* (*DI*). It is also known as the *dimensionless severity* and may be defined as:

$$DI = (LVOT_{tvi})/(AV_{tvi}) \text{ or}$$

$$DI = (LVOT_{velocity})/(AV_{velocity})$$

A *DI* of ≤ 0.25 for native valve AS is consistent with critical AS. As this flow ratio does not change with a reduced (severe cardiomyopathy) or elevated (severe

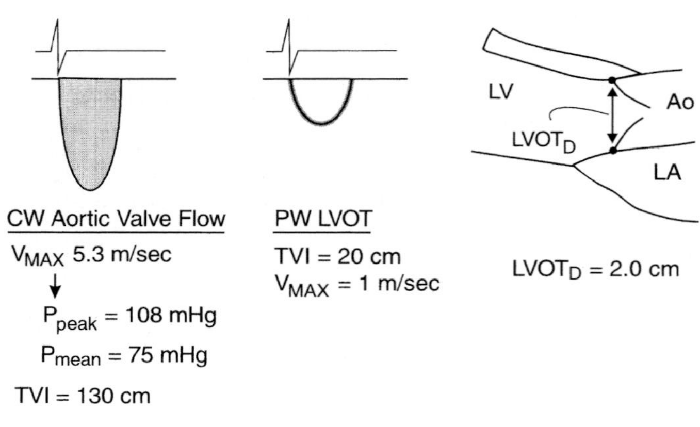

$$FLOW_{LVOT} = FLOW_{AV}$$

$$(TVI_{LVOT}) \times (Area_{LVOT}) = (TVI_{AV}) \times (AVA)$$

$$Area_{LVOT} = 3.14(D_{LVOT}/2)^2$$

$$(TVI_{LVOT}) \times [3.14(D_{LVOT}/2)^2] = (TVI_{AV}) \times (AVA)$$

Rearranging the equation leads to:

$$AVA = \frac{(TVI_{LVOT}) \times [3.14(D_{LVOT}/2)^2]}{(TVI_{AV})}$$

$$AVA = \frac{(20\ cm) \times [3.14(2.0\ cm/2)^2]}{130\ cm}$$

Fig. 7.17 Calculations of aortic valve area (AVA) from the TVI at the left ventricular outflow tract (LVOT), TVI of the aortic valve, and LVOT diameter.

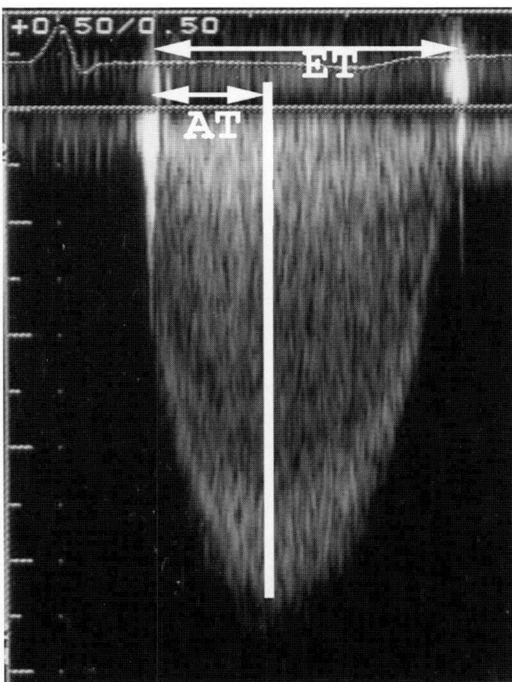

Fig. 7.18 CW Doppler waveform of aortic stenosis. The acceleration time (AT) and ejection time (ET) are noted. Note the delayed onset (compared to onset of the QRS) of aortic stenosis flow. Mitral regurgitation generally begins earlier (closer to the onset of the QRS) in comparison to the onset of AS.

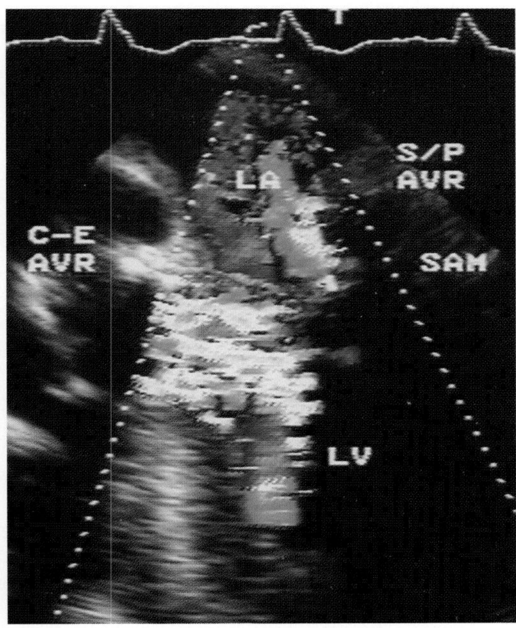

Fig. 7.19 TEE in the horizontal plane in a patient with a recent Carpentier–Edwards aortic valve replacement (C-E AVR) for aortic stenosis. The patient had a thickened septum and narrowed LVOT at the time of surgery. The patient presented with marked exertional dyspnea and had a systolic murmur noted. Systolic anterior motion (SAM) of the mitral valve with a resting subvalvular gradient of 70 mmHg by transthoracic echocardiography was noted. TEE revealed SAM and color flow turbulence starting in the LVOT at the site of SAM.

anemia) cardiac output, it is a useful tool in the evaluation of patients with AS (see also Chapter 10).

Mild AS generally has a rapid *acceleration time* (AT) and rapid *deceleration time* (DT). The AT is the time from the onset of aortic flow to peak velocity, and DT is the time from peak velocity to the end of aortic flow (Fig. 7.18). If a patient has significant aortic regurgitation (AR) with mild AS, the forward AS velocity gradient may be relatively high, but the AT and DT will be rapid. More severe AS is associated with a slower AT and DT. If the *AT divided by ejection time* (AT/ET) is ≥0.5, moderate-to-severe obstruction will probably be present. The LVOT PW waveform will correspondingly have a delayed peak also.

Other parameters of importance in patients with AS include:

- cardiac output calculation
- assessment of *mitral valve apparatus* integrity and MR
- TR jet velocity measurement for *pulmonary artery systolic pressure* calculation
- *diastolic filling* properties
- calculation of LV systolic pressure using MR velocity
- *LV ejection fraction* estimation
- determination of the degree of LVH, LV *mass*
- assessment of the *subaortic region*—1–2% of patients have significant *basal septal hypertrophy* requiring myectomy at the time of valve replacement (Fig. 7.19).
- assessment of *aortic annulus*/supravalvular portion of ascending aorta—select prosthesis size.

If a good quality echocardiogram result is available, coronary arteriography without LV angiography or hemodynamic measurements may be all that is needed during cardiac catheterization.

Potential "pitfalls" in the echo-Doppler evaluation of aortic stenosis

Potential pitfalls include:

- *Nonparallel Doppler/blood flow intercept angle*—angles less than 20° are generally acceptable, as this

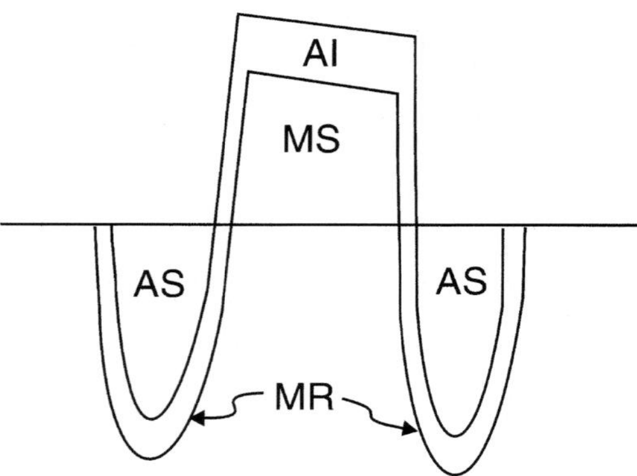

Fig. 7.20 Timing of stenotic and insufficient left heart flow. Left ventricular systole (and mitral regurgitation (MR)) begins before aortic valve opening. MR is also longer in duration than aortic stenosis (AS). Likewise, the duration of aortic regurgitation (AR) is longer than the duration of mitral stenosis (begins before and ends after mitral stenosis).

may lead to a 6% underestimation of true velocity, but higher angles dramatically underestimate true velocity (cosine of the angle).

- *Suboptimal LVOT diameter measurement*—when using the continuity equation the diameter is squared, therefore any error in measurement is squared in calculations.
- *Misidentification of mitral regurgitation (MR) as aortic stenosis (AS)* (Figs 7.18 & 7.20).
- *Variable heart rate*—atrial fibrillation, ventricular premature contractions (some laboratories will obtain simultaneous aortic valve stenotic flow and LVOT flow with the CW probe in the apical five-chamber position; either both TVIs from the same heartbeat are planimetered or the dimensionless index is calculated).
- *Inadequate search for the maximum jet envelope.*
- *Inadequate Doppler signal.*
- *Error in recording the LVOT velocity*—either the PW sample is too close to the aortic valve, in which case spectral broadening is noted, or the sample is too far down in the LV cavity (one should "inch" up toward the aortic valve, and stop at a level just before spectral broadening is noted).
- *Associated subaortic stenosis*—this will not allow use of the LVOT for continuity equation calculations.
- *Low output, low gradient aortic stenosis*—to obtain a more accurate measurement, one should perform mean and peak valve gradient measurements and calculate the valve area by the continuity equation after heart failure improves or with an inotropic challenge. Typically, one would cautiously infuse dobutamine to raise a patient's ejection fraction preferably into the ~30% range, and if the valve gradient significantly increases, then the etiology of the patient's LV dysfunction is probably at least in part due to aortic stenosis. The dimensionless index (*DI*) should theoretically reflect the degree of valvular stenosis despite severe LV dysfunction.
- *Measurement of only valvular gradients*—gradients will vary depending on stroke volume. If the patient has a depressed ejection fraction or significant MR (reduced forward stroke volume) the gradient will be lower than expected. If the patient has increased flow across the aortic valve (significant AR, anemia, fever), higher gradients than expected will be found.
- *Discrepancies with catheterization results*—in addition to the above "pitfalls" and measurement of instantaneous (echo) versus peak-to-peak (catheterization laboratory) pressures (Fig. 7.12), the phenomenon of *pressure recovery* may result in higher gradients measured by echo as opposed to catheterization results (see Chapter 3).

Aortic regurgitation

As with AS, one needs to not only quantify aortic regurgitation (AR), but evaluate for its etiology (Fig. 7.21). AR generally occurs secondary to an abnormality of the *aortic valve structure* itself, or due to an abnormality of the *aortic root* (hypertension with root dilatation, Marfan's and cystic medial necrosis, and aortic dissection). The etiologies of AR include the common causes of AS (bicuspid aortic valve, calcific valve disease, rheumatic valve disease), and also myxomatous valve disease (with myxomatous mitral valve disease) and endocarditis.

M-mode and two-dimensional features

Features of AR include:

- *Fine to usually coarse diastolic reverberations* on the aortic valve closure line (Fig. 7.3)—indicative of a fenestrated or flail leaflet.
- *Diastolic fluttering on the mitral valve* (Fig. 7.22)—usually the anterior leaflet.
- *Diastolic LV septum fluttering* (Fig. 7.23)—regurgitant jet through the noncoronary cusp.
- *Early mitral valve closure* (Fig. 7.24)—severe AR with an elevated LVEDP.
- *Early aortic valve opening*—severely elevated LVEDP.

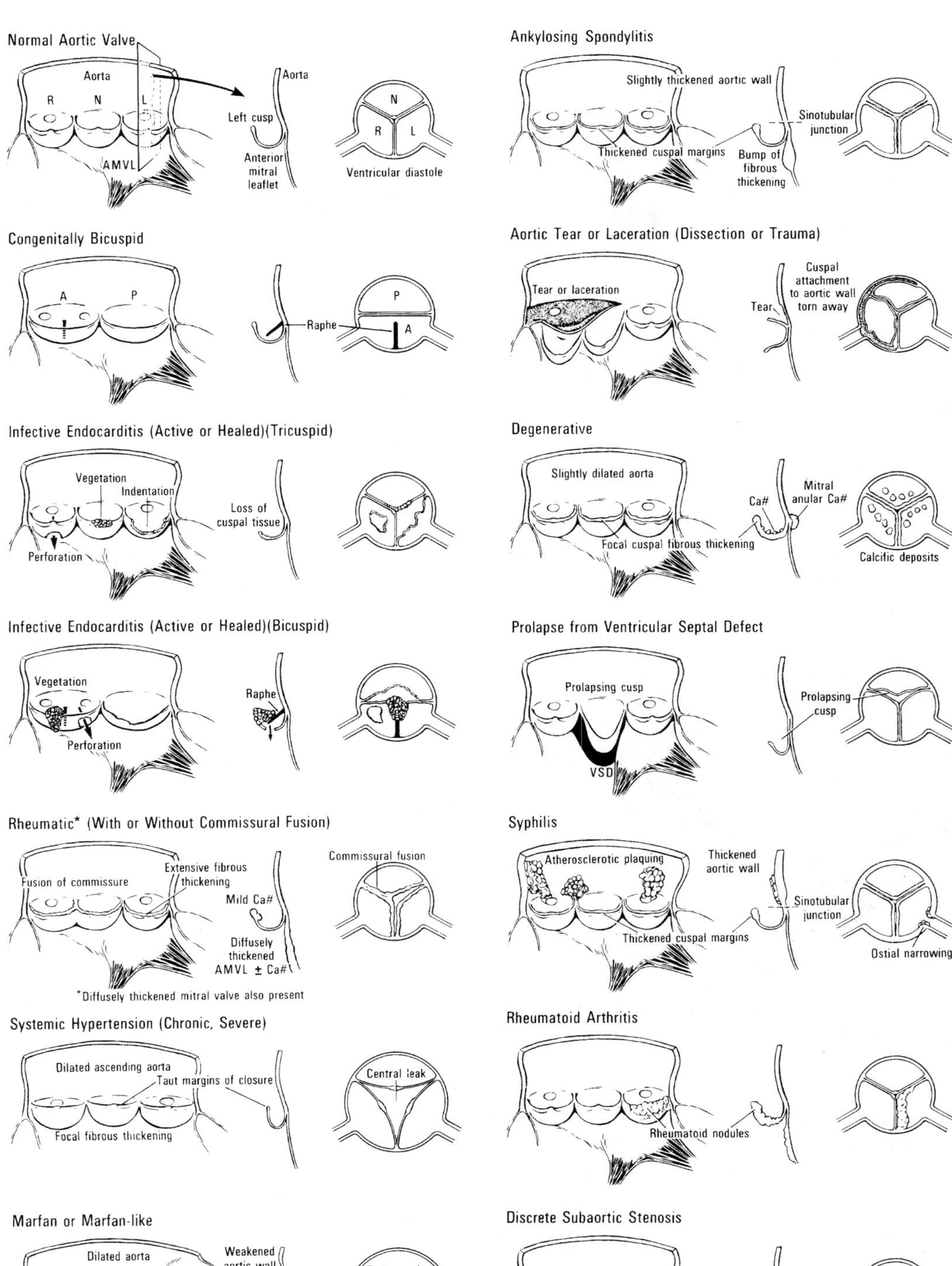

Fig. 7.21 The various causes of pure AR. (Reproduced with permission from: Waller BF, Block T, Barker BG, *et al.* Evaluation of operatively excised cardiac valves: etiologic determination of valvular heart disease, in Waller BF (guest ed) Symposium on Cardiac Morphology. Cardiology Clinics 1984; 2(4): 701.)

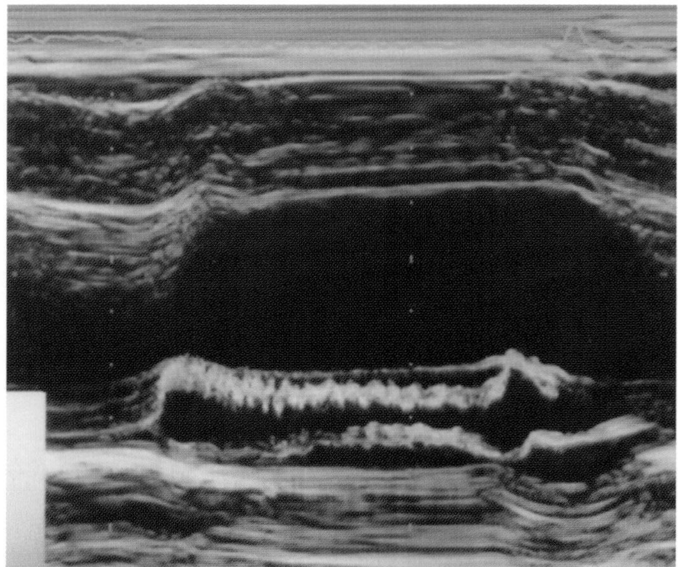

(a)

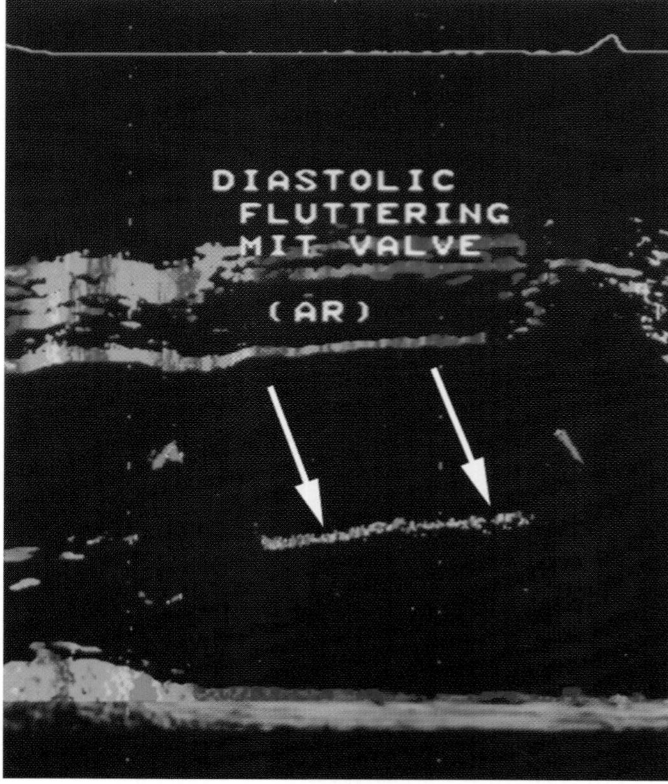

(b)

Fig. 7.22 Mitral valve M-mode (a) and M-mode with tissue Doppler imaging (b) in a patient with AR. TDI well demonstrates leaflet fluttering (arrows) during diastasis.

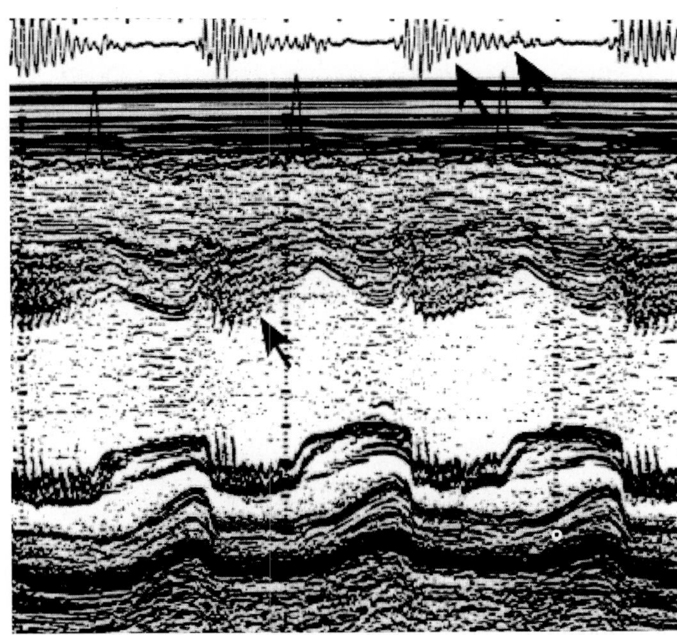

Fig. 7.23 M-mode through the LV in a patient with AR. Septal fluttering is noted (arrow). Double arrow (top right) is a phonocardiogram of the AR.

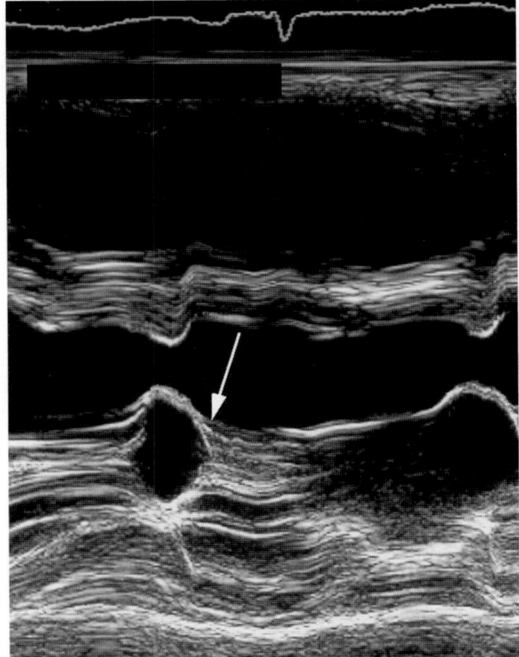

Fig. 7.24 M-mode of the mitral valve in a patient with severe AR demonstrates early mitral valve closure (arrow) secondary to a markedly elevated LVEDP.

- *Depressed or absent M-mode mitral E wave* (Fig. 7.25)—severe AR.
- *Reversed doming of the mitral valve* by 2-D imaging (Fig. 7.26)—regurgitant jet strikes the opening anterior mitral leaflet.
- *Left ventricular volume overload*—increased LV septal and posterior wall motion.

Doppler features of aortic regurgitation evaluation

Pulsed wave Doppler

Pulsed wave techniques were used before the advent of color flow Doppler to "map" the AR regurgitant jet into the LV cavity. Using apical five- and three-chamber views semiquantification of AR is "graded" as:

- *Trivial*—just below aortic leaflets.
- *Mild*—LVOT.
- *Moderate*—AR extends to mitral leaflet level.
- *Severe*—body of the LV.

With significant AR, *forward flow is increased* and therefore LVOT velocity is increased. A LVOT peak velocity of ≥1.5 m/s is consistent with marked AR.

Suprasternal notch PW Doppler of the descending aorta, just past the level of the left subclavian artery may reveal significant *diastolic flow reversal*. If the "initial velocity" is 0.6 m/s or greater and "holodiastolic

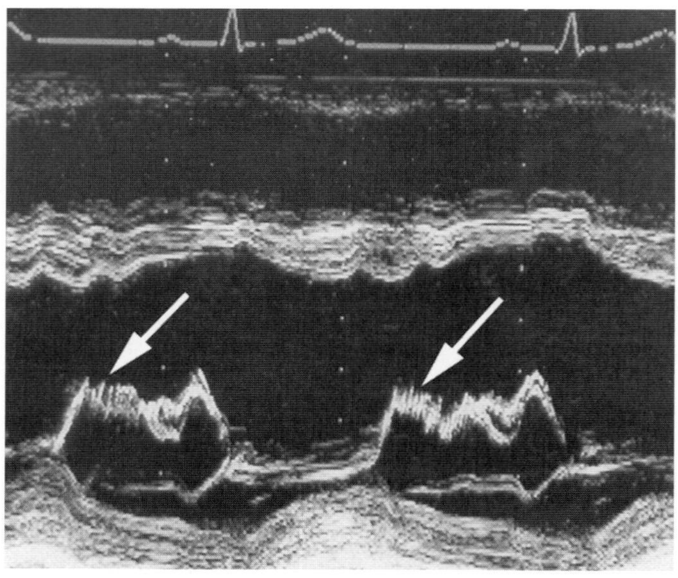
(a)

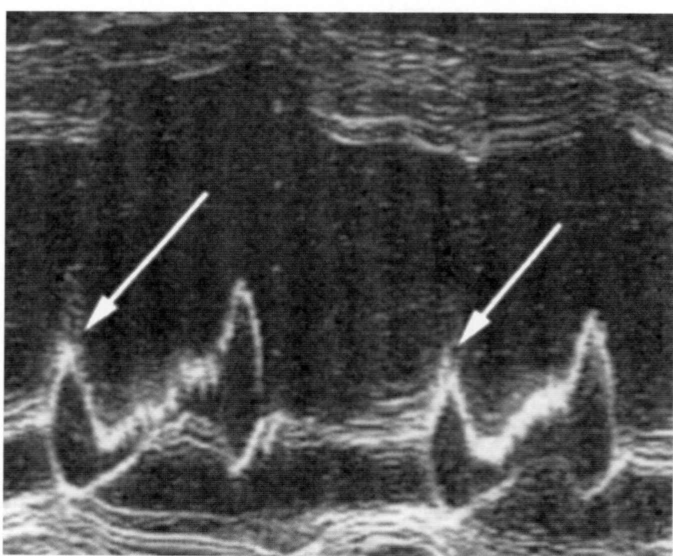
(b)

Fig. 7.25 Depressed E wave (arrows) noted by M-mode of the mitral valve (a & b) in two different patients with severe AR. Diastolic fluttering is also noted on the mitral valve leaflet.

velocity" is 0.2 m/s or greater, consider severe AR (Fig. 7.27). PW Doppler of the abdominal aorta may reveal diastolic reversed flow. If noted, this is consistent with severe AR.

Diastolic flow reversal may also be seen with other conditions that are associated with aortic diastolic "runoff." These include *aorto-pulmonary window*, *ruptured sinus of Valsalva*, *aorta-LV tunnel*, *patent ductus arteriosus*, and a large upper extremity *dialysis shunt*.

Mitral inflow patterns by PW Doppler will be a restrictive pattern with significant AR, as the LVEDP will quickly rise (see also Chapter 6). *Diastolic mitral regurgitation* may be seen with severe AR (Figs 7.28 & 6.9).

Continuous wave Doppler

Generally, the *intensity* of the aortic regurgitation CW waveform correlates with severity of regurgitation. The more red blood corpuscles that regurgitate, the more intense the Doppler signal. This principle applies to all regurgitant jets.

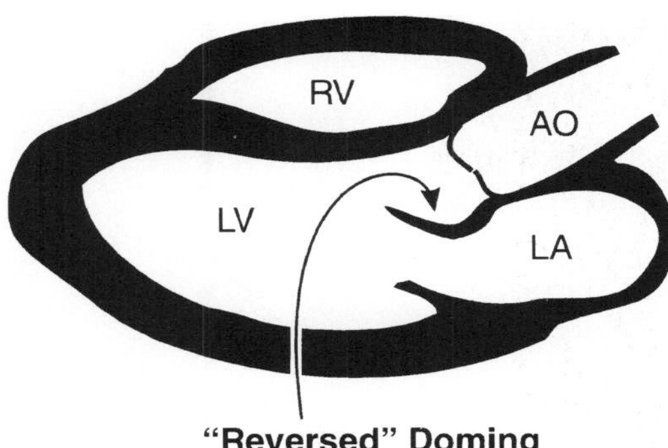

Fig. 7.26 Diagram of a 2-D image of a patient with AR. The regurgitant jet strikes the anterior leaflet of the mitral valve, not allowing it to open fully, giving the appearance of *"reversed doming."*

CW allows for calculation of the *pressure half-time* (PHT). The PHT is defined as the time (in ms) required for the peak initial pressure (P_1) to drop by one half (P_2). Keeping in mind that Doppler measures velocity, one must apply the modified Bernoulli equation to convert to pressure. The velocity (V_2) at which the corresponding pressure is one half the original pressure is $V_2 = (0.707)\ V_1$, where V_1 is the original velocity (see Chapter 3). Hence, *the PHT is the time for the maximum velocity to drop to approximately 70% of the initial velocity.* The more rapid the downslope of the AR profile (the shorter the PHT), the more severe the AR (Fig. 7.29). Color Doppler may help "line up" the regurgitant jet for the CW probe. If the CW probe is misaligned with respect to the AR, the *PHT may appear to be more rapid than it actually is* and one may think the AR is more severe than it truly is. Importantly, as patients with severe chronic AR will tend to have a compliant LV, the PHT may not be rapid, and subsequently, based on the PHT measurement, the patient may be thought to have less severe AR. Patients with acute severe AR will have a rapid PHT. The PHT method may be most useful to differentiate acute from chronic severe AR and less useful to differentiate moderate from severe AR.

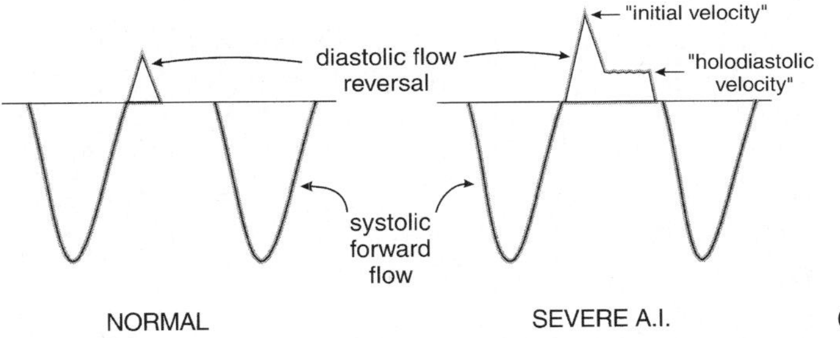

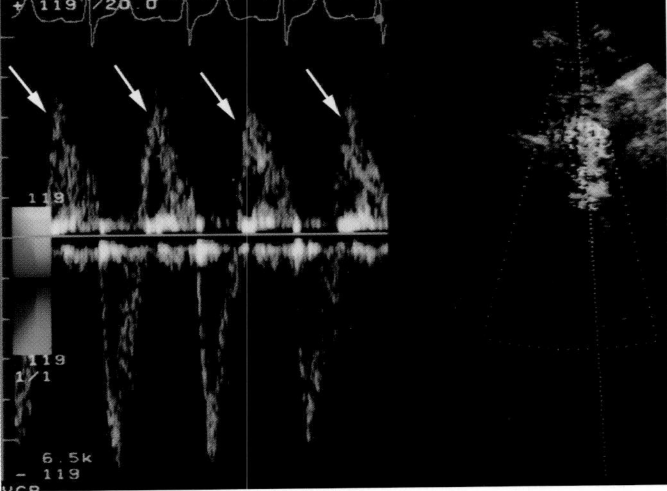

Fig. 7.27 Suprasternal notch PW Doppler of the descending aorta just distal to the left subclavian artery. (a) (left drawing) Diagram of normal diastolic flow reversal occurring in early diastole, and (right drawing) diastolic flow reversal associated with severe aortic regurgitation (severe AI). In (b) a patient with severe AR is studied from the suprasternal notch. Color flow Doppler is used (right panel) to help "line up" the PW Doppler probe. Note prominent holodiastolic flow reversal (arrows).

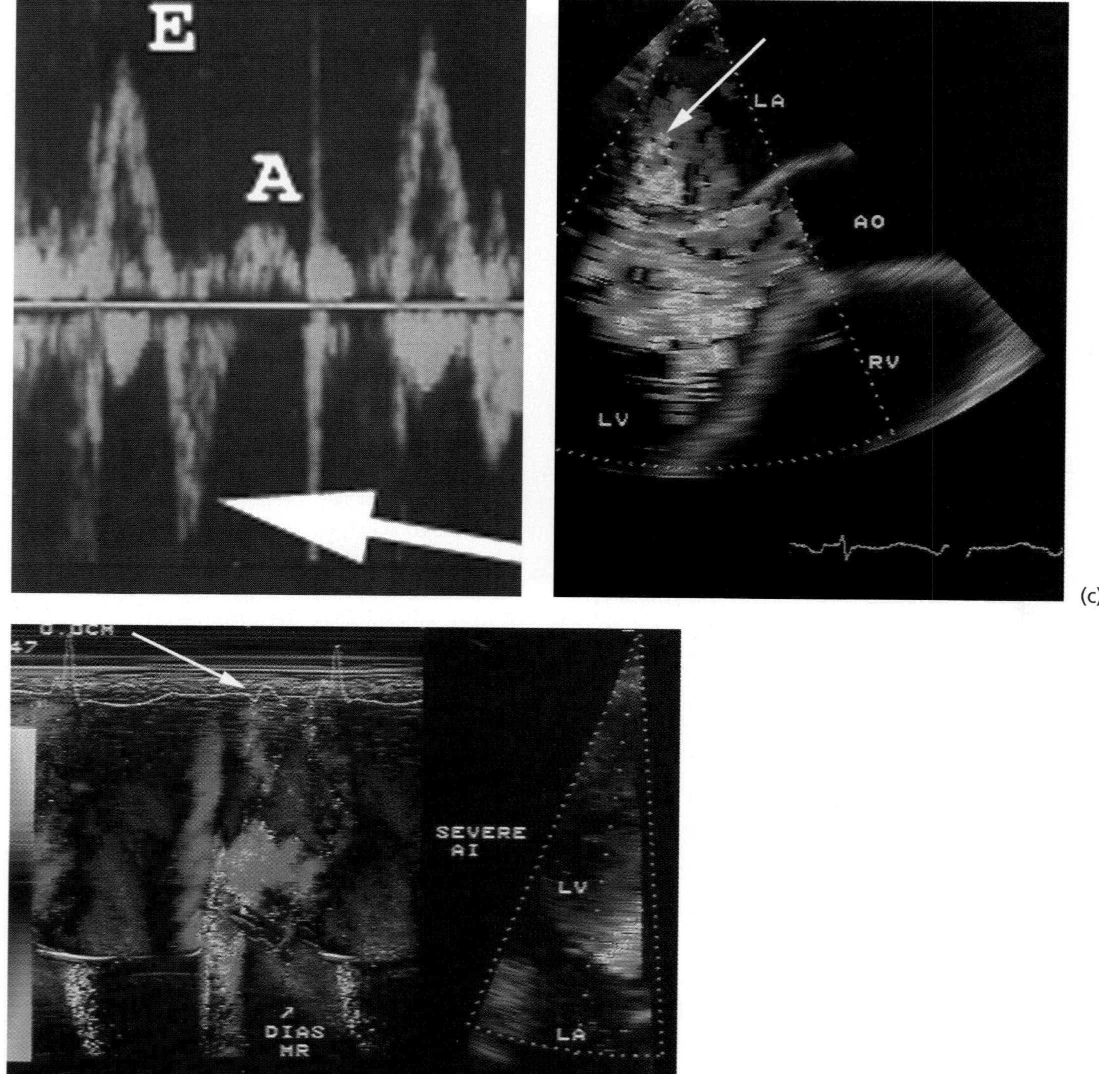

Fig. 7.28 Diastolic MR associated with severe AR. (a) Apical four-chamber view with PW Doppler at the level of the mitral valve reveals the typical low velocity (usually <1.5 m/s) diastolic mitral regurgitant jet (arrow). The E and A wave are labeled. (b) Apical four-chamber view with color M-mode in a patient with acute bacterial endocarditis of the aortic valve with severe AR and a prolonged PR interval. Diastolic MR is again noted (DIAS MR), but the diastolic MR occurs after the onset of the P wave (arrow). Although this patient had severe AR, diastolic MR may also occur secondary to a prolonged PR interval, therefore one must carefully evaluate and further quantify AR if the noted diastolic MR occurs solely after the PR onset. (c) TEE at 120° in a patient with severe AR. Note relatively low velocity diastolic MR (arrow).

The concept of *regurgitant volume* and *regurgitant fraction* was introduced earlier (see Chapter 3). For quantification of AR, one may use mitral inflow for the systemic flow component if there is no significant MR. Mitral flow (used as systemic flow) is the product of the annulus area and the MV time velocity integral (TVI). The MV annulus is an ellipse; therefore, the area is better defined as:

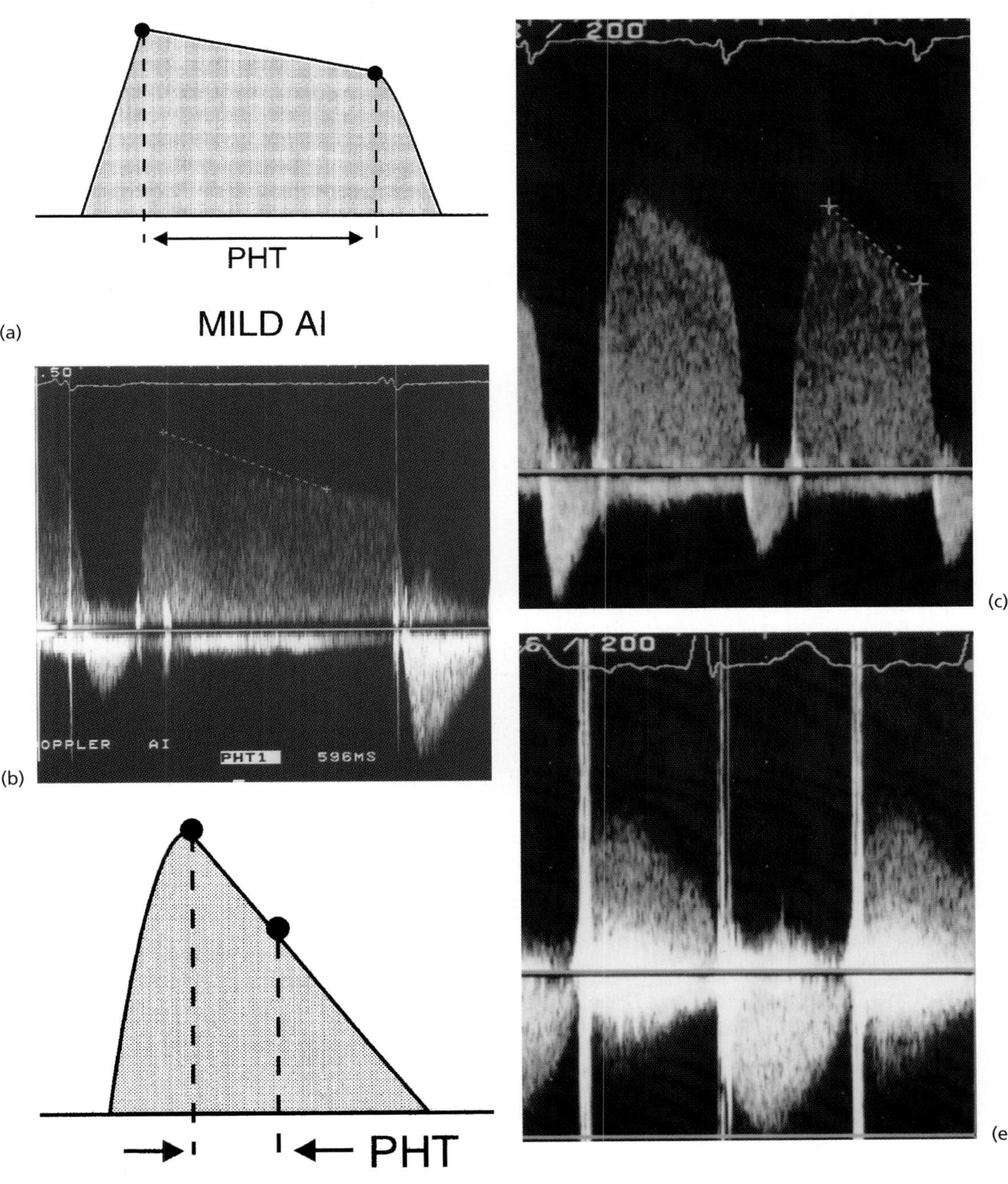

Fig. 7.29 Pressure half-time (PHT) measurements are helpful when quantitating AR. (a) Diagram of mild AR, and (b) a patient with mild AR and a PHT of 596 ms. (c) A patient with moderate AR and a PHT of 392 ms. (d) Diagram of severe AR, and (e) a patient with severe AR and a rapid PHT. A PHT of <300 ms is usually associated with severe AR, and a PHT >700 ms is usually mild AR. PHT values between 300 and 700 ms may be of limited help when quantitating AR severity.

(a)

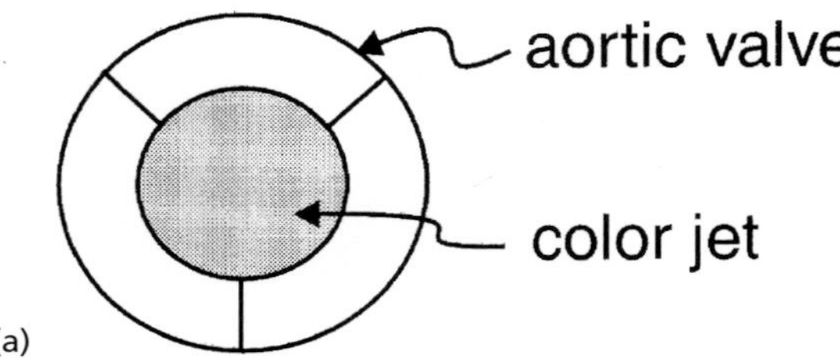

(b)

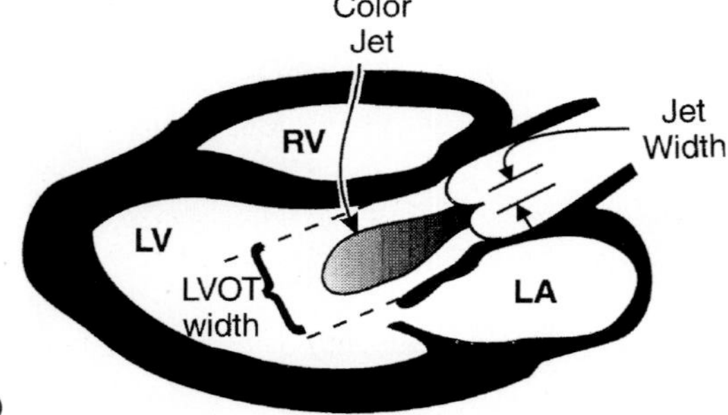

Fig. 7.30 Using color flow Doppler to semiquantify AR in the (a) parasternal short axis and (b) parasternal long axis views. From the aortic valve orifice in the short axis view, the ratio of the color jet area to aortic annulus is calculated. One must be careful to planimeter the color area of the regurgitant jet at the level of the valve, and not below the valve, as the jet will "fan out" below the valve, causing an erroneously large color area to be measured. From the long axis view, the color Doppler jet width at the valve orifice is compared to the width of the aortic annulus. The depth that the color jet extends into the left ventricular outflow tract (LVOT) is poorly correlated with AR severity.

$$MV_{area} = \pi[(D_1)/2 + (D_2)/2]$$

and

$$MV_{flow} = (MV_{area}) \cdot (MV_{tvi})$$

where MV_{area} is the calculated MV area, D_1 and D_2 are MV diameters in the apical two- and four-chamber views, and MV_{tvi} is the mitral TVI. RV for AR is flow through the LVOT minus flow through the MV orifice:

$$RV_{aortic} = LVOT_{flow} - MV_{flow}$$

where RV_{aortic} is aortic regurgitant volume and $LVOT_{flow}$ is stroke volume through the LVOT. A RV ≥60 mL is consistent with severe AR.

Table 7.2 Quantitation of aortic regurgitation using color Doppler.

Severity	Short axis (*jet area/LVOT area*)	Long axis (*jet width/LVOT width*)
1+	<20%	<25%
2+	20–40%	25–46%
3+	40–60%	47–64%
4+	>60%	>65%

Note: Using multiple methods of quantitating AR in an individual patient will improve accuracy.

The aortic regurgitant fraction (RF_{aortic}) is defined by the formula:

$$RF_{aortic} = [RV_{aortic}/LVOT_{flow}]$$

The *effective regurgitant orifice* (ERO) has been presented earlier (see Chapter 3). The ERO of AR may be calculated by one of two methods. The first is calculated as:

$$ERO = RV_{aortic}/AR_{TVI}$$

where AR_{TVI} is the TVI of the AR jet using CW Doppler. The second way to calculate the aortic ERO is to use the PISA profile of the AR jet (using color Doppler). PISA flow (see Chapter 3) is surface area $[2\pi(r)^2]$, where r is the radius of the PISA jet, multiplied by the PISA aliasing velocity (VEL_{pisa}). The ERO is the PISA flow divided by the peak AR velocity (AR_{peak}). Therefore:

$$ERO = \{[2\pi(r)^2] \times [VEL_{pisa}]\}/[AR_{peak}]$$

Color flow Doppler

Color Doppler methods are subjective when used for AR quantification. Color Doppler measures velocity information and not regurgitant volumes. The extent to which the AR jet extends back into the LV cavity is a poor method for AR quantification. The ratio of the regurgitant area at the valve orifice to the aortic orifice area in the parasternal short axis view is the best color technique for quantitating AR. Measuring the ratio of the jet width to the LVOT width (Fig. 7.30) in the long axis views is also good for quantification of AR (Table 7.2).

CHAPTER 8

Mitral Valve

The mitral valve structure involves the annulus, the anterior and posterior leaflets, chordae tendinae, papillary muscles, and the myocardial base of the papillary muscles (see Chapter 4). M-mode of the mitral valve contributes to evaluation of an echocardiographic study (Figs 8.1–8.5).

Mitral stenosis

Congenital

Several congenital forms of LV inflow obstruction may be noted in adulthood. These include mitral parachute valve, double orifice mitral valve, supravalvular ring, and cor triatriatum.

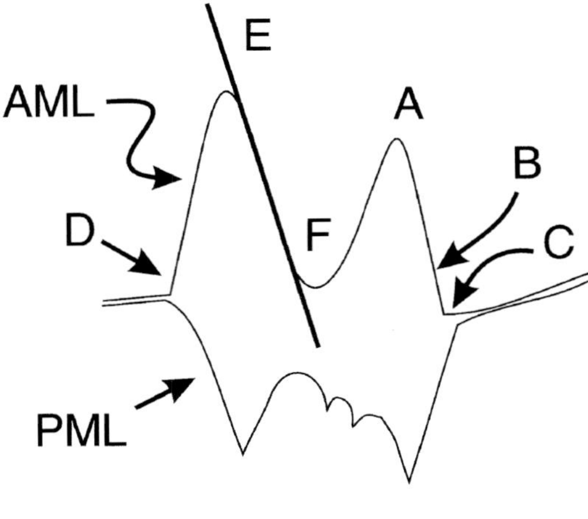

Fig. 8.1 M-mode of the mitral valve. D point, the position of leaflets at the onset of diastolic opening; E point, the peak of early diastolic opening; EF slope, the initial diastolic closing motion of the anterior mitral leaflet; A wave, leaflet re-opening in response to atrial systole; AC slope, the end-diastolic leaflet closure; C point, final leaflet coaptation; B point, position of mitral leaflets at the onset of ventricular systole; AML, anterior mitral leaflet; PML, posterior mitral leaflet.

Parachute mitral valve (Fig. 8.6) involves a single large papillary muscle (usually a posteromedial papillary muscle), but a rudimentary second papillary muscle may be present. This second papillary muscle will have no chordal attachments. Valve leaflets and chordae are usually normal. Inflow stenosis occurs at the valvular and/or chordal level. The most common associated abnormality is the *Shone complex* (multiple left heart obstructive lesions).

Double orifice mitral valve (Fig. 8.7) involves duplication of the mitral orifice, with or without subvalvular chordal fusion. Usually all chordae of the same orifice insert into the same papillary muscle. The valve may be stenotic, regurgitant, or normal. Associated defects include *atrioventricular septal defect, ventricular septal defect (VSD), atrial septal defect (ASD), Ebstein's anomaly, tetralogy of Fallot,* and *coarctation of the aorta.*

A *mitral supravalvular ring* involves tissue from the base of the atrial side of the mitral leaflets. The ring is located between the mitral annulus ring and the left atrial appendage (LAA) and foramen ovale. A calcified mitral annulus may simulate a supravalvular ring. A supravalvular ring will appear as a "band" in the left atrium at the mitral annulus, moving toward the mitral valve in diastole and away from the mitral valve in systole. In systole, the ring may not be able to be distinguished from the mitral annulus. Color flow Doppler acceleration and turbulence occurs at the mitral annulus level and not the valve level. A supravalvular ring should be suspected when a Doppler pattern of "mitral stenosis" occurs, but there is no mitral valve abnormality or doming seen by two-dimensional imaging. The most common associated lesions include an *ASD* and a *persistent left-sided superior vena cava*. Mitral supravalvular ring may be part of the *Shone complex.*

Cor triatriatum involves membranous tissue in the mid-portion of the left atrium. It is well seen in

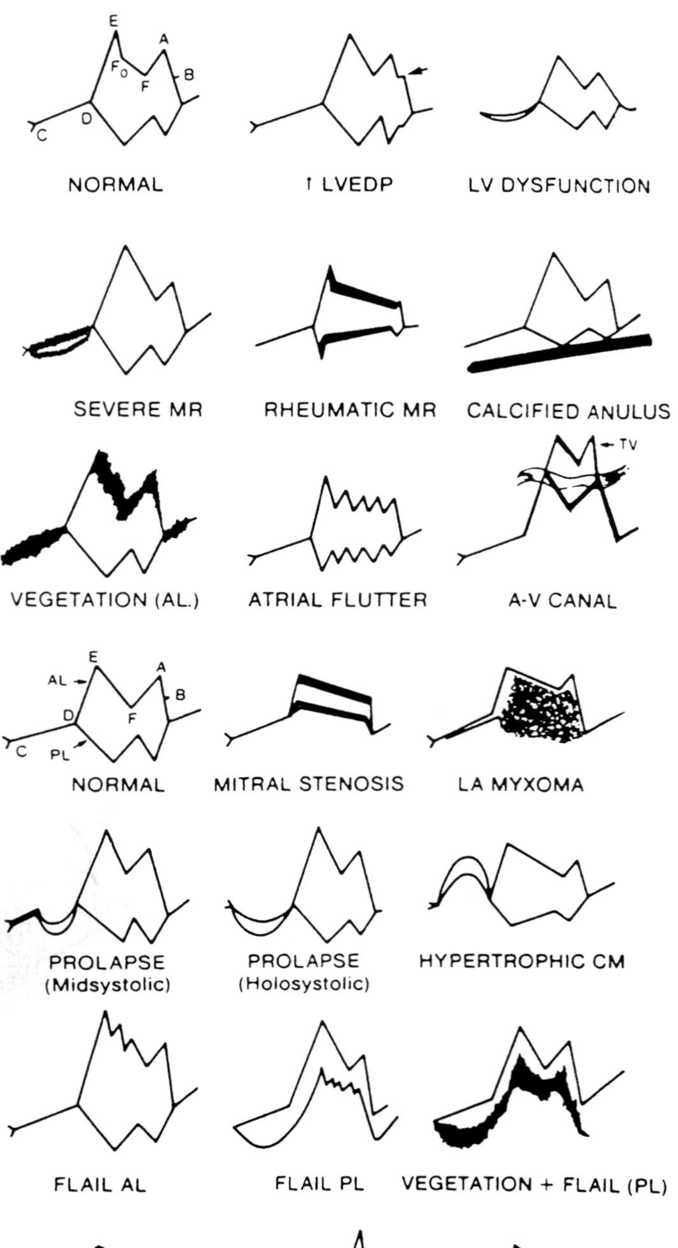

Fig. 8.2 Various M-mode patterns of the mitral valve. (Reproduced with permission from: Felner JM, Martin RP. The echocardiogram. In: Schlant RC, Alexander RW, eds. The Heart, 8th edn. New York: McGraw-Hill, 1994: 401.)

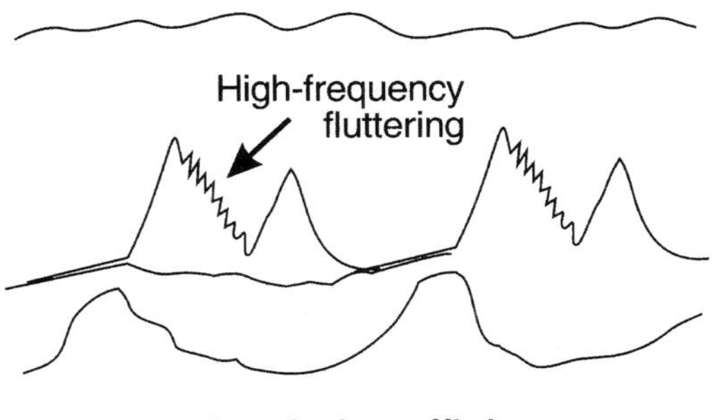

Fig. 8.3 M-mode diagram of the mitral valve in a patient with aortic regurgitation. Fluttering is often noted on the anterior leaflet and occasionally the posterior leaflet (see also Chapter 7).

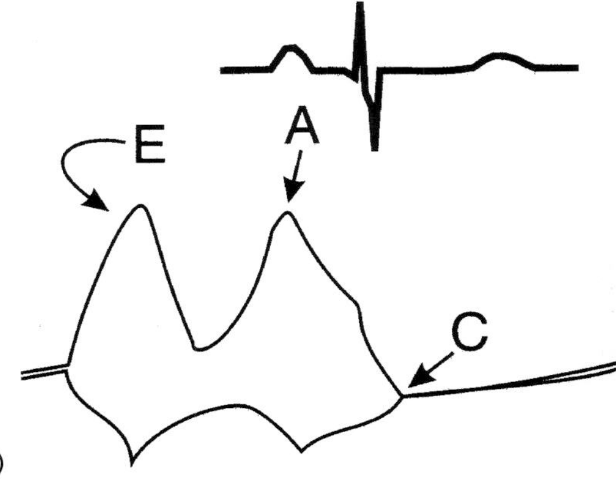

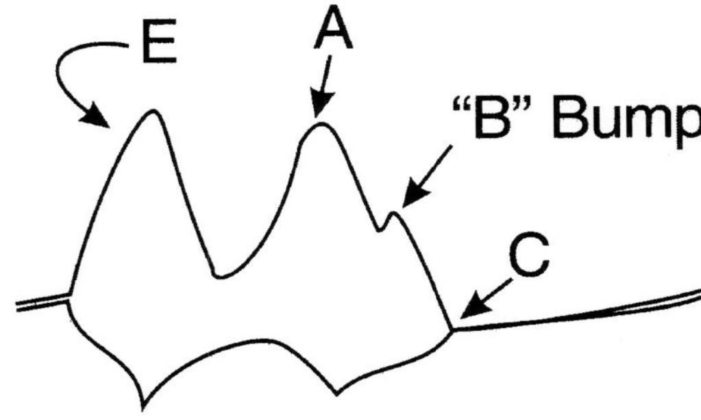

Fig. 8.4 Normal M-mode (a) and an M-mode of a patient with an elevated left ventricular end-diastolic pressure (b). A "B-Bump" suggests an LV end-diastolic pressure (LVEDP) >15 mmHg in patients with LV systolic dysfunction (see Chapter 6).

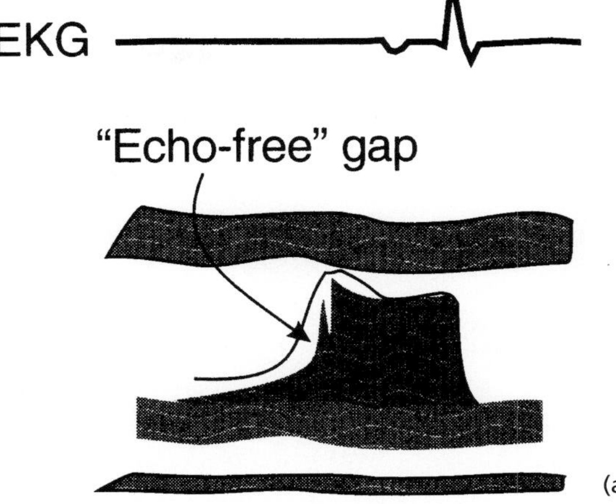

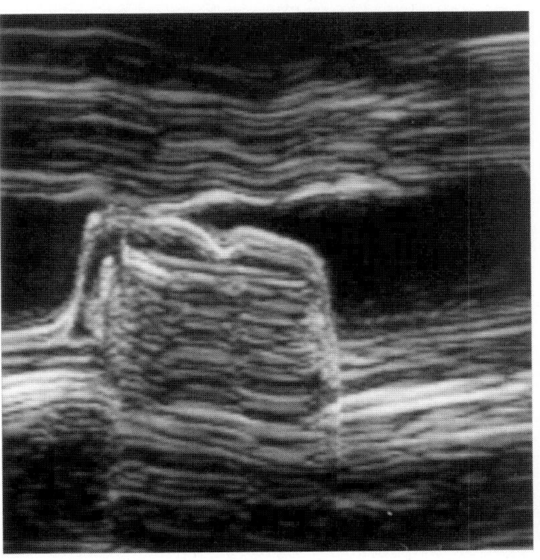

Fig. 8.5 M-mode of a patient with a left atrial myxoma. The diagram (a) and image (b) show an "echo-free" gap that helps to differentiate a mobile tumor, as illustrated, versus either a mass attached to the valve or heavy mitral annular calcification (MAC). This M-mode is typical of myxoma.

the parasternal long axis and apical four-chamber views (Fig. 8.8). The "superior" chamber receives the pulmonary veins, and the "inferior" chamber contains the LAA, foramen ovale, and mitral annulus. Tissue membrane perforation is usually posterior, but may be anterior, and obstruction may be minimal or absent.

An important differentiating factor between supravalvular ring and cor triatriatum is the relation of the left atrial membrane to the LAA and foramen ovale. With supravalvular ring, the membrane is located inferior in position to the foramen ovale and LAA, whereas with cor triatriatum the membrane is superior to these structures.

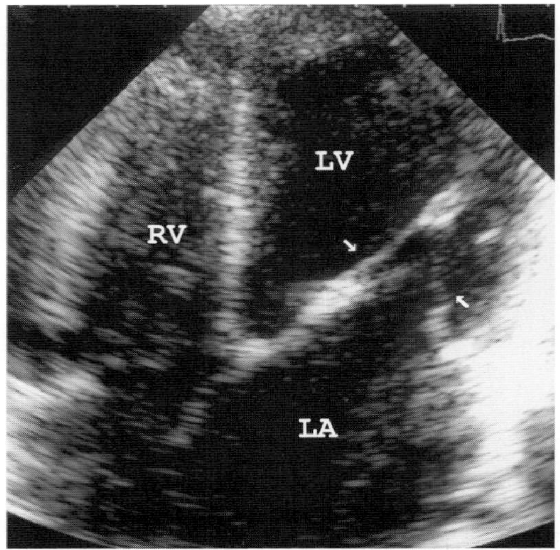

Fig. 8.6 Parachute mitral valve from an apical four-chamber view. Chordal apparatus (arrows) attach to a single papillary muscle. (Courtesy Gencie Bonnette, RDCS, Huey P. Long Hospital, Pineville, LA.)

The most common abnormality associated with cor triatriatum is an *ASD* (secundum type) or *persistent left-sided superior vena cava*. Other associated abnormalities include *atrioventicular septal defect*, *coarctation of the aorta*, and *anomalous pulmonary venous return*.

Mitral annular calcification

In addition to congenital forms, a markedly *calcified annulus* may cause some obstruction to LV inflow. Usually a calcified annulus leads to mitral regurgitation, but it may extend into the mitral leaflet base and cause obstruction.

Rheumatic

Rheumatic mitral stenosis is the most common (>99%) form of adult mitral stenosis. Rheumatic disease almost always involves the mitral valve. Features of a rheumatic mitral valve include *diffuse valve thickening*, *commissural fusion*, and *chordal fusion and shortening*. The leaflet tips will often appear thickened with the

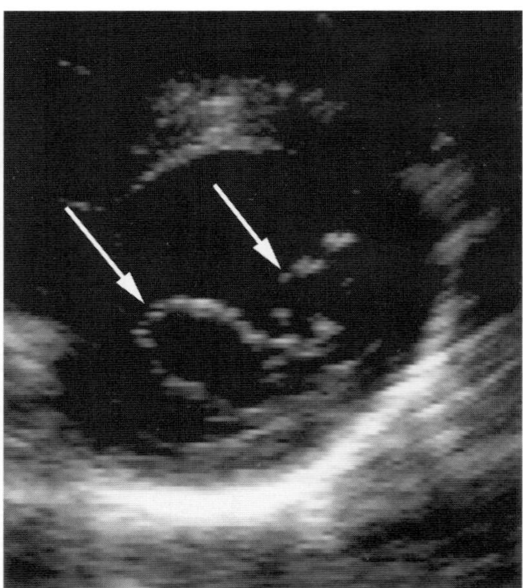

(a)

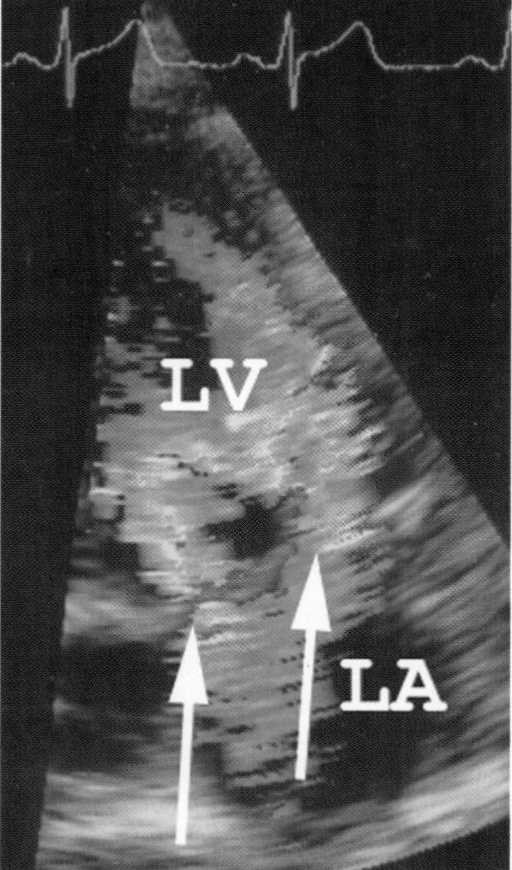

(b)

Fig. 8.7 (*right*) Double orifice mitral valve with (a) both orifices (arrows) simultaneously seen in the parasternal short axis view. (b) Modified apical four-chamber view with color Doppler demonstrates flow through both orifices (arrows). The patient is an asymptomatic physician without any mitral hemodynamic abnormality. (Courtesy Lisa Peters, RDCS, Natchez Regional Medical Center; Natchez, MS.)

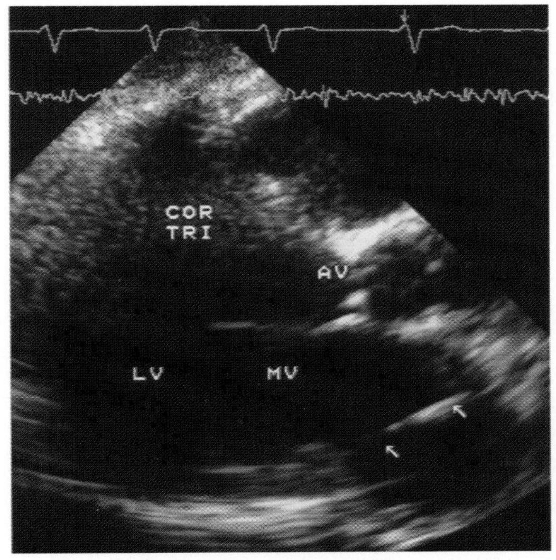

(a)

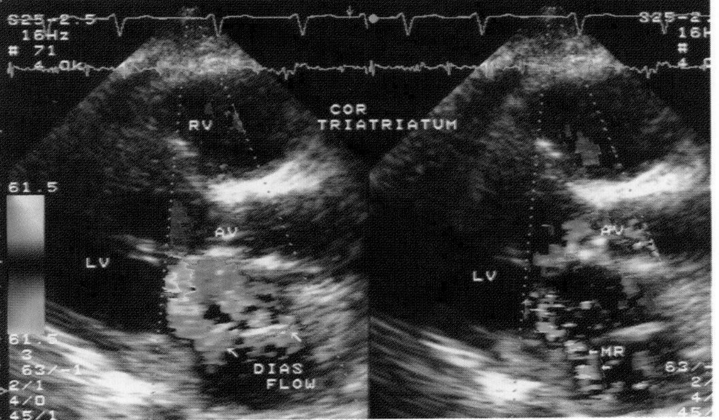

(b)

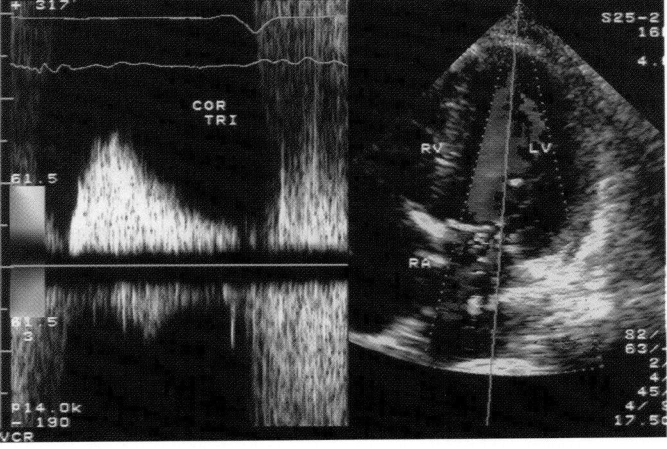

(c)

Fig. 8.8 A 62-year-old-female without any prior cardiac history presented with pulmonary edema and rapid atrial fibrillation. She was found to have cor triatriatum. (a) Modified parasternal long axis view reveals the LA membrane (arrows). (b) Parasternal long axis frames with color wave (CW) Doppler reveals diastolic flow (left panel) through the LA membrane, and systolic frame (right panel) coexistent mitral regurgitation. (c) Apical four-chamber view with CW Doppler reveals that the membrane is mildly stenotic (left panel) with a peak velocity of ~1.5 m/s and a slow deceleration time (DT).

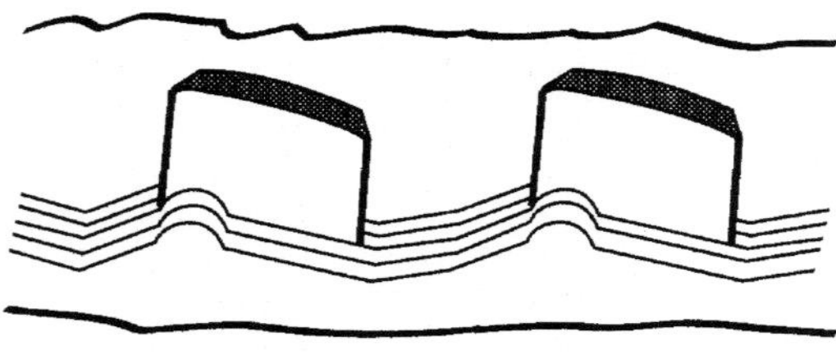
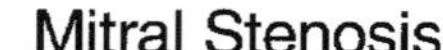

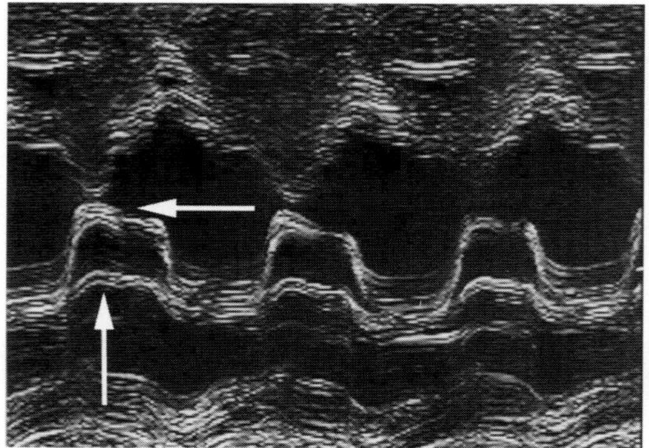

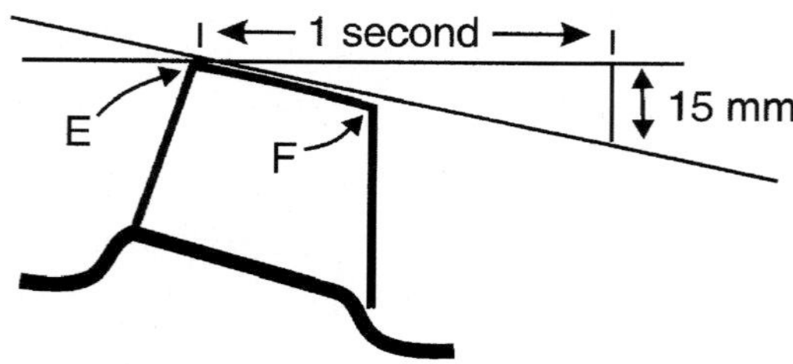

Fig. 8.9 (a,b) M-mode of mild mitral stenosis in a patient in normal sinus rhythm. Anterior motion (vertical arrow) of the posterior mitral leaflet, and a thickened anterior leaflet of the mitral valve (horizontal arrow) with a diminished EF slope. (c) The EF slope is the drop (in mm) of the EF, from baseline, over 1 s, which in this example is 15 mm.

mid and base sections of the leaflets demonstrating variable amounts of thickening and calcification. If the mid and base sections are uninvolved, then the commissures and chordae will only be involved with fusion. A feature of rheumatic valve disease is commissural fusion (see also Chapter 7). In contradistinction to rheumatic mitral stenosis, a calcified annulus with resultant *calcific mitral stenosis* will not involve the commissures and will spare the valve tips. Other rare causes of obstruction to LV inflow include *atrial tumors*, *iatrogenic* (mitral annulus valve ring), *thrombus*, and *vegetation*.

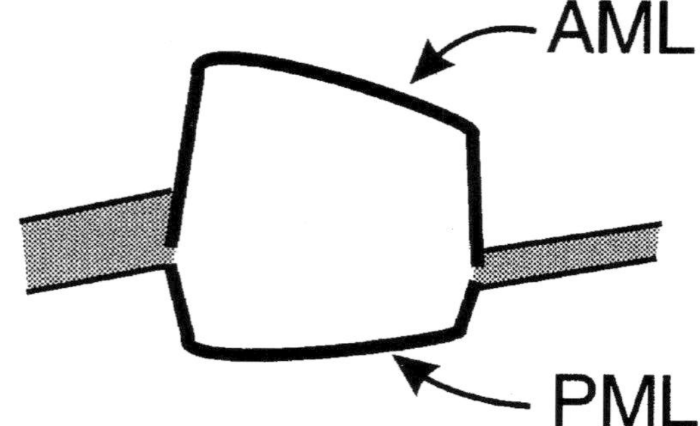

Fig. 8.10 Although this patient has a diminished EF slope, there is no mitral stenosis. Note the posterior directed motion of the PML and lack of thickening of the anterior mitral leaflet AML.

Mitral stenosis with an associated ASD is termed *Lutembacher's syndrome*. *Rheumatic tricuspid stenosis* has been reported to occur in 2–22% (probably <10%) of cases of rheumatic mitral stenosis (see Chapter 9). *Rheumatic aortic stenosis or regurgitation* may be associated with rheumatic mitral stenosis (see Chapter 7). Rheumatic aortic valve disease is nearly always associated with rheumatic mitral valve disease.

M-mode criteria of mitral stenosis

M-mode features of rheumatic mitral stenosis (Figs 8.9–8.11) include:

- *Thickened and calcified mitral leaflets.*
- *Posterior mitral leaflet immobility or anterior motion* due to cusp fusion—90% of patients with mitral stenosis have anterior motion of the posterior leaflet.
- *Loss of M-mode "A" wave.*
- *Decreased EF slope*—the EF slope is not reliable in quantification of mitral stenosis, but may be useful in serial follow-up studies in individual patients. Other causes of a diminished EF slope include reduced LV compliance, pulmonary hypertension, a markedly decreased LV preload, or an increased LV afterload.

Two-dimensional criteria of mitral stenosis

By two-dimensional (2-D) imaging, one should assess for the *level of obstruction* (supravalvular, valvular, subvalvular). For rheumatic mitral valve disease, one should evaluate for valve doming (Fig. 8.12), which may be present in any stenotic valve. In particular, evaluation for valve *mobility*, *thickness*, *calcification*, and *subvalvular thickening and fusion* should be car-

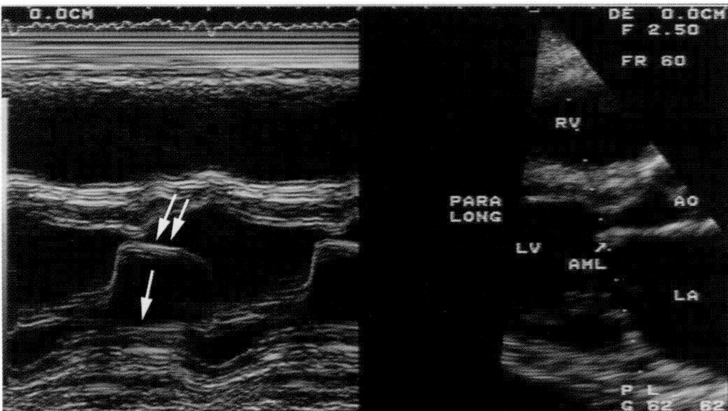

Fig. 8.11 M-mode and two-dimensional (2-D) imaging in a patient with mitral stenosis. Note an "immobile" posterior mitral leaflet (arrow) in this example, and the thickened and diminished EF slope (double arrow) of the anterior mitral leaflet.

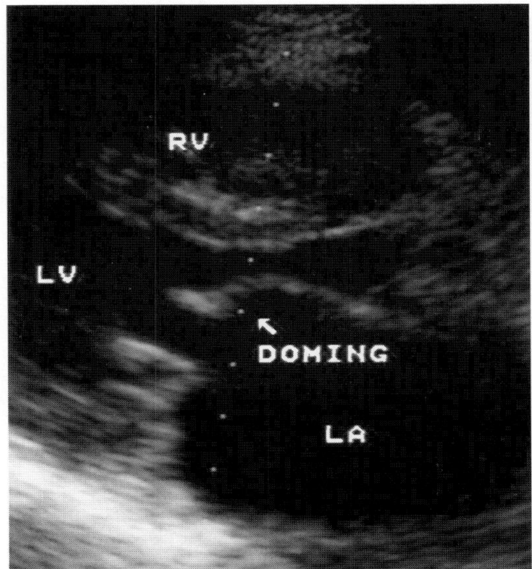

Fig. 8.12 Parasternal long axis 2-D image in diastole demonstrating mitral valve doming in a patient with mitral stenosis.

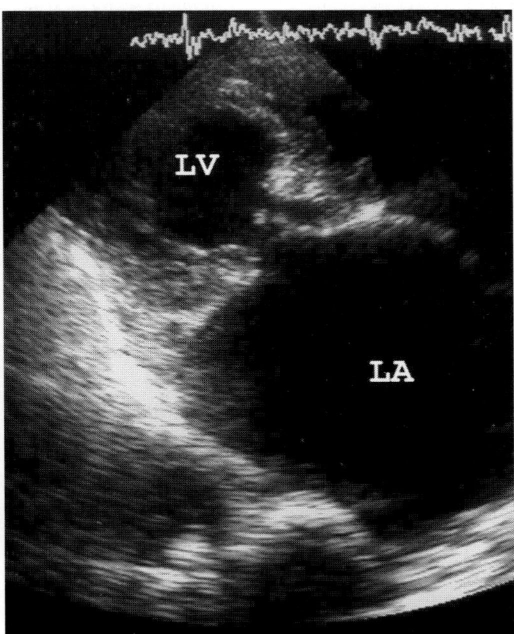

Fig. 8.13 An elderly patient with *giant left atrium*. A giant left atrium usually results from rheumatic mitral valve disease in which both longstanding stenosis and predominantly regurgitation are present. The left atrium may touch the *right* lateral chest wall (many define giant left atrium only when the LA does touch the right lateral chest wall). On occasion, an enlarged LA may cause the atrial septum to deviate toward the right heart and *impede IVC to RA inflow*. This may cause excessive venous congestion. Pulsed wave (PW) Doppler evaluation of the IVC–RA junction may reveal increased flow (>1 m/s) that varies with respiration.

ried out. These four features are used to "score" a valve for predicting success for *percutaneous mitral balloon valvuloplasty* (PMBV). Planimetry of the mitral valve orifice, from the parasternal short axis, may be performed, but one should be careful to find the smallest orifice area to trace. In addition to evaluation of the mitral valve structure, one should assess LA size (Fig. 8.13), right heart size and pressures, and evaluate for either rheumatic tricuspid (see Chapter 9) or aortic (see Chapter 7) valve involvement.

Table 8.1 Criteria for grading mitral stenosis for the PMBV procedure.

Grade	*Mobility*	*Subvalvular thickness*	*Thickening*	*Calcification*
1	Highly mobile valve with only leaflet tips restricted	Minimal thickening just below the mitral leaflets	Leaflets near normal in thickness (4–5 mm)	A single area of increased echo brightness
2	Leaflet mid and base portions have normal mobility	Thickening of chordal structures extending up to one third of the chordal length	Mid-leaflets normal, considerable thickness of margins (5–8 mm)	Scattered areas of brightness confined to leaflet margins
3	Valve continues to move forward in diastole, mainly from the base	Thickening extending to the distal third of the chords	Thickening extending through the entire leaflet (5–6 mm)	Brightness extending into the mid-portion of the leaflets
4	No or minimal forward movement of the leaflets in diastole	Extensive thickening and shortening of all chordal structures extending down to the papillary muscles	Considerable thickening of all leaflet tissue (>8–10 mm)	Extensive brightness throughout much of the leaflet tissue

Note: Each of the listed four features are scored (see text). Those patients with a score of less than 8 will benefit the most, with the least likelihood of complications.

Percutaneous mitral balloon valvuloplasty

As discussed above, mitral valve "scoring" can help determine who is a *candidate for PMBV*, who is at *risk for complications*, who should have a *good result*, and who will *likely restenose* (Table 8.1). Each of the four features is given a score based on grade (from 1 to 4), with 1 the least involvement, and 4 the most. Scores of less than 8 will tend to benefit the most. Complications of PMBV include that of severe MR from leaflet rupture, calcific and thrombotic emboli, LV perforation, and hemodynamically significant ASD formation especially in those with a suboptimal reduction in mitral valve obstruction (iatrogenic Lutembacher's syndrome).

TEE is routinely performed before and during the PMBV procedure for:

- *detection of possible thrombus in the LA and LAA*—procedure is contraindicated if thrombus is present
- *better definition of mitral anatomy*—but subvalvular structures may be difficult to visualize due to shadowing from calcification of the mitral valve and annulus
- *quantification of mitral regurgitation if present*
- *guiding the needle across the fossa ovalis for the transseptal puncture*
- *guide-wire and balloon placement across the mitral valve.*

During the first 24 h after PMBV, with dynamic left atrial and LV compliance changes, the pressure half-time (PHT) method for mitral valve area (MVA) calculation will be inaccurate. Measurement of the mitral mean gradient will remain accurate, as does the continuity equation for calculation of the resultant mitral valve area. Generally, small ASDs tend to close and the degree of MR may improve within 6 months after the PMBV procedure.

Doppler evaluation of mitral stenosis

Doppler findings consistent with mitral stenosis include:

- In normal sinus rhythm, the CW Doppler A wave is *increased* (opposite to that found on the M-mode tracing where the A wave is diminished).
- The diastolic slope (PHT) is prolonged.
- The PW Doppler demonstrates *spectral broadening.*
- The transmitral Doppler velocity is increased.

The mitral valve area and the mean valve gradient should be calculated. As is the case with aortic stenosis, the Doppler and catheterization mean valve gradient should be the same. The mitral mean valve gradient (MVG) is influenced by not only the mitral valve area (MVA), but by:

- *Heart rate*—slow heart rates may be associated with relatively low valve gradients and few symptoms.
- *Flow across valve*—there is an increased gradient with increased forward flow (increased cardiac output, mitral regurgitation).

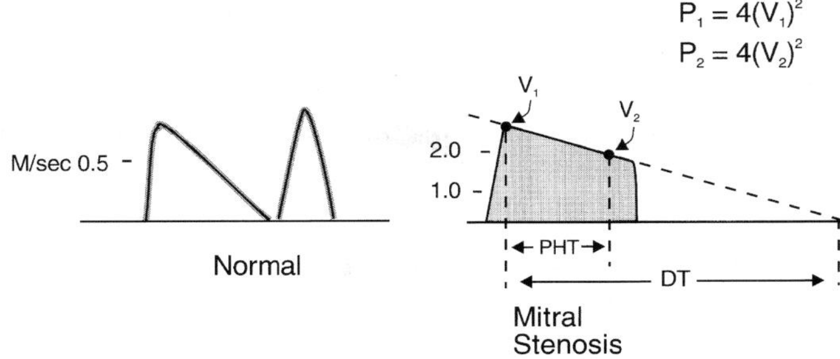

Fig. 8.14 Diagram of normal mitral inflow (left panel) and CW Doppler of mitral stenosis (right panel). The pressure half-time (PHT) is the time it takes for the pressure profile to decay by one half. The velocity profile must be converted to pressure, using the modified Bernoulli equation (see text). The DT is the time it takes for the initial velocity to decay (by extrapolation) to zero.

- *Exercise*—the gradient increases quickly with exercise (due to increased heart rate and increased cardiac output).

The two Doppler methods most often used for calculation of the mitral valve area are the *pressure half-time (PHT) method*, and the *continuity equation*.

To determine the PHT (Fig. 8.14), CW Doppler of mitral inflow from the apical four-chamber view is used. Color flow Doppler of mitral flow is usually used to help "guide" the CW probe directly into mitral flow. V_2 is the velocity at which P_2 is one half the value of P_1 (see Chapter 7). The MVA may be obtained from the PHT (Fig. 8.15) by using the experimentally derived equation:

$$MVA = 220/PHT$$

where *PHT* is in milliseconds. The deceleration time (*DT*) can be measured (Fig. 8.14), and the *PHT* then calculated as:

$$PHT = 0.29 \times DT$$

As above, the *PHT* is calculated by multiplying the *DT* by 0.29. A "simplified" method to calculate the *MVA* uses the following equation:

$$MVA = 759/DT$$

where *DT* is in milliseconds. For calculation of the *MVA*, the *PHT* method is valid with significant mitral regurgitation, but cannot be used in the following situations:

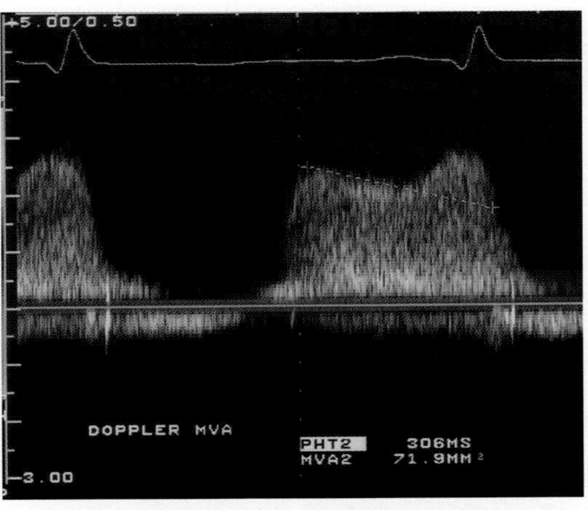

(a)

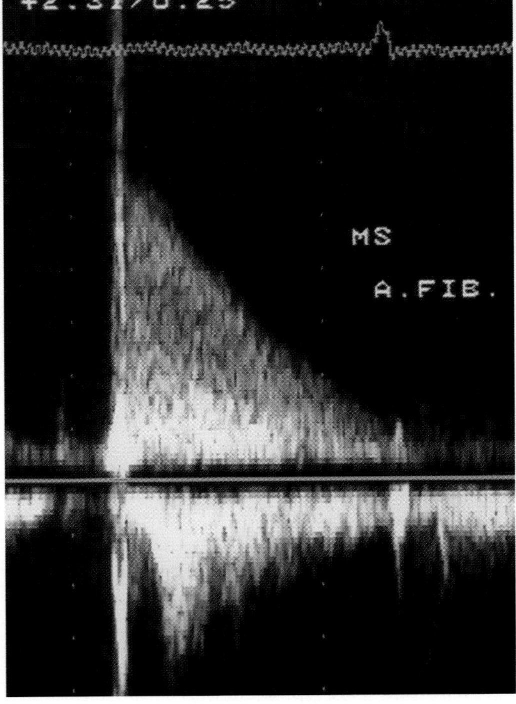

(b)

Fig. 8.15 (*right*) (a) CW Doppler of mitral inflow in a patient in normal sinus rhythm with mitral stenosis. Note the increased velocity and spectral broadening of the flow profile. A prominent A wave is noted. The PHT is 306 ms, and the mitral valve area (MVA) calculated to be approximately 0.7 cm^2 (b) CW Doppler of mitral inflow in a patient in atrial fibrillation with mitral stenosis. Note the absence of an A wave.

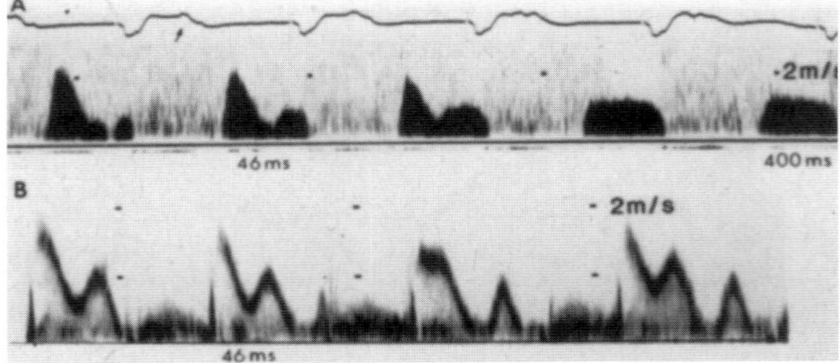

Fig. 8.16 (A) This patient has severe mitral stenosis. The rapid DT of the first three beats is due to *AV block* with the atrial contraction effect "on top of" the E-wave deceleration time. (B) Effect of *atrial flutter* on the decay pattern in a patient with mitral stenosis. (Reproduced with permission from: Hatle L. Doppler echocardiographic evaluation of mitral stenosis. Cardiology Clinics 1990; 8(2): 233.)

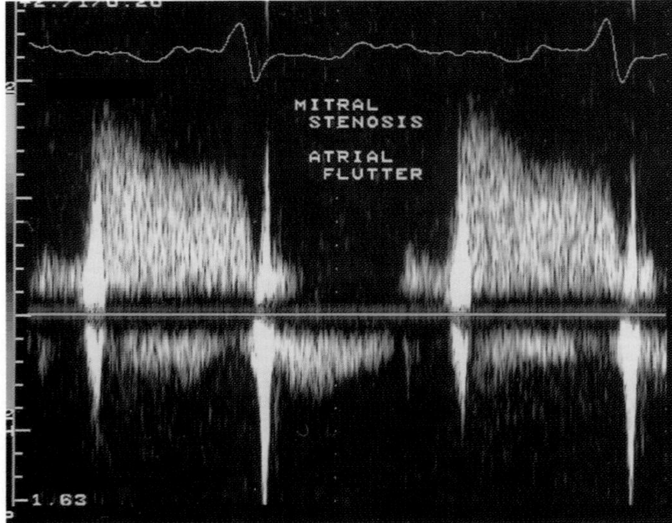

Fig. 8.17 A patient with mitral stenosis and atrial flutter. This example demonstrates why the PHT method cannot be used to calculate the MVA in patients with atrial flutter. The flutter "f" waves are superimposed over the mitral deceleration profile, therefore a valid PHT cannot be measured.

• Any situation in which the *LV diastolic pressure rises quickly* (restriction to filling), as with *significant aortic regurgitation* (AR), *marked LV diastolic noncompliance*, or *ischemia*. With marked AR, the PHT method may produce results suggesting less severe stenosis than is truly present (the LV cavity diastolic pressure rises quickly; therefore, the pressure difference between the LA and the LV quickly equilibrate, and the PHT is less than it should be).

• *Post-PMBV*—3–4 days after the procedure the PHT method is valid.

• *Merging of the E and A wave*—tachycardia, long PR interval, atrial flutter. The effect of atrial contraction is superimposed on the E-wave relaxation, and marked underestimation of MVA results. In atrial flutter, the flutter wave Doppler patterns may change the E-wave decay (PHT) pattern (Figs 8.16 & 8.17).

It is important to use the most "representative" slope of the CW profile for calculation of the MVA. With mitral stenosis, one should also have a significant gradient at end-diastole (Figs 8.18 & 8.19). With atrial fibrillation, one should avoid measurements

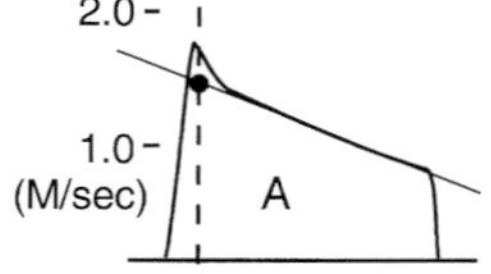

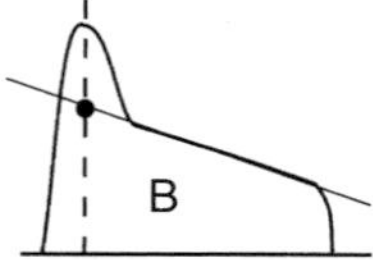

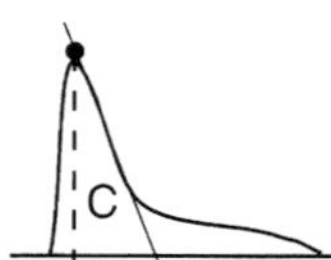

Fig. 8.18 The mitral Doppler curves in (A) and (B) reveal a "slow" decay in late diastole with a significant pressure gradient still present at end-diastole. The deceleration times shown are "most representative," and are consistent with significant mitral stenosis. In (C), although the late diastolic deceleration is "slow," not much pressure gradient is present, and therefore the initial part of the curve, as shown, is "most representative." In this case, the DT is normal with a normal end-diastolic gradient, indicating no evidence of mitral stenosis.

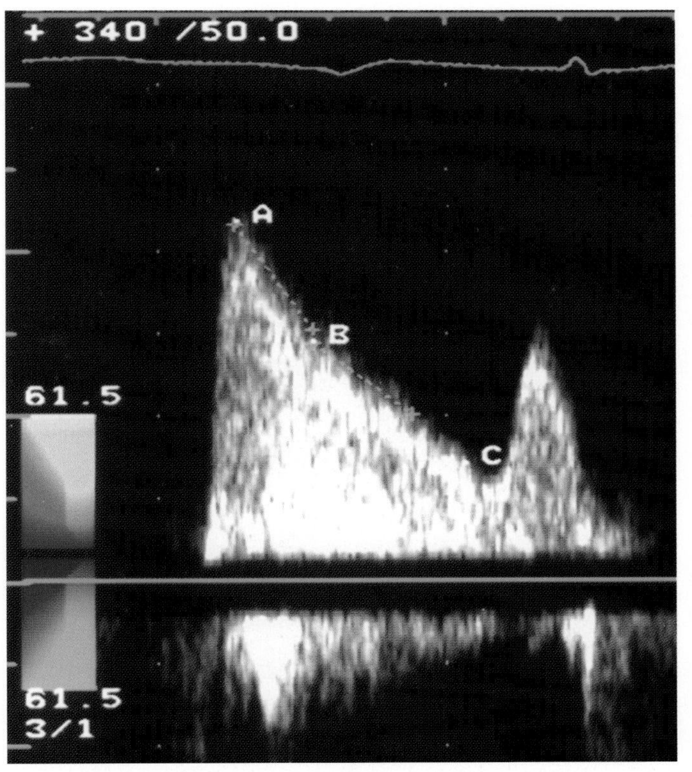

(a)

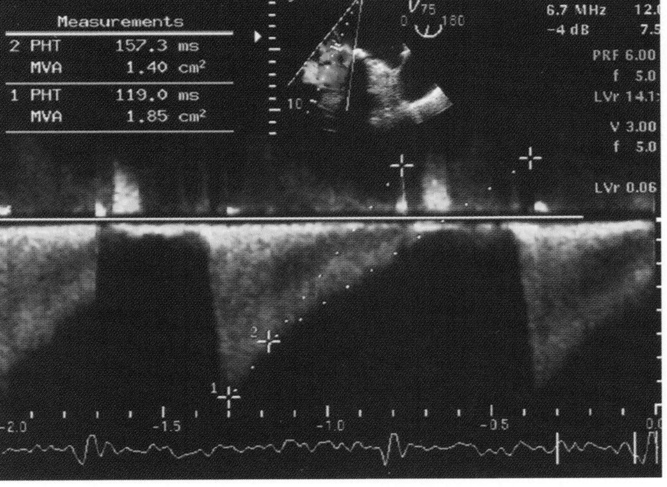

(b)

Fig. 8.19 CW Doppler patterns of mitral stenosis. (a) This CW pattern from the apex shows the most representative slope which is line segment BC. Segment AB is brief in early diastole, and not the most representative of pressure decay. (b) Transesophageal echocardiography (TEE) performed CW recording shows that slope number (1) has a PHT of 119 ms, and resultant MVA of 1.85 cm^2. The best pressure decay, however, is (2) and yields a PHT of 157 ms, and a MVA of 1.4 cm^2.

during short RR intervals because these will give shorter PHTs. It is also important to average several beats, as the gradient and DT will vary somewhat, dependent on the RR interval.

In the absence of significant mitral regurgitation, the *continuity equation* may be used to calculate the MVA (see Chapter 3). If there is no significant aortic regurgitation present, the LVOT may be used in calculations:

$$\text{Mitral flow} = LVOT_{\text{flow}}$$

$$(MV_{\text{tvi}}) \times MVA = (LVOT_{\text{tvi}}) \times LVOT_{\text{area}}$$

and

(a)

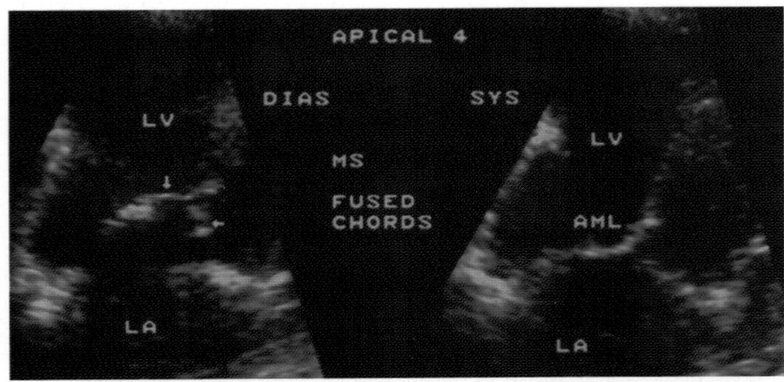

(b)

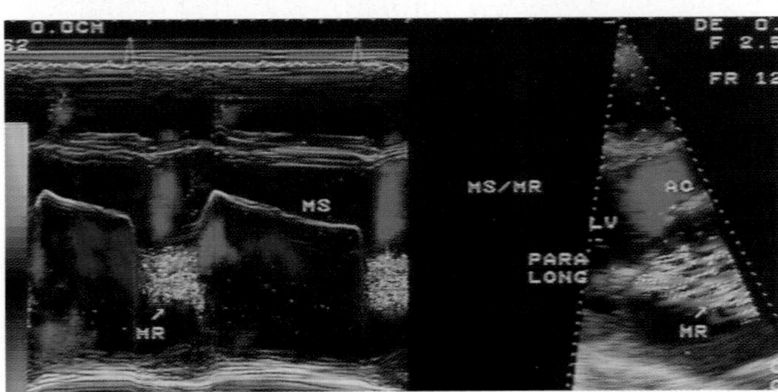

Fig. 8.20 (a) Apical four-chamber image in diastole (left panel) and systole (right panel) in a patient with rheumatic heart disease. The chords (arrows) have fused. The patient had mild mitral stenosis with predominantly mitral regurgitation. (b) Parasternal long axis view with M-mode color in a middle-aged male with mild rheumatic mitral stenosis and marked rheumatic mitral regurgitation.

$$MVA = [(LVOT_{tvi}) \times LVOT_{area}]/MV_{tvi}$$

If significant AR is present, the pulmonic valve may be used instead of the LVOT.

A third method for calculation of MVA uses the *proximal isovelocity surface area* (PISA) from color Doppler. This method, with examples using mitral regurgitation and also mitral stenosis is discussed elsewhere (see Chapter 3).

Mitral regurgitation

Mitral regurgitation, if diligently searched for, is found in up to 70% of normal people. The jet may be of a short duration and is found by color to not extend far from the closing mitral leaflets (see also Chapter 21 for a discussion of drug-related valvular disease and reproducibility/reliability of color Doppler assessment of valvular regurgitation).

Mitral regurgitation is generally grouped into three categories (see Chapter 15), based on functional etiology:

Type I—normal leaflet mobility:
- mitral annulus dilatation
- leaflet perforation
- cleft valve.

Type II—excessive leaflet mobility:
- elongated or ruptured chordae/papillary muscle.

Type III—Restricted leaflet mobility:
- rheumatic
- papillary apical displacement secondary to LV dilatation.

Relatively common etiologies of significant mitral regurgitation (MR) include:

- *Myxomatous degeneration* (mitral valve prolapse).
- *Rheumatic* (Fig. 8.20)—commissures fuse, chordae thicken and fuse, usually with some degree of mitral stenosis, but mitral regurgitation may be the predominant problem.
- *Dilated cardiomyopathy*—see Chapter 11.
- *Ischemic*—see Chapter 13.
- *Endocarditis*—see Chapter 18.
- *Calcific degeneration.*
- *Trauma*—chordal rupture with blunt chest trauma.
- *Cleft mitral valve* (Fig. 8.21)—involves the anterior leaflet, either isolated or as part of an AV canal. When isolated, however, the anatomy is distinct from that associated with AV canal. A *cleft septal leaflet of the tricuspid valve* may coexist.
- *Endomyocardial fibroelastosis*—may simulate rheumatic disease.

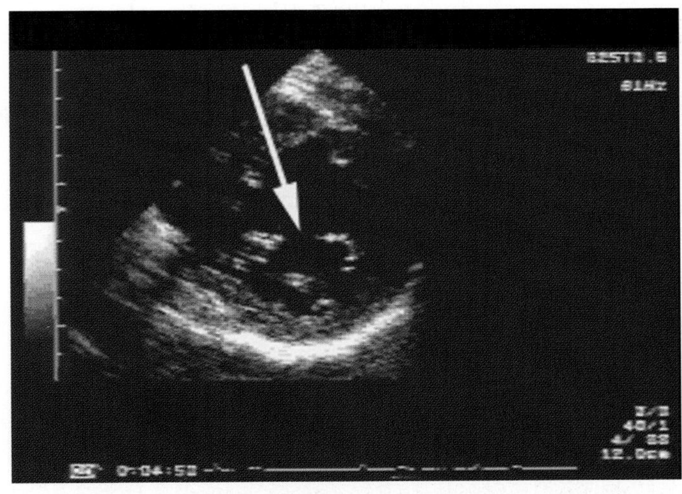

(a)

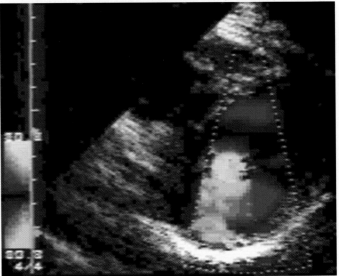

(b)

Fig. 8.21 Parasternal short axis image of a 22-year-old-female with exertional shortness of breath and a murmur of mitral regurgitation. (a) The patient has a cleft (arrow) in the anterior leaflet of the mitral valve. The valve will appear to have three leaflets when viewed in diastole. (b) Color Doppler demonstrates regurgitation through the cleft. In addition to a cleft septal leaflet of the tricuspid valve, other associated defects with a cleft mitral valve include *ventricular septal defect, coarctation of the aorta, double outlet right ventricle,* and *tricuspid atresia*. The valve was repaired.

Myxomatous degeneration is the most common etiology of MR in Western society (45%), having replaced rheumatic involvement (now 40%). Rheumatic involvement remains the most common etiology in many areas of the world. Ischemic heart disease (~10%) and endocarditis (~2%) are also relatively common.

Mitral valve prolapse

Myxomatous degeneration is the most common cause (see also Chapter 15) of pure mitral regurgitation (MR). When evaluating for mitral valve prolapse (MVP), one needs to evaluate for *functional* changes (leaflet prolapse) and for *structural* changes of the mitral valve.

Functional valve *prolapse* (see Fig. 15.6) involves one leaflet-free margin overriding another. *Billowing* is protrusion of the belly of the leaflet into the LA, but the free edges remain in apposition to one another. Localized portions of one or both leaflets are displaced posterosuperior to the mitral annulus plane, into the LA (Figs 8.22 & 8.24).

The mitral annulus assumes a somewhat "saddle" shape. The annulus attached to the posterior leaflet

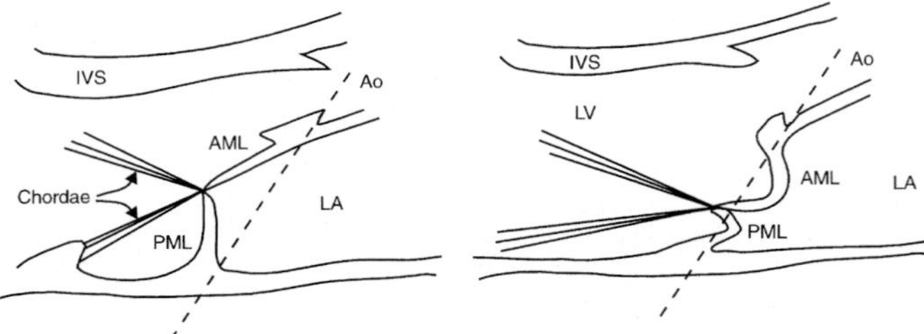

Fig. 8.22 Diagram of parasternal long axis with (left panel) normal mitral valve coaptation, and (right panel) billowing of both PMLs and AMLs beyond the mitral plane (dashed line) into the LA. Ao, aortic root; IVS, interventricular septum.

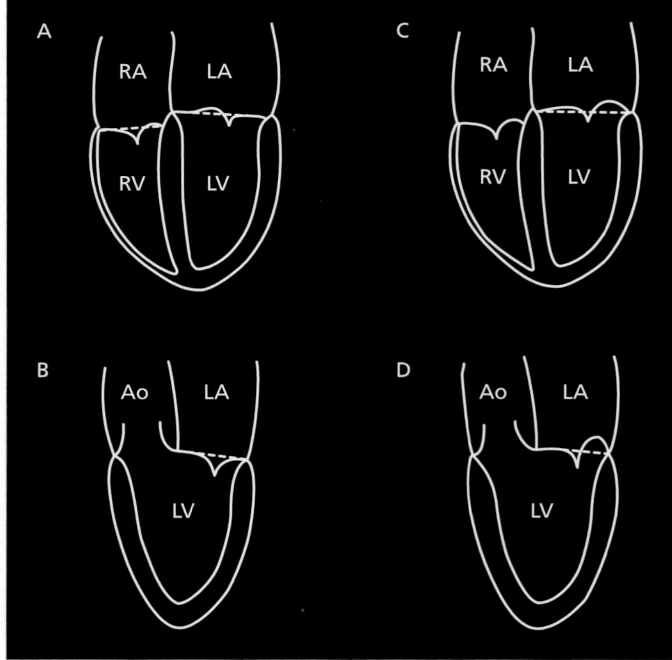

Fig. 8.23 As the annulus adjacent to the anterior leaflet of the mitral valve lies "out of plane" to the remainder of the mitral annulus and is "bowed" toward the apex, the anterior leaflet may appear to prolapse in apical views. (A) A normal mitral valve appears to prolapse in the apical four-chamber view. (B) A normal three-chamber (apical long axis) view. (C,D) True prolapse of the posterior leaflet is evident. (Reproduced with permission from: Shah PM. Echocardiographic diagnosis of mitral valve prolapse. Journal of the American College of Cardiology 1994; 7(3): 288.)

lies in one plane, but the portion of the annulus attached to the anterior leaflet "bows" toward the LV apex. When imaging the mitral valve from an apical view, this so-called "distortion" of the mitral annulus, may cause the anterior leaflet to appear to protrude into the LA during systole (Fig. 8.23). Diagnosis of anterior leaflet prolapse should not be made if anterior leaflet billowing is observed solely from an apical view. If, however, anterior leaflet billowing exceeds 1 cm, true leaflet billowing may be present (mitral valve anatomy is further discussed in Chapter 15). When prolapse occurs, most often the middle scallop of the posterior leaflet is involved. The lateral posterior scallop is next in frequency of occurrence, followed by the anterior leaflet. Infrequently, the medial scallop of the posterior leaflet will be involved (Fig. 8.24). Parasternal and apical long axis views image the *medial segment of the anterior leaflet* and *middle scallop of the posterior leaflet* (Fig. 8.25). The apical four-chamber view images the *medial segment of the anterior leaflet* and the *posterior lateral scallop*. The apical two-chamber view images the *anterior leaflet lateral segment* and the *medial scallop of the posterior leaflet*.

M-mode criteria for prolapse include posterior displacement of 2 mm or greater for late systolic prolapse or 3 mm or more for holosystolic prolapse (Fig. 8.26). Holosystolic posterior displacement may be seen but is not specific. It may be produced with a high interspace transducer position. Early anterior motion of leaflet chordae followed by late systolic posterior

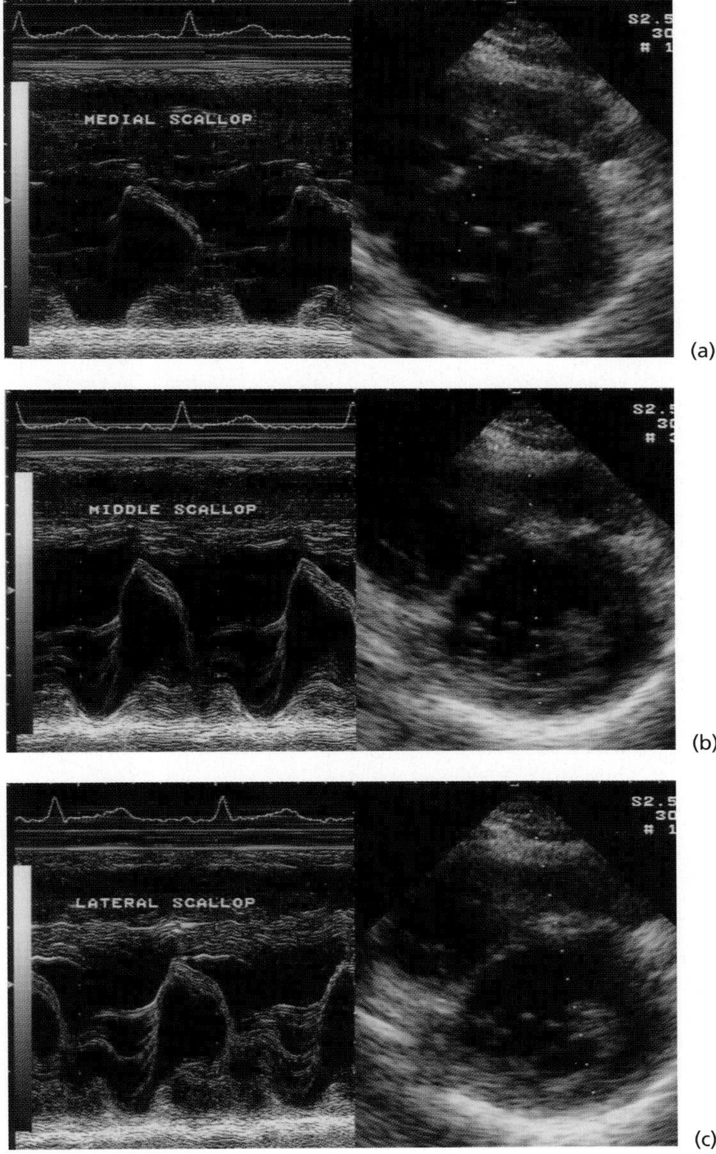

Fig. 8.24 M-mode (left panels) and 2-D parasternal short axis image level of the mitral valve (right panels) in a patient with mitral valve prolapse (MVP) involving the posterior leaflet. M-mode through the medial leaflet (a) does not suggest leaflet prolapse, but mid (b) and lateral (c) scallops are myxomatous as evidenced by M-mode late systolic prolapse.

motion may be seen with elongated chords and MVP (Fig. 8.27).

Coexistence of prolapse of other valves may occur. *Tricuspid valve prolapse* (TVP) is found in upwards of 50% of patients with MVP. TVP is best noted from the RV apex and from a parasternal short axis view. *Aortic valve prolapse* is uncommon. It is best seen in a parasternal or apical long axis view. Aortic valve prolapse may also occur with a bicuspid aortic valve.

Structural changes associated with myxomatous degeneration include *thickened mitral valve leaflets* and *tissue redundancy*. The anterior mitral leaflet is normally not as thick as the posterior aortic wall, and has a similar thickness to the aortic leaflets. The normal mitral leaflet may appear to have the same thickness as the LV endocardium. As an increased ultrasound gain setting will appear to increase the thickness of cardiac structures, this is

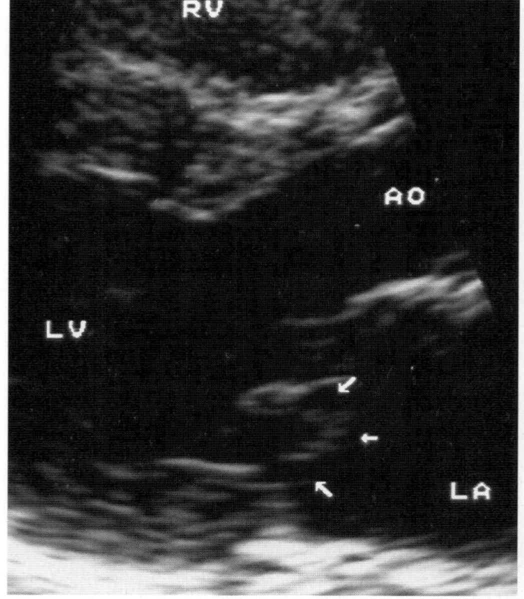

(a)

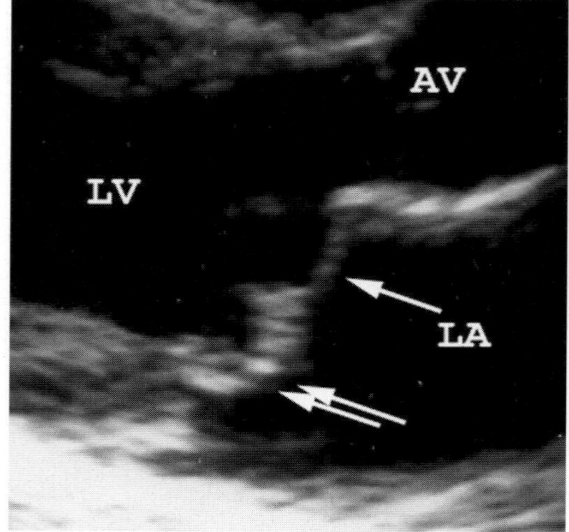

(b)

Fig. 8.25 Parasternal long axis image (a) of a patient with prolapse of the posterior leaflet of the mitral valve (arrows). (b) Both anterior (single arrow) and posterior (double arrow) leaflets prolapse into the LA. Note the thickened posterior mitral valve leaflet in this image.

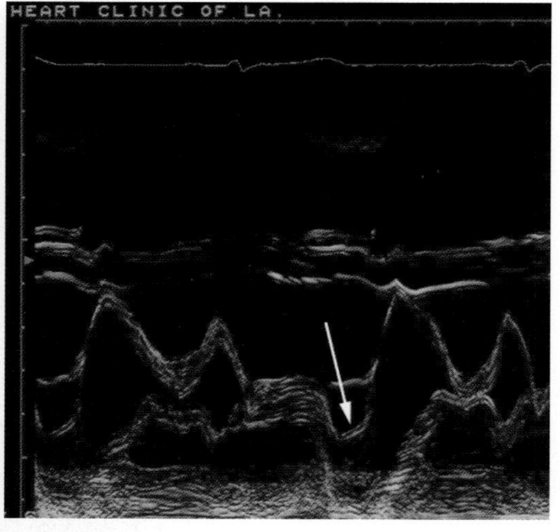

(a)

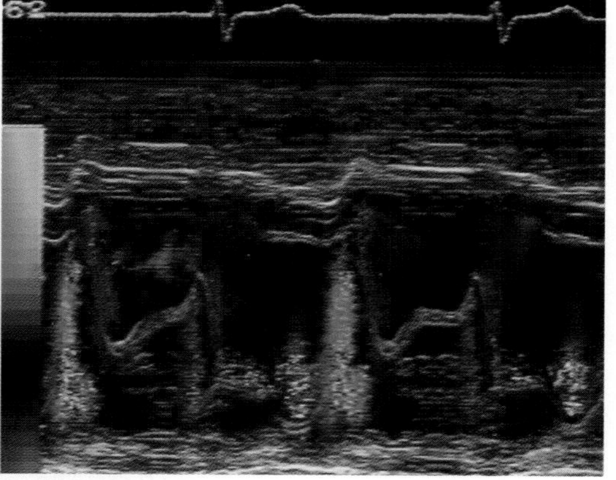

(b)

Fig. 8.26 (*above and right*) (a) M-mode of the mitral valve in a patient with late systolic mitral valve prolapse (arrow). Color Doppler (b) reveals mitral regurgitation occurs at the time of prolapse.

a good guideline to follow when evaluating mitral leaflet thickness. Thickened (myxomatous) leaflets (Figs 8.25 & 8.28) are probably associated with histologic changes within the valve. Although sometimes difficult to accurately measure, 5 mm is generally used as criteria to describe a thickened valve leaflet. These patients are at an increased risk of complications, such as endocarditis and the need for future mitral valve surgery.

Mitral annulus dilatation may occur with myxomatous mitral degeneration (Fig. 8.29). The mitral annulus area is calculated from the apical four- and two-chamber views, assuming the orifice is an oval. The equation for the mitral annulus area (A) is:

$$A = \pi\left[\frac{D_1}{2}\right]\left[\frac{D_2}{2}\right]$$

where D_1 and D_2 are diameter measurements in orthogonal views (apical four- and apical two-chamber).

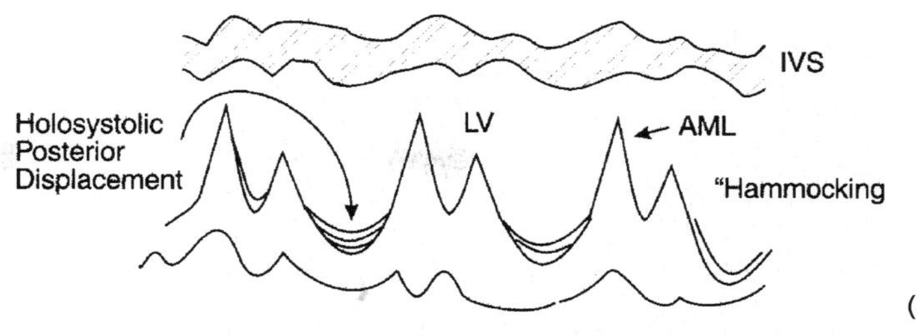

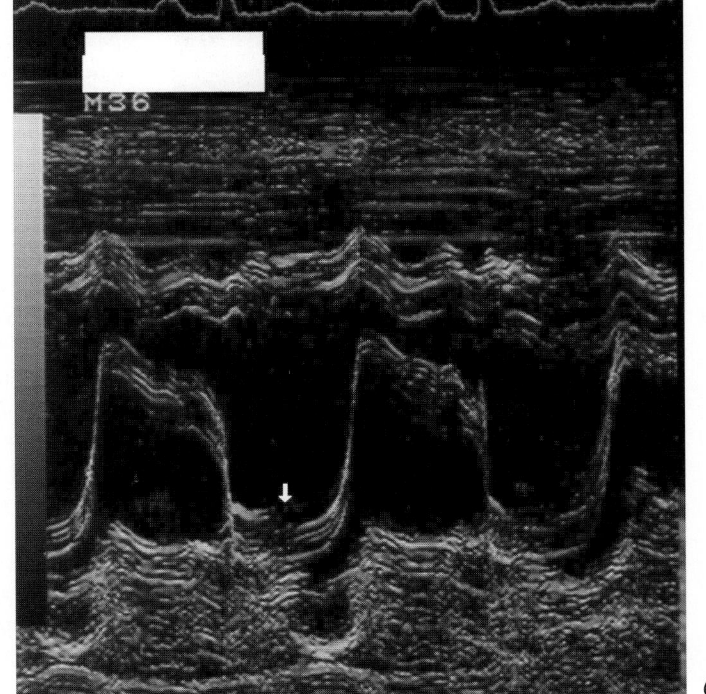

Fig. 8.26 *(cont'd)* (c,d) Holosystolic prolapse is noted (arrow).

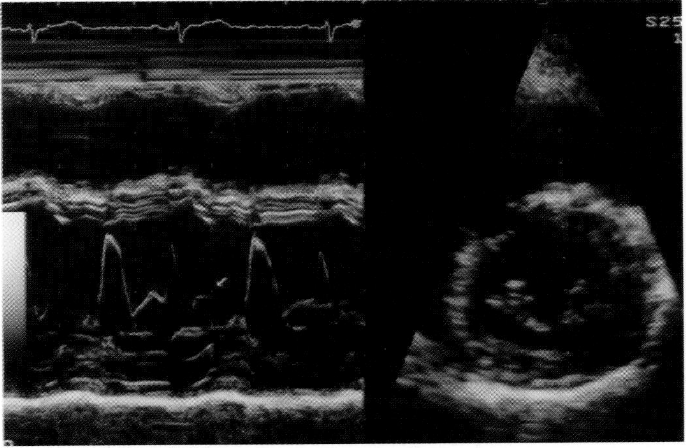

Fig. 8.27 M-mode (left panel) and 2-D parasternal short axis (right panel) images at the level of the mitral valve reveal early systolic anterior motion of mitral chordae (arrow).

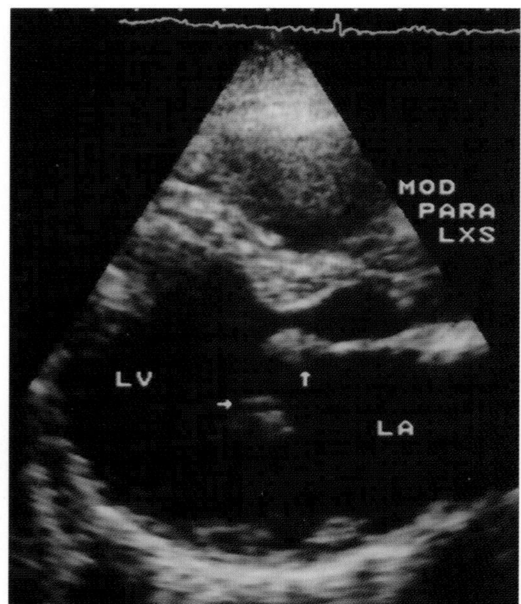

(a)

(b)

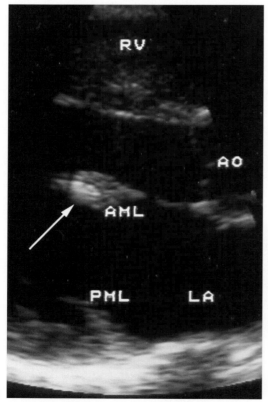

Fig. 8.28 Parasternal long axis images of myxomatous degeneration of the mitral valve. The leaflets are thickened, most notably near the leaflet edges (arrows).

Diameter measurements are made using the inner-edge to inner-edge technique in early diastole.

If the left ventricular cavity is reduced in size, such as with hypovolemia or a significant left-to-right shunt, the mitral chordal structures may become elongated relative to the small size of the LV and leaflet billowing may result.

Flail mitral valve

A *flail mitral valve* is most commonly caused by *chordae rupture*, and less commonly by a *ruptured papillary muscle*. Chordal rupture may occur as a result of myxomatous degeneration, blunt chest trauma, and infective endocarditis. Papillary muscle rupture (see Chapter 13) most commonly may result from trauma or myocardial infarction. M-mode criteria suggesting a flail mitral leaflet (Fig. 8.30) include:

- holosystolic posterior leaflet displacement
- posterior leaflet moves anteriorly in early systole
- coarse diastolic fluttering of the mitral leaflet
- fine systolic fluttering of the mitral leaflet
- valve echos noted in the left atrium in systole.

Two-dimensional criteria for diagnosis of flail mitral valve leaflet include:

- absence of mitral leaflet coaptation (note that this is the definition of prolapse according to the Carpentier surgical criteria—see Chapter 15)
- sudden whipping of chordae from the left ventricle to the left atrium (Fig. 8.31)
- prolapse of part of the leaflet into the left atrium just after the P wave (before the QRS onset) and continuing into systole
- systolic fluttering of the valve in the left atrium—about 20% of patients
- diastolic "chaotic" motion of leaflets best seen in the parasternal short axis view—about 65% of patients.

Transesophageal echocardiography (TEE) is the best method for diagnosis and evaluation of flail mitral leaflet (Fig. 8.32; see also Fig. 15.11). TEE also enables characterization of the resulting mitral regurgitant jet (see Fig. 15.11).

Diagnosis and quantification of mitral regurgitation

M-mode and 2-D echocardiographic diagnosis of mitral regurgitation (or any other regurgitant lesion) is somewhat limited. These modalities do help in

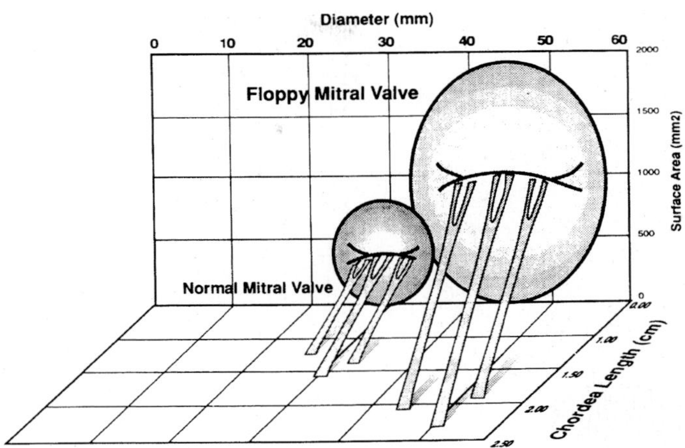

Fig. 8.29 The *mitral annulus diameter* and hence *mitral annulus area* may be increased with myxomatous degeneration. *Chordal elongation* may lead to leaflet billowing into the left atrium. Mitral regurgitation results when there is inadequate leaflet coaptation along the line of closure. (Reproduced with permission from: Fontana ME, Sparks EA, Boudoulas H, Wooley CF. Mitral valve prolapse and the mitral valve prolapse syndrome. Current Problems in Cardiology 1991; 16(5): 328.)

determination of the etiology of MR and the effect of the MR on LV size and function. M-mode and 2-D clues to the presence of MR (Fig. 8.33) include:

• incomplete valve closure in systole—rheumatic MR
• increased atrial emptying volume
• increased left ventricular diastolic volume—volume overload
• abnormal systolic aortic valve closure
• exaggerated left ventricular septal motion—volume overload
• increased systolic expansion of the left atrium posterior wall—not often present
• "bowing" of the atrial septum toward the right throughout the cardiac cycle.

The continuous wave (CW) Doppler *signal intensity* is generally proportional to the number of red blood cells in the regurgitant jet. As MR severity increases, the normal *pulmonary vein flow pattern* will change (Fig. 8.34; see also Fig. 6.16). Mild to moderate MR is associated with a diminished pulmonary vein (PV) systolic: diastolic ratio, and a prominent atrial reversal wave (see Chapter 6). With 4+ MR, PV systolic flow reversal may be seen. Although evaluation of PV flow is often possible with transthoracic echocardiography (TTE), evaluation is best obtained using TEE with PW Doppler about 1 cm deep into the PV. Unilateral PV flow reversal may occur with eccentric MR jets. This may be one mechanism of unilateral pulmonary edema. Usually PV systolic flow reversal is indicative of severe MR, but a relatively small volume jet directed into a single PV may cause systolic flow reversal.

With severe MR, *mitral inflow patterns* have a "restrictive" pattern due to elevated pressure in the LA. "Significant" MR has been associated with a mitral E wave of more than 1.3 m/ s. Severe MR may be associated with a mitral inflow E wave greater than 1.5–1.8 m/s and a deceleration time (DT) less than 150 ms. Although initial E velocities are also high with mitral stenosis, the DT is relatively slow.

A CW *peak velocity* of 4 m/s or less suggests an elevated LA pressure. A higher CW velocity tends to correlate with a normal LA pressure and a large gradient between LV and LA. The *"cut-off" sign* is indicative of a rapid rise in LA pressure in systole often seen in acute severe MR (Fig. 8.35). The rapid rise in pressure in a normal-sized LA will decrease the gradient between LV and LA and cut off the pressure gradient during late systole.

Evaluation of systolic function (dp/dt) is discussed in Chapter 5 (see Fig. 5.11).

By comparing the total pixel intensity of the CW mitral regurgitant jet to the total pixel intensity of forward LVOT flow, one may theoretically calculate the regurgitant fraction (RF) of MR. The total pixel intensity of a CW jet is termed *backscatter power*, and is proportional to the number of objects that an ultrasound beam reflects off, back to the transducer; that is, for a larger number of red corpuscles in a jet, the more intense the CW Doppler signal. If the transmit power and gain are held constant, then the intensity of the LVOT and MR flow (by CW Doppler) are proportional to the number of red corpuscles in each jet, and the following equation may be applied:

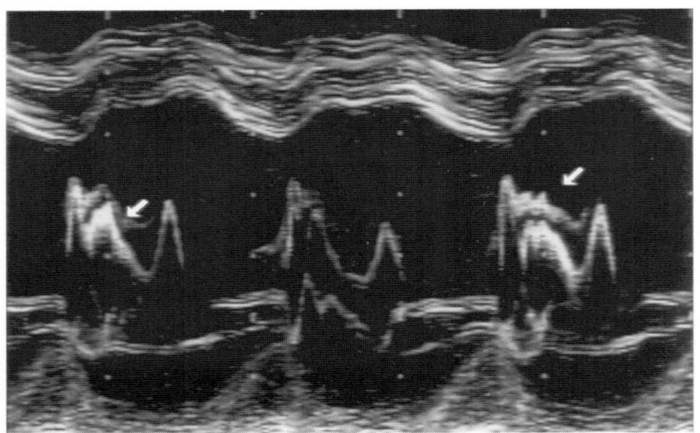
(a)

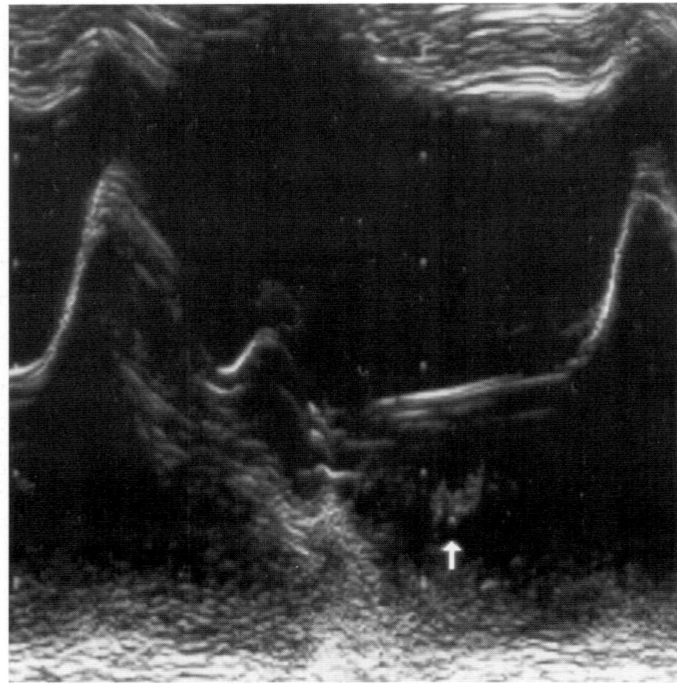
(b)

Fig. 8.30 (a) M-mode image of a flail chordal attachment to the anterior leaflet of the mitral valve. Note diastolic fluttering (arrows). (b) M-mode image of a patient with a flail mitral leaflet. Note echos within the left atrium during systole.

$$RF = (MR - LVOT_{flow})/MR$$

$$RF = 1 - LVOT_{flow}/MR$$

and

$$RF = 1 - (LVOT_{total\ pixel\ intensity})/(MR_{total\ pixel\ intensity})$$

(As the signal intensity gray-scale display is usually logarithmically compressed, each sequential pixel intensity value is not linearly related as to returning ultrasound beam intensity, and must be mathematically adjusted.)

Color flow Doppler helps in characterizing and quantitating MR. The *jet direction* into the LA helps identify the mitral abnormality causing the MR (see Chapter 15 & Fig. 15.7) (Table 8.2).

Evaluation of the *regurgitant jet area* is helpful in semiquantification of MR (Fig. 8.36). Color Doppler measures velocity, however, and not regurgitant

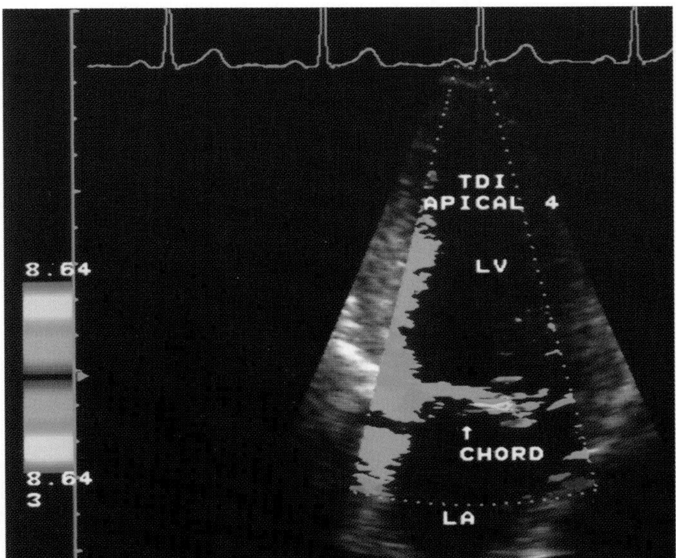

Fig. 8.31 Tissue Doppler imaging (TDI) in an apical view of a patient with a flail mitral chordae. TDI helped identify the chordae "whipping" into the LA during systole.

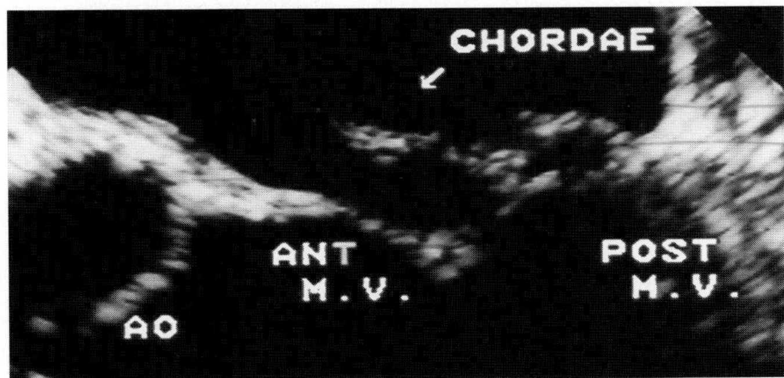

Fig. 8.32 TEE in the horizontal plane in a patient with a flail posterior mitral valve leaflet. Chordae are noted to extend into the LA during systole. Note the lack of apposition of the valve leaflets. ANT M.V., anterior mitral valve leaflet; POST M.V., posterior mitral valve leaflet; AO, aortic valve.

volume. Therefore, this technique is only an approximation. To avoid underestimation of the regurgitant jet (low gain settings), one should turn the gain initially maximally, then "dial down" the gain setting slowly until a good color image is obtained, with the maximal color gain setting possible used.

The MR *jet width* at the mitral leaflet level (best visualized with TEE) seems to correlate with severity of regurgitation. A width of less than 0.4 cm is mild, and a width greater than 0.6 cm moderate to severe MR.

A regurgitant jet may wrap around and "hug" the left atrial wall. The severity of MR is easily underestimated when this occurs, in that energy is dissipated when a jet contacts adjacent structures. This loss of momentum and velocity is termed the *Coanda effect.*

The principle of using *PISA* for the calculation of mitral valve area in mitral stenosis, and the effective orifice area for mitral regurgitation, is discussed in Chapter 3 (see Figs 3.12 & 3.13). *Jet momentum* is based on the *law of conservation of momentum.* The principle of jet momentum as it may potentially be applied to quantification of mitral regurgitation is discussed in Chapter 3.

The following is a list of several signs of severe mitral regurgitation (adapted from Dr Nelson Schiller) and things to watch out for when evaluating a patient with mitral regurgitation:

- the jet is wall hugging—Coanda effect
- the jet enters the LAA
- the jet enters the pulmonary veins (PV) and PV systolic flow reversal is noted

(a)

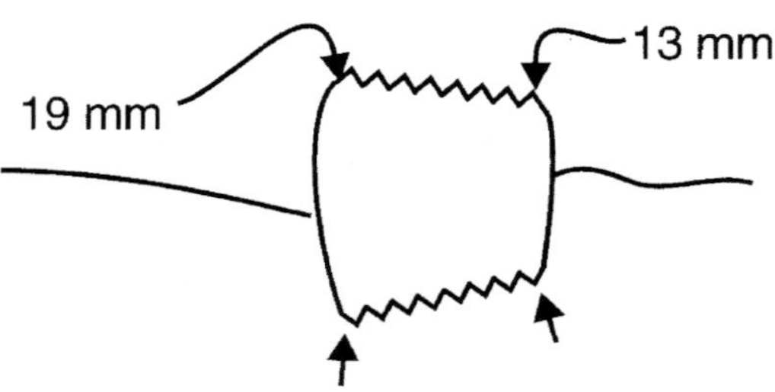

(b)

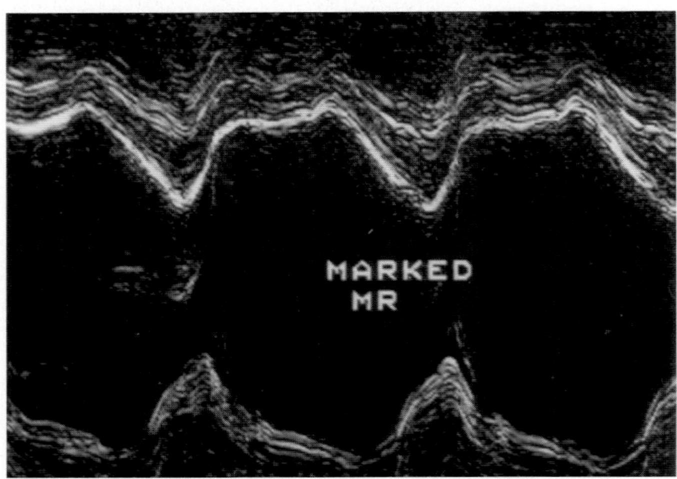

Fig. 8.33 (a) An M-mode image of an aortic valve in a patient with severe mitral regurgitation (MR). The aortic valve leaflet opens normally, but gradually closes during systole due to a low forward stroke volume. This pattern may be also seen with marked LV systolic dysfunction and reduced stroke volume. Early systolic aortic valve closure, similar to that of *subaortic stenosis*, may also be seen. (b) M-mode image of the LV in a patient with sudden severe MR demonstrating exaggerated posterior wall and septal motion, consistent with LV volume overload.

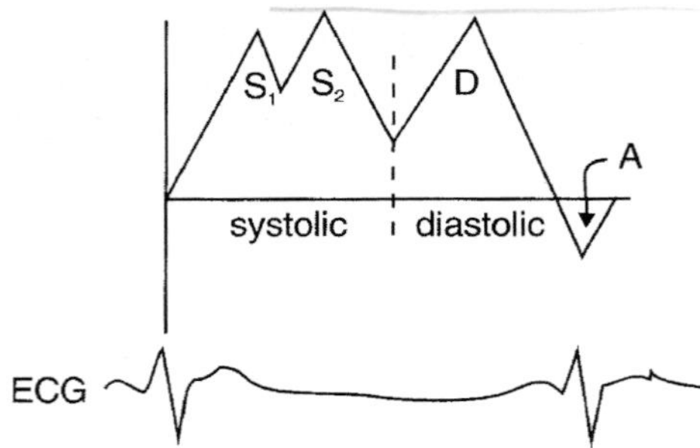

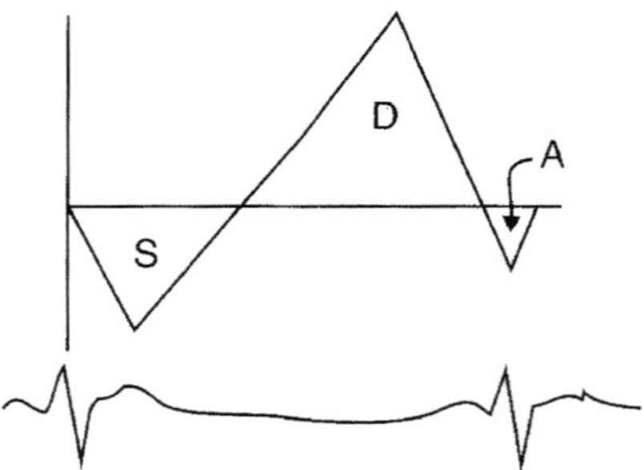

Fig. 8.34 Pulsed wave Doppler of pulmonary vein flow normally, and with 4+ mitral regurgitation.

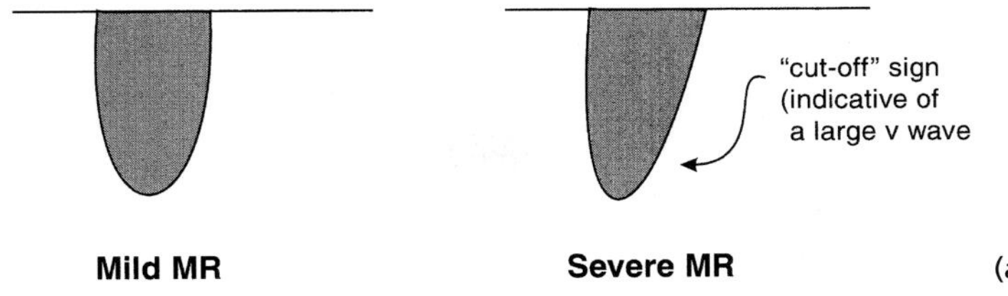

Fig. 8.35 The "cut-off" sign is indicative of a rapid equalization of LA and LV pressures due to severe MR. (a) The usually symmetric waveform (left panel) becomes asymmetric (right panel) with severe MR. (b) CW Doppler through the mitral annulus, from the apical four-chamber view, in a patient with a recent myocardial infarction and sudden shock. 2-D echo revealed rupture of an entire papillary muscle. Note that the MR jet has only a peak velocity of 2.5 m/s, and a very prominent cut-off sign (arrow), consistent with severe MR.

Table 8.2 Utility of jet direction in identifying etiology of MR.

Defect	*Jet direction*
Prolapse/flail	
Posterior leaflet	Anterior direction
Anterior leaflet	Posterior direction
Papillary muscle infarction	
Posteromedial	Posteromedial commissure → posterolaterally
Anterolateral	Anterolateral commissure → posteromedially
Mitral annulus dilatation	Central
Rheumatic	Posterior (posterior leaflet restriction to opening)

- the jet circles the entire left atrium
- "agitated" flow is seen in the left atrium—simultaneous appearance of multiple colors in the left atrium
- spontaneous echo contrast is almost never seen, except in a very large left atrium
- CW demonstrates a cut-off sign or at least a very "strong" signal
- mitral inflow demonstrates an increased TVI
- mitral inflow E velocity is greater than 1.5–1.8 m/s
- if the mitral inflow demonstrates A wave predominance (abnormal relaxation), it is unlikely that severe or even moderate MR is present
- LA size expands with systole
- the LA is dilated (not necessarily in acute MR)
- a diminished forward stroke volume is noted by pulsed wave Doppler in the aorta
- in the most severe forms spontaneous echo contrast is noted in the thoracic aorta

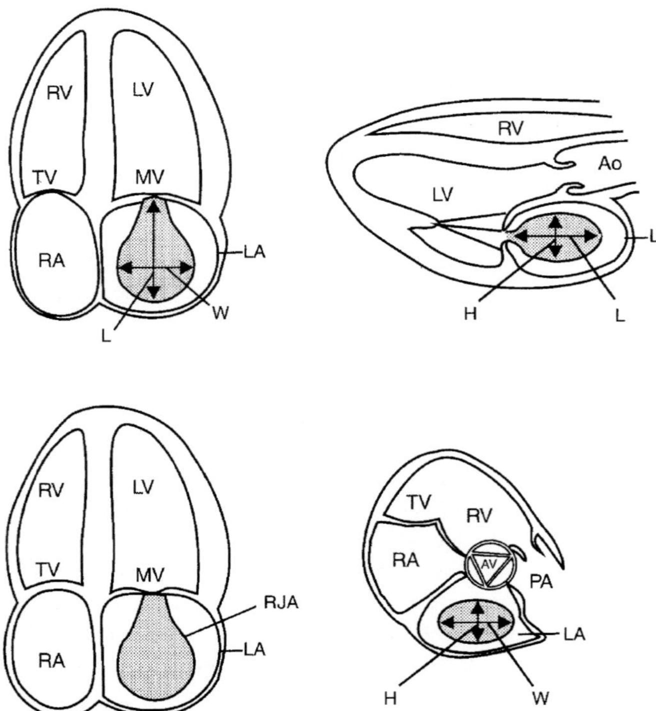

Fig. 8.36 Color flow images of MR are compared with the LA size. The maximal regurgitant jet (RJA) to left atrial area (LA) ratio correlates with severity. Mild <25%, moderate 25–50%, and severe >50%. Multiple factors including gain settings affect the color jet.

• the LV appears "globular" with an increased end-diastolic volume and preserved or increased ejection fraction

• PISA radius is prominent

• pulmonary artery flow is diminished (TVI <15 cm)

• width of the MR jet is greater than 0.6 cm (color Doppler) at the mitral valve

• large regurgitant jet (color) area is visualized—be careful!

• the atrial septum bulges toward the RA with no diastolic reversal

• especially with TEE evaluate valve anatomy for vegetations, ruptured chordae, or leaflet.

CHAPTER 9

Right Heart, Pulmonary Artery, and Ventricular Septum

Echo-derived *right ventricular volumes* from biplane two-dimensional (2-D) echocardiograms seem to underestimate the volumes obtained using biplane angiography. Calculation of the *RV ejection fraction* is also made difficult by the presence of marked RV trabeculations, resulting in a problem tracing the endocardial border. Evaluation of *right ventricular hypertrophy* (RVH) is accurate, however. The *right ventricular free wall*, usually best measured from a parasternal long axis and sometimes a subcostal position, is used. An end-diastolic free wall thickness of less than 5 mm is considered normal. The shape of the interventricular septum may be accurately described using an *eccentricity index*, defined from a short axis parasternal view as the ratio of the length of two perpendicular diameters through the LV, one of which bisects the mid-ventricular septum. The ratio is normally 1 : 1 in end-diastole and end-systole. With *RV pressure overload* the index is greater than 1 in both end-diastole and end-systole, whereas with *RV volume overload* only the end-diastolic ratio is less than 1 (Fig. 9.1), with the end-systolic ratio normal.

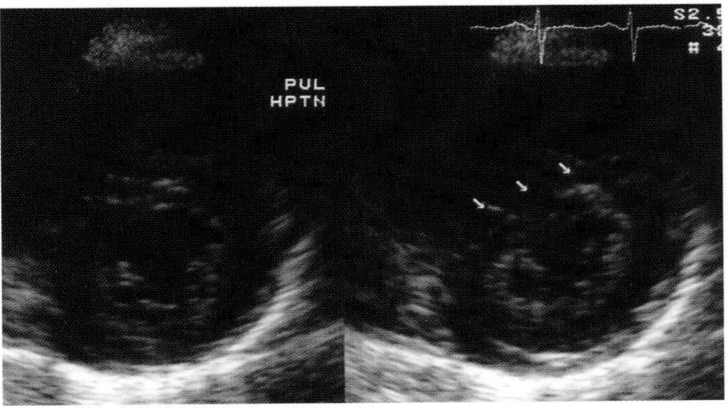

(a)

(b)

Fig. 9.1 (a) Parasternal short axis view in (right panel) end-systole, and (left panel) end-diastole in a patient with pulmonary hypertension and right heart pressure overload. Having septal flattening in systole suggests *right heart pressure overload*, whereas ventricular septal flattening in diastole suggests *right heart volume overload.* Septal flattening in both systole and diastole (b) is suggestive of right heart pressure and volume overload.

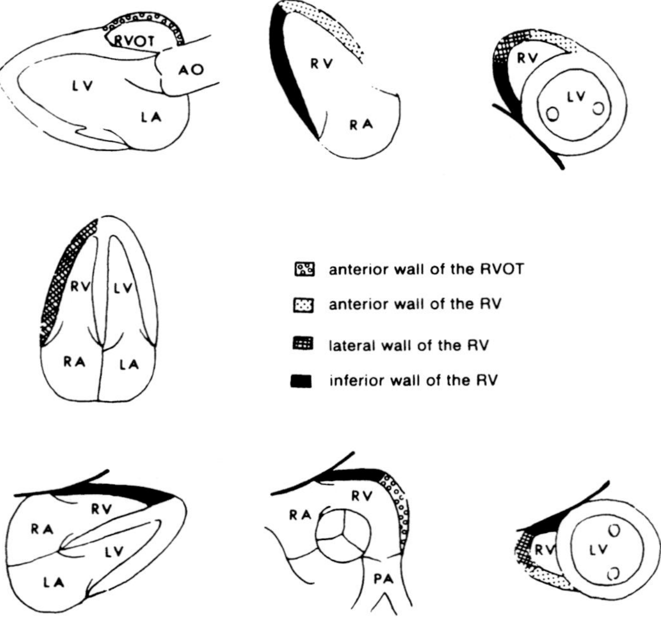

Fig. 9.2 System for identifying and evaluating right ventricular segments. Parasternal (upper three images), apical (middle image), and subcostal (lower three images) may all characterize these segments for hypertrophy, thinning, and function. (Reproduced with permission from: Jiang L, Wiegers SE, Weyman AE. Right ventricle. In: Weyman AE, ed. Principles and Practice of Echocardiography, 2nd edn. Philadelphia: Lea and Febiger, 1994: 916.)

The *right ventricle* may be divided into four segments and these are readily identified from various transthoracic windows (Fig. 9.2). The *tricuspid valve* is made of the *anterior leaflet* (from the infundibulum to the inferolateral wall), the *septal leaflet* (attached to membranous and muscular septum and *apically displaced relative to anterior mitral leaflet*), and the *posterior leaflet* (septum to inferolateral wall). The *posterior papillary muscle* and *septal papillary muscle* are attached to the RV wall, and the *anterior papillary muscle* originates from both the moderator band and the RV wall.

Right ventricular dysplasia (*arrhythmogenic right ventricular dysplasia*) involves adipose infiltration of right ventricular myocardium, either diffusely or focally. Echo reveals RV enlargement with diffuse or local dysfunction of the RV free wall. The free wall thickness may be thin or normal. *Local aneurysms* are classic but not always present. Other causes of RV enlargement should be ruled out (Ebstein's, partial anomalous pulmonary venous return, atrial septal defect (ASD), and congenital partial absence of the left pericardium).

Tricuspid stenosis

Tricuspid stenosis (TS) is unusual and is most often due to *rheumatic* heart disease (see Chapter 8). It is associated with rheumatic mitral valve disease and probably occurs in less than 5% of patients with mitral stenosis. TS is easily missed when evaluating a patient with rheumatic heart disease. A markedly dilated right atrium should serve as a clue to possible TS. As with the mitral valve, commissural fusion and diastolic leaflet doming occur secondary to the rheumatic process. *Doming*, *thickening*, and *restricted motion* of the tricuspid leaflets are usually noted. Doming is best seen in the modified parasternal long axis or apical views. M-mode may reveal a decreased EF slope with anterior motion in diastole of the posterior leaflet similar to that noted in mitral stenosis (Figs 9.3 & 9.4).

Doppler evaluation for TS may be difficult. The tricuspid gradient may be as low as 2 mmHg, but it may rise to 5 mmHg or more after saline infusion. Usually rheumatic TS will have associated significant tricuspid regurgitation (TR). Whereas patients with TR alone generally have a high initial continuous wave (CW) E velocity (almost 1 m/s) and a rapid deceleration time, those patients with TS, however, will have a slow deceleration time. (Fig. 9.5). It is important to obtain the tricuspid maximum E velocity, mean valve gradient, and deceleration time. A pressure half-time formula has not been verified for tricuspid stenosis, and therefore cannot be used in the calculation of tricuspid valve area (normal tricuspid valve area is 6–7 cm^2).

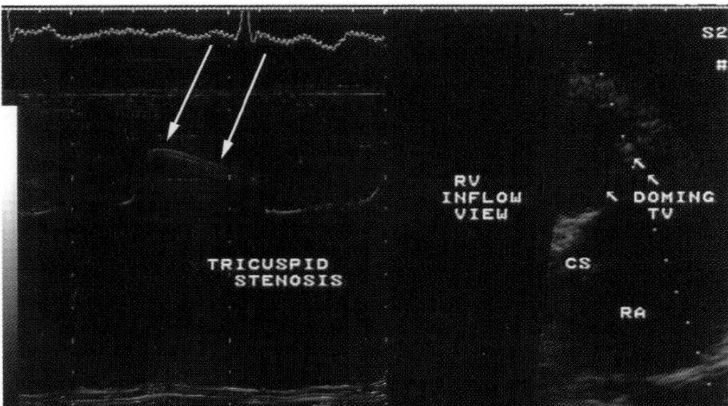

Fig. 9.3 Rheumatic tricuspid stenosis in a patient with right heart failure. M-mode of the tricuspid valve (left panel) reveals a diminished EF slope and valve thickening (double arrow). Two-dimensional echo from the parasternal RV inflow view (right panel) reveals tricuspid valve doming.

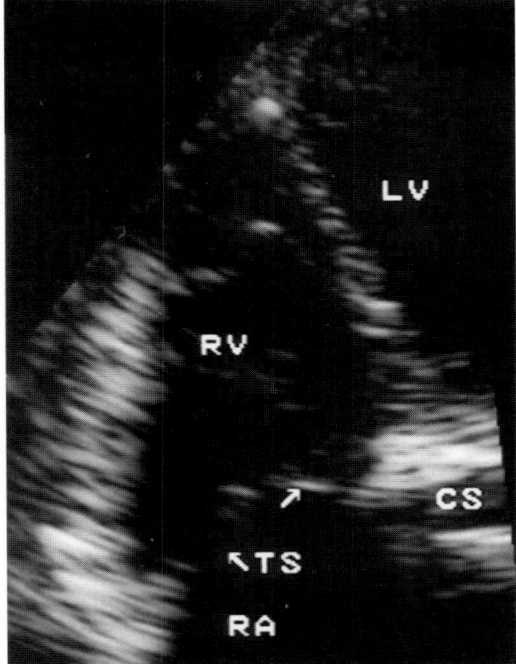

Fig. 9.4 2-D echocardiogram from the four-chamber view of tricuspid stenosis with noted valve doming (arrows) and leaflet thickening. CS, coronary sinus.

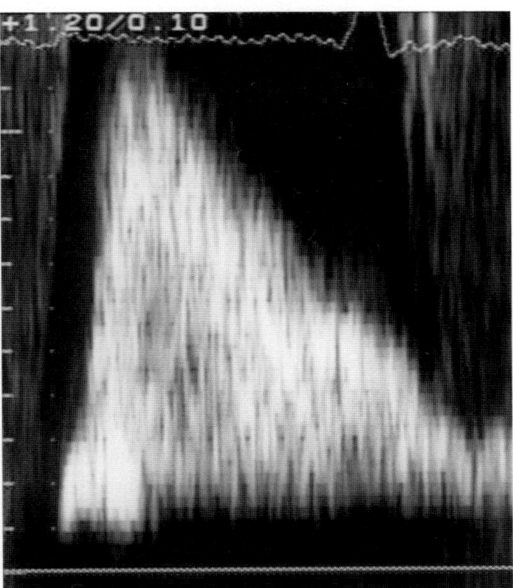

Fig. 9.5 Continuous wave (CW) Doppler of a patient with significant tricuspid stenosis. The maximum velocity is 1.2 m/s and the deceleration time is delayed. The patient is in atrial fibrillation. A patient with tricuspid regurgitation and no tricuspid stenosis may have an increased initial E wave velocity, but the deceleration time will be rapid.

Other causes of tricuspid stenosis include:

- a result of a *foreign body* such as a transvenous pacemaker wire across the tricuspid annulus causing fibrosis of the wire and valve (rare)
- *right atrial tumor* causing obstruction of tricuspid flow (primary cardiac tumor or metastatic lesion)
- *carcinoid heart disease*, but the patient usually will have predominately tricuspid regurgitation with some element of tricuspid stenosis (see Chapter 21)
- *prosthetic heart valve* as thrombus may form despite adequate anticoagulant therapy (mechanical heart valve) because of low right heart flow. Annuloplasty rings may be stenotic from the time of insertion (Fig. 9.6).

Tricuspid regurgitation

Tricuspid regurgitation (TR) causes volume overload of the RA and RV, and will cause right heart dilatation.

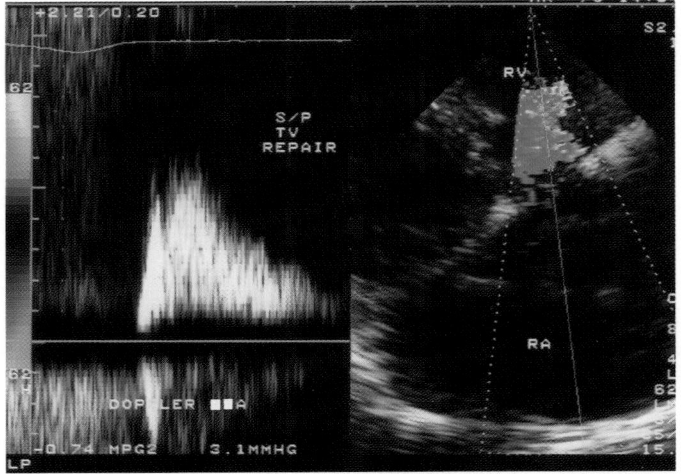

Fig. 9.6 Parasternal RV inflow with color Doppler and CW Doppler of a patient several months post tricuspid annuloplasty ring placement. The patient's RA is markedly dilated, and CW Doppler confirms tricuspid stenosis. The maximum velocity is 1.1 cm/s and the deceleration time is prolonged.

The RV shape will change, with a "D" shape (flattened ventricular septum) noted in diastole (see Fig. 9.1). Right ventricular hypertrophy (RVH) may be seen, and occasionally asymmetric septal hypertrophy, a dilated and pulsatile IVC and hepatic vein, a dilated coronary sinus, and systolic bowing of the interatrial septum toward the LA (severe TR) will be noted. A rapid anterior motion of the interventricular septum is seen at the onset of systole (isovolumic contraction) in RV volume overload (seen with any cause of RV volume overload), and this is one form of *paradoxical ventricular septal motion.* Injection of agitated saline contrast into a peripheral vein with subsequent systolic appearance (and persistence) in the IVC or hepatic veins indicates severe TR.

Color flow Doppler may be used to help quantify TR. One can calculate the ratio of the color Doppler tricuspid regurgitation jet area (TRJ) to the right atrial area (RAA). If the TRJ/RAA ratio is less than 20% the TR is considered mild, if the ratio is 20–34% the TR is considered moderate, and if the ratio is higher than 35% the TR is considered severe. By pulsed wave Doppler, reproducible systolic retrograde flow into the hepatic vein during suspended respiration is consistent with moderate to severe TR.

A dark and intense continuous wave Doppler signal usually indicates at least moderate TR. A duration of longer than 100 ms is usually considered significant. Marked TR is associated with an increased forward tricuspid flow velocity (but usually <1 m/s) and a rapid tricuspid inflow deceleration time. An early peaking TR jet by CW with a TR "cut-off" sign (similar to that seen with acute severe MR) is consistent with severe TR and is associated with early equalization of RA and RV pressures. A large "*V*" *wave* in the jugular venous pulsation may be seen on physical examination. Marked respiratory variation with a decreased TR velocity with inspiration suggests an elevated RA pressure with inspiration (decreased pressure gradient from RV to RA with resultant decreased TR velocity jet)—*Kussmaul's sign* on physical examination (Fig. 9.7).

TR results from either *functional changes* (normal tricuspid leaflets with an enlarged tricuspid annulus most commonly secondary to pulmonary hypertension) or *structural changes* (altered tricuspid valve anatomy). Structural etiologies of tricuspid regurgitation include:

• *Rheumatic*—(see "Tricuspid stenosis" above). Tricuspid regurgitation is commonly associated with tricuspid stenosis.

• *Tricuspid valve prolapse*—occurs in ~20% of mitral valve prolapse, associated with *Marfan's syndrome, secundum type atrial septal defect*, and *Ebstein's anomaly.* A 2-mm posterior displacement in mid–late systole by M-mode or seen by 2-D imaging, usually involves the *anterior tricuspid leaflet.*

• *Ebstein's anomaly*—(see Chapter 16). Apical displacement of the tricuspid valve with the color regurgitant jet originating closer to the RV apex.

• *Carcinoid*—(see Chapter 21). Tricuspid regurgitation will usually predominate over tricuspid stenosis.

• *Infective endocarditis*—(see Chapter 18). Tricuspid vegetations are often larger than aortic or mitral vegetations. Often the organism is *Staphylococcus* sp. or *Candida* sp.

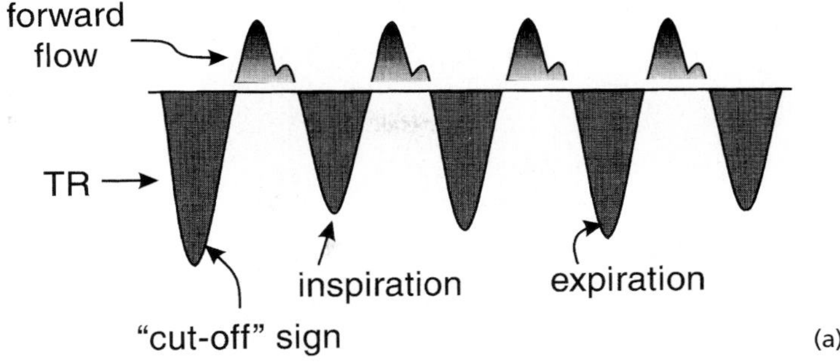

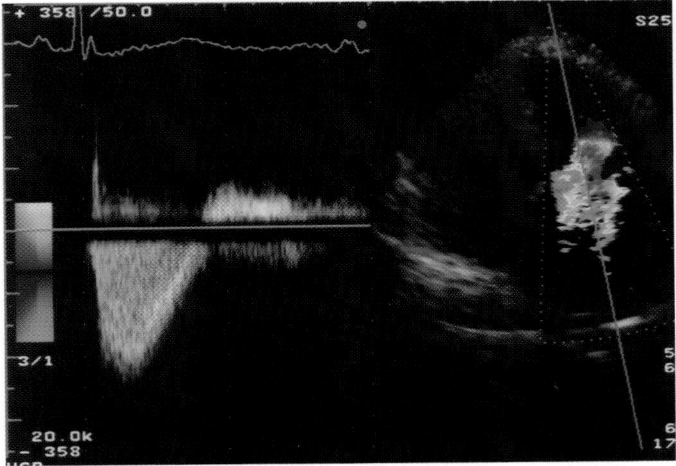

Fig. 9.7 (a) Severe tricuspid regurgitation (TR) by CW Doppler demonstrating respiratory variation and a "cut-off" sign. (b) Right panel is a four-chamber view with color Doppler demonstrating tricuspid regurgitation. CW Doppler (left panel) reveals an early peaking TR jet and a prominent "cut-off" sign, indicative of severe TR with equalization of RV and RA pressures.

- *Papillary muscle dysfunction*—may occur with right ventricular infarction, chordal rupture or papillary rupture. LV function may be relatively preserved.
- *Trauma*—tricuspid regurgitation may result from blunt chest trauma with chordal or papillary injury. The patient may present several years after the original injury.
- *Foreign body*—electrodes may injure the tricuspid apparatus by inhibiting chordal motion or occasionally the tricuspid leaflet.

Infundibulum and pulmonic valve

Valvular pulmonic stenosis (PS) accounts for 80% of right ventricular outflow tract (RVOT) obstruction. PS is usually congenital, but may rarely occur with rheumatic valvulitis or with carcinoid (see Chapter 21). RVOT obstruction may be classified as the following:

- *Subvalvular pulmonary stenosis*:
  discrete subpulmonary stenosis—obstruction between the RV and conus with a ridge at the level of the infundibular ostium; the infundibulum and pulmonic valve (PV) is usually normal
  double chambered right ventricle—muscle band across the RV; color Doppler helps localize turbulent flow; commonly associated with a ventricular septal defect (VSD) and sometimes valvular PS or discrete subaortic stenosis.
- *Valvular and infundibular stenosis*:
  pulmonic stenosis (PS)—80% of RVOT obstruction; usually tricuspid leaflets with valve cusp fusion
  tetralogy of Fallot—commonly associated with unicuspid or bicuspid pulmonic valve
  valvular and infundibular stenosis—hypertrophy of RV walls/conus; pulmonic annulus is normal; no poststenotic pulmonary artery dilatation
  hypoplastic valve annulus/conus—usually manifest in infancy with critical pulmonic stenosis; narrowed and hypoplastic trabeculated pulmonic valve annulus; small hypertrophied RV; usually dependent on a PDA for circulation; TV abnormalities may be associated.

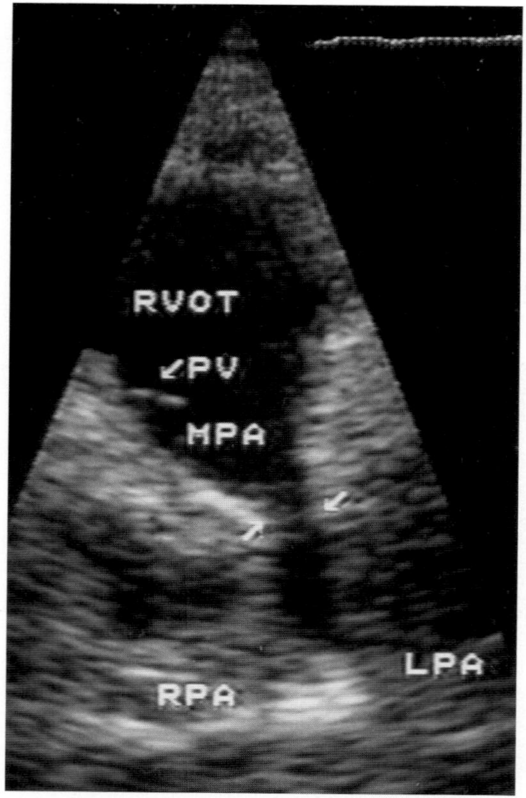

(a)

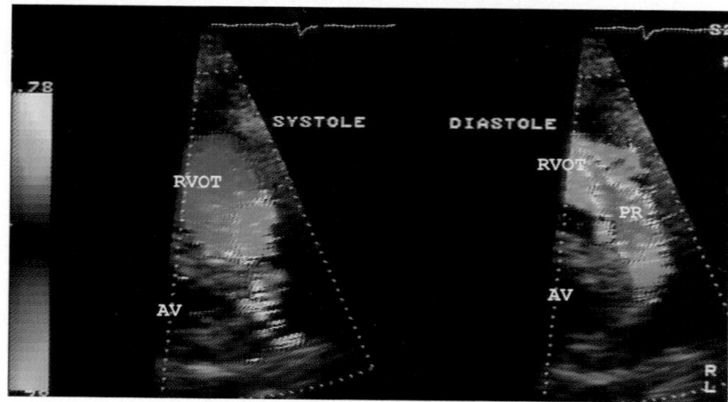

(b)

Fig. 9.8 Parasternal short axis two-dimensional (2-D) image of a patient with repaired tetralogy of Fallot. (a) The 2-D image demonstrates supravalvular pulmonic stenosis. (b) Color Doppler in systole reveals flow turbulence at the level of obstruction, and in diastole significant pulmonic regurgitation. MPA, main pulmonary artery; RPA, right pulmonary artery; LPA, left pulmonary artery; PV, pulmonic valve; RVOT, right ventricular outflow tract.

- *Supravalvular (pulmonary artery stenosis)* (Fig. 9.8) —most have several stenotic areas; discrete stenosis or tubular hypoplasia; involves the main pulmonary artery or branches; unexplained marked RVH and marked pulsation of the proximal pulmonary arteries are suggestive—pulsation is caused from diastolic runoff into the branch pulmonary arteries with a resultant low PA diastolic pressure and widened PA pulse pressure; tubular hypoplasia of the main PA is associated with rubella and Williams syndrome.

The *Noonan Syndrome* may demonstrate:

- PV leaflets thickened/myxomatous with stenosis
- PV dysplasia (<10%)
- PS without dysplasia (<20%)

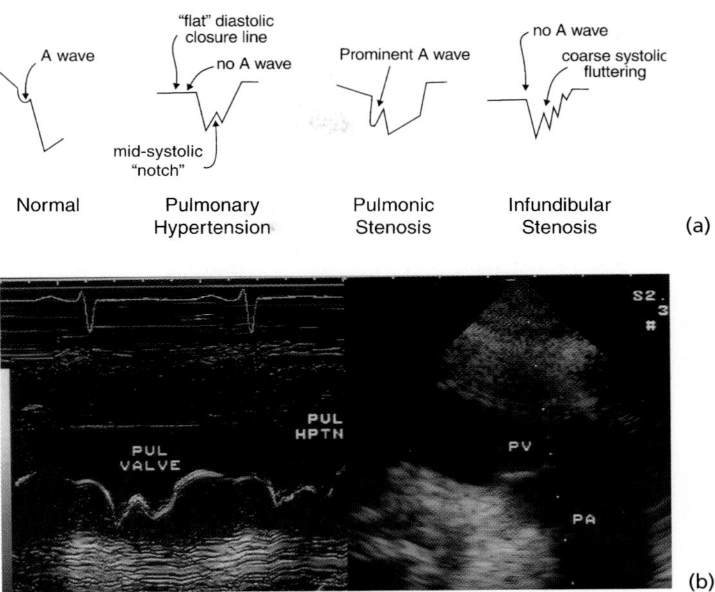

Fig. 9.9 (a) M-mode patterns of the pulmonic valve taken from a high parasternal view. With pulmonary hypertension, the diastolic closure line is generally "flat," but the "A" wave may reappear with development of coexistent right ventricular failure. *Idiopathic dilated pulmonary artery* may be also associated with a mid-systolic "notch." Infundibular stenosis may not exhibit coarse systolic fluttering of the pulmonic valve with coexistent valvular pulmonic stenosis, and the A wave may be present. (b) M-mode (left panel) with 2-D guidance of a patient with pulmonary hypertension. Note a "flat" diastolic line of closure, "A" wave present (suggestive of right heart failure), and a prominent mid-systolic notch.

- left ventricular hypertrophy (LVH) resembling asymmetric septal hypertrophy (ASH) with mostly anterior septal thickening (25%)
- other abnormalities with secundum type ASD most common (10%).

M-mode pulmonic valve patterns will differ with various RVOT obstructive lesions (Fig. 9.9). The mid-systolic pulmonic valve "notch" may not always be found with *pulmonary hypertension. Idiopathic dilated pulmonary artery* (defect in pulmonary artery elastic tissue, sometimes seen in patients with Marfan's syndrome) with normal pulmonary artery pressures may be also associated with this notch. In pulmonary hypertension, the "A" wave may reappear in patients with development of coexistent right ventricular failure.

Pulmonic valve motion may be observed in the parasternal short axis, parasternal long axis through the RVOT, the subcostal four-chamber, and the subcostal short axis views. Two-dimensional signs of *pulmonic valvular stenosis* include: a pulmonic valve annulus of normal size, restricted pulmonic valve leaflet mobility (valve doming), thickened leaflets, leaflets not parallel to the pulmonary artery vessel wall in systole, and RV pressure overload. RV systolic overload is manifested by RV free wall hypertrophy and ventricular septal flattening in systole. Pulmonic leaflets may prolapse into the RVOT in diastole. Usually the pulmonary artery will be dilated with the left pulmonary artery preferentially dilated as compared with the right pulmonary artery (the jet is directed into the left pulmonary artery). Poststenotic dilatation does not correlate with the severity of valve obstruction. The RV should be of normal size, and with severe PS there will be concentric RVH (RV anterior wall thickness does not correlate with the PV gradient) and the infundibulum will be normal or slightly narrowed (hypertrophy). The RA will be dilated with severe PS and the atrial septum will bow to the left (elevated RA pressure from a noncompliant RV). After relief of PS obstruction, RVH regression may not occur for years.

With *infundibular stenosis*, a coarse systolic fluttering due to a high velocity jet striking the pulmonary valve leaflets may extend into diastole. This fluttering may be absent with coexistent valvular pulmonic stenosis. Early closure of the pulmonic valve may be seen. In addition, an "A" wave may be noted on the M-mode pattern.

In patients with *valvular pulmonic stenosis* (PS) the instantaneous peak gradient by CW Doppler may be used to quantify severity (Fig. 9.10). As opposed to that obtained for aortic valvular stenosis, this seems to correlate with the peak-to-peak gradient obtained by

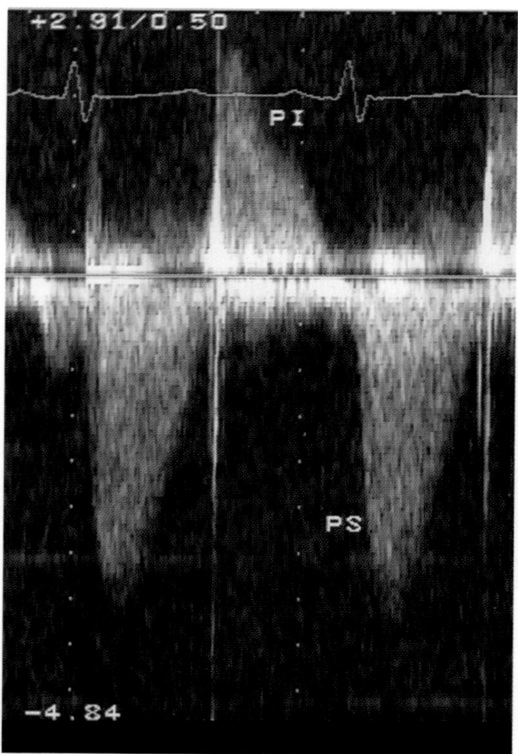

Fig. 9.10 CW Doppler from a high parasternal window of a patient with valvular pulmonic stenosis (PS) with coexistent significant pulmonic regurgitation (PI).

invasive cardiac catheterization. The pulmonary valve area is usually not calculated. Use of color flow Doppler to guide the CW Doppler beam will help obtain the maximum gradient. The jet is usually directed toward the left PA or left lateral main PA. One should use multiple windows including the parasternal short axis (sometimes an intercostal space lower than the best 2-D image will yield a higher gradient), the parasternal long axis of the RVOT, the subcostal short axis, and the subcostal four-chamber view. Subcostal views are generally best in patients with marked poststenotic dilatation. As PS severity increases, the pulmonary acceleration time (AT) to ejection time (ET) ratio (AT/ET) will increase (see also Chapter 7).

Often valvular pulmonic stenosis will coexist with right ventricular infundibular obstruction, secondary to chronic increased pressure in the RVOT. Color Doppler reveals increased and turbulent velocities within the RVOT, as opposed to normal flow in the RVOT with pure valvular PS. By CW Doppler a "concave" mid-late peaking velocity profile will be seen (Fig. 9.11). Because of the phenomenon of pressure recovery, the Doppler gradient by CW may overestimate the catheter-derived gradient.

"Physiologic" *pulmonary regurgitation* (PR) is very common. Pathologic etiologies of PR include: pulmonary artery dilatation, endocarditis (uncommon), malignant carcinoid (usually PS more significant), rheumatic, postoperative PS repair, tetralogy of Fallot, and pulmonary hypertension (Fig. 9.12). PR is considered significant if: the PR jet is "wide," there is pandiastolic regurgitation, and the color jet extends more than 2 cm into the RVOT.

Pulmonary artery and right heart pressure, hepatic vein evaluation

M-mode and 2-D signs of elevated pulmonary artery pressures are discussed earlier. Just as a "B" bump on the M-mode of the MV (see Fig. 6.2) indicates an elevated LV end-diastolic pressure (LVEDP), a "B"

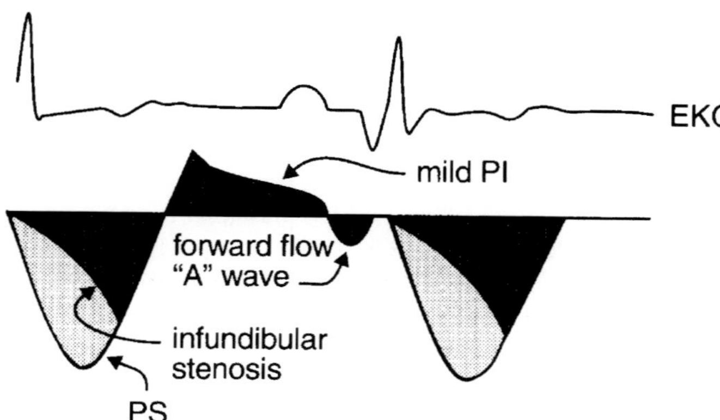

Fig. 9.11 Diagram showing combined pulmonic valvular (PS) and infundibular stenosis. Infundibular stenosis is late-peaking (dynamic obstruction). The "A" wave is forward (out of the pulmonary artery (PA)) and prominent secondary to right ventricular hypertrophy (RVH) and diminished RV compliance.

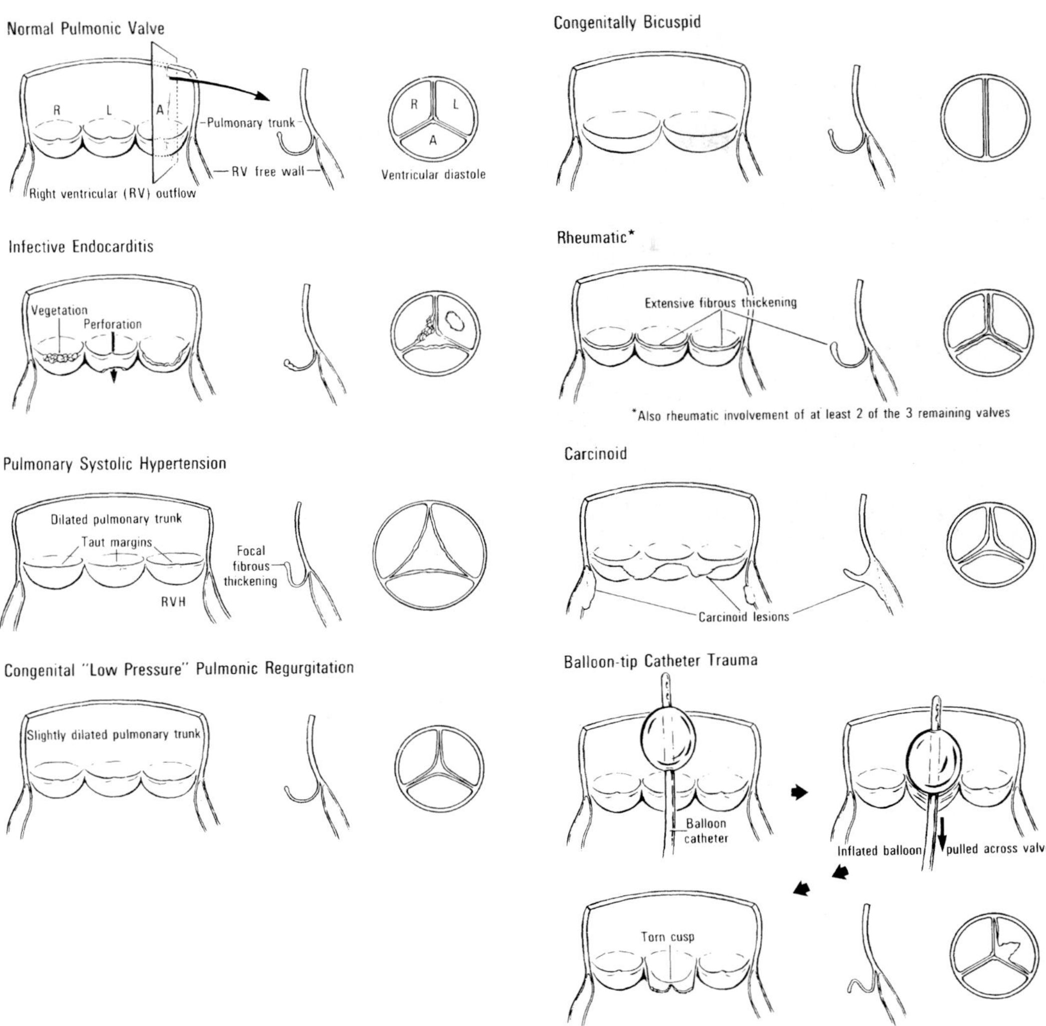

Fig. 9.12 The various etiologies of pure pulmonary regurgitation. (Reproduced with permission from: Waller BF, Block T, Barker BG, *et al*. Evaluation of operatively excised cardiac valves: etiologic determination of valvular heat disease, in Waller BF (guest ed), Symposium on Cardiac Morphology. Cardiology Clinics 1984; 2(4): 703.)

bump on the tricuspid valve indicates an elevated RV end-diastolic pressure (RVEDP) (Fig. 9.13). The most accurate way to calculate pulmonary artery pressures is by Doppler techniques. *Pulmonary artery systolic pressure* (PASP) is calculated using the tricuspid regurgitation CW waveform. PASP estimation should be performed as part of the routine echocardiographic examination. As an adequate TR jet may be obtained in over 90% of patients, this measure should be routinely reported. *Pulmonary artery diastolic pressure* (PADP) may be calculated from the pulmonary regurgitation CW waveform (Fig. 9.14). These calculations use the modified Bernoulli equation.

To calculate the PASP, one should first calculate the RV–RA systolic pressure gradient $[4 \times (TR)^2]$ and add the estimated right atrial pressure (RAP) to that. One should make sure that the maximum TR jet envelope is obtained, as any underestimation of the TR jet velocity will result in an underestimation of the pressure by a "squared" factor (the TR velocity is squared

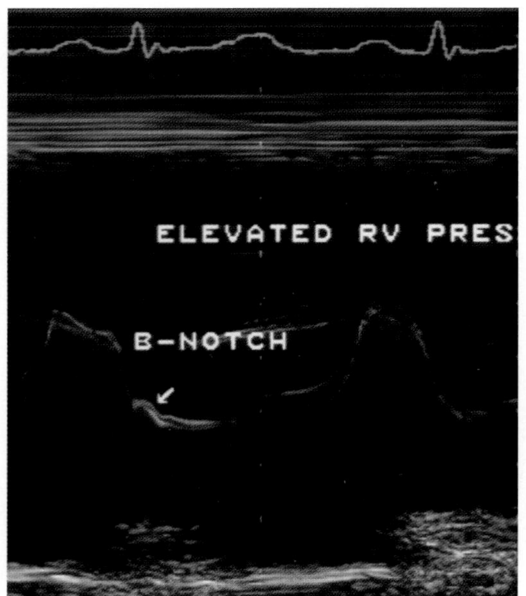

Fig. 9.13 M-mode of the tricuspid valve from a parasternal window demonstrates a tricuspid valve B-notch, consistent with an elevated right ventricular end-diastolic pressure.

in the modified Bernoulli equation). This calculation assumes there is no gradient in systole between the RV and PA (such as infundibular or valvular pulmonic stenosis).

Use of color flow Doppler to image the regurgitant jet helps in proper placement of the CW jet. The sonographers should make sure to always use all possible imaging windows for obtaining the maximum velocity jet (parasternal short axis, parasternal RV inflow, apical four-chamber, and subcostal views). When imaging from the apical four-chamber view, moving the transducer several centimeters toward the midline may help "lineup" the flow jet. One should *avoid crossing the upper ventricular septum with the CW jet* as aortic flow may be inadvertently obtained.

The severity of TR does not equate with the pulmonary artery pressure. If a primary tricuspid valve abnormality exists, the patient may have severe TR but have normal pulmonary artery pressures with relatively low velocities (Fig. 9.15). Likewise, a patient with severe pulmonary hypertension may have a high velocity TR jet, yet only mild TR.

To calculate the PADP, calculate the PA–RV end-diastolic pressure gradient $[4 \times (PA_{ED})^2]$ and add the RA pressure to that. The PA early diastolic pressure gradient (PA_{ear}) between the PA and RV (using the modified Bernoulli equation) seems to correlate with the *PA mean pressure* (PA_{MP}) as:

$$PA_{MP} = 4 \times (PA_{ear})^2$$

Pulmonary vascular resistance (PVR) can be determined by catheterization as:

$$PVR = (PA_{MP} - PC_{WP})/CO$$

where PA_{MP} is pulmonary artery mean pressure, $PA_{MP} = [PA_{DP} + 1/3(PA_{SP} - PA_{DP})]$, PC_{WP} is pulmonary capillary wedge pressure, CO is cardiac output, PA_{DP} is pulmonary artery diastolic pressure, and PA_{SP} is pulmonary artery systolic pressure.

PVR has been described in the echo laboratory using the pulsed wave Doppler signal of pulmonary artery flow at the level of the pulmonic valve. The derived Doppler equation for PVR in the echo laboratory is:

$$PVR = -0.156 + \{1.154 \times [(PEP/AT)/TT]\}$$

where PEP is pulmonic preejection period, AT is pulmonary acceleration time, and TT is total pulmonary systolic time (PEP + ejection time). This equation has been found to correlate with catheter-derived values of PVR in patients with severe heart failure undergoing evaluation for cardiac transplantation.

RV systolic pressure (RV_{SP}) may be calculated from a ventricular septal defect (VSD) jet as:

$$RV_{SP} = LV_{SP} - 4 \times (V_{vsd})^2 + RAP$$

where LV_{SP} is LV systolic pressure and V_{vsd} is peak VSD velocity. The systolic blood pressure (blood pressure cuff) may be substituted for LV_{SP} if there is no LVOT obstruction. The PA_{SP} is obtained in the same way as the RV_{SP} if no obstruction exists between the RV and pulmonary artery. As with TR jets, one should use color Doppler to optimally line up the VSD jet for CW Doppler measurement. When using the VSD method for RV_{SP} measurement, errors may occur, especially in the presence of electrocardiogram conduction delay patterns. The RV and LV peak pressures may occur at a significant time difference, and therefore the instantaneous pressure gradient may be markedly different from the peak RV and peak LV systolic pressure difference.

With pulmonary hypertension the *pulmonary acceleration time* (AT) as measured by PW Doppler at the pulmonic valve annulus level, will shorten. An AT <100 ms is consistent with pulmonary hypertension.

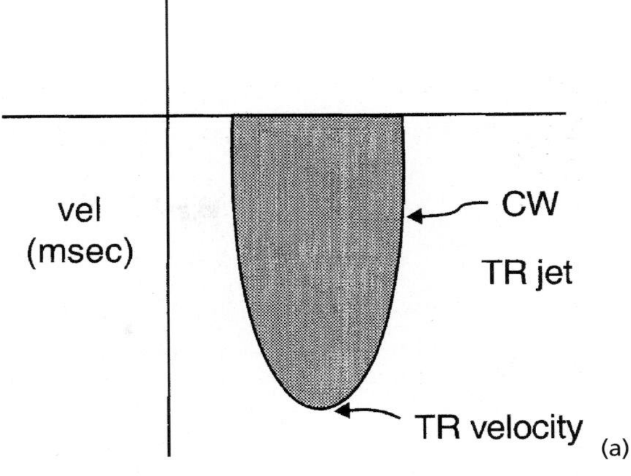

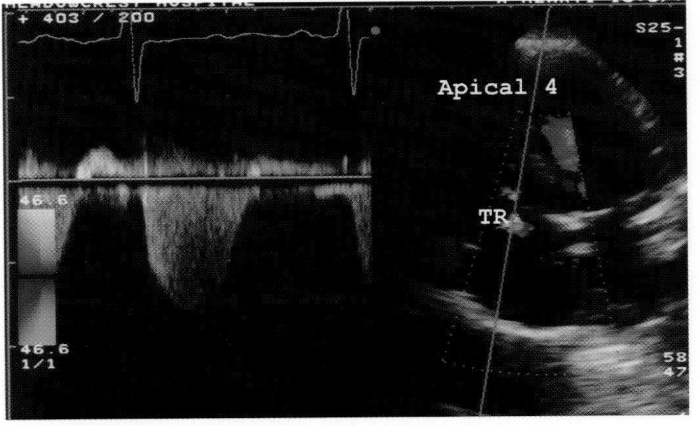

PA Early-Diastolic Velocity (PAEarD)

PA End-Diastolic Velocity (PAED)

vel (msec)

CW

$PADP = [4 \times (PAED)^2] + RAP$

vel (msec)

PAED

"A" wave

(c)

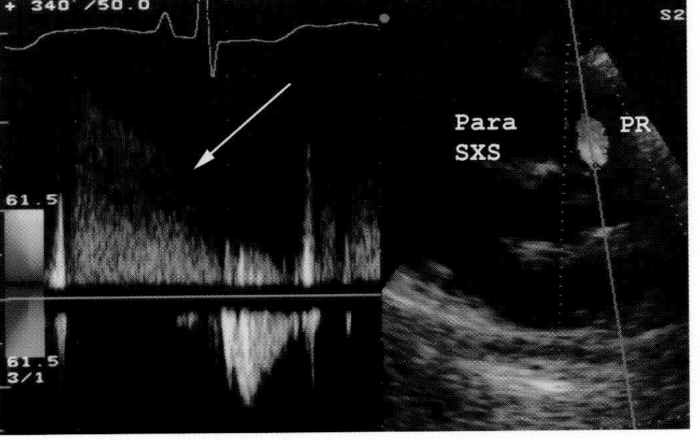

Fig. 9.14 (a) Tricuspid regurgitation (TR) using continuous wave (CW) Doppler. Pulmonary artery systolic pressure (PA_{SP}) is derived using the modified Bernoulli equation as $PA_{SP} = [4 \times (TR)^2] + RAP$, where TR is the maximum TR velocity and RAP is estimated right atrial pressure (see text). (b) Apical four-chamber image with color Doppler to help "line-up" the CW jet to obtain the TR velocity profile. (c) CW Doppler of pulmonary regurgitation used to obtain the pulmonary artery diastolic pressure (PA_{DP}) using the modified Bernoulli equation. $PA_{DP} = [4 \times (PA_{ED})^2] + RAP$, where PA_{ED} is the pulmonary artery end-diastolic velocity. When an "A" wave is present, use the velocity as noted in the right panel. (d) High parasternal short axis with CW Doppler helps obtain a CW Doppler waveform of pulmonary regurgitation (PR). The end-diastolic velocity (arrow) is used to obtain the PA_{DP}.

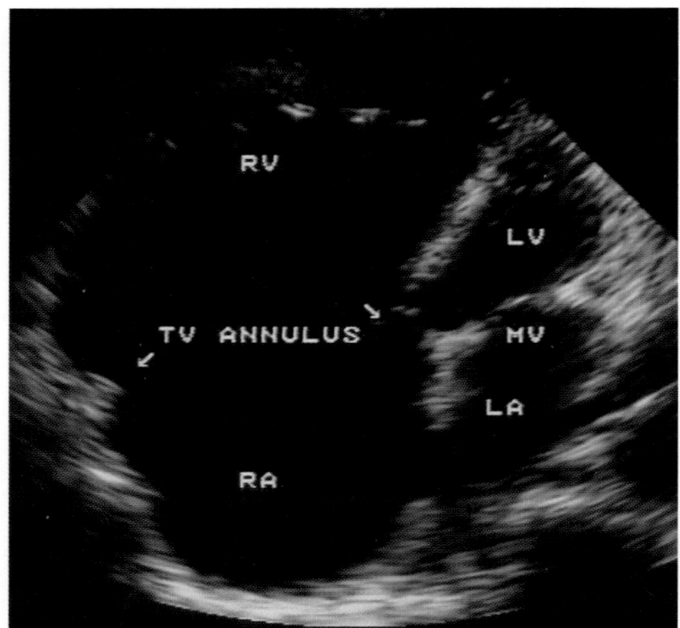

(a)

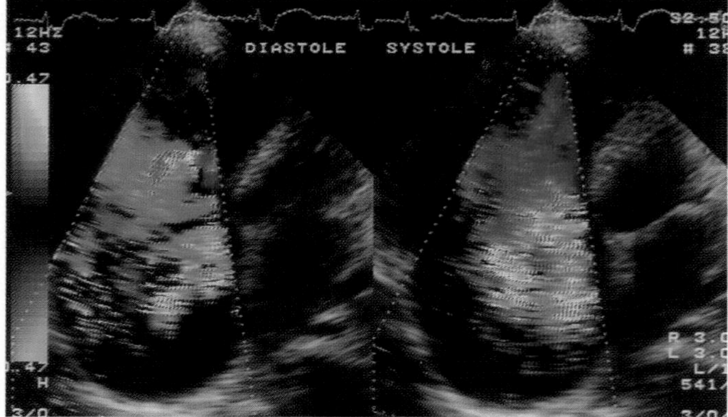

(b)

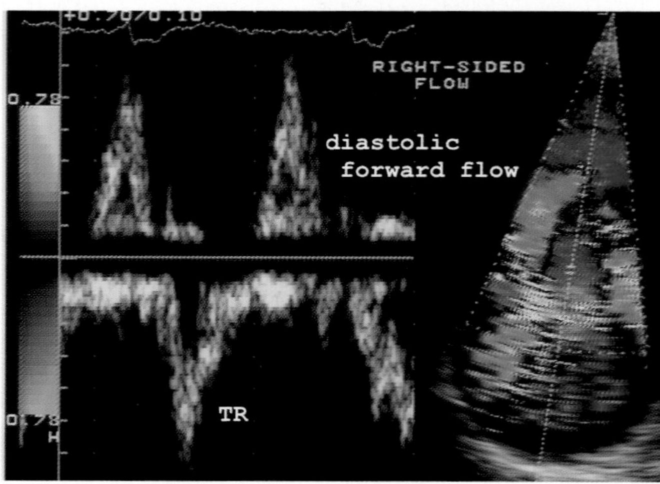

(c)

Fig. 9.15 Apical four-chamber imaging in a patient several years post tricuspid valve resection for bacterial endocarditis. (a) 2-D image reveals a large right heart. The annulus (arrows) is noted. (b) CW Doppler reveals diastolic forward flow (red color in left panel), and systolic severe regurgitant flow (blue mosaic in right panel). (c) PW Doppler at the level of the tricuspid annulus reveals systolic reversed flow with a low maximum velocity and prominent "cutoff sign". This patient has normal pulmonary artery pressure with severe TR.

Table 9.1 IVC size and dynamics for estimation of RA pressure.

(a) IVC size

Size		↓ *IVC size with inspiration (sniff)*
		IVC collapse
Small	<1.5 cm	Normal >50%
Normal	1.5–2.5 cm	Abnormal <50%
Dilated	>2.5 cm	Dilated IVC: no change

(b) IVC findings

Findings	*Estimated RAP*
Small & collapse	0–5 mmHg
Normal & normal ↓ size	5–10 mmHg
Normal & abnormal ↓ size	10–15 mmHg
Dilated & abnormal ↓ size	15–20 mmHg
Dilated & no change in size	>20 mmHg

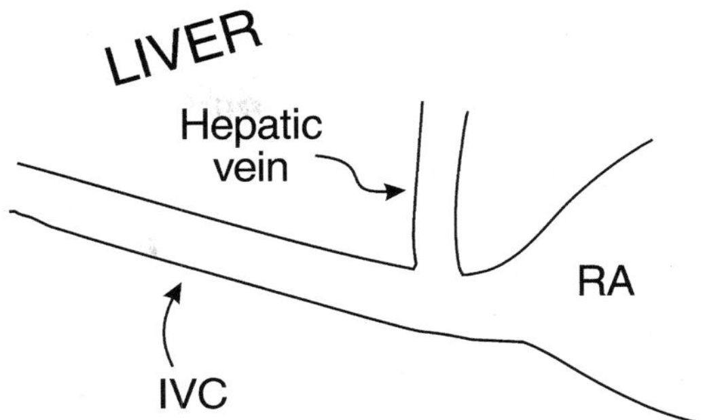

Fig. 9.17 Subcostal image of the IVC and hepatic vein. As hepatic vein flow is parallel to a Doppler beam in the subcostal position, it is ideal for assessment of flow patterns. Pulsed wave Doppler is typically used. Normally, flow is noted in systole and diastole toward the RA, and there may be mild reversed flow (toward the transducer) after the systolic wave (end-systole) and after the diastolic wave (atrial systole). With inspiration, flow toward the RA increases, and reversed flow will diminish.

This is in distinction from valvular pulmonic stenosis (PS) where the AT is prolonged. With pulmonary hypertension, the peak of the PW Doppler waveform will be more sharply peaked and with severe pulmonary hypertension, a notch may appear on the downslope of the waveform.

Accurate estimation of RA pressure is helpful to accurately calculate PA pressures (Table 9.1). Physical evaluation of jugular venous distention is not very reliable. The IVC diameter will change with inspiration (or a "sniff") and helps estimate RA pressure. With normal RA pressure, the IVC will be less than 1.5 cm diameter and will collapse by more than 50% with inspiration or sniff. One should observe the IVC about 0–2 cm from the orifice of the RA, between the hepatic vein and the RA (Figs 9.16 & 9.17).

Many but not all echo laboratories use IVC findings to estimate RA pressure. Some laboratories use a

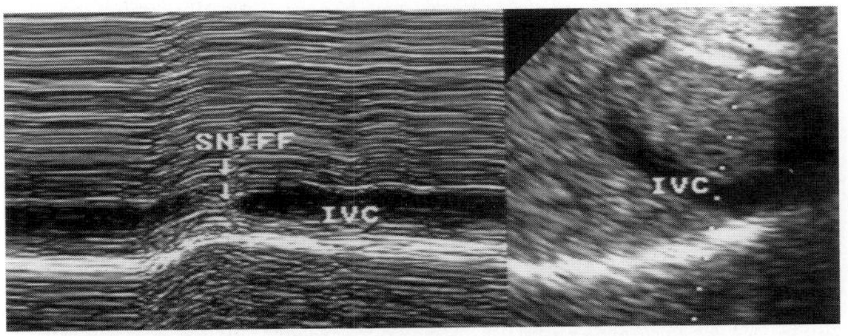

(a)

(b)

Fig. 9.16 Subcostal 2-D and M-mode of the IVC. (a) Normal sized IVC and normal collapse >50% with a "sniff". (b) In this case the IVC is moderately enlarged and there is <50% collapse with a "sniff." The RA pressure is estimated to be ~15 mmHg.

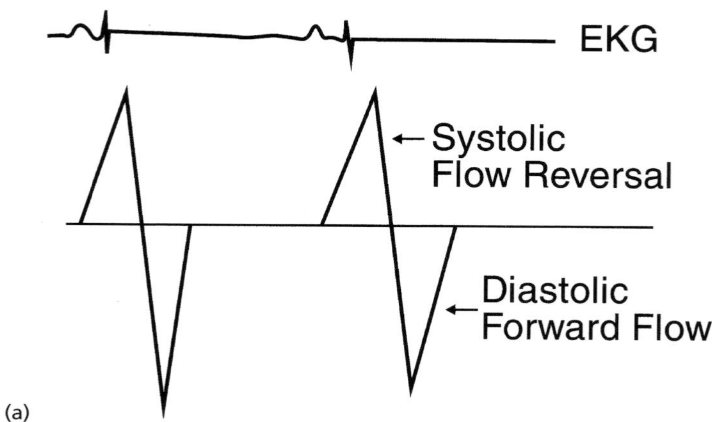

(a)

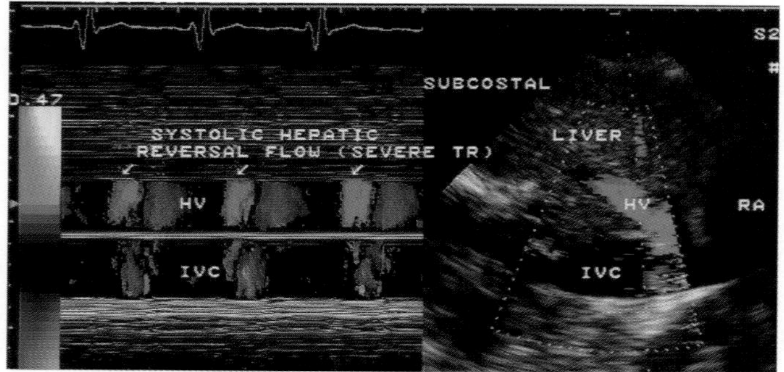

(b)

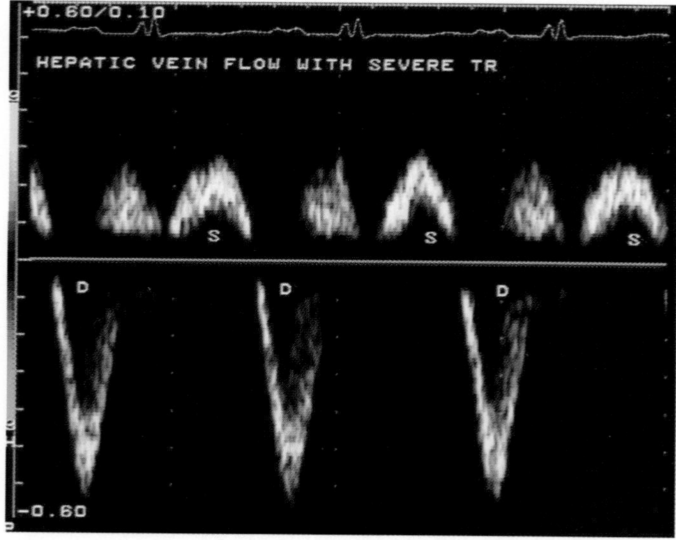

(c)

Fig. 9.18 (a) PW Doppler flow pattern in the hepatic vein, from the subcostal position. With severe TR, there is noted systolic flow reversal, with flow away from the RA and toward the transducer. (b) 2-D and M-mode color image from the subcostal window of a patient with severe TR. Color Doppler demonstrates systolic flow reversal (M-mode red jet). Note a dilated and plethoric IVC by M-mode. (c) PW Doppler of the hepatic vein in a patient with severe TR. Note systolic flow reversal (S). The only forward flow towards the RA occurs during diastole (D).

single assumed RA pressure (usually ~10 mmHg) in the calculation of PA pressure.

Hepatic vein flow (Fig. 9.17) helps in attempting to quantify TR and in assessment for restrictive, constrictive and tamponade physiology (see Chapter 12). With increasing tricuspid regurgitation the systolic component decreases until there is hepatic systolic reversed flow with 4+ TR (Fig. 9.18).

The ventricular septum

Normally the interventricular septum (IVS) contracts as part of the LV. Motion is dependent on forces acting from the RV and LV. During systole, the IVS thickens and moves toward the LV centroid. IVS movement occurs secondary to contraction/relaxation of septal muscle and total heart motion. IVS motion is usually best evaluated by M-mode echocardiography near the mitral valve level and is classified as either normal or abnormal.

Normal

The LV retains its circular shape during contraction/relaxation.

Abnormal

A *Septal hyperkinesis*

1 LV volume overload (see Fig. 8.33b).

2 Compensatory hyperkinesis—secondary to hypokinesis/infarction of other LV segments.

3 Anomalous origin of left coronary artery—basal septal hyperkinesis and anterolateral hypokinesis.

B *Septal hypokinesis/akinesis*

1 Infarction/ischemia, cardiomyopathy, infiltrative disorders.

2 Abnormal electrical activation.

C *Paradoxical septal motion*

1 Systolic paradoxical septal motion:

(a) ischemic dyskinesis—no septal thickening/possibly thins

(b) exaggerated LV motion—pericardial effusion, congenital absence of left pericardium (normal systolic septal thickening)

(c) post open-heart surgery—etiology not definitely known.

2 Systolic and diastolic paradoxical septal motion.

(a) RV volume overload—most prominent septal flattening (2-D) in late diastole

(b) RV pressure overload—most prominent septal flattening (2-D) in early diastole—the septum appears to retain its flattening through systole.

3 Diastolic paradoxical septal motion:

(a) mitral stenosis—prominent early diastolic notch (RV filling precedes LV filling resulting in the IVS bulging toward the LV in early diastole)

(b) aortic regurgitation—end-systolic abrupt anterior motion followed by an early diastolic notch

(c) pericardial constriction (see Chapter 12).

With pericardial constriction or tamponade, respiration affects IVS motion. With inspiration the M-mode LV end-diastolic dimension decreases and the IVS moves toward the LV. With expiration the LV end-diastolic dimension increases and the IVS moves toward the RV.

A left bundle branch block (LBBB) electrocardiogram pattern causes an abrupt rapid posterior IVS motion at the onset of the QRS, the so-called "septal beak." Differentiating abnormal septal motion due to an ECG conduction defect or ischemia/injury may be difficult. However, abnormal IVS motion due only to a conduction abnormality will demonstrate septal thickening whereas with ischemia/injury IVS thickening diminishes.

10

CHAPTER 10

Prosthetic Heart Valves

Prosthetic heart valves are classified as either biologic (tissue) or mechanical. Biologic valves are subdivided into homografts (allografts) or heterografts (xenografts). Mechanical valves are subdivided into ball-in-cage, single-tilting disk, or double-tilting disk. Annular rings are classified in the mechanical group. Normal Doppler parameters for prosthetic valves are provided in the Appendix. Basic hemodynamics and its application to prosthetic valves are introduced in Chapter 3. Commonly used prosthetic valves are categorized as shown in Table 10.1.

Homograft valves

Homografts are preserved cadaver human valves, most often preserved aortic valves used in the aortic position. They may be stented or nonstented. Homografts are relatively resistant to infection, do not need anticoagulation, and have good hemodynamics, even in patients with a small aortic root size. Development of aortic stenosis is generally not a problem. Homografts generally fail from gradually progressive aortic regurgitation. Severe AR may develop in up to 4% of patients (due to valve dehiscence, cusp rupture, rarely endocarditis). *Aortic nonstented homografts* generally appear by echocardiography to be the same as a native aortic valve. The aortic annulus may appear brighter and thicker than normal due to sutures. The aortic homograft is typically inserted as an aortic valve, annulus, and proximal aorta. Coronary arteries are reimplanted to the donor root. The homograft is inserted within the patient's original root, therefore a potential space exists between the original and cadaveric aortic root. As a homograft is stored in a deep-freezer and thawed before use, preoperative transesophageal (TEE) is helpful to measure the aortic annulus diameter. A homograft 1–2 mm smaller than the measured size is then used. Homografts are often used in cases of aortic valve endocarditis, especially when an abscess is present. Pulmonic and mitral valves have also been used for homografts in those positions.

Table 10.1 Classification of prosthetic valves.

Biological	*Mechanical*
Homograft	Ball-and-cage
Aortic	Starr–Edwards
Pulmonary	
Mitral	Single-tilting disc
	Medtronic–Hall
Heterograft (stented)	Lillhehi–Kaster
Porcine	Omniscience
Hancock	Bjork–Shiley
Carpentier–Edwards	
Ionescu–Shiley	Double-tilting disc
Bovine	St Jude Medical
Ionescu–Shiley	Carbomedics
Heterograft (nonstented)	Annular ring
Medtronic Freestyle	Carpentier (stiff)
Toronto SPV	Duran (flexible)
CryoLife–O'Brien	Puig Massana–Shiley (adjustable)

Heterograft valves

Heterografts (bioprosthetic) may be either stented (Fig. 10.1) or nonstented (Fig. 10.2). Most are porcine (pig), but the Ionescu–Shiley pericardial valve is bovine (cow). The latter was removed from production because of valve dehiscence. A small percentage of stented valves (~10%) may have minimal "backflow" upon closing. Nonstented valves have improved hemodynamics (larger effective valve orifice for an annulus size) and have been used mostly in older males (>60 years) in the aortic position. Calcification of the stented bioprosthetic valve has been problematic, with calcific degeneration and leaflet failure beginning 5 years post implantation in some patients.

(a)

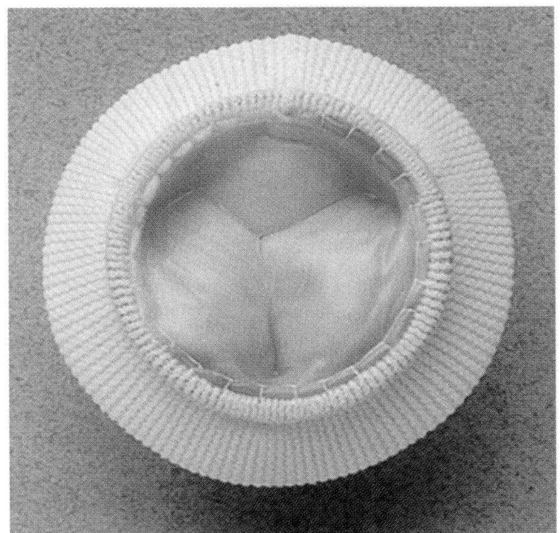

(b)

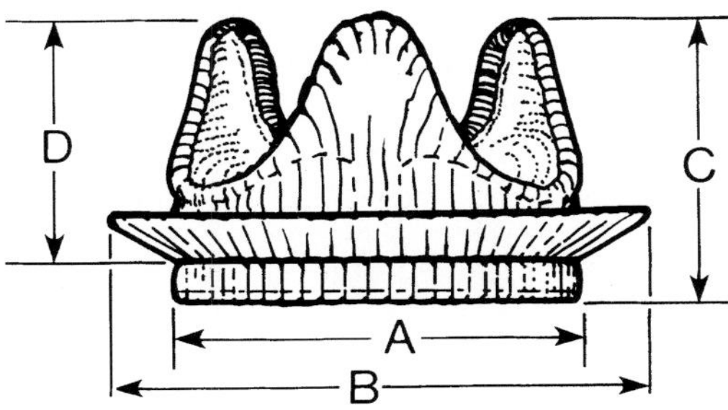

Fig. 10.1 (a) Example of a stented bioprosthesis: the Hancock aortic porcine valve. (b) The valve size is determined by its annulus diameter (A). The suture ring diameter (B), valve height (C), and aortic profile (D) are noted. (Courtesy of Medtronic, Inc.)

Calcification may develop rapidly in young adults and patients with metabolic problems involving calcium, causing valvular stenosis. Up to 90% of patients over 70 years, however, may be free from reoperation 12–15 years after implantation. The nonstented valve may have less of a problem with calcification and failure. Heterografts have a low incidence of thromboembolism. Other heterograft problems include torn cusps (valvular regurgitation) and valve dehiscence. Nonstented valves may be used as: (i) a valve with an aortic root requiring coronary reimplantation; (ii) an aortic root replacement preserving the native coronaries; or (iii) a subcoronary attachment, where the coronary arteries remain attached to the native aortic root.

The CryoLife–Ross valve is a *pulmonary nonstented heterograft valve* composed of three noncoronary porcine aortic cusps. It is used to replace the pulmonic valve, and may be used during the Ross procedure.

Mechanical valves

The Starr–Edwards valve is a *ball-and-cage* valve. It is a Silastic ball with a circular sewing ring with a "cage" to hold the ball. Doppler assessment of these valves must be made around the sides of the ball, as the highest velocities occur around the ball (Fig. 10.3). Larger size valves should be implanted in the mitral position (Figs 10.4 & 10.5); smaller valves are implanted in the aortic position. They are associated with significant turbulence, transvalvular gradients and hemolysis with an increased tendency toward thrombosis.

The first *single tilting disk valve* was the Bjork–Shiley (Figs 10.6 & 10.7), but was removed from the market because a certain percentage of valves developed sudden leaflet escape followed by sudden death. Presently, the Medtronic–Hall is often used. These valves have a single ring (sewing ring and leaflet orifice) and a disk attached eccentrically by a single hinge. Therefore, they have a "major" and "minor" orifice for forward flow, and an effective valve orifice area that is not the area of the sewing ring, but is a function of these two orifices. In the mitral position, the major orifice is toward the lateral wall of the LV, which allows blood to enter the LV laterally. If the major orifice is toward the LV outflow tract, blood will enter the LV towards the septum. Leaflet closure occurs by fluid pressure on the largest part of the disk. Blood may stagnate behind the disk, leading to thrombus formation. Also gradual pannus formation may impinge on inflow through the orifices or affect the leaflet hinge. Color flow Doppler will demonstrate a prominent central regurgitant jet and a small amount of flow between the closing disk and the sewing ring.

The *double tilting disk valve* is composed of two semicircular disks with a midline hinge (Figs 10.8 & 10.9). There are two openings of equal size, and a smaller central rectangular opening. The effective orifice area is relatively large for the sewing ring size. With color flow Doppler, the St Jude mechanical valve will demonstrate from three to five small "candle flames" upon closure. The Carbomedics valve will have four small closing "pivotal washing jets" noted by color Doppler. During insertion, pledgets may stick

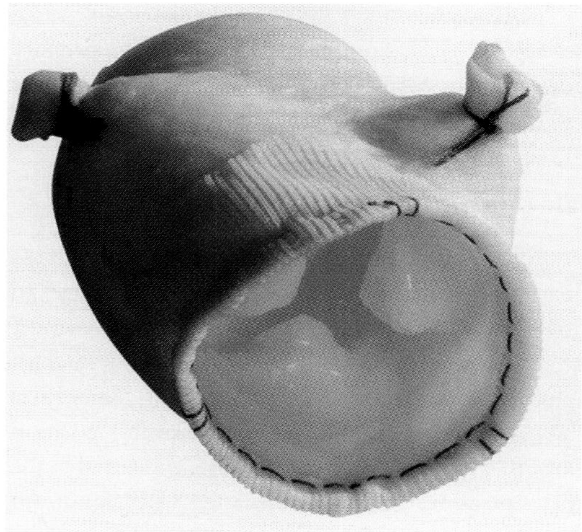

(a)

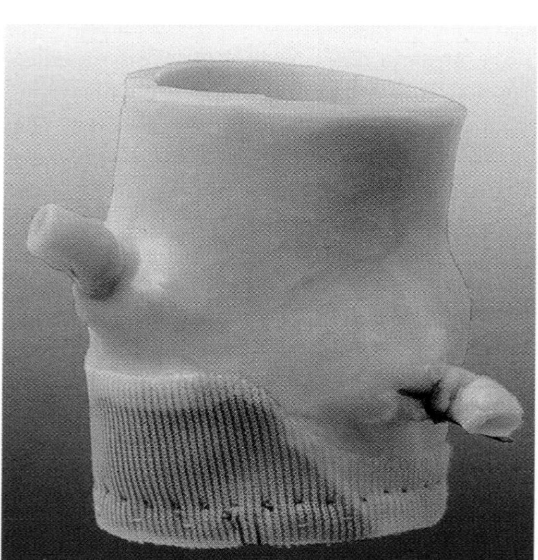

(b)

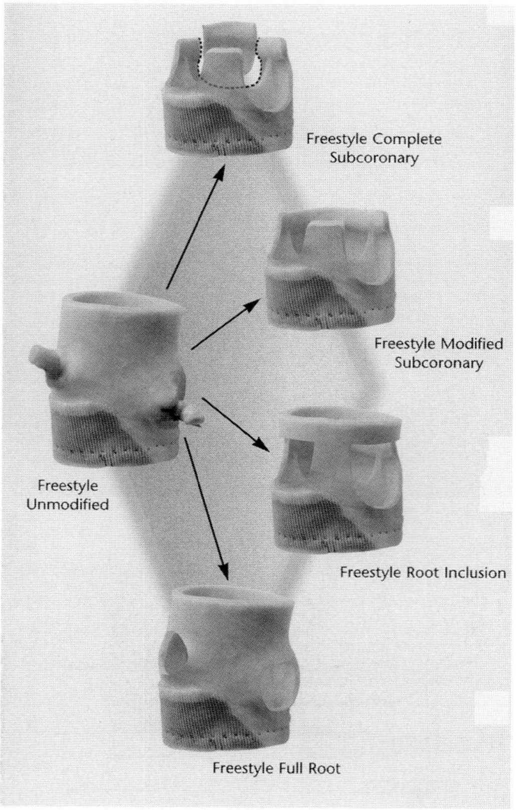

(c)

Fig. 10.2 Three stentless tissue heterografts (Toronto SPV—St Jude Medical; Freestyle—Medtronic Heart Valves; CryoLife—O'Brien) are commonly used for aortic valve replacement. They are porcine aortic root, and implanted without a rigid sewing ring or support struts. The stentless valve will allow one to two sizes larger for implantation than that of a stented valve (important in patients with a small aortic root). Unlike the stented valve, stentless valves have two suture lines. The proximal suture line is circular and close to the level of the native aortic valve annulus. The distal suture line is along the line of the distal edge of the prosthesis. The Toronto SPV valve distal suture line is between the native sinuses of Valsalva and the three semilunar valve cusps below the native sinus of Valsalva. The Freestyle aortic root may also be implanted as a *subcoronary valve* (as in the Toronto SPV), but also a *modified subcoronary valve*, where the noncoronary porcine sinus of Valsalva is retained in the prosthesis. The Freestyle valve may also be implanted as a *full aortic root* or as a *root inclusion* (these two are used in patients with significant aortic root disease). The full aortic root allows resection of the patient's proximal aortic root and insertion of the Freestyle porcine valve with root. Coronaries are reimplanted. The root inclusion technique includes the cylinder portion of the porcine aortic root, but the patient native coronaries do not need to be reimplanted. (a,b) The stentless Freestyle unmodified porcine aortic root. (c) The (complete) subcoronary, modified subcoronary, root inclusion, and full root. By echocardiography the Freestyle *full root* will appear normal (thin leaflets, normal leaflet motion, possibly mild aortic regurgitation—valvular or paravalvular), the *subcoronary* may have increased paravalvular echodensity, the *modified subcoronary* an increased paravalvular echodensity at the noncoronary cusp, and the *root inclusion* an increased paravalvular soft tissue appearance that is circumferential. (Courtesy Medtronic, Inc.)

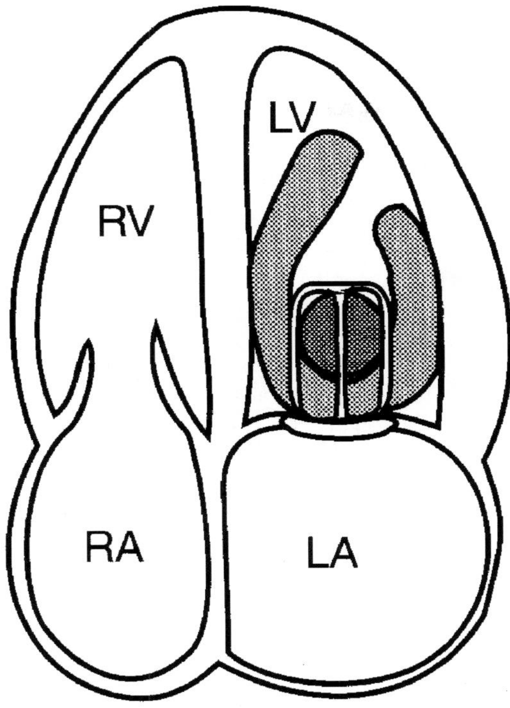

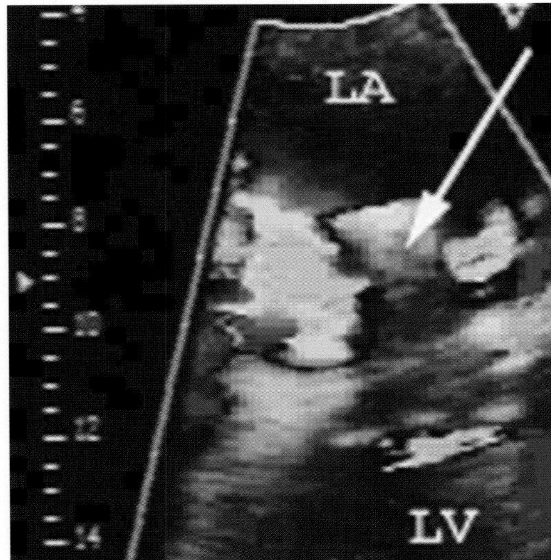

Fig. 10.3 (a) Diagrammatic and (b) 2-D imaging with color Doppler from an apical window of the Starr–Edwards ball-and-cage prosthesis in the mitral position. Flow occurs around the prosthesis, therefore Doppler interrogation should be performed laterally. Use of color flow helps "line up" the Doppler transducer for best results. Arrow in (b) points to the prosthesis ball.

within a leaflet, as the disks are relatively close to the narrow sewing ring. Chronically, thrombus or tissue growth may involve the hinge, causing the leaflets to acutely stick in a partially open position, with sudden severe regurgitation resulting.

Annular rings (see also Chapter 15) are in the category of mechanical valves. Systolic anterior motion (SAM) with dynamic obstructive hemodynamics may occasionally occur with the stiff Carpentier ring and rarely with the flexible Duran ring. SAM may be noted immediately post mitral valve repair and often resolves with fluids. Other complications include annular ring dehiscence and orifice stenosis.

Other prosthetic valves

The *Ross procedure* involves replacing the abnormal aortic valve with the patient's own native pulmonic valve and placing a nonstented homograft or porcine bioprosthesis in the pulmonic position. Early problems include continuing endocarditis (for which the operation was performed), and late problems include aortic annulus dilatation, endocarditis, valvular degeneration, and obstruction in the distal part of the pulmonic conduit.

Valved conduits (usually employing bioprosthetic valve) are often used to connect right heart flow to the pulmonary artery terrritory. Conduits with a Hancock bioprosthetic valve are used to connect the LV apex to the descending aorta in patients with critical calcific aortic stenosis who have a *porcelain aorta* (an ascending aorta that is heavily calcified), as the risk of embolism is increased with cross-clamping of the ascending aorta during aortic valve replacement (Fig. 10.10).

Echo techniques in evaluation of prosthetic valves (see Chapters 3, 7, and 8)

A complete echo examination should be performed. In particular, one should assess *left ventricular size* and *function*, and calculate *pulmonary artery pressures*. A baseline echocardiogram should be obtained on all patients 4–6 weeks after valve surgery.

M-mode opening and closing of ball-and-cage and bioprosthetic valves should be *vertical* and of *large amplitude*. Tissue Doppler imaging (TDI) may help identify rapid opening and closing of the prosthetic

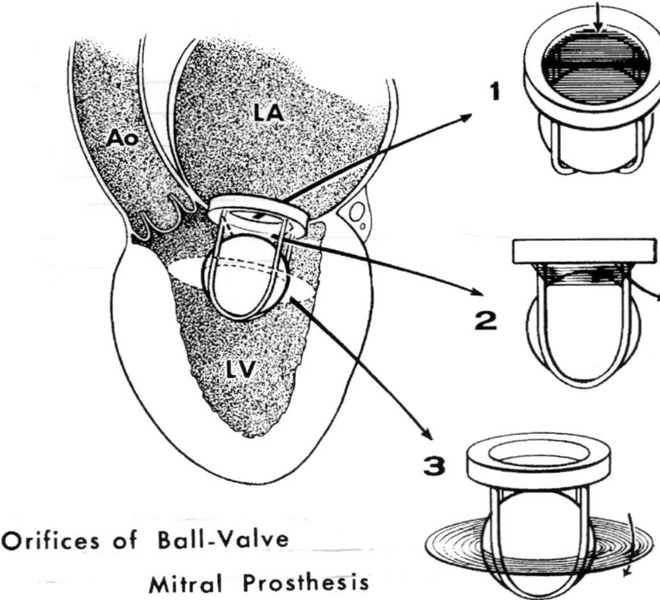

Fig. 10.4 The Starr–Edwards valve in the mitral position. Three potential levels of functional valve obstruction are noted. (Reproduced with permission from: Glancy DL, O'Brien KP, Reis RL, Epstein SE, Morrow AG. Hemodynamic studies in patients with 2M and 3M Starr–Edwards prostheses: evidence of obstruction to left atrial emptying. Circulation 1969; 39,40(suppl 1): I117, figure 8.)

valve. A normal bioprosthetic mitral valve rarely demonstrates proto-diastolic closure (it is mildly stenotic). Prosthetic valve dysfunction is hard to evaluate with M-mode and two-dimensional (2-D) echo. Masking of structures or flow behind the valve is due to the inability of the ultrasound beam to travel past the artificial valve. Bioprosthetic valves (especially in the mitral position) can be best evaluated for cusp thickness, masses, valve rocking motion due to dehiscence, and flail leaflets with TEE.

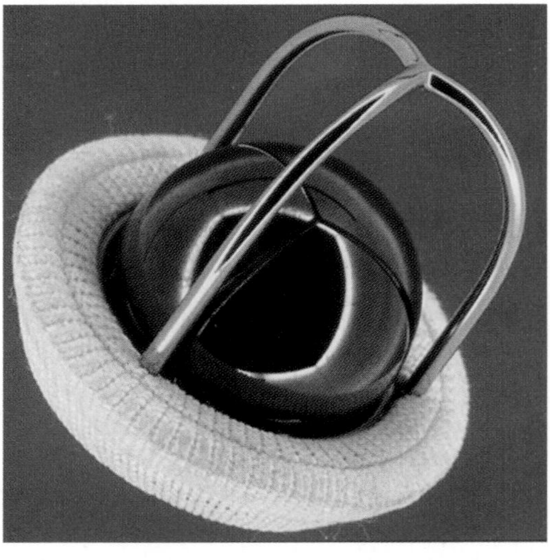

Fig. 10.5 The Debakey–Surgitool aortic position ball-and-cage prosthesis. This valve was first implanted in 1969. (Courtesy of CarboMedics, Inc.)

As with native valves, calculation of the time velocity integral (TVI), pressure gradients (instantaneous peak-to-peak, mean valve gradient), effective valve orifice area, and quantification of regurgitation can be performed. Ball-and-cage valves produce flow around the sides of the ball. Doppler at the sides of the ball should be performed for accurate results. Tilting disk valves produce eccentric flow patterns into the LV, mostly coming through the large (major) orifice. Bioprosthetic valves flow centrally and therefore should be interrogated at the center of the valve.

Mitral valve

Doppler measurements of a mitral prosthesis should be performed in a manner similar to that of a native mitral valve. Calculation of the *mean pressure gradient* (correlates with catheterization derived mean pressure gradient) and *effective orifice area* should be performed in all prosthetic mitral valves. The mitral prosthesis may become stenotic due to thrombus formation in mechanical valves. Calcific degeneration in stented bioprosthetic valves may lead to valve stenosis or cusp tears with valve regurgitation.

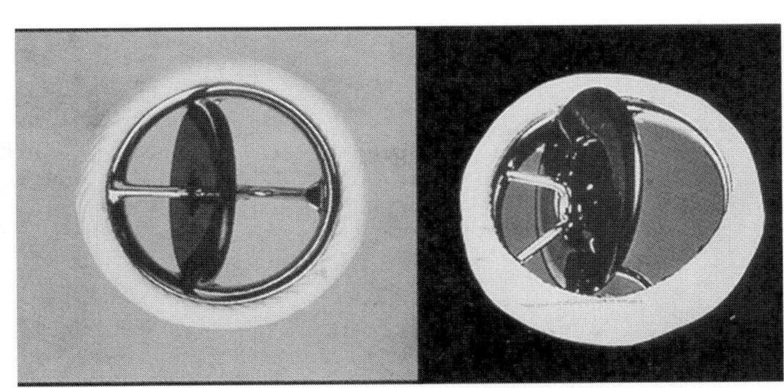

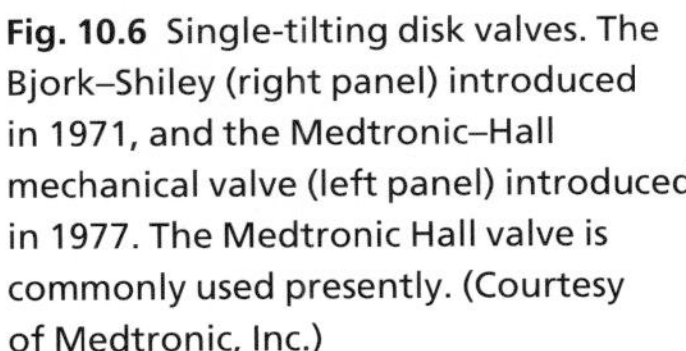

Fig. 10.6 Single-tilting disk valves. The Bjork–Shiley (right panel) introduced in 1971, and the Medtronic–Hall mechanical valve (left panel) introduced in 1977. The Medtronic Hall valve is commonly used presently. (Courtesy of Medtronic, Inc.)

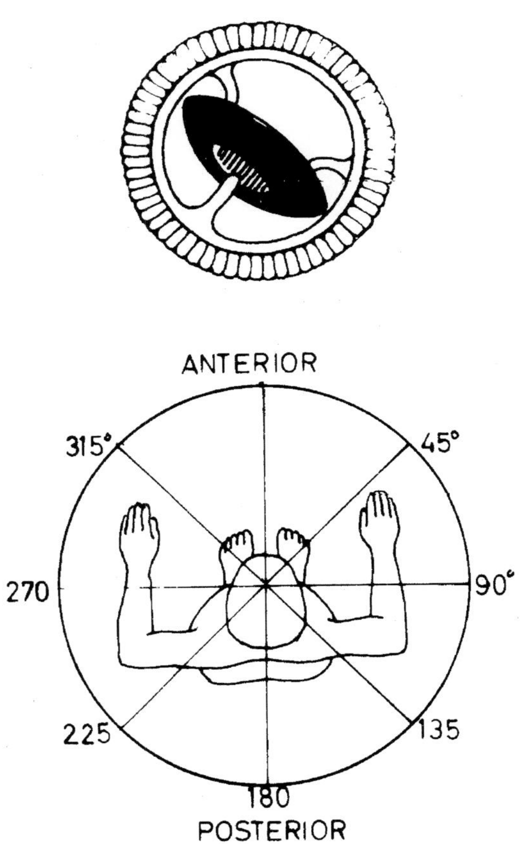

(a)

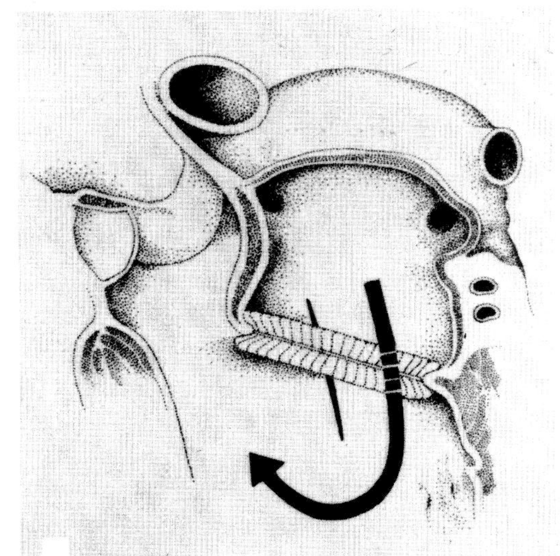

(b)

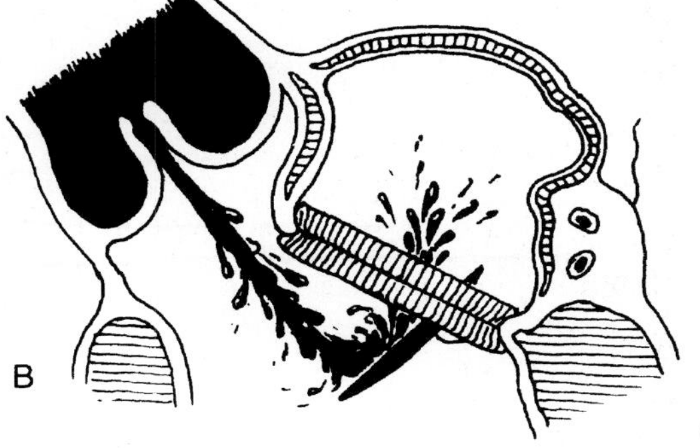

(c)

Fig. 10.7 (a) Desired implantation rotation angle in the aortic position for the Bjork–Shiley mechanical prosthesis. (b) In the mitral position the single-tilting disk valve should ideally have the large orifice directed away from the aortic orifice. (c) If the disk points toward the aortic valve, aortic regurgitation may hit the disk and cause marked diastolic mitral regurgitation. (Reproduced with permission from: Bjork VO, Lindblom D. Monostrut Bjork–Shiley Heart Valve. Journal of the American College of Cardiology 1985; 6(5): 1142–1148.)

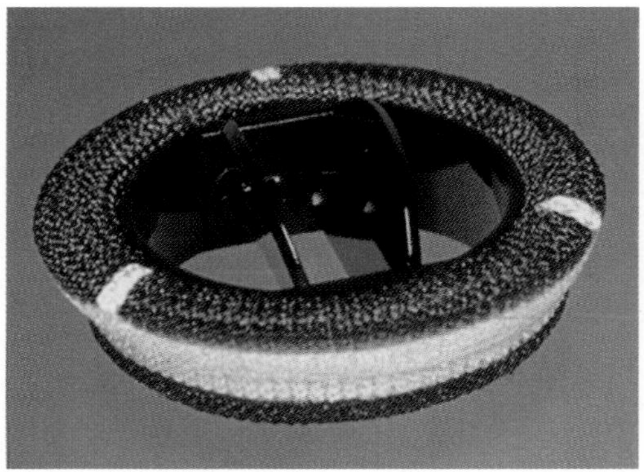
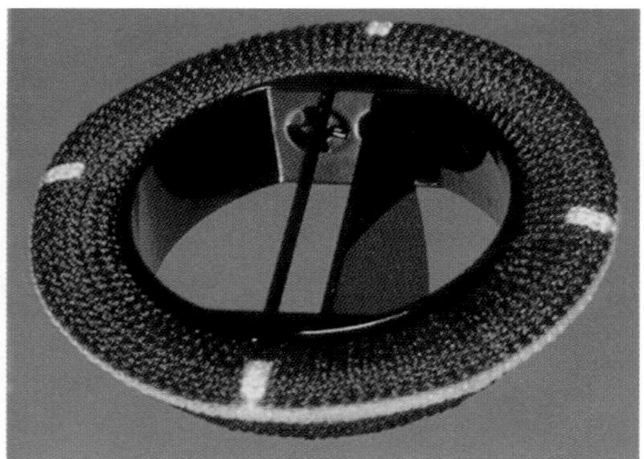

(a)

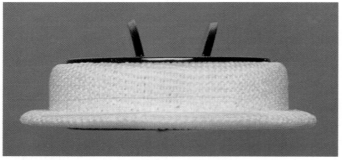

(b)

Fig. 10.8 (a) CarboMedics bileaflet aortic (left panel) and mitral (right panel) mechanical prostheses. (b) The supra-annular "Top Hat" valve for implantation in the aortic position. This valve allows for implantation of a larger orifice valve in patients with a small aortic root (usually one size larger than standard). The manufactured valve size approximates the tissue annulus diameter in the "Top Hat" model, and is about 1 mm smaller than the tissue annulus diameter of the standard valve. The internal diameter (orifice diameter) is several millimeters smaller than the tissue annulus diameter. (Courtesy of CarboMedics, Inc.)

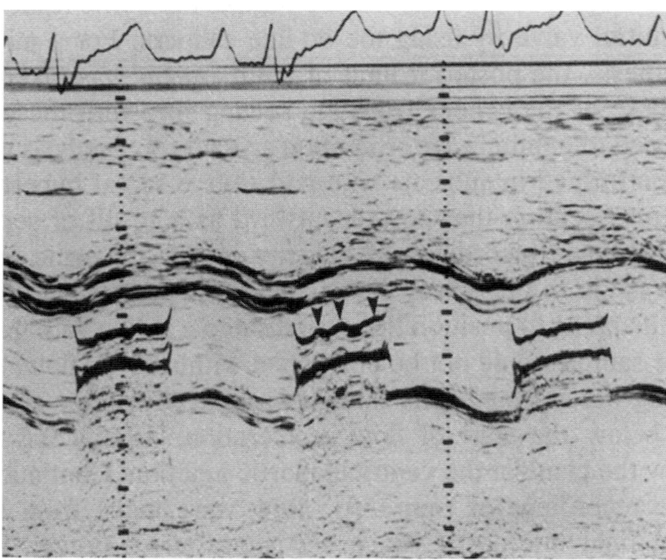

Fig. 10.9 M-mode through the tips of the leaflets of an aortic position CarboMedics prosthesis. Note normal course systolic fluttering (arrows). (Reproduced with permission from: Chambers J, Cross J, Deverall P, Sowton E. Echocardiographic description of the CarboMedics bileaflet prosthetic heart valve. Journal of the American College of Cardiology 1993; 21: 398–405.)

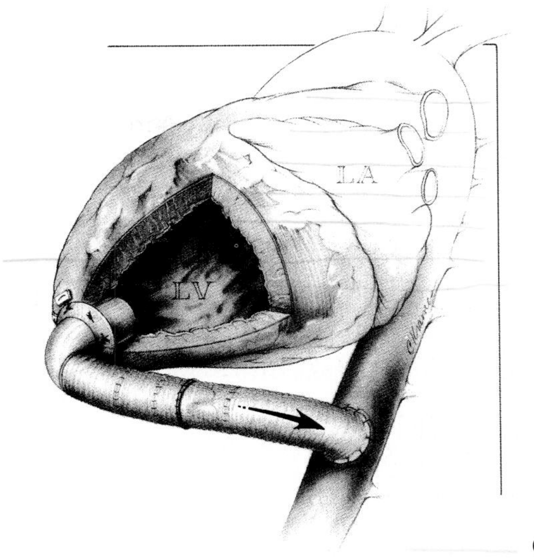

(a)

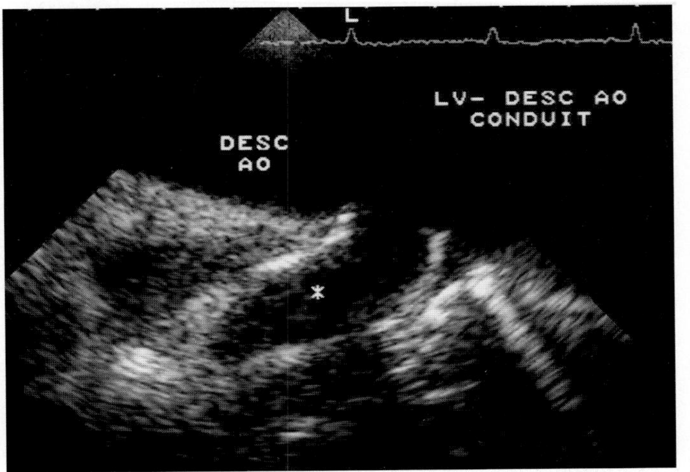

(b)

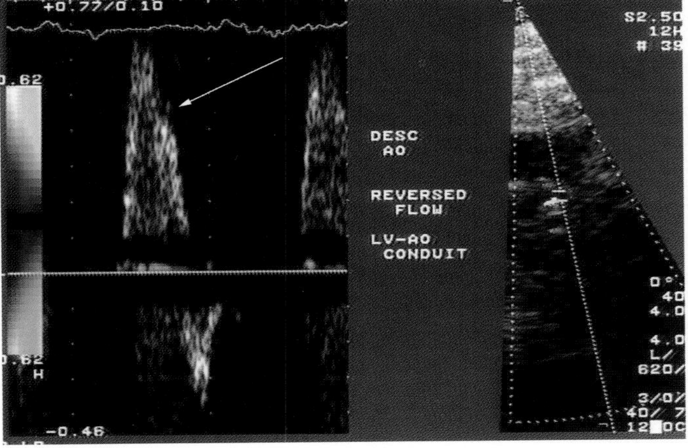

(c)

Fig. 10.10 (a) The Hancock Apical Left Ventricle Connector with Valved Conduit. The connector is curved at a 90° angle in order to facilitate anastomosis to the descending aorta (DESC AO). (b) Transesophageal (TEE) imaging in the vertical plane demonstrating the junction between the conduit (*) and descending aorta. (c) Transthoracic (TTE) imaging from the suprasternal notch demonstrates "reversed" systolic flow within the descending aorta, along with a brief early diastolic flow reversal. ((a) Reproduced with permission from Medtronic, Inc. (b,c) Reproduced with permission from: Kerut EK, Hanawalt C, Everson CT, Frank RA, Giles TD. Left ventricular apex to descending aorta valved conduit. Echocardiography 2001; 18(6): 463–468.)

When evaluating for *prosthetic mitral valve stenosis*, the following should be obtained:

- early peak velocity
- mean valve gradient
- end-diastolic gradient
- pressure half-time (PHT)
- pulmonary artery pressure
- mitral valve area (MVA)—PHT technique, continuity equation, PISA method (see Chapters 3 and 8).

As with native mitral stenosis, calculation of the MVA using the PHT method is inaccurate with significant aortic regurgitation or with a noncompliant LV. The continuity equation is inaccurate with significant mitral regurgitation (MR). If significant aortic regurgitation (AR) is present, the pulmonary TVI must be used instead of the LVOT TVI. Calculation of the mitral *mean valve pressure gradient* is important with prosthetic stenosis. All "normal" prosthetic valves have some restriction to flow with initial mitral velocities as high as 1.5–1.9 m/s but have a rapid PHT (in contrast to an obstructed valve, which will have a prolonged PHT). TEE can help to determine the etiology of valve obstruction. Thrombi usually form on the atrial side and pannus formation may be difficult to find (Figs 10.11 & 10.12). The valve may appear relatively normal despite definite obstruction by CW Doppler. Normally functioning MV prostheses have an effective valve area greater than 1.8 cm^2, with the St Jude prosthesis having the largest area. "Normal" values may vary considerably among various types and sizes of valves.

High-profile mitral prostheses (Carpentier–Edwards, Starr–Edwards) may cause *LVOT obstruction* in systole. The valve stents or cage may protrude into the left ventricular outflow tract (LVOT), causing a "fixed" LVOT obstruction pattern by Doppler (aortic valve stenosis and also subaortic membrane cause a "fixed" obstruction pattern, whereas hypertrophic obstructive cardiomyopathy (HOCM) is associated with dynamic LVOT obstruction, having a dagger appearance on the CW Doppler LVOT waveform). Symptoms related to obstruction may not present until years after implantation. An uncommon complication of mitral valve replacement with a high profile prosthesis is development of a *LV posterobasal pseudoaneurysm* (Carpentier–Edwards mitral prostheses) (Fig. 10.13). It occurs at the time of valve implantation, where the valve stent appears to perforate the LV during valve insertion.

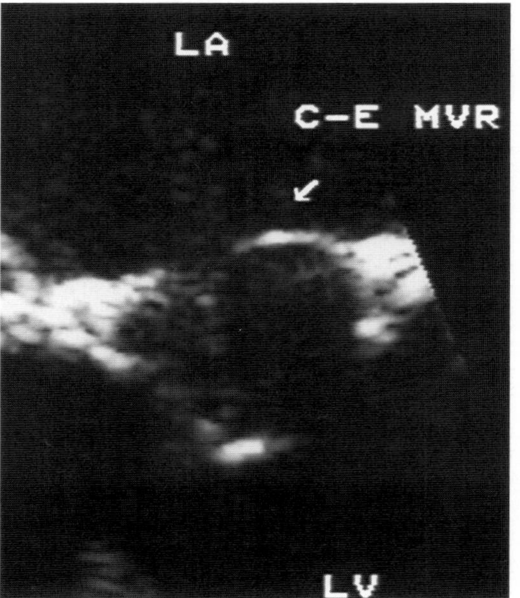

(a)

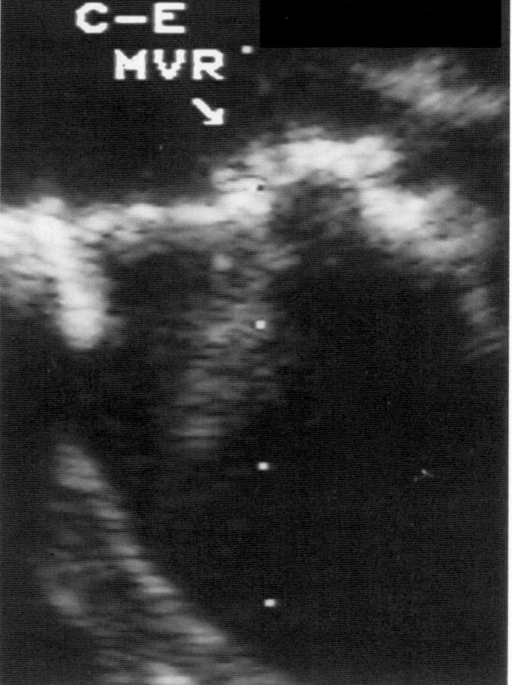

(b)

Fig. 10.11 (a) TEE of a normal Carpentier–Edwards mitral prosthesis. Note the thin leaflet structure. (b) TEE of a 42-year-old-female with a Carpentier–Edwards mitral prosthesis inserted 12 years earlier. The calculated valve area using the pressure half-time method was 0.8 cm^2. At surgery the valve was thickened with pannus formation.

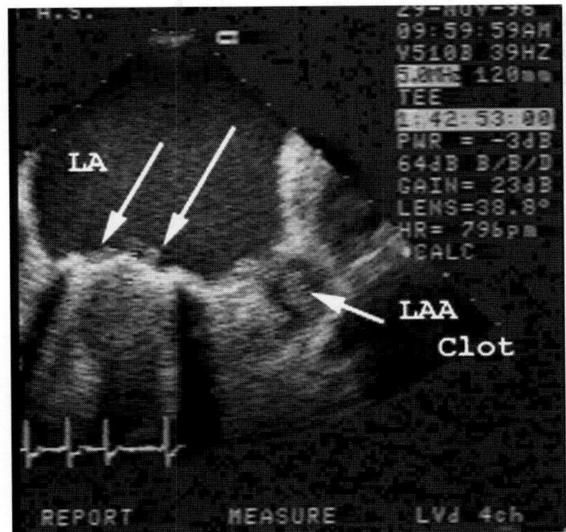

(a)

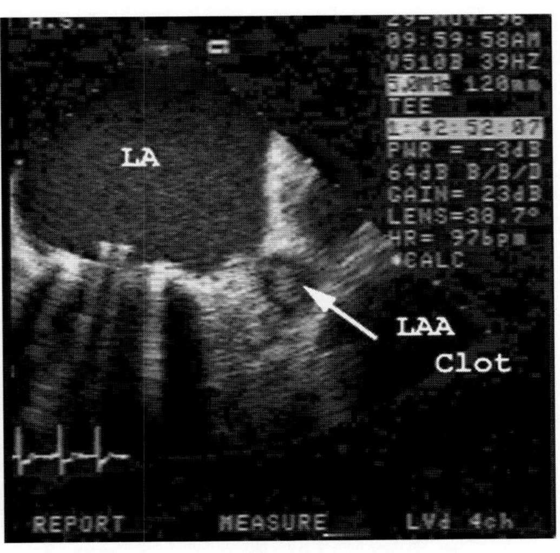

(b)

Fig. 10.12 TEE of a patient with a mitral position St Jude prosthesis with suboptimal anticoagulation. A thrombus was found within the valve apparatus, but was nonobstructive. (a) Systolic frame reveals thrombus (arrows) on the atrial side of the prosthesis. (b) In diastole both disks are noted to fully open (parallel vertical lines of valve disks). A left atrial appendage (LAA) thrombus was noted (arrow to LAA clot) in both frames.

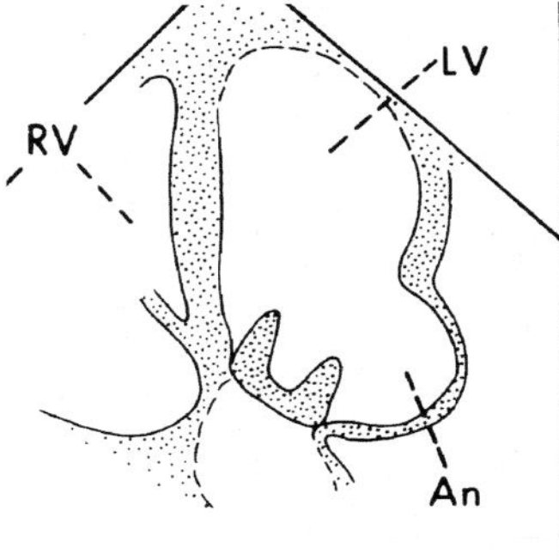

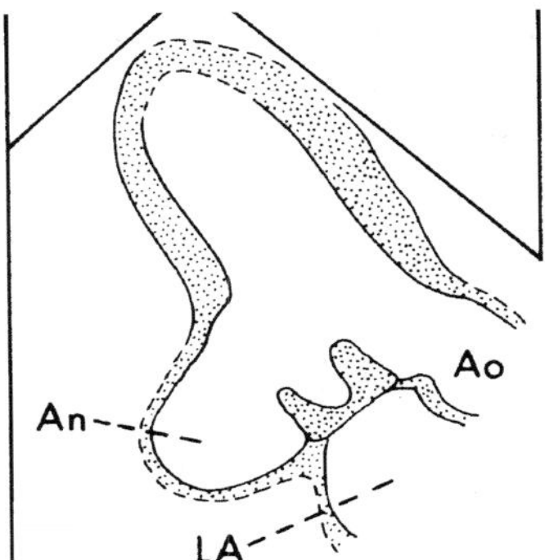

Fig. 10.13 Development of a LV pseudoaneurysm (An) in a patient 3 years post mitral valve replacement with a #29 Carpentier–Edwards prosthesis. As opposed to what would be expected for a LV pseudoaneurysm, this one had a wide mouth. Apical four-chamber (left panel) and apical two-chamber (right panel) views are shown. Ao, aortic root. (Reproduced with permission from: Carlson EB, Wolfe WG, Kisslo J. Subvalvular left ventricular pseudoaneurysm after mitral valve replacement: two-dimensional echocardiographic findings. Journal of the American College of Cardiology 1985; 6: 1164–1166.)

"Normal" (minimal to mild mitral regurgitation) prosthetic mitral regurgitation occurs in 15–30% of mitral prostheses, with a higher incidence occurring in mechanical (Fig. 10.14) as compared to bioprosthetic valves. Grading of severity, by transthoracic echo, using color Doppler is similar to that of native valve regurgitation. *Physiologic backflow* (Fig. 10.15) associated with mechanical valves tends to be of short duration and generally appears nonturbulent (a small "flame") by color Doppler, whereas pathologic regurgitation is longer in duration and appears turbulent. Using TEE, the St Jude mechanical valve will normally have from three to five small "flames" noted in the left atrium, whereas the Medtronic–Hall valve will have a larger single flame in the center of the valve (Fig. 10.16). Evaluation may be very difficult by transthoracic echocardiography (TTE) due to acoustic shadowing of the ultrasound beam by the prosthetic valve. TEE helps determine prosthetic versus periprosthetic regurgitation, the etiology of regurgitation, and complications of endocarditis. If a bioprosthetic leaflet (mostly noted in the mitral position) is torn, it may demonstrate a musical quality by PW Doppler. The Doppler spectrum may have *"tiger stripes"*—horizontal striations in systole (Fig. 10.17).

Indicators of significant prosthetic MR include:

- peak early mitral inflow diastolic velocity >2.0 m/ s
- PHT <100 ms (shortened deceleration time)
- mitral inflow TVI >40 cm
- mean mitral diastolic gradient >5–7 mmHg
- short isovolumic relaxation time (IVRT) indicative of high LA pressures
- pulmonary hypertension (new or increasing)
- pulmonary vein diastolic flow predominance and systolic flow reversal (systolic flow reversal is more likely with acute vs. chronic MR, as the LA is smaller and stiffer with acute MR)
- diminished aortic (also gradual closure of aortic valve by M-mode) and pulmonary TVIs, indicative of diminished forward cardiac output
- detection of a systolic PISA jet (TTE from an apical window) along an aspect of the prosthetic valve ring

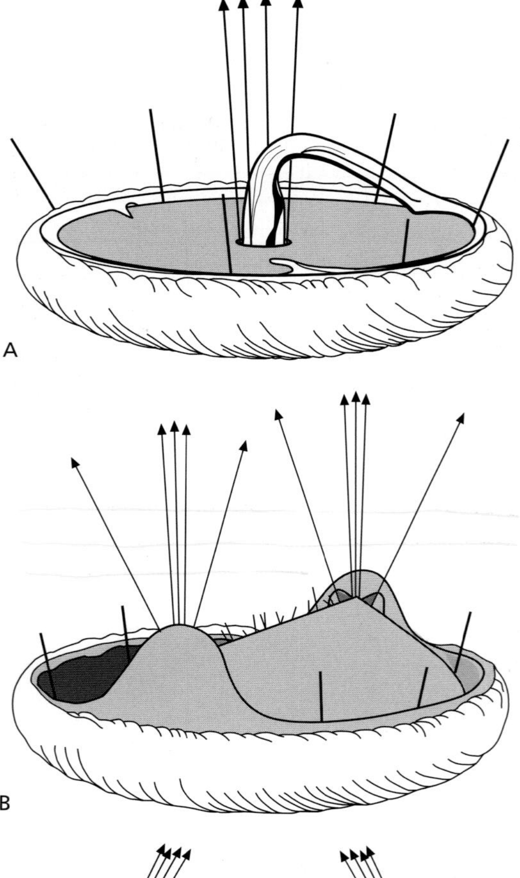

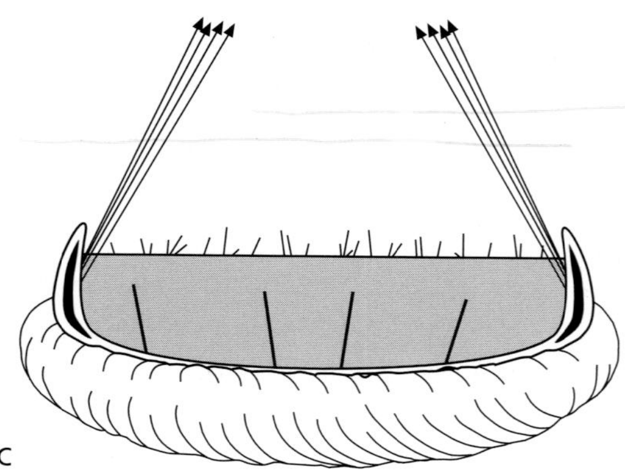

Fig. 10.14 (*left*) Direction of normal regurgitant jets of mechanical prostheses. (A) The single disk valve (Medtronic–Hall) has a predominant jet around the central strut. This jet extends further than the smaller peripheral jets. Therefore, a peripheral jet of the same size or larger than the central jet suggests a possible paravalvular leak. (B,C) A bileaflet valve (St Jude, CarboMedics). Depending on the plane of imaging, the prominent hinge point jets will exhibit either a diverging V pattern or a converging pattern. (Reproduced with permission from: Flachskampf FA, O'Shea JP, Griffin BP, *et al*. Patterns of normal transvalvular regurgitation in mechanical valve prostheses. Journal of the American College of Cardiology 1991; 18: 1493–1498.)

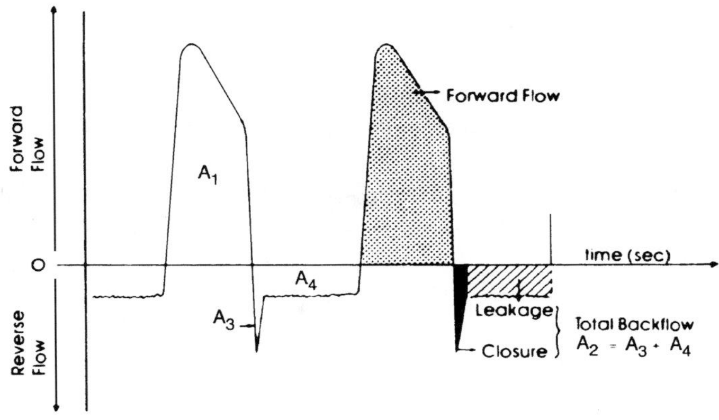

Fig. 10.15 Flow across a mechanical prosthesis. A1 represents forward flow, and A2 total backflow. Valve closure (A3) and leakage (A4) compromise total backflow. (Reproduced with permission from: Dellsperger KC, Wieting DW, Baehr DA, *et al.* Regurgitation of prosthetic heart valves: dependence on heart rate and cardiac output. American Journal of Cardiology 1983; 51: 321–328.)

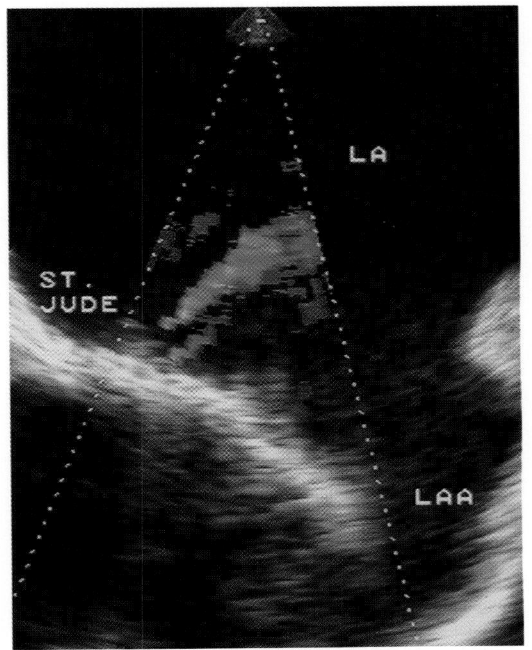

(a)

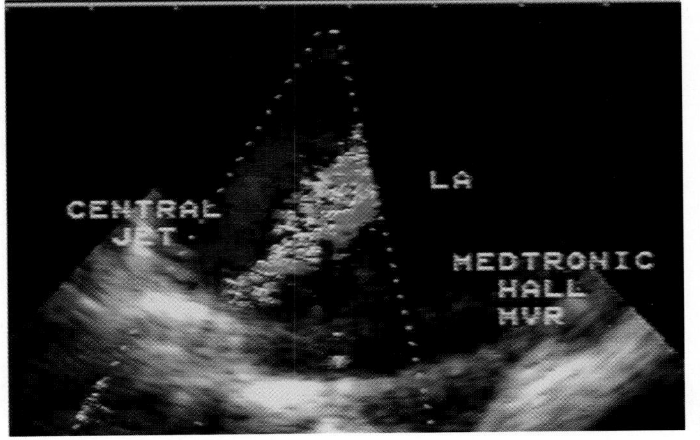

(b)

Fig. 10.16 TEE of mechanical prostheses in the mitral position. (a) The St Jude mitral prosthesis may have from three to five relatively small "candle-flame" jets noted upon closing, whereas (b) the single-tilting disk Medtronic–Hall prosthesis will have a prominent central jet upon closing.

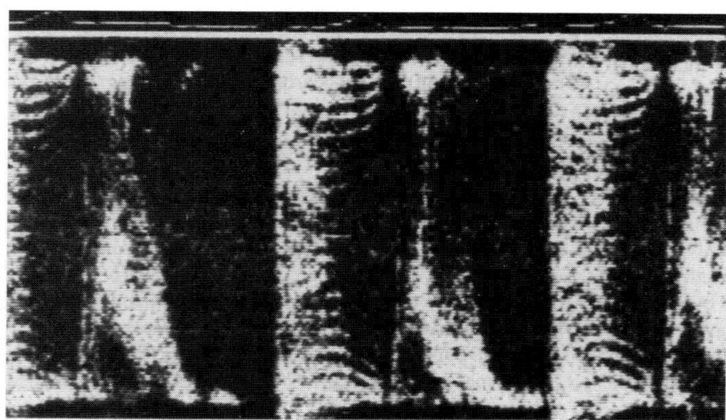

Fig. 10.17 Pulsed wave Doppler of mitral regurgitation in a patient with a flail bioprosthetic leaflet. Horizontal striations are noted, termed "tiger stripes". (Reproduced with permission from:Alam M, Rosman HS, Lakier JB, *et al*. Doppler and echocardiographic features of normal and dysfunctioning bioprosthetic valves. Journal of the American College of Cardiology 1987; 10: 851–858.)

• an eccentric MR jet is usually more significant than the color Doppler would suggest (Coanda effect)—color flow into the LAA suggests severe MR (Fig. 10.18).

Generally, signs indicating increased forward flow through the mitral prosthesis, with evidence of decreased forward cardiac output across the aortic valve, point to severe MR (Figs 10.19–10.21).

Aortic valve

Prosthetic aortic valve measurements should include *peak velocity*, *mean valve gradient*, *effective orifice area*, and the *dimensionless index* (DI). The LVOT should be evaluated (Fig. 10.22) for obstruction (narrow LVOT, dynamic LV obstruction). Normally functioning aortic prostheses have a peak instantaneous gradient of usually less than 45 mmHg, with the Starr–Edwards valve having the highest gradients. Peak velocities upwards of 3.5–4.0 m/s may be noted, but the mean gradient will be normal for the particular valve type and size.

High Doppler velocities with a normal prosthesis may be present with coexistent AR, increased cardiac output, or anemia. *Patient–prosthesis mismatch* may also cause an elevated aortic valve gradient. This problem is defined as an inability of the LV operating at a stable inotropic level to maintain a normal stroke volume against the present loading systolic conditions. The prosthetic valve functions as designed but hemodynamics are less than ideal compared with a normal valve. Inappropriately high pressure gradients may be evident only during or following exercise. Clinically, the patient post aortic valve replacement will have exertional dyspnea or heart failure, and regression of left ventricular hypertrophy (LVH) (usually noted by 6 months postoperatively) will not occur. Diagnosis requires that a primary problem with the prosthetic valve is excluded. An aortic prosthetic valve gradient is proportional to the prosthetic effective orifice area (EOA) and cardiac output (CO). CO is related to a patient's body surface area (BSA). A patient is at risk for mismatch when the *indexed EOA* implanted is ≤0.85–0.90 cm²/m². The indexed EOA of a particular prosthetic valve is determined as:

$$\text{Indexed } EOA = EOA_{\text{prosthesis}}/BSA$$

$EOA_{\text{prosthesis}}$ is the effective orifice area of the prosthetic valve (provided by the manufacturer). In order to determine the "needed" *EOA* of a valve for a particular patient, the following is performed:

$$\text{“Needed” } EOA = 0.85 \times BSA$$

The formula for calculating BSA is:

$$BSA = (Wt \times 10^{0.425}) \times (Ht \times 10^{0.725}) \times 0.007184$$

Wt is weight in kilograms and Ht is height in centimeters. Patients at risk for patient–prosthesis mismatch are usually older, have smaller prostheses inserted, and usually have native valve aortic stenosis (as opposed to native valve aortic regurgitation). Mechanical valves tend to be larger than bioprostheses, but stentless bioprostheses may have a larger EOA than mechanical valves.

Prosthetic aortic stenosis may be evaluated in a similar manner as native valve aortic stenosis (see above). Stenosis will develop with thrombus formation (mechanical valves) or with progressive invading fibrous

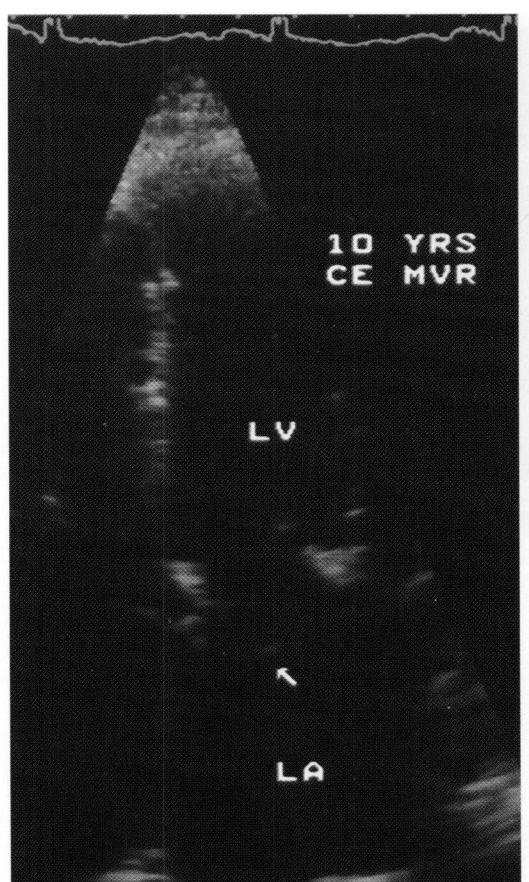

(a)

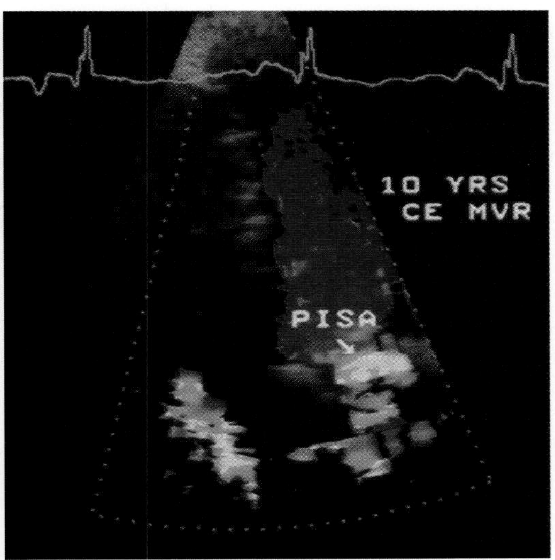

(b)

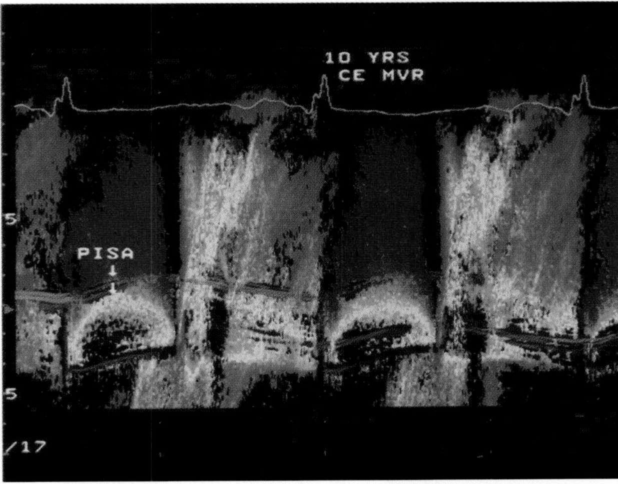

(c)

Fig. 10.18 An 80-year-old-male with a 10-year old Carpentier–Edwards mitral bioprosthesis presented with severe progressive dyspnea and heart failure. He had no symptoms or physical findings suggesting endocarditis. A loud murmur of mitral regurgitation was noted by auscultation. Continuous wave (CW) Doppler of the prosthetic valve revealed a high mitral inflow velocity (peak 2.47 m/s) and a rapid pressure half-time (76 ms). Although the mean pressure gradient was 10.9 mmHg, the patient had no evidence of valve stenosis. (a) Apical four-chamber view suggests a possible flail prosthetic leaflet (arrow) noted within the left atrium during systole. (b) With color Doppler there is noted PISA (arrow) in systole at the bioprosthetic valve orifice, suggesting valvular (not perivalvular) MR. (c) M-mode with color Doppler again reveals PISA (arrow) occurring within the prosthesis orifice, during systole. (*Continued on pp. 152–153.*)

(d)

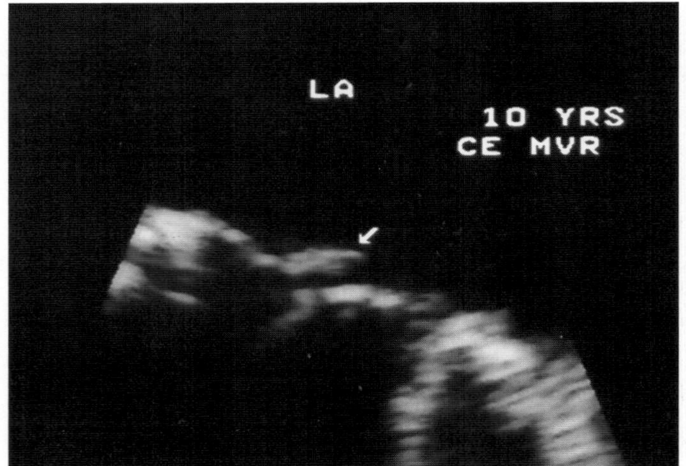

(e)

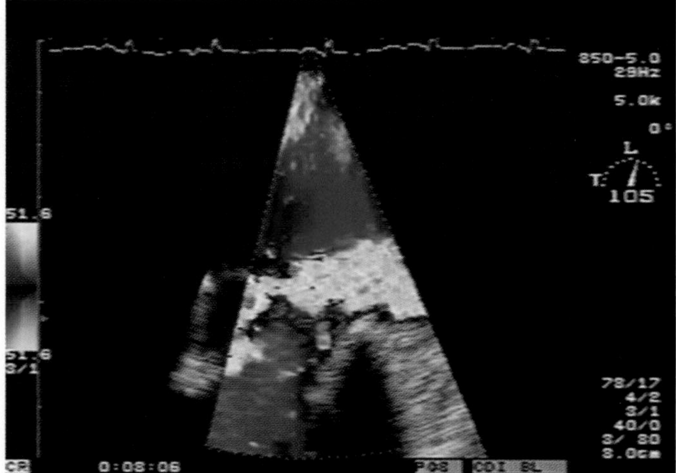

(f)

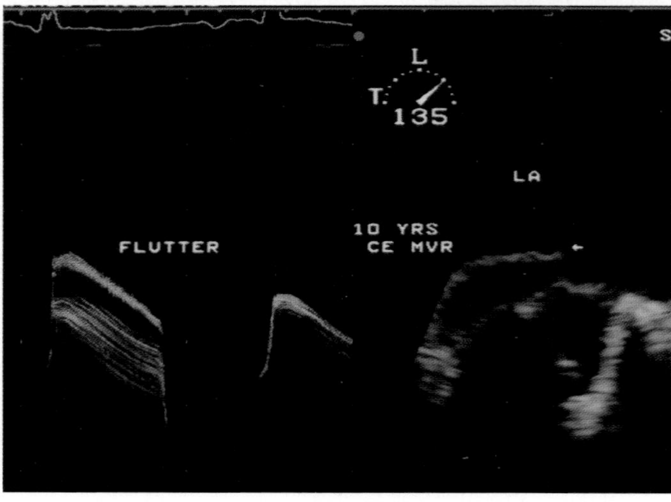

Fig. 10.18 (*cont'd*) (d) TEE at 105° reveals a flail prosthetic leaflet (arrow). (e) TEE at 105° with color Doppler demonstrates severe MR, having an eccentric jet. (f) M-mode and 2-D imaging at 135°. Note fine systolic fluttering of the flail leaflet.

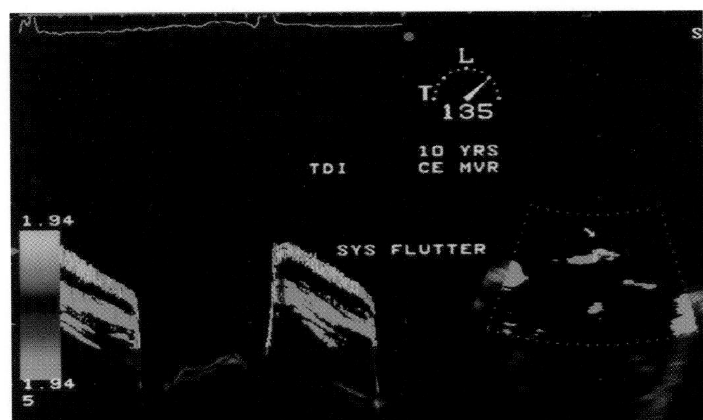

(g)

Fig. 10.18 (*cont'd*) (g) Image as in (f) but with tissue Doppler imaging (TDI). TDI helps highlight the flail leaflet fluttering.

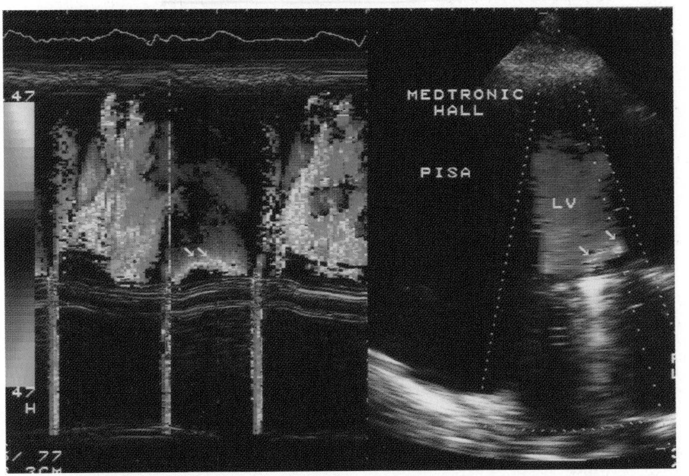

(a)

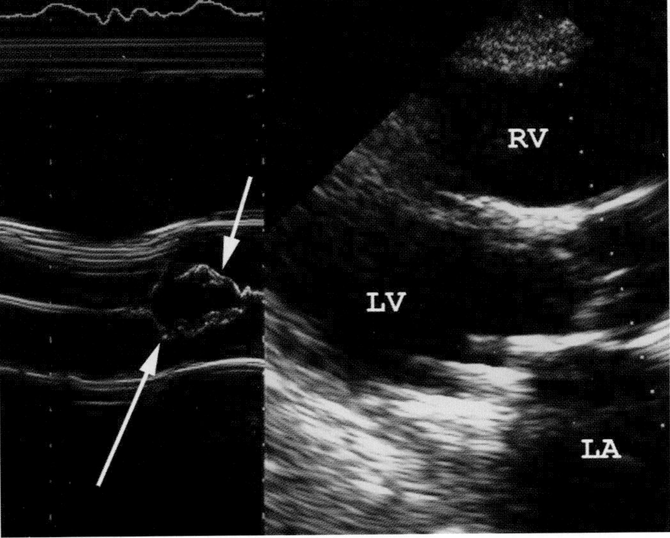

(b)

Fig. 10.19 A middle-aged male with progressive dyspnea and a loud mitral murmur. The patient had a Medtronic–Hall mitral valve prosthesis placed 6 months earlier. (a) Apical four-chamber view with color Doppler. Both 2-D (arrows) and M-mode (arrows) imaging reveals PISA in the lateral prosthetic annulus. From an apical window, slowly rotating the imaging transducer will often reveal an area of PISA within the valve annulus, at the site of periprosthetic leak. (b) Parasternal long axis imaging with M-mode through the aortic valve reveals gradual aortic closure (arrows), consistent with severe MR.

(a)

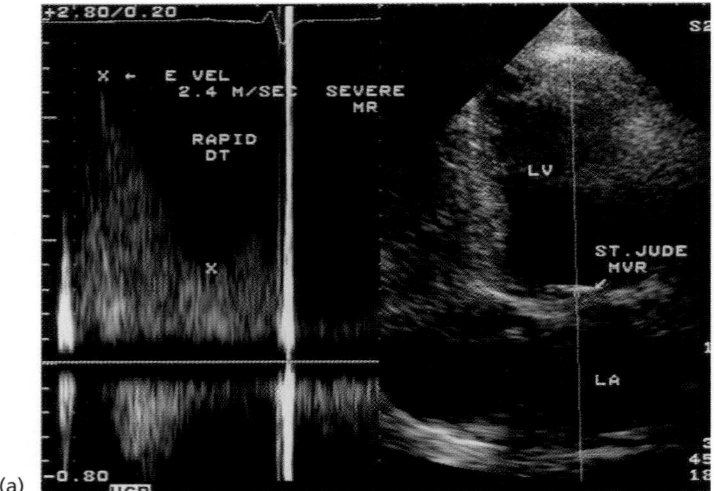

(b)

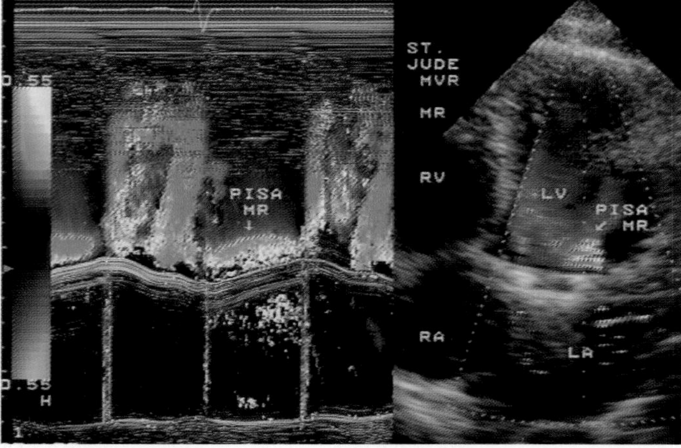

(c)

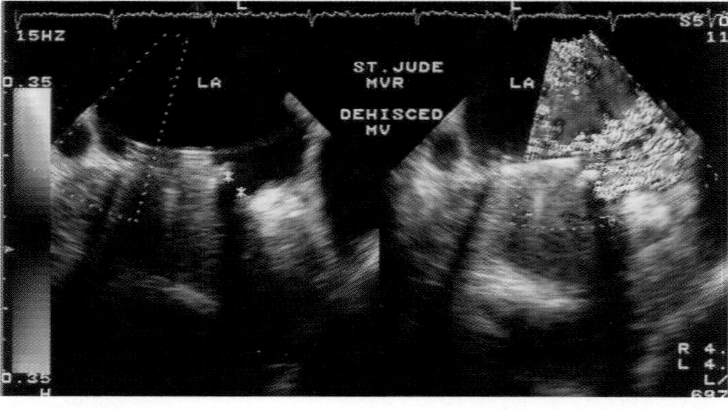

Fig. 10.20 A young male with a history of St Jude mitral valve replacement presents with severe dyspnea and a mitral regurgitation murmur. (a) Continuous wave Doppler from an apical four-chamber view reveals an increased mitral inflow velocity (2.4 m/s) and a rapid deceleration time. Although the velocity across the mitral prosthesis is high, the rapid deceleration time suggests the valve is not obstructed. (b) Apical four-chamber with color Doppler (M-mode and 2D) demonstrate systolic PISA through the prosthetic annulus. (c) TEE at 90° reveals a partially dehisced (left panel) mitral prosthesis (*), and color Doppler (right panel) mitral regurgitation (MR) through the dehisced portion of the valve annulus.

tissue (pannus formation). With severe prosthetic AS, the dimensionless index (DI) will be ≤0.20 across a mechanical valve or ≤0.15 for a bioprosthetic valve (<0.25 suggests severe native valve AS). The DI is theoretically not dependent on physiologic conditions, that is, it will not change with the development of a high cardiac output (as with severe anemia or fever) or a drop in cardiac output (large myocardial infarction). For cases of *low output, low gradient prosthetic aortic stenosis*, presumably one should apply similar methods as those for evaluation of native aortic valve stenosis (see Chapter 7).

Doppler methods for *prosthetic aortic regurgitation* evaluation are similar to that for native aortic regurgitation (AR). TEE is reserved for difficult transthoracic studies, to better determine the etiology of AR, and to evaluate the aortic root for associated pathology. "Normal" minimal AR may occur in up to 25–50% of aortic prostheses (most common in mechanical valves). Complications of endocarditis such as annular abscess and fistula formation are better diagnosed by TEE (see Chapter 18).

Tricuspid and pulmonic valve

Because of relatively low flow across the tricuspid valve, there is an inordinately high incidence of mechanical valve thrombosis, despite adequate anticoagulation. If a tricuspid prosthetic valve is required,

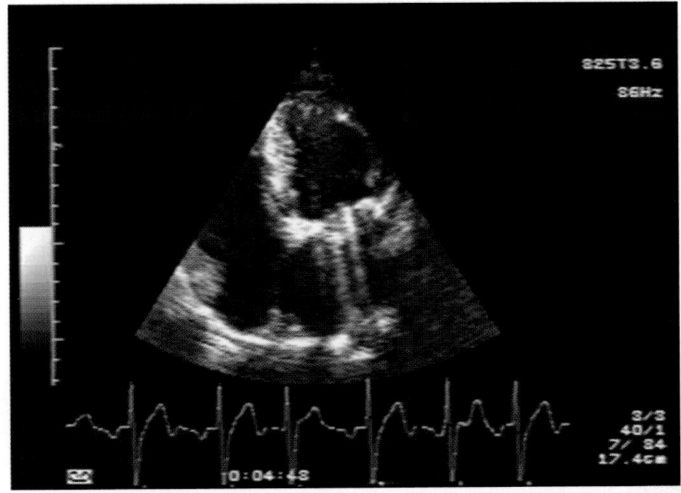

(a)

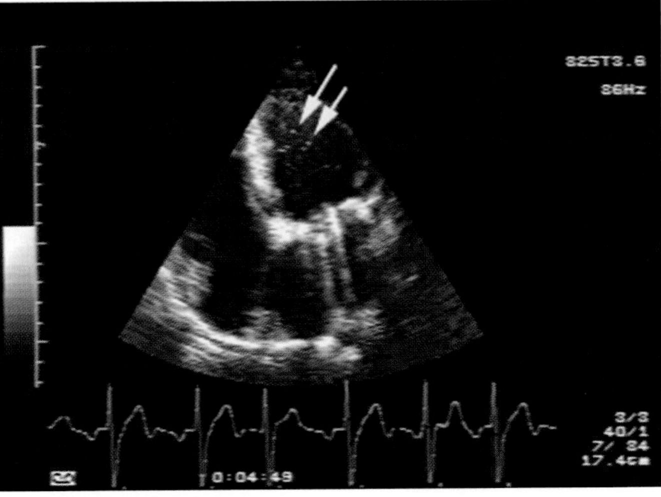

(b)

Fig. 10.21 Four diastolic frames from an apical window in an asymptomatic 40-year-old male with a double leaflet tilting disk mechanical valve. (a) As diastole begins the LV cavity is unremarkable, but several milliseconds later (b) quickly moving so-called "sparkles" are noted (arrows) to enter the LV. In (c) the sparkles (arrow) are still present, but by end-diastole (d) they have disappeared. These "sparkles" are thought to be a result of gas bubble formation resulting from a local (at the disk–annulus line of closure) rapid decrease in pressure as the mechanical disk opens. These "sparkles" are not suggestive of valve dysfunction or of any abnormality of clotting mechanisms. (*Continued on p. 156.*)

(c)

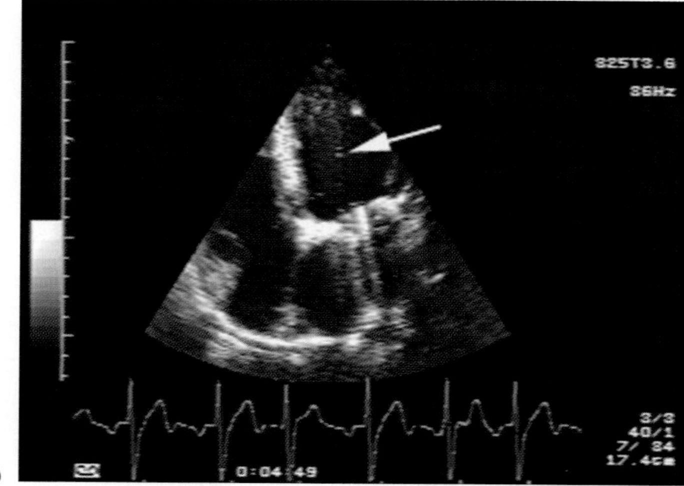

(d)

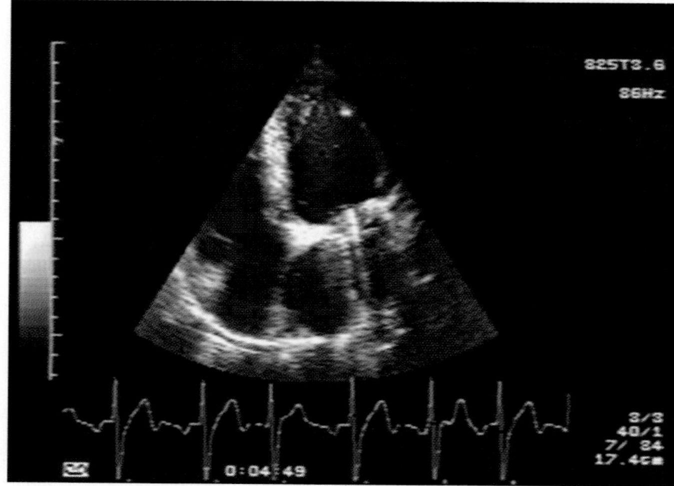

Fig. 10.21 *(cont'd)*

a biologic tissue valve is usually selected. Because marked tricuspid regurgitation (TR) is most often due to tricuspid annulus dilatation, an annuloplasty ring repair is often performed. One needs to document preoperatively the anatomic integrity of the tricuspid valve structure. Doppler methods of evaluation of prosthetic tricuspid stenosis and regurgitation are similar to those of native tricuspid valve disorders (see Chapter 9). When recording from an apical window, one needs to be careful not to confuse severe pulmonic regurgitation (PR) with prosthetic tricuspid stenosis. The PR jet may cross in front of the tricuspid valve. One needs to record at least 10 cardiac cycles, as significant respiratory variation occurs with flow across the prosthetic tricuspid valve. An average (from the 10 cycles) E wave velocity, mean valve gradient, and pressure half-time should be noted. As the native tricuspid annulus is relatively large, a relative high mean gradient may be noted across the tricuspid prosthesis. This may represent patient–prosthesis mismatch in the tricuspid position. Patients having an average (averaged over 10 cycles) mean gradient greater than 5.3 mmHg and PHT longer than 238 ms may have pathologic prosthetic valve stenosis.

Doppler evaluation of a prosthetic pulmonic valve is similar to that of native pulmonic valve stenosis and regurgitation.

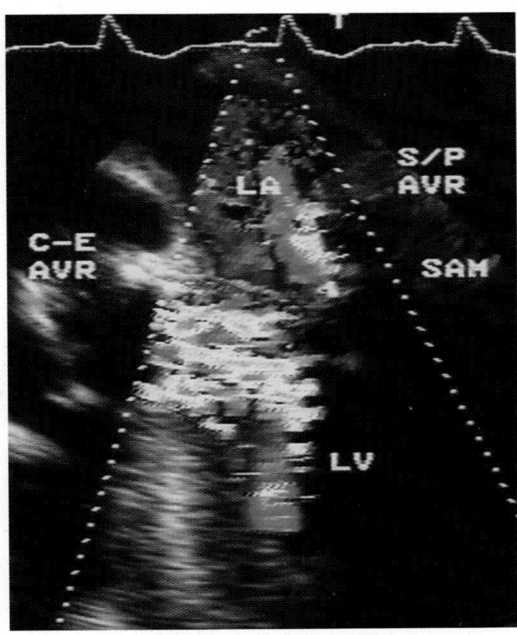

Fig. 10.22 TEE in the horizontal plane in a patient several weeks after aortic valve replacement with a Carpentier–Edwards bioprosthesis (C-E AVR). The patient presented with progressive exertional dyspnea and a loud systolic murmur along the left sternal border. Because of a difficult transthoracic acoustic window, a TEE was performed revealing a normally functioning aortic bioprosthesis, but an 80-mmHg dynamic gradient through the LVOT. Systolic anterior motion (SAM) was well documented along with the development of color flow turbulence within the LVOT. Preoperatively, patients with a relatively small LVOT, especially with aortic stenosis and significant LV hypertrophy, are at risk of postoperative dynamic LVOT obstruction. The cardiovascular surgeon may perform a septal myectomy along with the aortic valve procedure to reduce the possibility of postoperative LVOT dynamic obstruction.

Complete, partial and intermittent prosthetic valve obstruction

Mechanical disk valves may demonstrate *complete obstruction*, *partial obstruction*, or *intermittent obstruction* (Figs 10.23–10.25). Complete obstruction of a single-tilting disk valve may result in the disk becoming immobile in a partially open position. Marked elevation of gradients will be noted, and valve regurgitation may coexist. If the disk is "frozen" in the open position, severe prosthetic valve regurgitation will occur, and there may be no forward flow obstruction. One needs to be careful, as the regurgitation velocities may be low, and equalization of pressures may quickly occur across the prosthesis. With a double-disk mechanical valve, often only one disk will be "frozen". One needs to document full motion

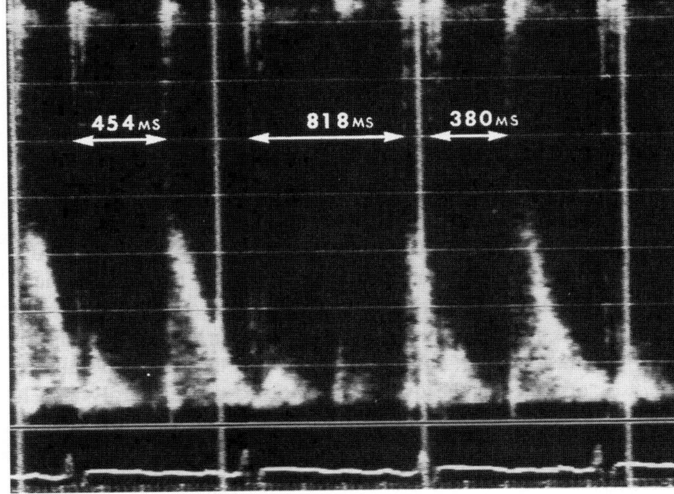

Fig. 10.23 Doppler interrogation of an intermittently "sticking" Bjork–Shiley mitral single disk mechanical valve. The patient had normal sinus rhythm. The numbers (arrows) are the time in milliseconds from valve closure to subsequent valve opening (opening interval). The third inflow is markedly delayed with flow beginning after atrial systole. (Reproduced with permission from: Mann DL, Gillam LD, Marshall JE, King ME, Weyman AE. Doppler and two-dimensional echocardiographic diagnosis of Bjork–Shiley prosthetic valve malfunction: importance of interventricular septal motion and the timing of onset of valve flow. Journal of the American College of Cardiology 1986; 8: 971–974.)

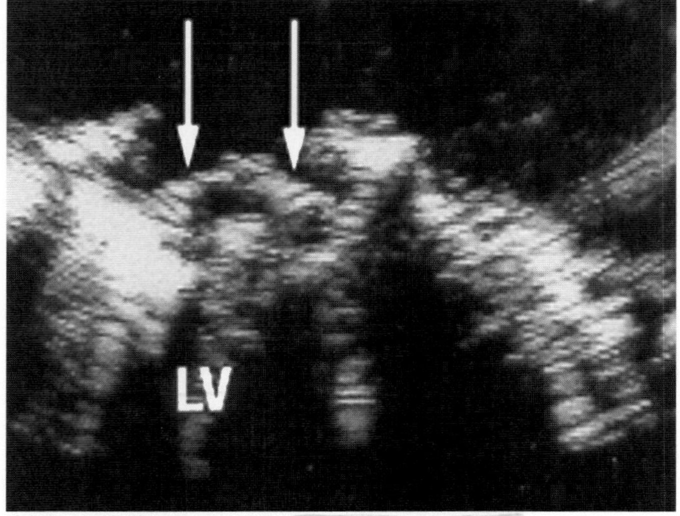

(a)

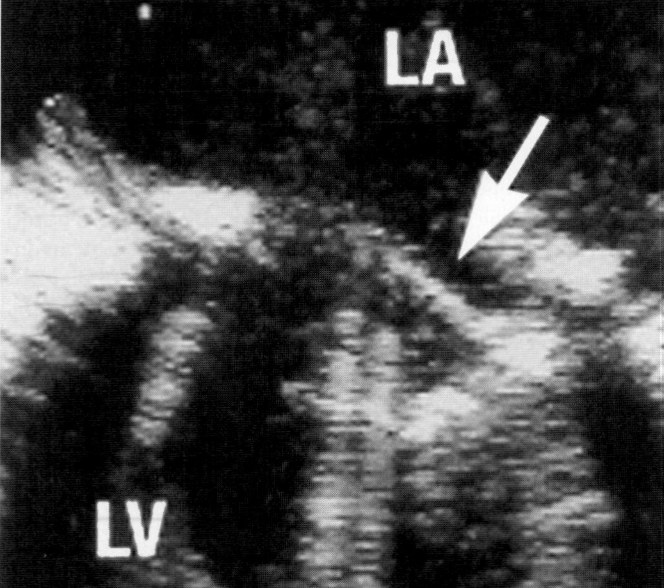

(b)

Fig. 10.24 TEE of a CarboMedics bileaflet mechanical valve with a single obstructed leaflet. (a) In systole both leaflets appear normal (arrows), but in diastole (b) one of the leaflets remains closed (arrow). (Courtesy of CarboMedics, Inc.)

of both disks to avoid missing this problem. Use of thrombolytic agents for thrombotic occlusion of mechanical valves has been used in patients generally at high risk for surgical intervention or in critically ill patients who it is felt would not survive the preparation involved in going to the operating room, and in whom immediate intervention is needed. Risks of thrombolytic therapy in these patients include arterial embolism.

Intermittent prosthetic valve opening may be seen either with a primary prosthetic valve problem, or with severe ventricular dysfunction. With a partially obstructed valve, the gradient across the abnormal valve will be elevated. In cases of severe ventricular dysfunction and a normal prosthetic valve (Fig. 10.26), the valve gradient will be low (in this case the ventricle is unable to normally open the normal prosthetic valve—seen usually with aortic prosthetic valves).

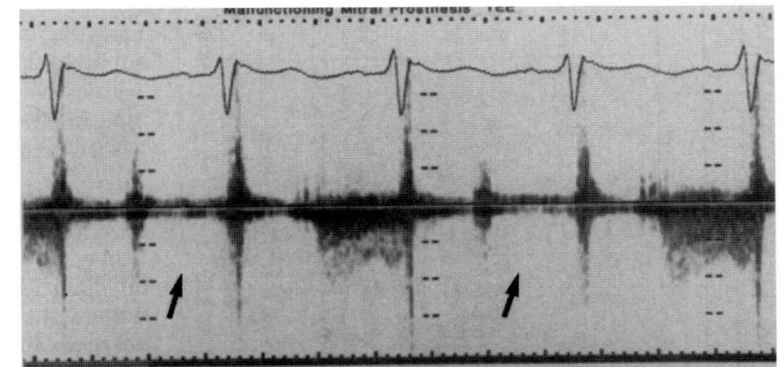

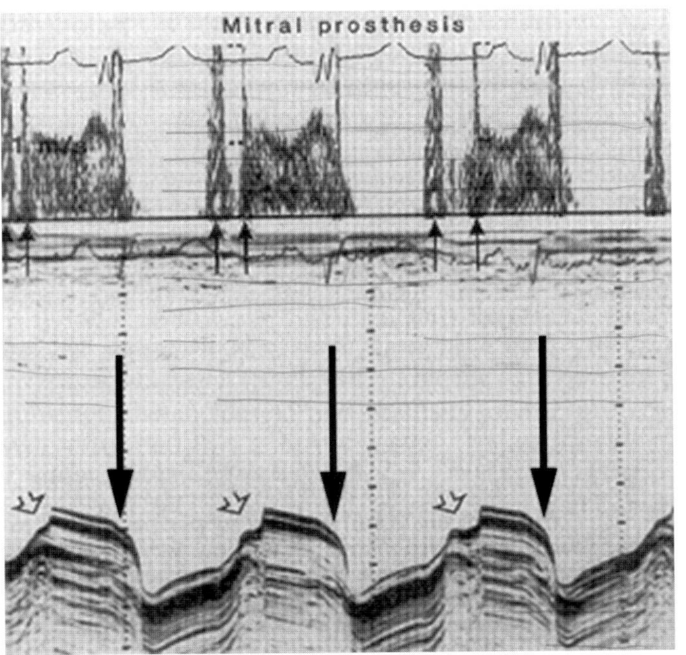

Fig. 10.25 Examples from an excellent paper by Shahid, Sutherland and Hatle (1995: see Further reading, p. 366) of Doppler patterns of intermittent obstruction of mechanical mitral valve prostheses. (a) A Bjork–Shiley single-tilting disk leaflet with no flow across the prosthesis in the second and fourth beats (arrows). *Increased* flow velocity, due to partial obstruction, is noted during the other beats. Each double dash represents 1 m/s. (b) M-mode and Doppler of a Bjork–Shiley mitral prosthesis from the apical window. The patient has intermittent obstruction, and is in normal sinus rhythm. Intermittently delayed opening of the disk is noted, as documented by Doppler (vertical arrows). By M-mode, restriction to disk opening, with a "rounded" pattern (oblique open arrows), and also a rounded disk closure pattern (single vertical arrows), are noted. (Reproduced with permission from: Shahid M, Sutherland G, Hatle L. Diagnosis of intermittent obstruction of mechanical mitral valve prostheses by Doppler echocardiography. American Journal of Cardiology 1995; 76: 1305–1309.)

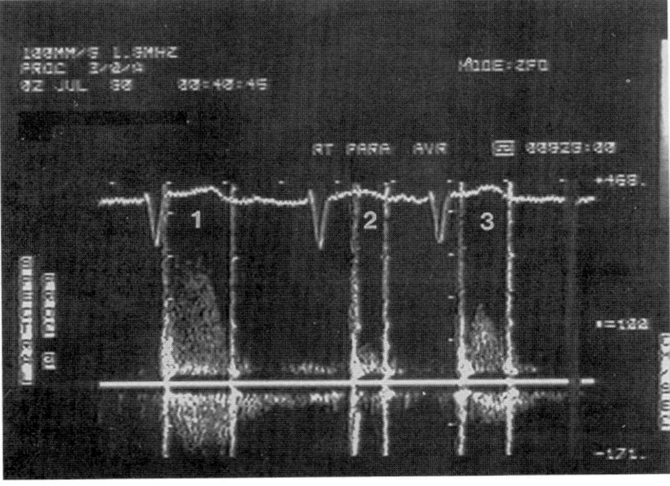

Fig. 10.26 CW Doppler from the right parasternal window in a patient with an aortic mechanical prosthesis. The second complex reveals delayed opening and decreased LVOT velocity. In the third beat there is mild delay in valve opening and mild reduction of flow velocity through the LVOT. This pattern of delayed valve opening (second and third complexes) is due to left ventricular dysfunction, as the velocity associated with delayed opening is reduced. The mechanical valve is normal. If the mechanical valve was abnormal, LVOT velocities would be increased. (Reproduced with permission from: Weyman AE. Principles and Practice of Echocardiography, 2nd edn. Philadelphia: Lea & Febiger, 1994: 1226, figure 38.45.)

11

CHAPTER 11

Cardiomyopathy and Heart Failure

Cardiomyopathy (idiopathic) is defined as a primary disease of heart muscle, as opposed to those attributed to other components of the cardiovascular system (ischemic, valvular, congenital, systemic, or pulmonary hypertension). The term *idiopathic* or *primary* is used when the cause is neither suspected nor known. Cardiomyopathy (CMP) is characterized by systolic or diastolic dysfunction. Categories of cardiomyopathy include *dilated, hypertrophic, restrictive,* and *arrhythmogenic right ventricular cardiomyopathy*. The *World Health Organization* (WHO) categorizes CMP as the following:

- dilated—idiopathic, familial, viral, immune, toxic/alcohol
- hypertrophic
- restrictive—idiopathic, secondary
- arrhythmogenic RV—autosomal dominant, recessive
- unclassified—noncompaction
- specific—ischemic, valvular, hypertensive, inflammatory, metabolic, general system disease, muscular/neuromuscular, toxic.

It may be convenient to classify CMP by dividing it into dilated and nondilated types, based on ventricular volume: increased versus normal or decreased. The dominant physiologic disturbance in dilated CMP is systolic ventricular dysfunction with secondary diastolic dysfunction, whereas in the nondilated types of CMP, isolated diastolic dysfunction predominates. Nondilated CMP may be divided further into hypertrophic and nonhypertrophic (restrictive, obliterative) types (after T.D. Giles, MD, p. 367).

Echocardiography is an important tool in patients with a clinical diagnosis of *congestive heart failure*, as up to 50% of these may have a normal LV ejection fraction (EF). Most heart failure patients with a normal EF have hypertension with *hypertensive heart disease* and may have *ischemic heart disease* concurrently. A few patients will have hypertrophic cardiomyopathy or a restrictive form of cardiomyopathy (see Fig. 5.7).

Dilated cardiomyopathy

Dilated cardiomyopathies generally manifest a uniform reduction of LV systolic function, with increased systolic and diastolic volumes and a decreased *relative wall thickness* (see Chapter 5 & Fig. 5.7). Patients with a greater LV wall thickness and smaller LV radius-to-thickness ratio appear to have a better prognosis. M-mode and two-dimensional (2-D) characteristics of dilated cardiomyopathies include (Figs 11.1–11.3):

- Biventricular uniform reduction in systolic function, but may appear to have segmental wall motion abnormalities.
- Increased systolic and diastolic chamber volumes.
- Wall thickness usually normal but may be increased or decreased. The increase in thickness is not proportionate to the increased chamber volume (diminished relative wall thickness).
- Increased cardiac mass.
- Dilated atria.
- Apically displaced papillary muscles with subsequent mitral valve coaptation apically displaced (relative chordal shortening) and reduction of contact between the mitral leaflets, thus reducing valvular competence.
- E-point to septal separation (EPSS) indicative of an enlarged left ventricle, a distance of greater than 6 mm is abnormal.
- Decreased aortic root motion and early aortic valve closure, indicative of low cardiac output.
- B-bump is indicative of an elevated end-diastolic pressure (occurs on either mitral or tricuspid valve).
- Increased risk of intracavitary thrombus formation.

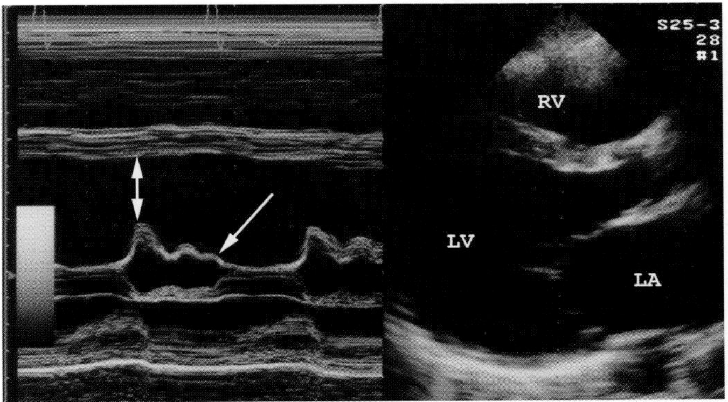

Fig. 11.1 Parasternal long axis two-dimensional (2-D) (right panel) and "2-D guided" M-mode (left panel) of a 50-year-old-female with an idiopathic dilated cardiomyopathy. All four cardiac chambers were dilated. Note the increased E-point to septal separation (EPSS) (double-headed arrow) and the prominent B-bump (single headed arrow) on the mitral tracing. A B-bump is usually noted with systolic dysfunction, and suggests an elevated LV end-diastolic pressure of ≥15 mmHg.

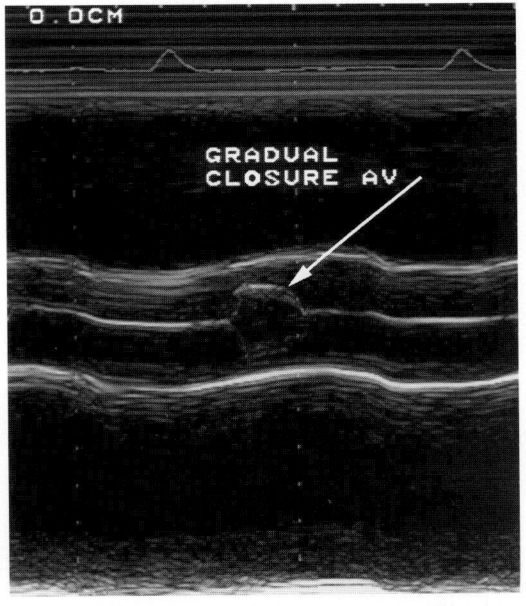

(a)

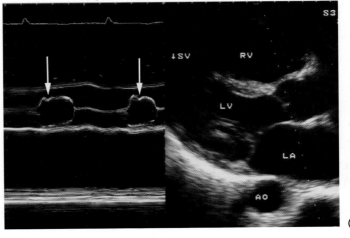

(b)

Fig. 11.2 (a) M-mode through the aortic valve in a patient with a dilated cardiomyopathy and poor forward stroke volume. Note a gradual leaflet closure prior to the completion of systole (arrow). (b) This patient also has a dilated cardiomyopathy and a low stroke volume. On occasion the M-mode pattern may demonstrate early or mid-systolic closure (arrows). This patient had no evidence of dynamic subaortic obstruction, but the pattern was due to a low stroke volume. AO, descending aorta.

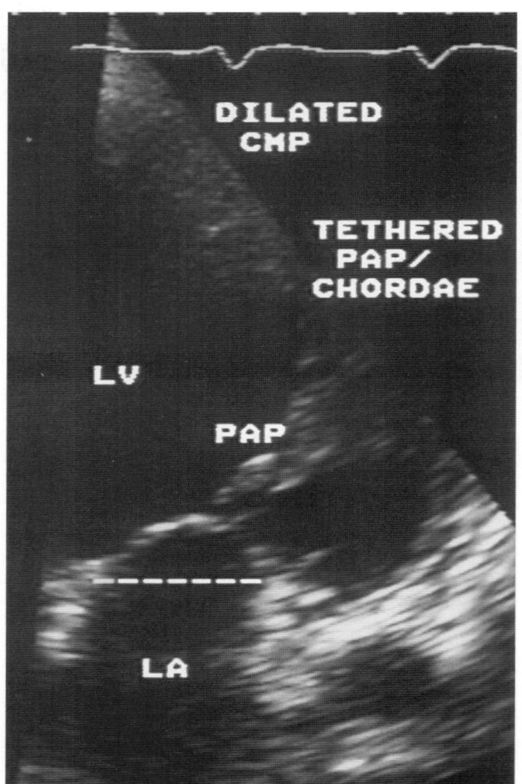

(a)

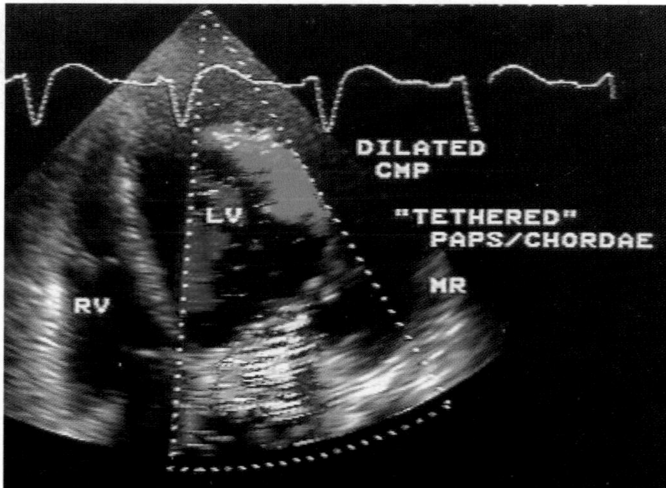

(b)

Fig. 11.3 Apical image of a patient with a dilated cardiomyopathy. Relative displacement of papillary muscles toward the LV apex, secondary to the altered LV geometry (the LV assumes a more globular shape), results in inadequate mitral valve coaptation and often marked mitral regurgitation. (a) The dashed line indicates the mitral valve plane, but valve closure occurs within the LV cavity, not at the mitral annulus as normally occurs. (b) Color Doppler demonstrates mitral regurgitation (MR) beginning well within the cavity of the left ventricle.

- Reduced EF, stroke volume (SV), cardiac output (CO).

Doppler methods are used to evaluate hemodynamics (see Chapters 4 & 5) and include the following:

- Calculation of stroke volume and cardiac output (often best to use the left ventricular outflow tract (LVOT)).
- Evaluation for coexistent mitral regurgitation (primary MR) and also MR secondary to the dilated LV (relative apical displacement of papillary muscles) (Fig. 11.3). The degree of MR (secondary to the dilated LV) is affected by loading conditions. With bicycle exercise echo-Doppler, those patients who develop marked increases in MR also have reduced functional capacity and develop a more spherical LV (sphericity index) during both systole and diastole.
- Estimation of left heart filling pressures using mitral and pulmonary vein flow, and tissue Doppler of the mitral annulus.
- Calculation of right heart pressures—tricuspid regurgitation and IVC dynamics.
- Assessment of response to medical therapy.

Differential diagnosis of forms of cardiomyopathy with systolic dysfunction

With *ischemic cardiomyopathy*, segments of akinesis or thinning/scarring are typically present, but in some patients the ventricle may appear diffusely hypokinetic. Patients with an idiopathic dilated cardiomyopathy may have segments of akinesis along with segments that appear to have normal contractility (usually the basal inferior and posterior segments). At end-stage, ischemic and nonischemic cardiomyopathy may be essentially impossible to differentiate. If, however, some regions have normal wall motion and others are akinetic to dyskinetic, the etiology is most likely ischemic.

Chronic volume overload may appear similar to dilated (idiopathic) cardiomyopathy. Often valvular (aortic regurgitation, mitral regurgitation) or an uncorrected congenital defect (patent ductus arteriosus, ventricular septal defect (VSD), atrial septal defect (ASD)) will simulate a dilated cardiomyopathy. One should look for a primary structural abnormality or abnormal Doppler flow pattern. Differentiating *primary mitral regurgitation* from that secondary to a dilated left ventricle (*functional mitral regurgitation*) may be difficult at "end-stage." Primary MR may have an observed structural abnormality (ruptured chordae or papillary infarction), whereas functional MR is suggested by apical and posterior displacement of papillary muscles, secondary to the LV assuming a spherical shape (Fig. 11.3).

The right ventricle is often spared (normal size) with ischemic cardiomyopathy and is often dilated with idiopathic cardiomyopathy, but there is too much overlap to use this as a strong differential point. In patients with dilated cardiomyopathy, patients with an equal degree of RV and LV dilatation appear to have a worse prognosis than those with relative RV sparing. In those with a *dilated RV*, there is generally more marked mitral and tricuspid regurgitation.

In patients with dilated cardiomyopathy, it appears that a greater *LV wall thickness* is associated with longer survival, and a smaller *LV radius-to-thickness ratio* appears to be "protective". Other echo predictors of a poor prognosis include a depressed *LV ejection fraction*, *increased LV chamber size* with progressive dilatation, and *abnormal LV shape* (increased LV sphericity).

Doppler parameters may also be predictive of survival. A *restrictive mitral filling pattern*, especially one that cannot revert to abnormal relaxation with medical therapy, has a much higher mortality rate than those with mitral abnormal relaxation. Maneuvers that alter LV preload are predictive of prognosis in patients with LV systolic dysfunction (Fig. 11.4). Also, a *tricuspid regurgitant jet of 2.5 m/s* or more is associated with increased mortality.

Bicycle stress testing with color Doppler identifies patients with a marked increase in MR during exercise. MR associated with a dilated cardiomyopathy is secondary to relative apical displacement of papillary muscles and apical displacement of mitral leaflet coaptation, reducing the contact between the two leaflets and compromising valvular competence—*functional mitral regurgitation*. Exercise tolerance, particularly symptoms of dyspnea, seems to be related to the degree of exercise-associated MR. An exercise-associated rise in pulmonary artery pressure also appears to be correlated with exercise-associated MR.

Arrhythmogenic right ventricular cardiomyopathy (ARVC) affects primarily the RV and involves gradual myocyte replacement with adipose and fibrous tissue. It may be difficult to differentiate from dilated cardiomyopathy in its most advanced form, when involvement progresses to both the RV and LV with

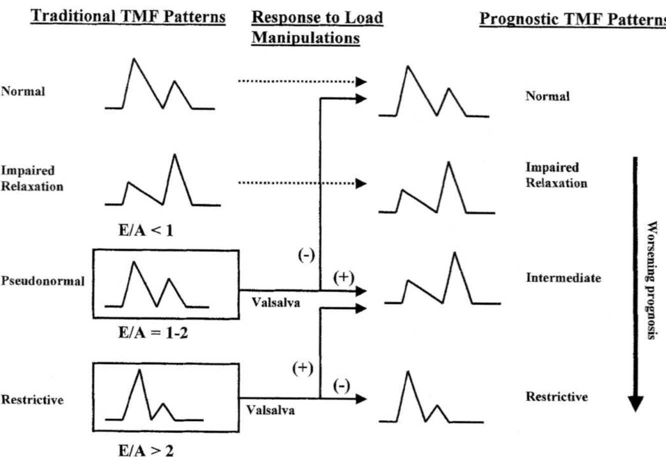

Fig. 11.4 Classification methodology from pulsed wave Doppler mitral inflow patterns (TMF) to assess prognosis in patients with congestive heart failure and LV systolic dysfunction. Patients with a pseudonormal and restrictive filling pattern (shown in boxes) are challenged with LV preload reduction by performing the *Valsalva maneuver*. Those who revert to an impaired relaxation pattern have a better prognosis than those who remain unchanged. *Sodium nitroprusside* infusion has been used by others to reduce LV preload and assess its effect on mitral inflow patterns. Also, in patients who have impaired relaxation, *leg lifting* (increasing preload) seems to identify patients with a worse prognosis, if the inflow pattern becomes pseudonormal or restrictive. (Reproduced with permission from: Xie G, Smith MD. Pseudonormal or intermediate pattern? Journal of the American College of Cardiology 2002: 39: 1796–1798.)

development of biventricular heart failure. ARVC often presents in young males (up to age 40) with symptoms related to ventricular tachycardia (usually a left bundle branch block morphology), and may present as sudden death with physical activity (the most common cause of sudden death in young Italian athletes) or heart failure. Diagnosis requires histologic confirmation of fatty replacement of RV muscle, but the disease process is segmental and the interventricular septum is usually not involved (the area usually biopsied), making diagnosis difficult. Because of this difficulty, criteria for diagnosis have been established (McKenna *et al.* 1994: see Further reading, p. 368). Echocardiographic features of ARVC may be easily missed. Findings include a hypokinetic and dilated RV, but the RV may appear normal. The most suggestive features include dilatation of the RV with localized aneurysms noted during diastole and dyskinesis in the inferior basal region. A RV/LV end-diastolic diameter ratio greater than 0.5 is suggestive of ARVC, with a value less than 0.5 having a significant negative predictive value. Extreme RV dilatation is better predictive of ARVC. Other findings include increased echo reflectivity of the RV moderator band and prominent RV apex trabeculations. Electron-beam computerized tomography (EBCT) and magnetic resonance imaging also appear to be useful for diagnosis of ARVC.

Hypertrophic cardiomyopathy

Hypertrophic cardiomyopathy (HCM) is a primary disorder of myocardium manifested by hypertrophy of a nondilated ventricle (usually the left ventricle), usually with histologic myocardial fiber disarray. The pattern of hypertrophy is usually asymmetric. Its incidence has been described as occurring in anywhere from 0.07% to 0.5% of the general population. Diagnosis is determined by finding hypertrophy (usually LV hypertrophy) without another etiology, such as aortic stenosis or hypertension. HCM is often associated with excessive LV systolic function, but no single "pattern" of hypertrophy is typical or classic. Hypertrophy may range from localized mild hypertrophy to involvement of multiple myocardial segments or all segments. Hypertrophy, however, nearly

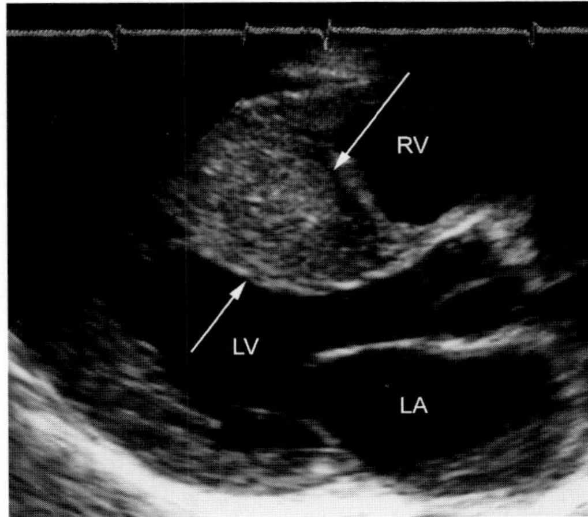

Fig. 11.5 Asymmetric septal hypertrophy (ASH) with prominent septal hypertrophy evident in the parasternal long axis view (arrows).

always involves some part of the ventricular septum, and most frequently the anterior septum. Asymmetric hypertrophy is most commonly found but symmetric hypertrophy may be occasionally noted. Heterogeneity of thickening from segment to segment is commonly noted with abrupt changes between thickened and nonthickened segments (Fig. 11.5).

HCM is categorized as:

Asymmetric septal hypertrophy (ASH; incidence in parentheses):

ventricular septal (90%)

mid-ventricular (1%)

apical (3%)

posteroseptal and lateral wall (1%).

Symmetric (concentric) hypertrophy 5%.

Right ventricular:

isolated or with associated left-sided hypertrophy.

ASH is the most common form of HCM, with an M-mode septal-posterior LV wall thickness ratio >1.3 associated, and a ratio >1.5 highly associated. An interventricular septal thickness (IVS) ≥15 mm is also suggestive. *Symmetrical hypertrophy* is an uncommon form of HCM. This may lead to difficulty in differentiating hypertensive or athlete's heart from HCM. Generally with ASH:

- The hypertrophic pattern is variable.
- The more extensive the hypertrophy, generally the more severe the functional impact.
- Upper septal hypertrophy with hypertrophy elsewhere is often associated with high LVOT gradients.
- Usually hypertrophy "spares" the basal posterior wall, but exceptions exist.
- Obstruction is associated with an LVOT diameter less than 20 mm and with the degree/duration of mitral systolic anterior motion (SAM).

ASH occurs in other situations (not all ASH is HCM). Other etiologies of ASH include:

- normal variants—elderly, athletes
- LV hypertrophy (LVH)—hypertension or aortic stenosis may have focal septal hypertrophy
- RV hypertrophy (RVH)—pulmonic stenosis, pulmonary hypertension
- infiltrative disorders—amyloid, tumors
- inferior myocardial infarction with LV scar formation
- hemodialysis
- LV free-wall infarction
- infant—diabetic mothers (transient)
- fetus—normal.

Asymmetric apical hypertrophy was first reported in Japan. Classic findings include *deep T wave inversions* over 10 mm across the precordium by ECG, and an "*ace of spades*" LV imaged by left ventriculography or echocardiography. Characteristics of asymmetric apical hypertrophy (Figs 11.6–11.8) include:

- Hypertrophy of apical LV segments—hypertrophy may start with a single apical segment and progress to all four segments with the "ace of spades" configuration.
- Usually absence of LVOT obstruction, unless hypertrophy extends toward the LVOT.
- "Spade-like" appearance at end-diastole, often noted by left ventriculography.
- Often deep T wave inversions across the precordium by ECG.
- Intracavitary LV Doppler flow during the isovolumic relaxation time (IVRT) toward the LV base (IVRT flow is directed toward the apex with most other forms of HCM).

Midventricular hypertrophy with obstruction from the mid-ventricle is uncommon. In this condition, hypertrophy occurs in the mid-portion of the LV with obstruction at the same level. Dynamic LVOT obstruction is usually not associated (no SAM or aortic mid-systolic closure). An apical infarction with aneurysm and hypercontractile function of the

(a)

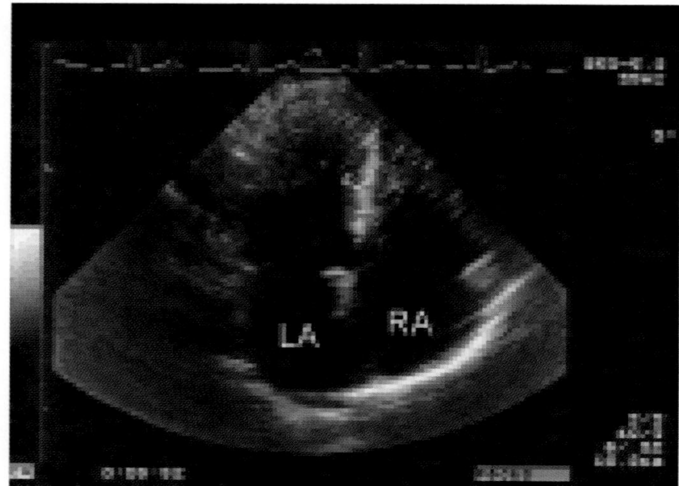

(b)

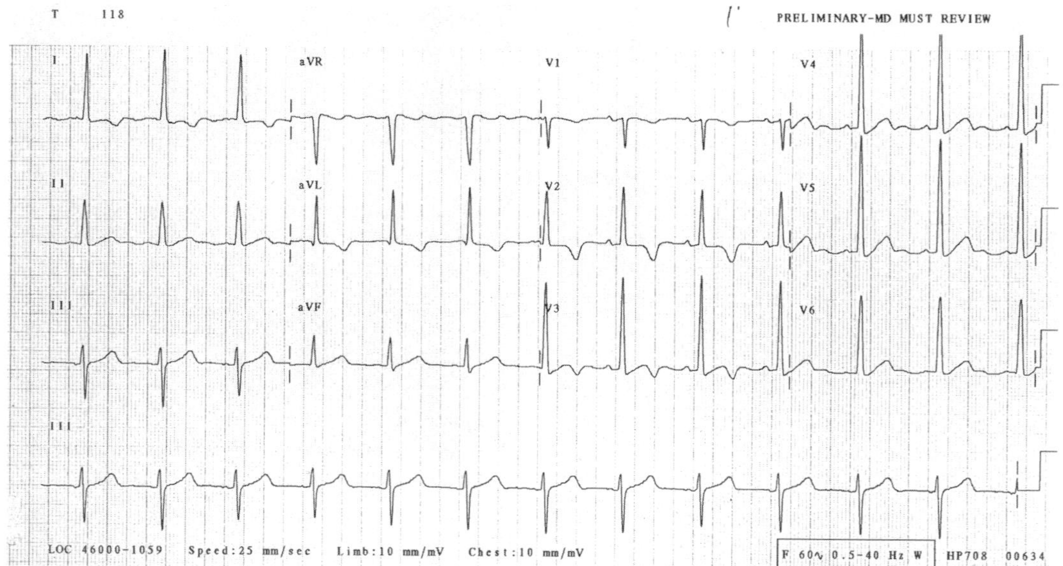

Fig. 11.6 A 64-year-old-female with exertional dyspnea is found to have apical hypertrophy (a) by apical four-chamber imaging. Significant LV cavity narrowing is noted toward the apex, associated with marked thickening from the mid LV segments toward the apex. She also has an abnormal ECG (b) with precordial T wave inversions. Coronary arteriography revealed normal epicardial coronary vessels.

midportion of the LV may functionally behave as midventricular hypertrophy.

Left ventricular cavity obliteration (Figs 11.9 & 11.10) is associated with vigorous LV systolic function, and with LV cavity obliteration at end-systole. Cavity obliteration is noted particularly in elderly patients and is more notable with relative volume depletion. It is also often noted with a hyperdynamic state, and with hypertension and aortic stenosis (concentric LVH).

Echocardiographic features (M-mode and 2-D) of *hypertrophic cardiomyopathy* (Figs 11.11–11.14) include:

1 Ventricular hypertrophy:

(a) Measure ventricular wall thickness, and look for regional wall thickness variations.

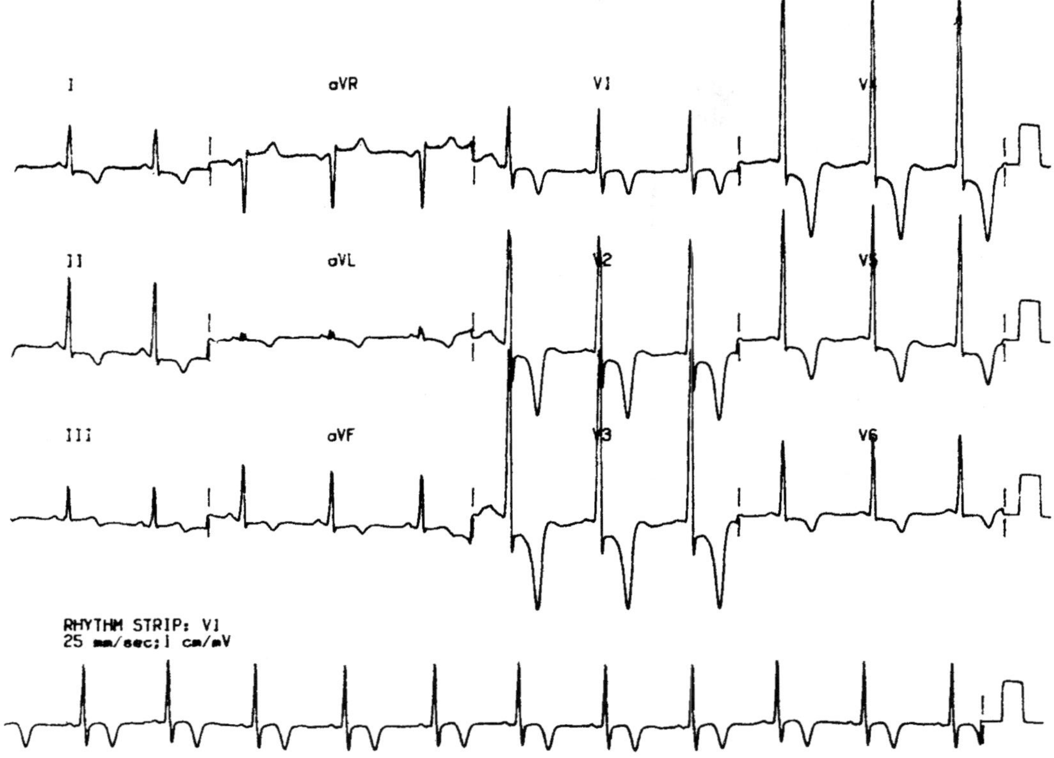

Fig. 11.7 "Typical" ECG pattern in a patient with apical hypertrophy highlights giant T wave inversions with high voltage QRS waveforms across the precordium. This ECG is from a classic paper describing apical hypertrophy. (Reproduced with permission from: Keren G, Belhassen B, Sherez J, *et al.* Apical hypertrophic cardiomyopathy: evaluation by noninvasive and invasive techniques in 23 patients. Circulation 1985; 71(5): 45–56.)

(b) Measure from the parasternal short axis basal, mid-papillary and LV chamber levels. Wall thickness may change abruptly from one segment to the next (it is important to evaluate and measure the end-diastolic thickness of each myocardial segment to evaluate for the extent of myocardial involvement).

(c) Avoid paraseptal (RV and LV) bands and chords in measuring septal thickness.

2 Systolic anterior motion (SAM):

(a) Anterior displacement of mitral valve and chordae in the LVOT.

(b) Involves mitral leaflet coaptation point to the valve tips.

3 Mid-systolic closure/notching of the aortic valve.

4 Normal or reduced LV chamber size.

5 Normal LV systolic function or an increased ejection fraction secondary to a small ventricular cavity.

6 Abnormal septal motion/systolic thickening.

7 Abnormal myocardial echo reflections:

(a) Unusual myocardial textural appearance of involved segments.

8 Mitral anterior leaflet:

(a) Often longer than normal.

(b) 10% have anomalous papillary insertion into the mitral leaflet.

9 SAM, outflow obstruction and the associated murmur will increase with a decrease in preload, a decrease in afterload or an increase in contractility.

10 SAM, outflow obstruction and the associated murmur will decrease with an increase in preload, an increase in afterload or a decrease in contractility.

SAM should be distinguished from "*chordal SAM,*" which is generally nonobstructive. "*Pseudo-SAM*" is systolic anterior leaflet motion that parallels the motion of the posterior LV wall. Most commonly

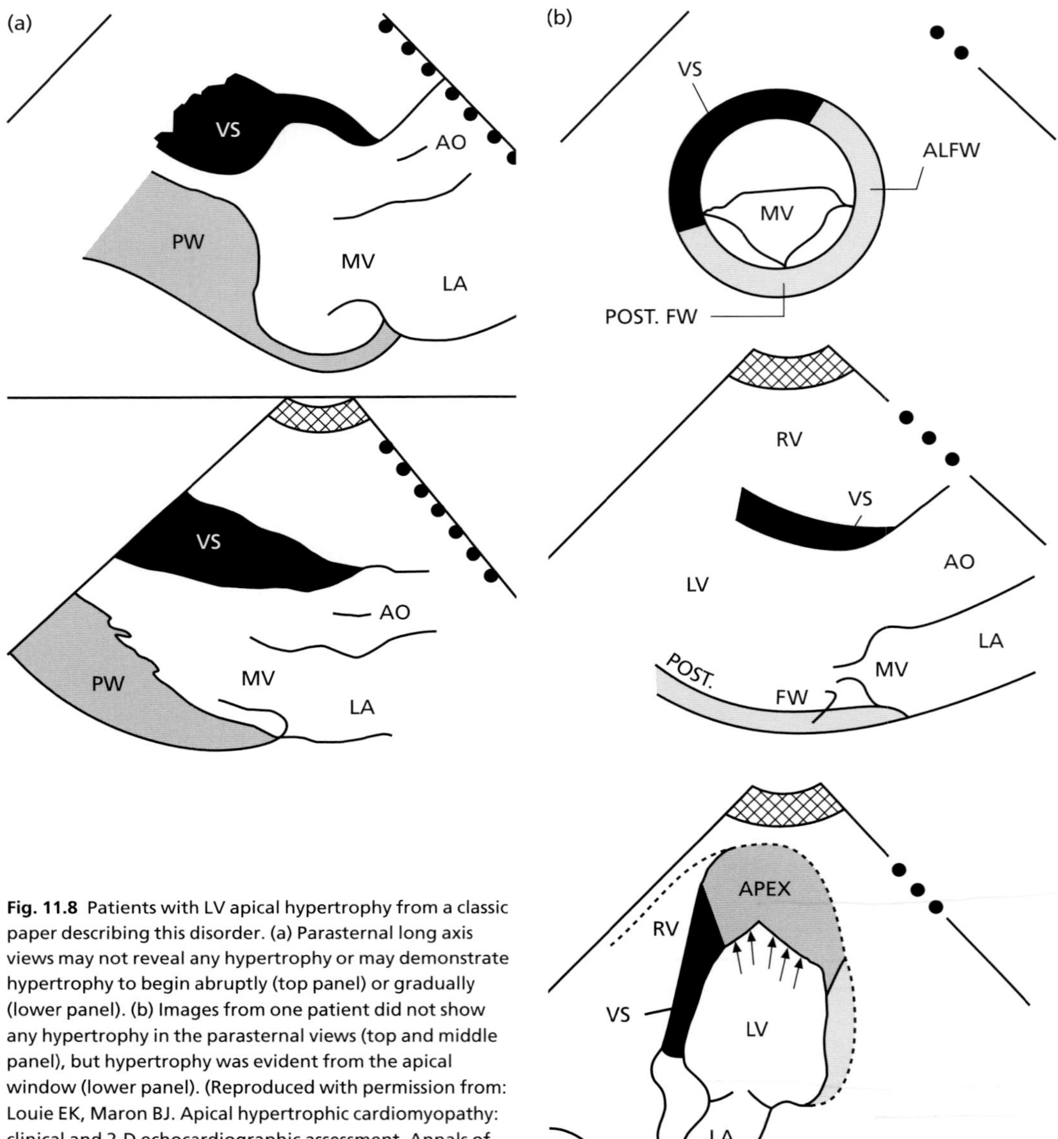

Fig. 11.8 Patients with LV apical hypertrophy from a classic paper describing this disorder. (a) Parasternal long axis views may not reveal any hypertrophy or may demonstrate hypertrophy to begin abruptly (top panel) or gradually (lower panel). (b) Images from one patient did not show any hypertrophy in the parasternal views (top and middle panel), but hypertrophy was evident from the apical window (lower panel). (Reproduced with permission from: Louie EK, Maron BJ. Apical hypertrophic cardiomyopathy: clinical and 2-D echocardiographic assessment. Annals of Internal Medicine 1987; 106: 663–670.)

pseudo-SAM is seen with pericardial effusion, atrial septal defect, or a hyperdynamic state. Some patients with elongated mitral chords will have early systolic anterior motion of the chords noted. This is also nonobstructive (see Fig. 8.27).

Other causes of LVOT obstruction include:

- discrete subaortic stenosis—a "fixed" obstruction Doppler pattern (see Chapter 16);
- mitral valve replacement with a strut or cage impeding the LVOT—a "fixed" obstruction (Fig. 11.15);
- mitral valve repair with a fixed ring and resultant SAM;
- anomalous papillary insertion into the anterior leaflet of the mitral valve.

Patients post aortic valve replacement for aortic stenosis may occasionally develop SAM. This is due to the combination of a hypertrophied LV with a sudden reduction in afterload. In addition, anemia, use of inotropes, hypovolemia, and a high catecholamine state may increase systolic function and be associated

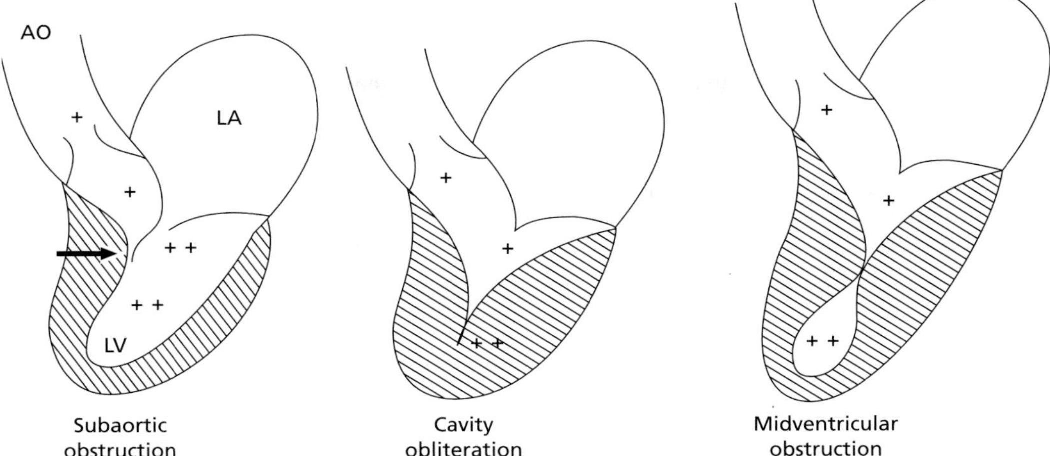

Fig. 11.9 The three levels of systolic obstruction. With *subaortic obstruction*, pressure proximal to the left ventricular outflow tract (LVOT) obstruction (due to mitral leaflet–septum contact) is increased. With *cavity obliteration*, an increase in flow is noted only at end-systole, and with *midventricular obstruction* an increased flow gradient is noted in mid-late systole. Only the subaortic obstructive form is associated with classic M-mode features of dynamic obstruction (systolic anterior motion (SAM) and mid-systolic aortic valve closure). (+), area of relatively low pressure; (+ +), areas of high pressure. (Reproduced with permission from: Wigle ED. Hypertrophic cardiomyopathy: a 1987 viewpoint. Circulation 1987; 75: 311–322.)

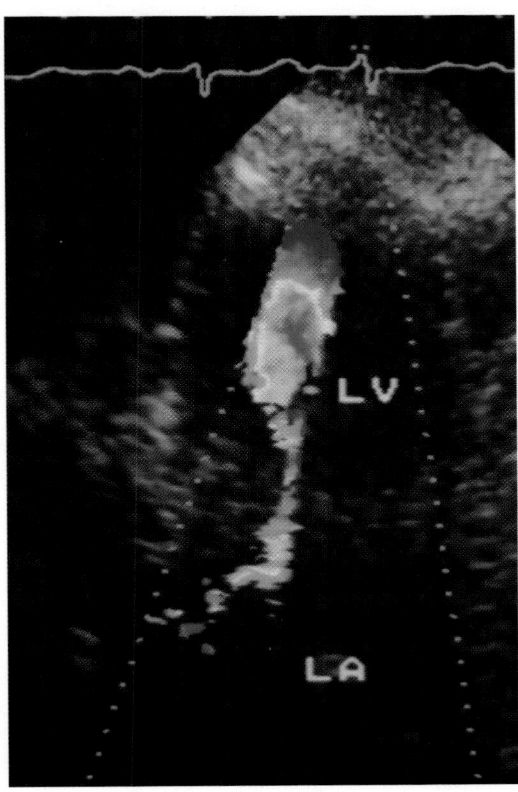

Fig. 11.10 Apical four-chamber image with color Doppler of a patient near end-systole with LV cavity obliteration.

with a small end-systolic volume (see Chapter 10 & Fig. 10.22).

In the elderly with hypertrophic cardiomyopathy (*hypertrophic cardiomyopathy of the elderly*), there appears to be a different LV morphology and mechanism of SAM. Elderly patients have relatively small hearts with a modest amount of hypertrophy which is usually localized to the anterior or posterior interventricular septum. Marked mitral annular calcification is a prominent feature. In relatively young patients dynamic obstruction occurs because of abrupt systolic anterior motion of the mitral valve motion toward the ventricular septum, with leaflet–septal contact made by the distal part of the mitral valve (most often anterior leaflet). The anterior leaflet will form an "L" shape as it touches the septum (Fig. 11.16), and posterior excursion of the ventricular septum contributes very little to the narrowed LV outflow tract. In contradistinction to this, elderly patients have relatively equal contributions of anterior mitral leaflet excursion and posterior motion of the ventricular septum toward the mitral leaflet. The mitral leaflet is almost flat in systole. In the elderly patient the LV cavity is ovoid with a normal septal curve (concave with reference to the LV cavity), but in younger patients a crescent-shaped LV cavity and convex septum (reversal of septal curvature) is noted (Fig. 11.17).

(a)

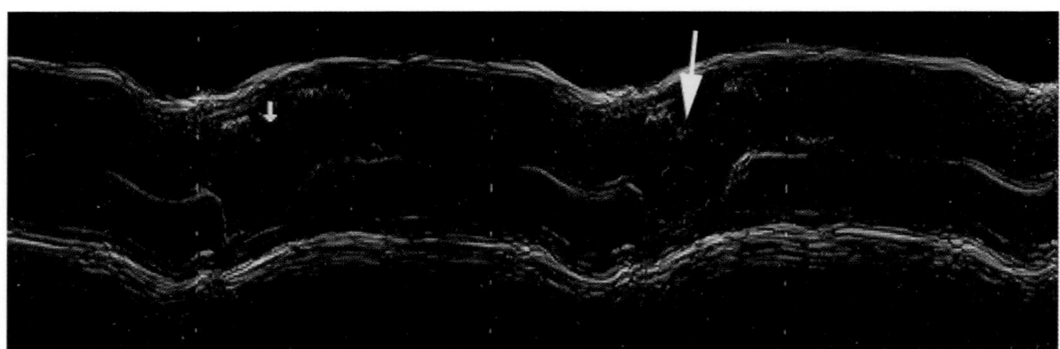

(b)

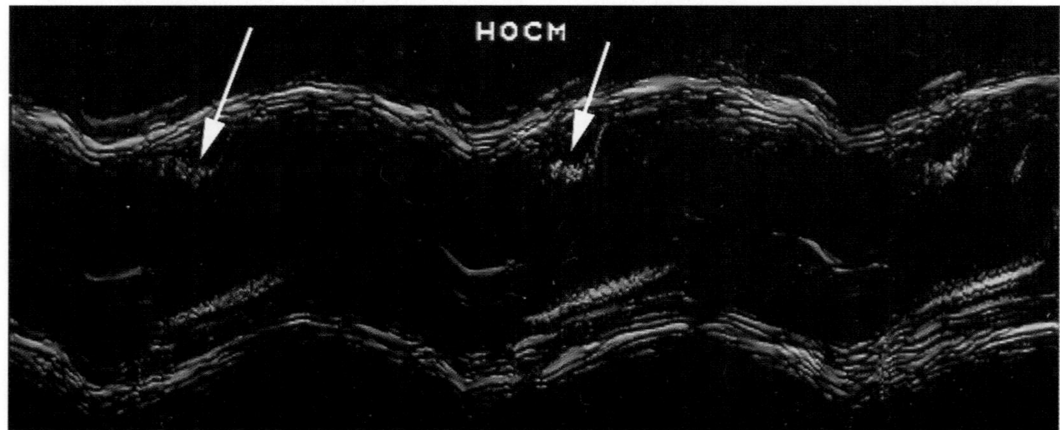

Fig. 11.11 M-mode through the aortic valve in two different patients (a,b) with hypertrophic cardiomyopathy (HCM) and dynamic LV outflow tract obstruction. Note mid-systolic closure (arrows).

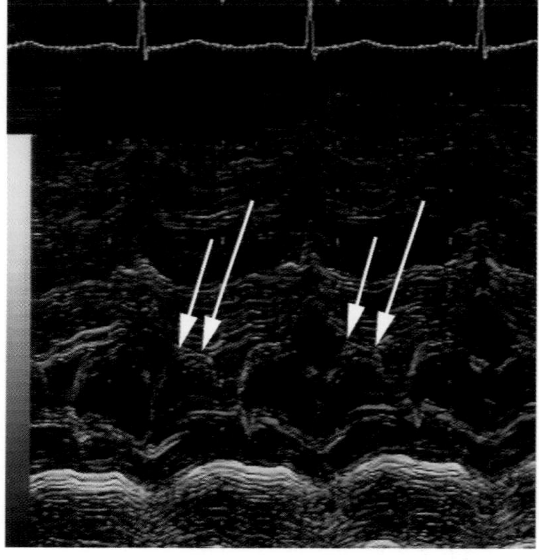

Doppler features of hypertrophic cardiomyopathy include evaluation to determine *the level and severity of obstruction* (and its dynamic nature), evaluation of mitral *regurgitation*, and evaluation of *diastolic properties*.

Dynamic LV obstruction may occur at basically three LV levels: LVOT obstruction, mid-ventricular obstruction, and LV cavity obliteration (Fig. 11.9). Some features to help distinguish the three levels of dynamic systolic obstruction are given in Table 11.1.

Distinguishing the level of obstruction may be difficult. The highest Doppler velocities will generally

Fig. 11.12 (*left*) SAM (arrows) of the mitral valve in an M-mode through the mitral valve in a patient with HCM and dynamic LV outflow tract obstruction.

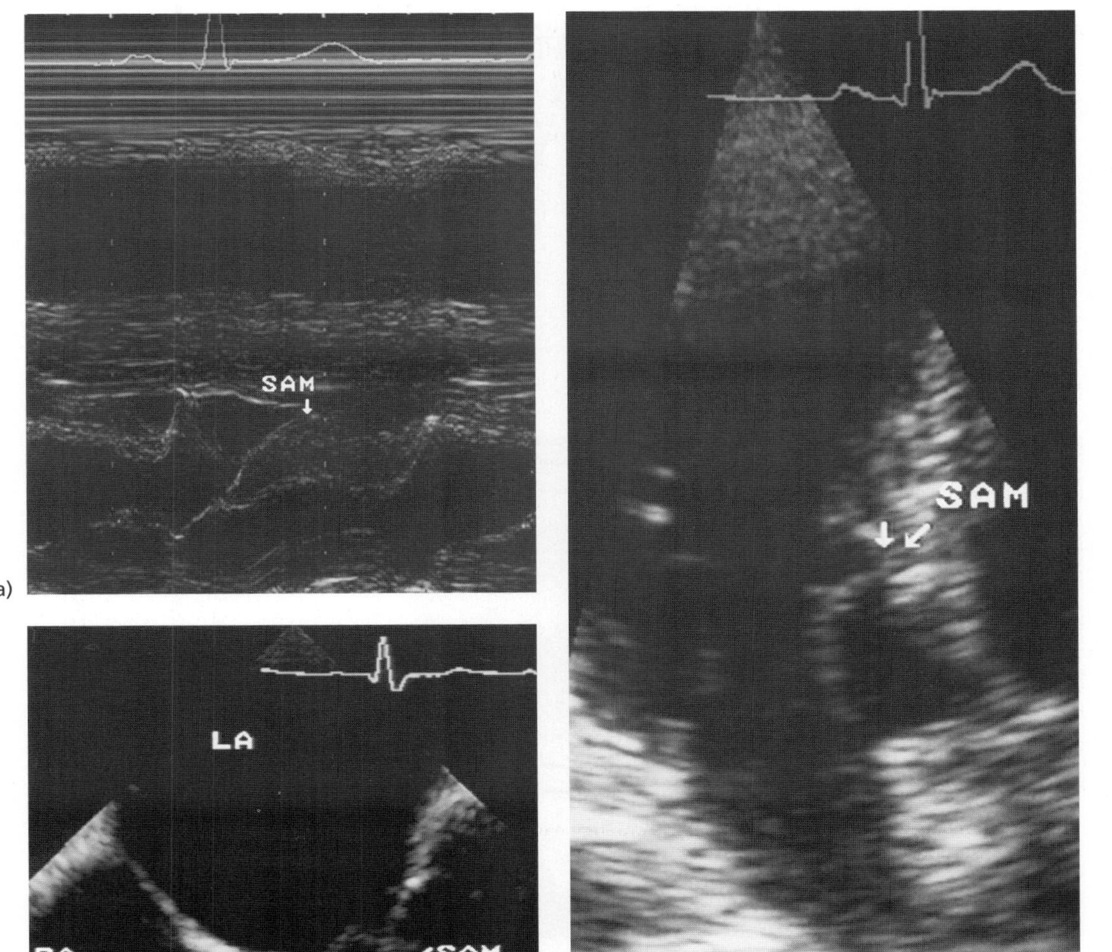

Fig. 11.13 (a) M-mode through a parasternal view of a patient with HCM and SAM. (b) 2-D apical four-chamber view of a patient with HCM and SAM of the mitral valve. (c) The same patient as in (b); imaging by transesophageal echocardiography (TEE). IVS, interventricular septum.

occur with LVOT obstruction (Figs 11.18–11.20). Each of the three "levels" of dynamic obstruction has a concave "dagger-shaped" systolic waveform. The peak velocity occurs in mid to late systole with LVOT obstruction, later in systole with mid-ventricular obstruction, and occurs in very late systole for LV cavity obliteration. The late systolic peak of LV cavity obliteration tends to be of relatively brief duration and

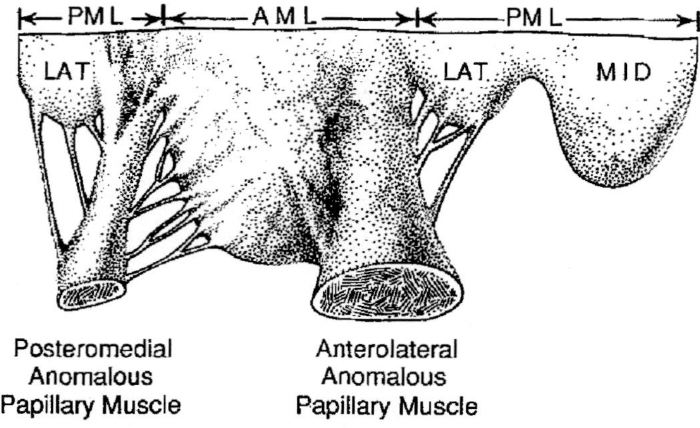

(a)

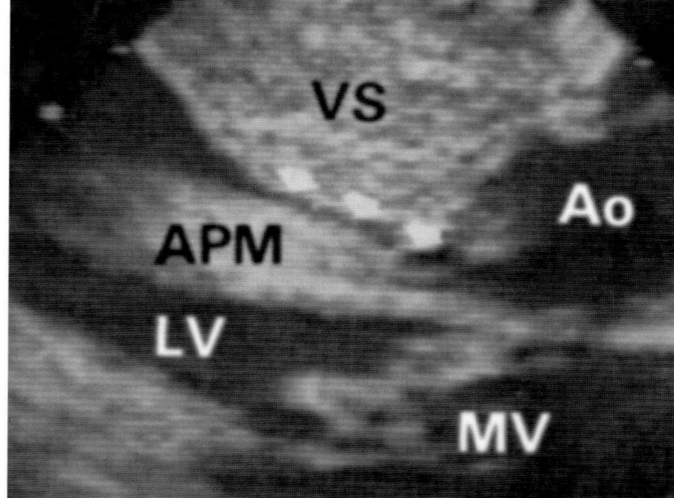

(b)

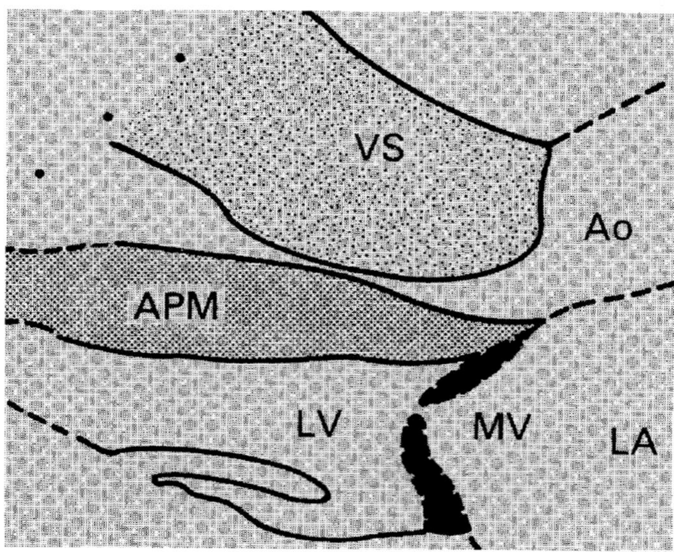

(c)

Fig. 11.14 Anomalous insertion of one or both left ventricular papillary muscles directly into the anterior mitral leaflet may be responsible for dynamic LVOT obstruction. (a) Representation of an opened mitral valve looking up from the left ventricle. The posteromedial and/or anterolateral papillary muscles may insert directly into the anterior mitral leaflet. There will be no chordae between the anomalous papillary muscle and the anterior leaflet of the mitral valve. The anomalous anterolateral papillary muscle is larger than the posteromedial papillary muscle and involves a larger portion of the anterior mitral leaflet. Photograph (b) and diagram (c) from a parasternal long axis view of a patient with an anomalous insertion of the anterolateral papillary muscle into the anterior mitral leaflet. (Reproduced with permission from: Klues HG, Roberts WC, Maron BJ. Anomalous insertion of papillary muscle directly into anterior mitral leaflet in hypertrophic cardiomyopathy. Circulation 1991; 84: 1188–1197.)

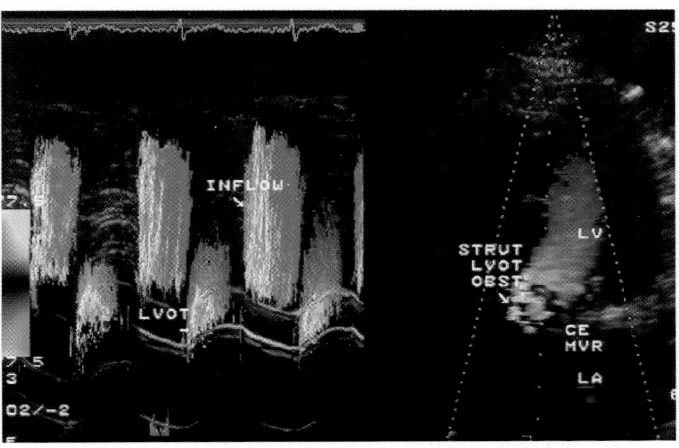

Fig. 11.15 Apical five-chamber view with color Doppler (right panel) and color M-mode (left panel) through the LVOT in a patient with a Carpentier–Edwards mitral valve replacement (C-E MVR). The strut touches the interventricular septum during systole and color flow turbulence is noted to begin at that site (LVOT in left panel and STRUT LVOT OBST in right panel). The resting CW gradient was 45 mmHg. The patient presented with exertional dyspnea and had a systolic murmur.

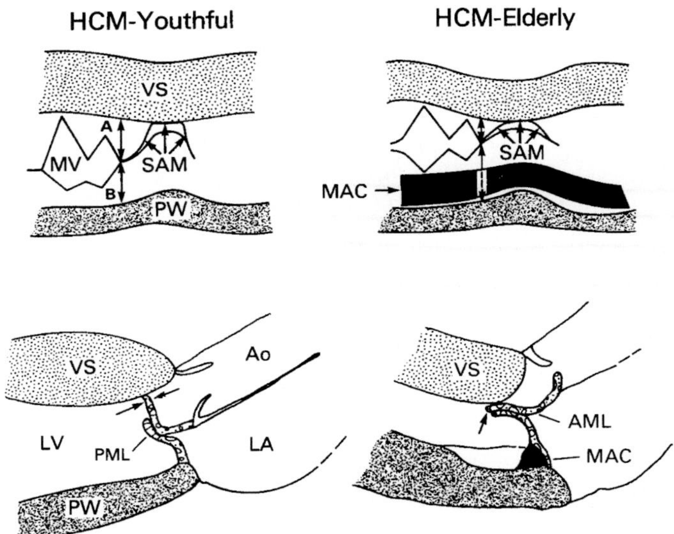

Fig. 11.16 The etiology of SAM and dynamic LV outflow obstruction in the (left panel) "Youthful" patient and the (right panel) "Elderly" patient. M-mode (upper panels) and parasternal long axis (lower panels) images are shown. In the "Youthful" patient (upper left panel) at end-diastole the distance from the mitral leaflets to the septum (A) is about the same as the distance from the mitral leaflets to the posterior wall (B). With systole, there is an abrupt anterior motion of the mitral leaflets noted. The interventricular septum contributes very little posterior motion toward the mitral leaflets in systole. The 2-D image of the "Youthful" patient (lower left panel) in mid-systole reveals an "L" shape bend in the anterior mitral leaflet as its tip contacts the interventricular septum. In the "Elderly" patient (right upper panel), the mitral valve–interventricular septum distance, in end-diastole, is less than that from the mitral valve to the posterior wall (arrows). The anterior leaflet is more anteriorly displaced, as compared to the "Youthful" patient, and marked mitral annulus calcification (MAC) is noted. In mid-systole, posterior motion of the interventricular septum and only mild anterior motion of the mitral leaflet (the mitral leaflet is already displaced anatomically toward the septum) cause the development of SAM. The anterior leaflet continues to have a flat appearance (lower right panel) with very little leaflet bend. (Reproduced with permission from: Lewis JF, Maron BJ. Elderly patients with hypertrophic cardiomyopathy: a subset with distinctive left ventricular morphology and progressive clinical course late in life. Journal of the American College of Cardiology 1989; 13: 36–45.)

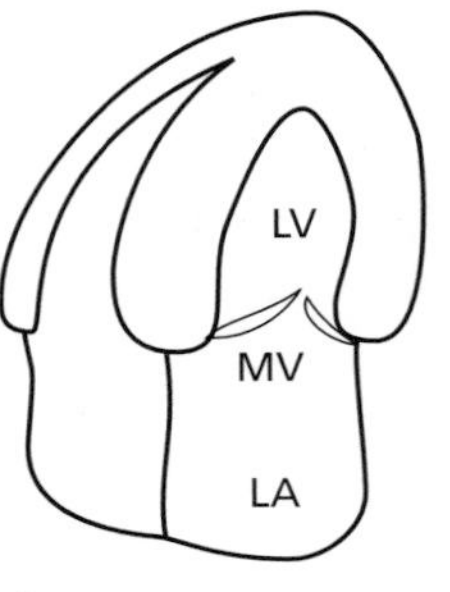

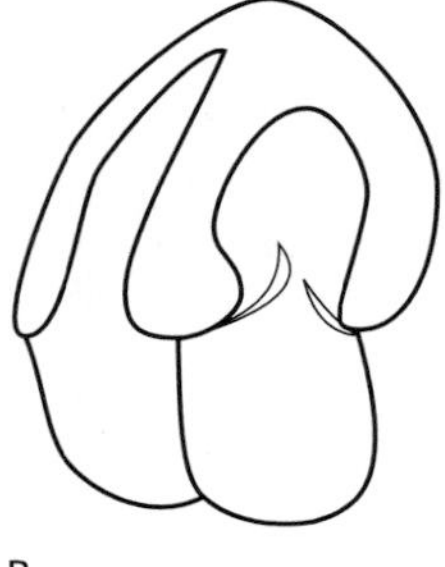

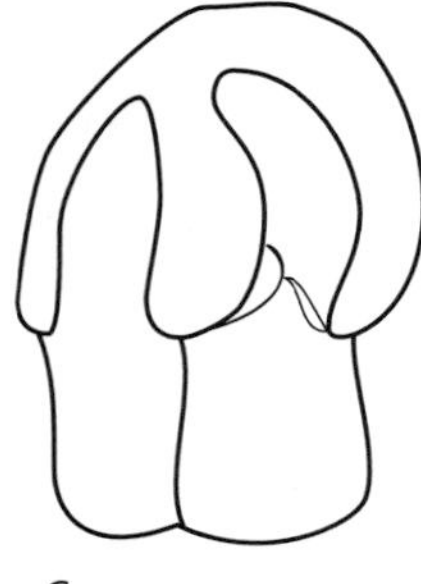

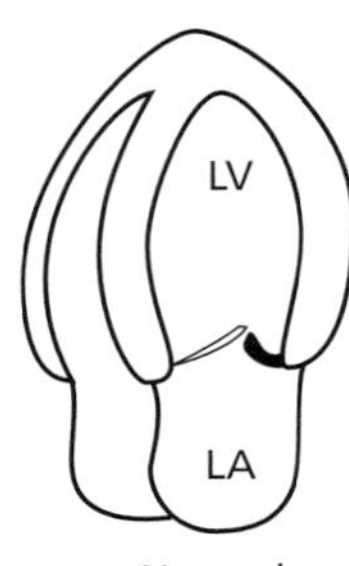

Fig. 11.17 Various LV shapes. In (D) a normal LV is shown. An ovoid LV shape is noted in an elderly patient with concentric left ventriclur hypertrophy (LVH) (A), and also an elderly patient (B) with LVH and a basal septal bulge. A typical young patient (C) with HCM demonstrates a convex direction of the interventricular septum. Note that the basic interventricular septal contour (concave) of the normal LV and elderly patient with hypertrophic cardiomyopathy is similar. (Reproduced with permission from: D'Cruz IA, Rouse CC. The hypertrophied ventricular septum: anatomic variants and their echocardiographic diagnosis. Journal of Noninvasive Cardiology 1997; Summer: 9–15.)

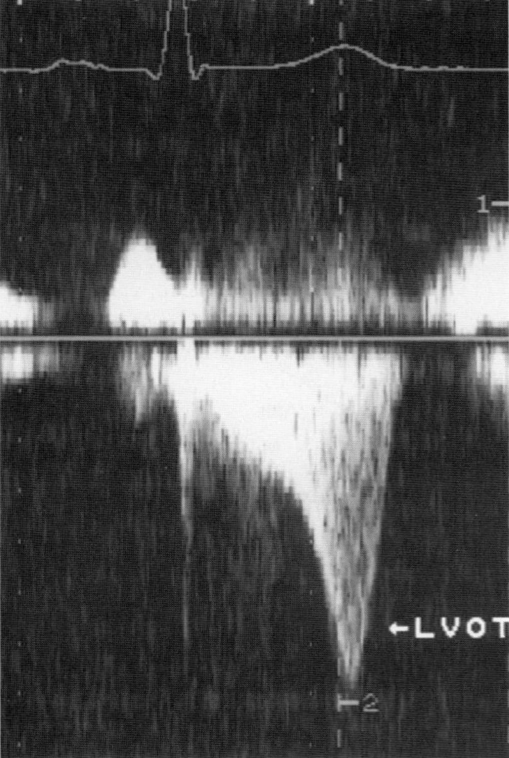

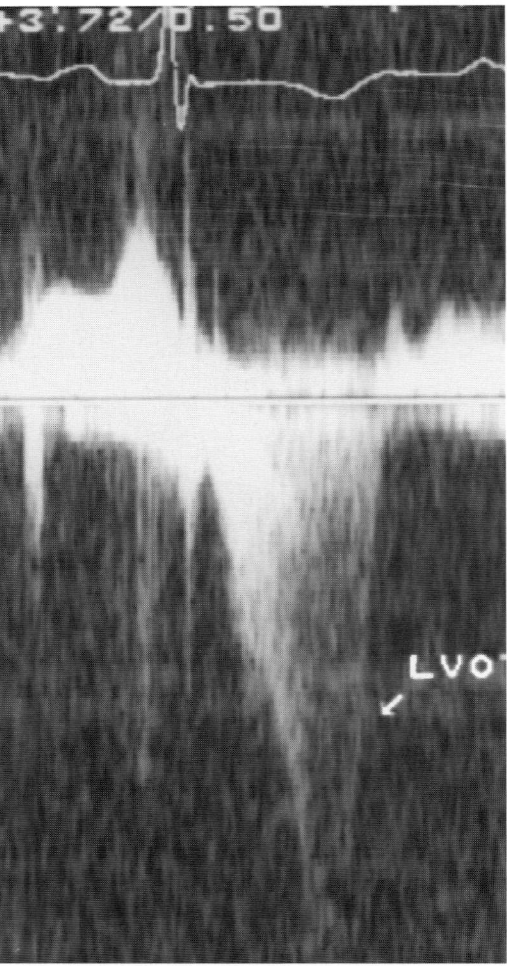

Fig. 11.18 Concave CW Doppler appearance of dynamic LVOT obstruction in two different patients with HCM.

Table 11.1 Features that will help in distinguishing the three levels of dynamic systolic obstruction.

	LVOT obstruction	*Mid-ventricular obstruction*	*LV cavity obliteration*
Hypertrophy	Upper or mid septum	Asymmetric interventricular septal thickness and free walls (papillary level)	Concentric with hyperkinesis
Systolic anterior motion (SAM)	Present	Absent	Absent
Aortic valve mid-systolic closure	Present	Absent	Absent
Mitral regurgitation	Present	Not associated	Not associated
Color flow turbulence	Level of SAM	Mid-cavity	
CW Doppler	Mid-late concave	Mid-late concave	Brief late concave (usually <2 m/s)

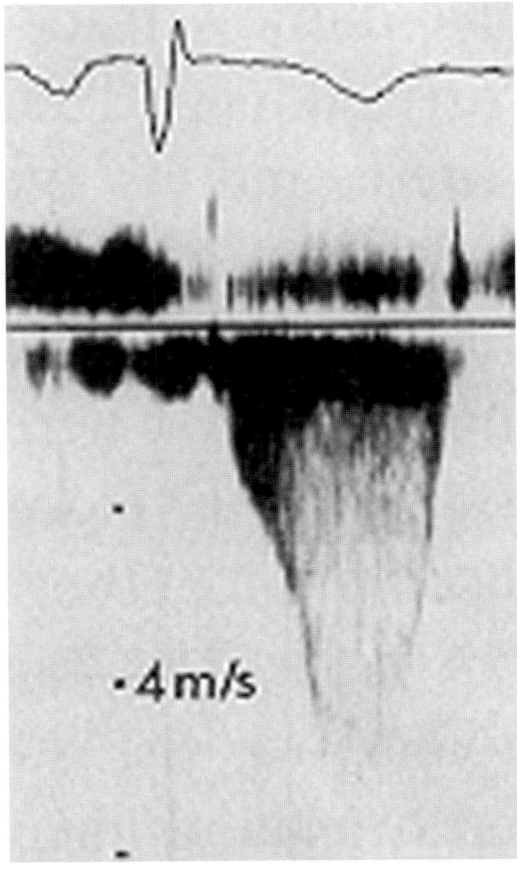

Fig. 11.19 Typical CW Doppler signal from the LVOT in a patient with HCM as first reported in 1988. Mid-systolic acceleration with a late systolic peak of flow is noted. (Reproduced with permission from: Sasson Z, Yock PG, Hatle LK, Alderman EL, Popp RL. Doppler echocardiographic determination of the pressure gradient in hypertrophic cardiomyopathy. J Am Coll Cardiol 1988; 11: 752–756.)

low velocity, but may be seen to approach 5 m/s on occasion (Fig. 11.21). Both LVOT obstruction and LV cavity obliteration may coexist with both Doppler patterns present.

The best method to obtain the continuous wave (CW) waveform of dynamic LVOT obstruction is from an apical window. Transesophageal echocardiography (TEE) may obtain the profile from a deep transgastric view. The magnitude of the velocity gradient may be somewhat higher than that obtained by catheterization, as pressure recovery may yield a lower gradient by catheterization.

Mitral regurgitation (MR) is associated with SAM and LVOT obstruction. MR generally coincides with mitral closure, but the MR intensifies following SAM (Fig. 11.22). The mitral leaflets during SAM are directed toward the ventricular septum, and a mitral "funnel" results, with a *posteriorly* directed MR jet. MR is a function of the amount of anterior leaflet SAM and the length and mobility of the posterior leaflet. In 10–20% of patients with HCM with LVOT obstruction, the MR is due to an "*independent*" valve abnormality (mitral annulus calcification, leaflet fibrosis, rheumatic, mitral valve prolapse or ruptured chordae, anomalous insertion of a papillary muscle into the anterior mitral leaflet), which is important to know if surgery is to be performed. Provocative maneuvers (Valsalva maneuver, amyl nitrate inhalation, post premature ventricular contraction (PVC)) that accentuate the LVOT gradient will also accentuate MR (Fig. 11.23). Angiotensin infusion will relieve the obstruction and MR, but in patients with "independent" MR, the MR will worsen.

Patients with HCM have impaired diastolic properties. Patients have *delayed relaxation* (abnormal active

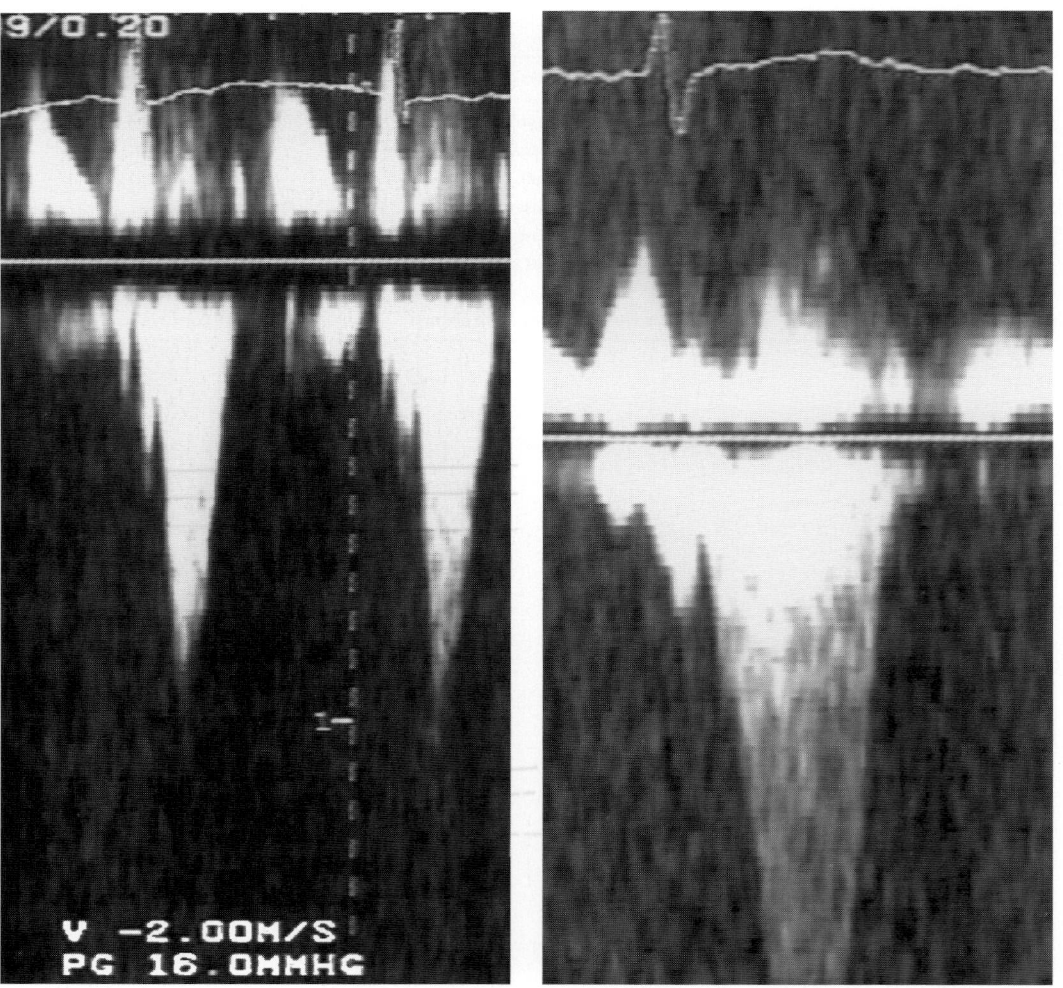

Fig. 11.20 CW Doppler of a patient with HCM and SAM who had severe exertional dyspnea. (a) The resting gradient of 16 mmHg increased (b) to 102 mmHg with repeated deep knee bends. The patient developed marked dyspnea.

relaxation) and *increased chamber stiffness* (passive component of relaxation). Chamber stiffness is proportional to LV mass and myocardial fibrosis, and inversely proportional to LV chamber volume. The pattern of abnormal relaxation is most often noted (↑IVRT and DT (deceleration time), and ↓E and E/A ratio). The E wave increases and DT decreases as LV compliance diminishes and the LA filling pressure increases; however, there appears to be no significant relationship of the DT with LA filling pressures. As filling pressures continue to rise, there appears to develop the typical patterns of mitral inflow pseudonormalization and restriction to filling, along with corresponding pulmonary vein flow changes (see Chapter 6). Tissue Doppler Imaging (TDI) of the mitral annulus may help in estimation of LV filling pressures in patients with HCM. Left atrial filling pressure (LAP) may be estimated by the following equation:

$$LAP = [1.25 \times (E/Ea)] + 1.9$$

where E is the mitral inflow E wave peak velocity, and Ea is the mitral annulus early diastolic peak velocity (see also Chapter 6).

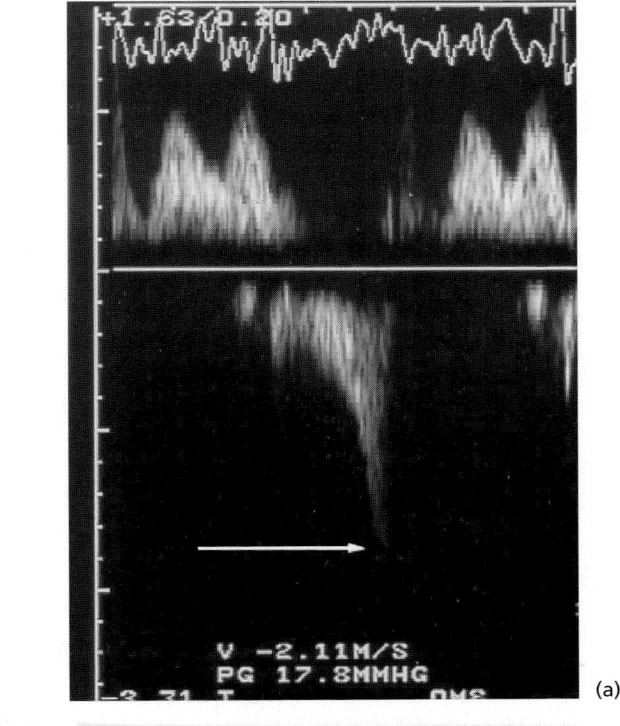

(a)

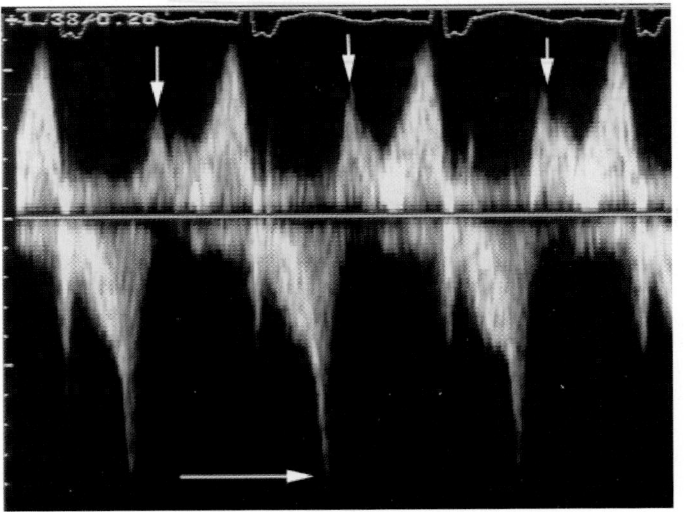

(b)

Fig. 11.21 CW Doppler in two patients with vigorous LV systolic function and cavity obliteration. (a) Peak velocity occurs at end-systole (arrow) and is ~2 m/s. (b) Peak velocity again occurs at end-systole (horizontal arrow) and is <2 m/s. Note conspicuous isovolumic relaxation time (IVRT) flow (vertical arrows) toward the LV apex (toward the transducer).

During the isovolumic relaxation time (IVRT) there may be noted Doppler flow toward the LV apex due to dyssynchronous LV relaxation (recording in the apical four-chamber view with flow recorded toward the transducer). With mid-cavity or in particular apical hypertrophy, IVRT flow may be toward the base. This flow may persist into early diastole (Fig. 11.21b; see Figs 6.17 & 6.18).

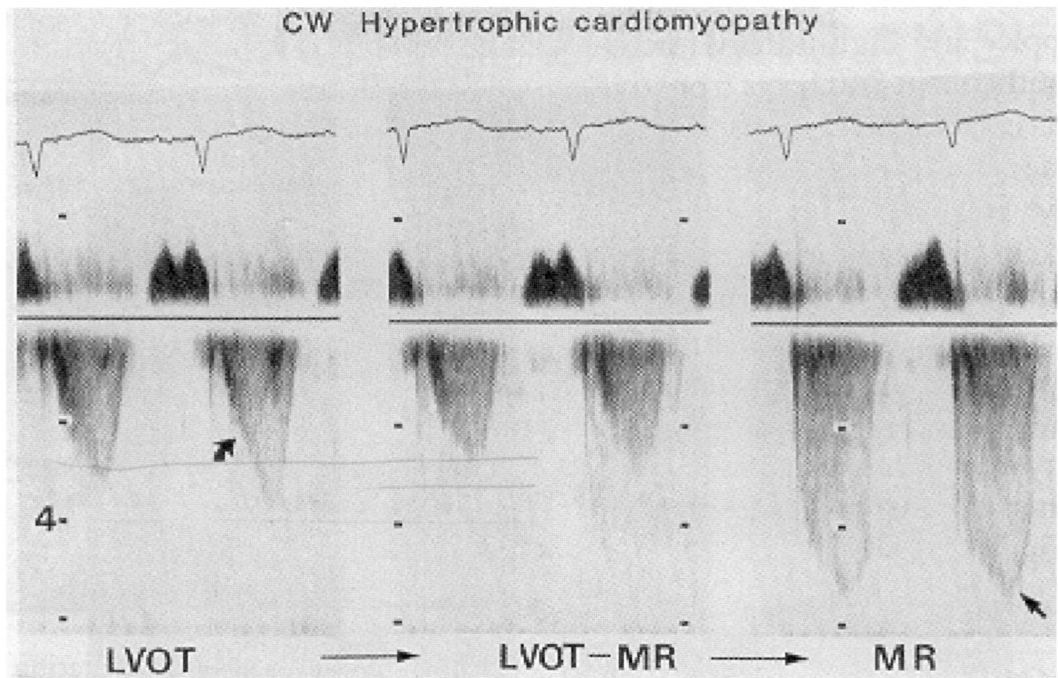

Fig. 11.22 CW Doppler from the LV apex in a patient with HCM. A typical pattern of LVOT dynamic obstruction is noted (left panel). (right panel) Shows mitral regurgitation in the posterior left atrium, and a mixed pattern (middle panel) of LVOT obstruction and MR is noted. Usually MR begins earlier in systole, but when associated with HCM, it increases as the LVOT obstruction increases later in systole. Color Doppler will help one to avoid contaminating the CW LVOT signal with the CW signal from MR. (Reproduced with permission from: Rakowski H, Sasson Z, Wigle ED. Echocardiographic and Doppler assessment of hypertrophic Cardiomyopathy. Journal of the American Society of Echocardiography 1988; 1: 31–47.)

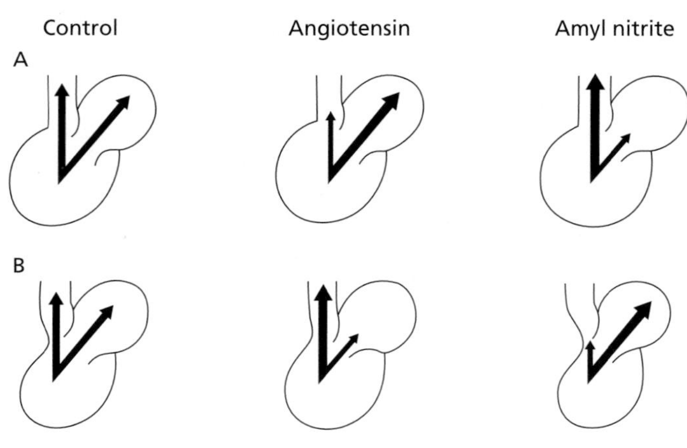

Fig. 11.23 Pharmacodynamics of MR. (A) Primary mitral valve disease. (B) MR secondary only to HCM. (Reproduced with permission from: Wigle *et al.* Hypertrophic cardiomyopathy. the importance of the site and the extent of hypertrophy: a review. Progress in Cardiovascular Disease 1985; XXVIII(Jul/Aug): I30.

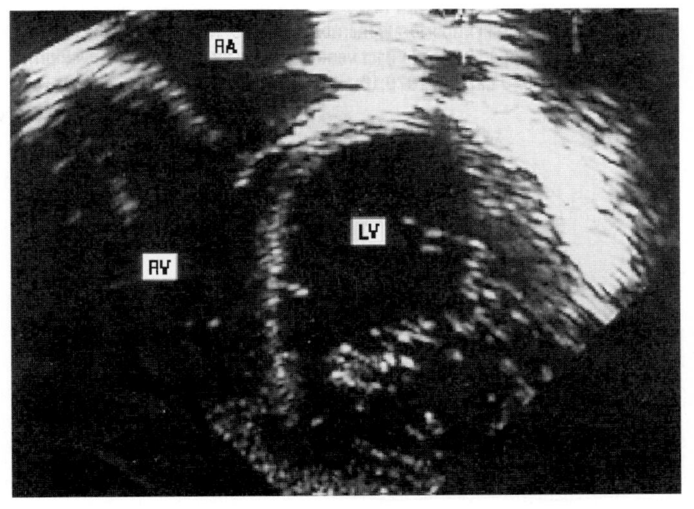

(a)

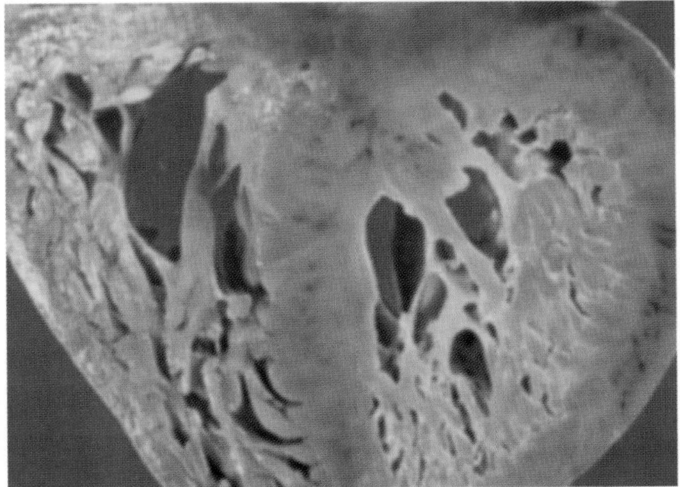

(b)

Fig. 11.24 Noncompaction of the left ventricle in a 6-year-old boy. (a) Echocardiogram in an apical four-chamber view (inverted view). (b) Corresponding pathologic specimen. At autopsy a globular heart with trabeculations in both the LV lateral and septal segments were noted. *Fibroelastosis* (development of a thick fibroelastic coat) of adjacent endocardium is secondary to abnormal blood flow in the LV chamber.

Restrictive cardiomyopathy

Nondilated cardiomyopathies may be divided into hypertrophic and nonhypertrophic types. Of the nonhypertrophic types, restrictive and obliterative types exist. Restrictive cardiomyopathy is a nondilated ventricle (normal or small), the absence of myocardial hypertrophy, and the presence of restrictive physiology. Reduced ventricular compliance is a characteristic hemodynamic abnormality. Thus, for the ventricle to expand to a sufficient volume, high filling pressures are required. Atrial dilatation is therefore a characteristic, as high atrial filling pressures will occur.

Examples of restrictive cardiomyopathy include *idiopathic restrictive cardiomyopathy*, *endocardial fibrosis*, and *Loeffler's cardiomyopathy*. Other examples include interstitial disease such as *amyloidosis*, *sarcoidosis*, *hemochromatosis*, *glycogen storage disease*, *lipid storage disease* (*Fabry's disease*, *Gaucher's disease*, *Niemann–Pick's disease*), *mucopolysaccharidoses* (*Hurler's* and *Hurler–Scheie syndrome*), *scleroderma*, and *radiation*. *Diabetic cardiomyopathy* may also display restrictive physiology.

Noncompaction of the left ventricle (Fig. 11.24) (*persistence of spongy myocardium*) is a form of cardiomyopathy, sometimes categorized in the restrictive

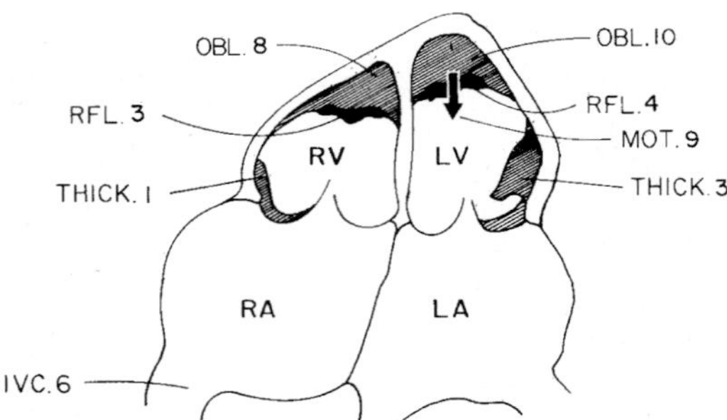

Fig. 11.25 2-D echo features of endomyocardial fibrosis. MOT, preserved or enhanced inward systolic motion of the apex; RFL, increased reflectivity of the obliterative surface; THICK, increased thickening of the basal papillary muscle ± posterior atrioventricular valve; OBL, obliteration. Numbers indicate the number of patients (out of a total of 10) with the described finding. (Reproduced with permission from: Acquatella H, Schiller NB, Puigbo JJ, *et al*. Value of 2-D echocardiography in endomyocardial disease with and without eosinophilia. Circulation 1983; 67: 1219–1226.)

type. Echocardiography reveals prominent LV trabeculations and deep intertrabecular recesses, with color Doppler often revealing flow within the trabeculations. The RV may also be involved. Serial echocardiography may reveal progressive LV dilatation. The LV endocardium fails to "smooth out" as it normally does during the first 2 months of embryonic development, with a resultant two-layered wall (thin compacted epicardium and a thick, noncompacted endocardium). The patient is predisposed to thrombus formation with systemic embolism, ventricular arrhythmias, and also diastolic and systolic heart failure. Screening of siblings is recommended.

Endomyocardial fibrosis (with or without hypereosinophilia) echo features include (Figs 11.25 & 11.26):

- apical obliteration of either one or both ventricles with material suggesting fibrosis or thrombosis
- bright and specular echoes on the endocardial surface of the apical obliteration suggestive of patchy calcification
- LV systolic inward motion (as opposed to dyskinetic motion of a thrombus in an apical aneurysm—either ischemic or Chagas in origin)
- papillary muscle and posterior AV valve involvement
- preserved ventricular systolic function in most patients
- normal or small ventricles with enlarged atria.

Pseudoxanthoma elasticum (*Gronblad–Strandberg syndrome*) is an inherited connective tissue disorder with clinical features of a thickened, yellowish, sagging skin ("plucked-chicken" appearance). Endocardial fibrosis with intimal coronary artery fibrosis may be present. Autopsy findings similar to endomyocardial fibrosis may be found.

Sarcoid granulomas in the heart have been found at autopsy in up to 25% of sarcoid patients. Lesions are usually found in the superior aspect of the ventricular septum, contributing to conduction disturbances. Local aneurysms may be present within the myocardium. Pericardial effusions and echo-Doppler evidence of cor pulmonale may be evident. Tissue characteristics of granulomatous involvement and scar formation may appear as bright echoes, particularly in the

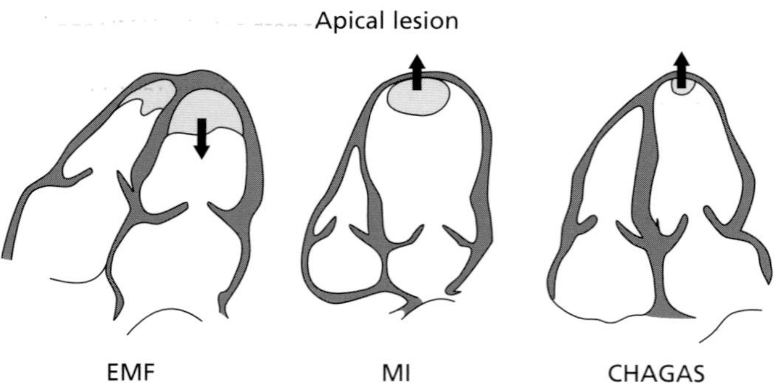

Fig. 11.26 Apical lesions with endomyocardial fibrosis (EMF), myocardial infarction (MI) with apical aneurysm, and Chagas' disease. Although the apex is "filled" with all three disorders, with EMF the systolic motion of the apex is toward the base. In chronic Chagas' disease, a small neck aneurysm may be present, but large aneurysms, as found with ischemic heart disease, may be evident. (Reproduced with permission from: Acquatella H, Schiller NB. Echocardiographic recognition of Chagas' disease and endomyocardial fibrosis. Journal of the American Society of Echocardiography 1988; 1: 60–68.)

septum and LV free wall. On rare occasion, restrictive physiology will be evident in patients with extensive involvement of myocardium. A dilated cardiomyopathy, with or without segmental wall motion abnormalities, may be found.

Iron storage disease (*hemochromatosis*)—both primary (idiopathic where excess iron is dietary in origin) and secondary (excess iron from multiple long-term blood transfusions)—results in iron deposition within myocardial cells, particularly the subepicardium, subendocardium, papillary muscles, and less often the myocardium and atria. In contrast with sarcoid and amyloid, deposition is less common in the conduction system. Echocardiographic findings typically include increased LV dimensions and mass, with LA enlargement. Those with systolic dysfunction have a poorer prognosis, as systolic dysfunction appears to progress with disease involvement.

Glycogen storage disease (type 2 or *Pompe's disease* as an example) may reveal significant LVH, and even asymmetric septal hypertrophy with dynamic LVOT obstruction. Less often these findings are noted with type 3 glycogen storage disease (*Cori's disease*).

Lipid storage disorders (*Fabry's disease, Gaucher's disease, Niemann–Pick's disease*) may have echo features similar to that of amyloidosis. Biventricular hypertrophy with a granular, sparkling texture appearance of the myocardium, normal ventricular cavity size, and mildly reduced systolic function may be evident. Pericardial effusions may also be present.

A restrictive cardiomyopathy with the *mucopolysaccharidoses* (*Hurler's, Hunter's, Sanfilippo's* and *Hurler–Scheie syndrome* are the most common of these rare disorders) may reveal upper interventricular septal thickening (termed *pseudohypertrophy*). Marked mitral leaflet thickening with MR may be evident. With *Maroteaux–Lamy syndrome* marked mitral leaflet thickening with mitral stenosis and also aortic valve disease (aortic stenosis) may be evident (Fig. 11.27).

Pericardial involvement is commonly found with *scleroderma*, but up to 50% of autopsied hearts will reveal areas of myocardial fibrosis. Restrictive physiology is often found by echo-Doppler evaluation.

Diabetic cardiomyopathy is defined as heart muscle disease not due to that from epicardial coronary atherosclerosis. Autopsy findings reveal an increased cardiac weight, pale appearance, and firmness. Increased myocardial collagen with thickened capillaries, focal myocardial fibrosis with intimal proliferation of arterioles, and interstitial glycoprotein and collagen accumulation, are noted histologically. Coexistence of hypertension markedly increases these findings. Echo and Doppler findings of diastolic abnormality are found even in adolescents.

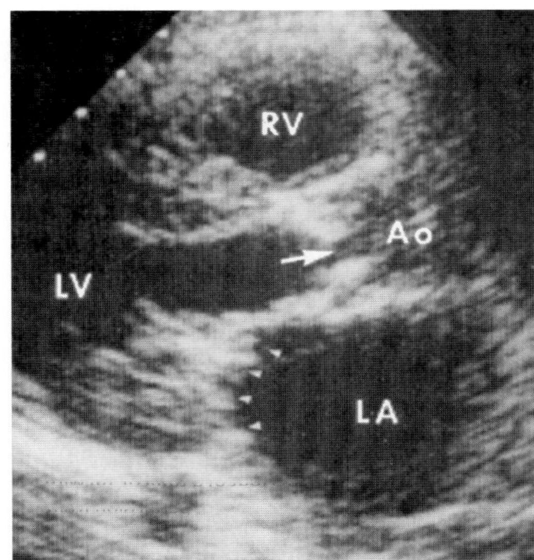

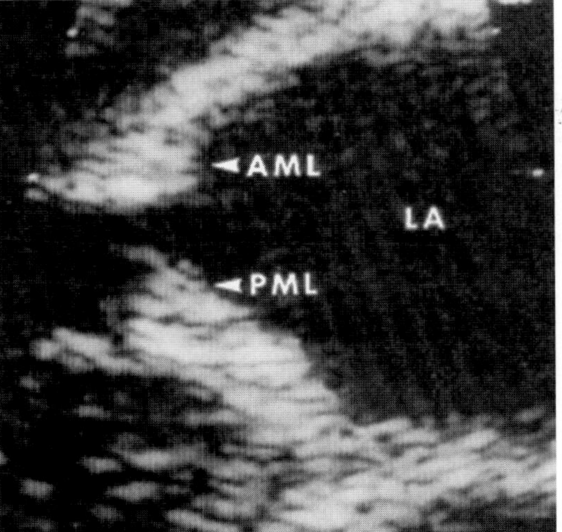

Fig. 11.27 Valvular involvement in Maroteaux–Lamy syndrome includes: (a) thickening and stenosis of the aortic valve (arrow); (b) thickening of both anterior (AML) and posterior (PML) leaflets of the mitral valve (arrows) with stenosis. (Reproduced with permission from: Tan CTT, Schaff HV, Miller FA, *et al.* Valvular heart disease in four patients with Maroteaux–Lamy syndrome. Circulation 1992; 85: 188–195.)

Radiation therapy may result in acute or delayed pericarditis, myocardial fibrosis, and accelerated coronary disease. Myocardial fibrosis results in a restrictive process and may present as intractable heart failure. Mediastinal irradiation may involve the right ventricle more extensively, probably reflecting higher radiation doses to that ventricle from the anterior radiation field. Restrictive cardiomyopathy secondary to irradiation should be differentiated from pericardial constriction, as constrictive symptoms may improve after pericardiectomy.

Carnitine deficiency may be associated with progressive skeletal myopathy; either hypertrophic or a dilated cardiomyopathy may be evident.

Carcinoid syndrome (see Chapter 21), in which hepatic metastases are present, is associated with endocardial plaques, usually involving the right heart. Valvular involvement with predominantly functional tricuspid regurgitation (mild tricuspid stenosis) and pulmonic stenosis (some pulmonic regurgitation) is evident. Following valvular replacement, physiology of restrictive cardiomyopathy may become evident, often leading to death.

Amyloid cardiomyopathy is the most common form of restrictive cardiomyopathy in the Western world. Amyloid material accumulates within the myocardium. Amyloidosis may result from four general etiologies:

1 *Immunocytic dyscrasias*—an amyloid protein is produced which is an immunoglobulin light chain, associated with monoclonal gammopathy or plasma cell myeloma. The heart, tongue, skin, gastrointestinal tract, and carpal ligaments may become involved.

2 *Systemic reactive type*—associated with chronic inflammatory disorders such as tuberculosis or rheumatoid arthritis. Cardiac involvement is unusual.

3 *Heredofamilial amyloidosis*—at least 50% of patients have an associated cardiomyopathy.

4 *Senile amyloidosis*—associated with advancing age, cardiac involvement rarely occurs without the initial involvement of other organs. At autopsy, the heart is firm, rubbery, and nondilated.

Amyloid should be considered in patients, particularly over 60 years old, with intractable heart failure, restrictive hemodynamics, and low voltage on the electrocardiogram. Progressive biventricular heart failure is the usual presentation. The combination of low electrocardigraphic voltage and an increase in LV mass by echocardiogram is very suggestive of the diagnosis, and appears to correlate with disease severity (Fig. 11.28). Cardiac amyloid involvement is progressive. Wall thickness and Doppler of mitral inflow are prognostic. With severe involvement (wall thickness >15 mm and restrictive filling pattern), the 1-year survival is low, whereas in patients with wall thicknesses of 12–15 mm the survival is better, and in those with a wall thickness less than 12 mm and abnormal relaxation the survival is best. Serial follow-up of patients with early amyloidosis may reveal progressive LV thickening and changes from normal diastolic flow to LV abnormal relaxation, progressing to "pseudonormalization," and finally to that of restriction to filling (Fig. 11.29).

M-mode and 2-D echocardiographic features of amyloid include:

- Increased right and left ventricular wall thickness.
- "Speckled" appearance throughout the myocardium (abnormal reflections in HCM are usually localized to the ventricular septum). A speckled appearance may also be seen in the hypertrophy of patients with renal disease.
- Significant biatrial enlargement (due to elevated filling pressures).
- Cardiac valves, papillary muscles, and atrial septum are thickened (probably more evident with senile amyloid as opposed to amyloid secondary to blood dyscrasias).
- Small to moderate pericardial effusion.
- Pleural effusions.
- Generally normal ventricular chamber dimensions.
- Systolic dysfunction may develop, but ventricles will usually not dilate (with hypertension and hypertrophic cardiomyopathy, by comparison, systolic dysfunction is associated with ventricular dilatation).

Doppler features of restrictive cardiomyopathy (see also Chapter 12 for echo and Doppler differentiation of tamponade, constriction, and restriction) include:

- Variable mitral inflow patterns based on the amount of myocardial infiltrative involvement (see earlier discussion).
- Patients with a classic "dip-and-plateau" pattern in the cardiac catheterization laboratory have a Doppler end-stage restrictive filling pattern.
- No respiratory variation of tricuspid and mitral inflow patterns, as is noted with constrictive pericarditis and tamponade.
- Valvular regurgitation is usually rather mild.

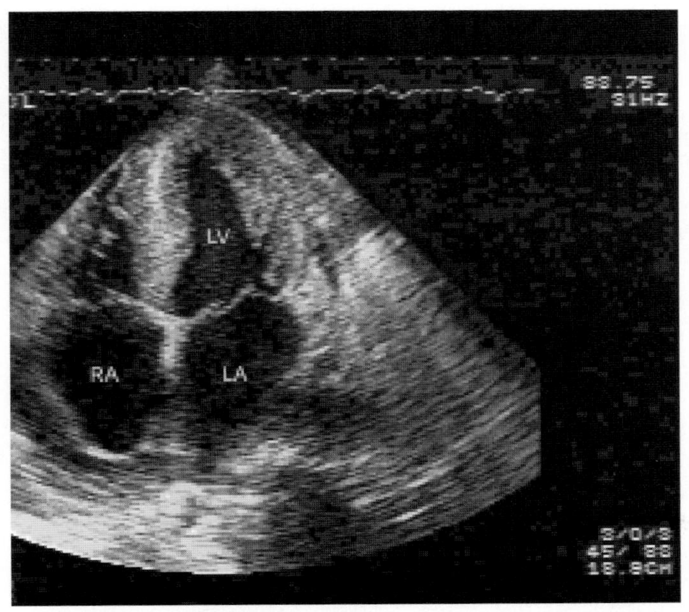

(a)

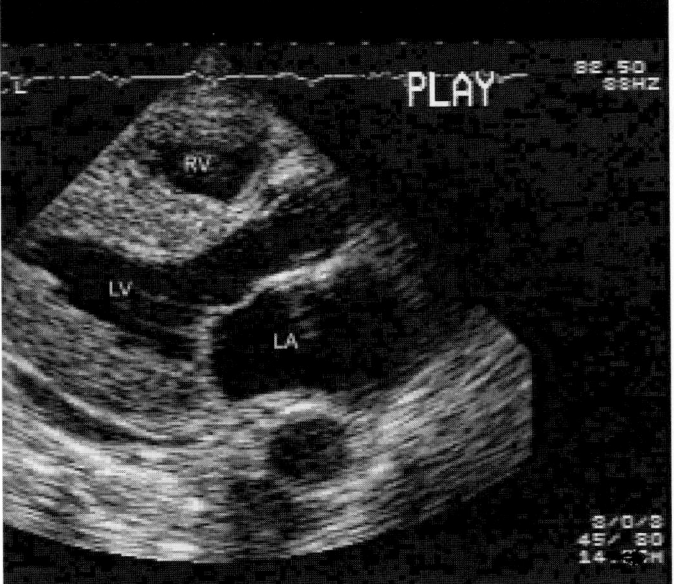

(b)

Fig. 11.28 A 37-year-old female presented with severe biventricular heart failure. (a) Apical four-chamber view. (b) Parasternal long axis view. The patient was documented to have cardiac amyloid secondary to light chain disease with multiple myeloma. There was no history of hypertension, but the ventricles were thickened and atria enlarged. The patient had pericardial and pleural effusions, and low voltage on electrocardiogram.

Differential diagnosis of forms of cardiomyopathy with normal systolic function

Differentiating *hypertensive heart* (see also Chapter 5), *hypertrophic cardiomyopathy* (HCM), and *restrictive cardiomyopathy* may be difficult. With HCM and amyloid there may not be a history of hypertension. The pattern of hypertrophy with HCM is usually asymmetric, whereas with restriction and hypertension it is usually symmetric. However, in hypertension, the hypertrophy may sometimes be asymmetric.

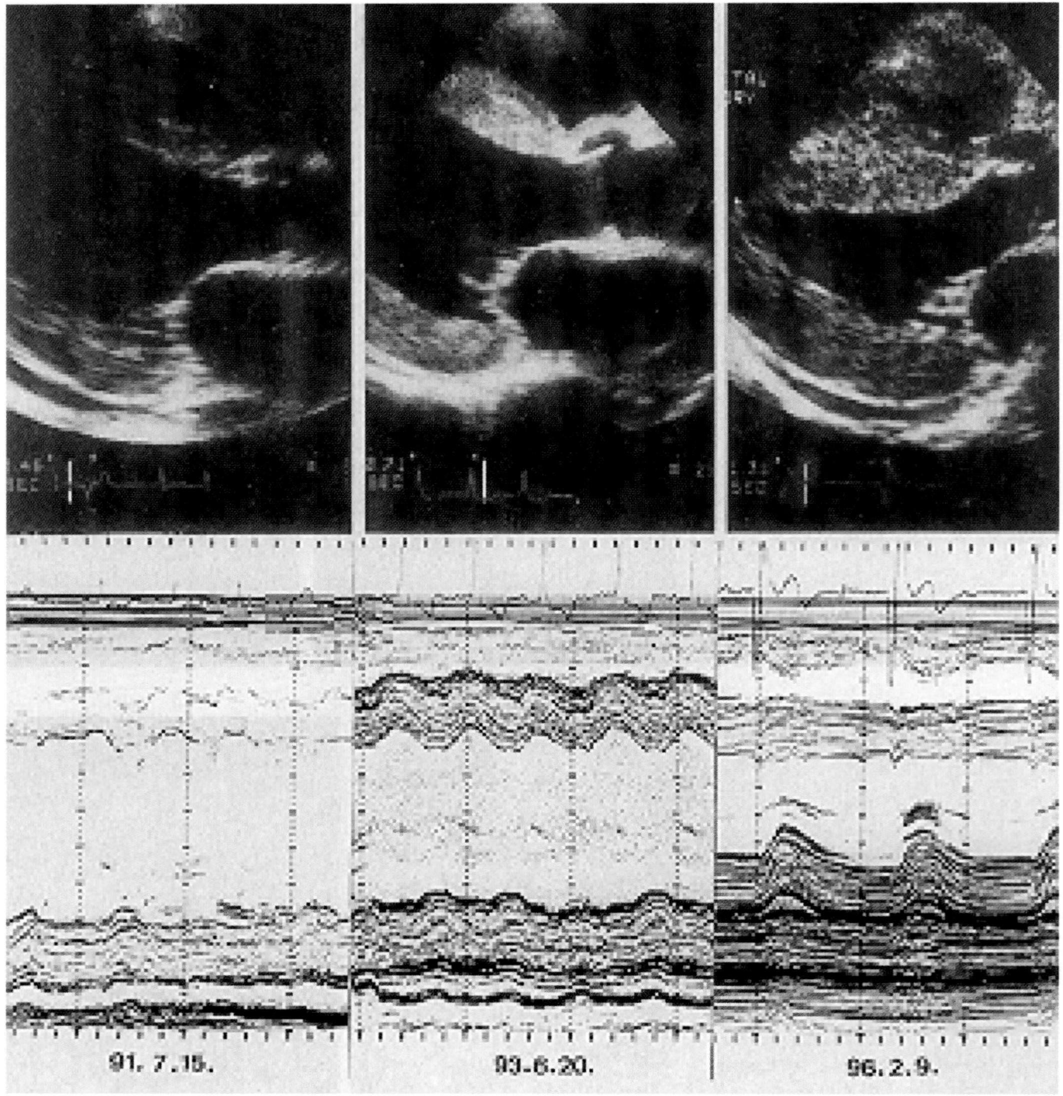

Fig. 11.29 Serial echocardiograms from a patient over the course of 5 years. A gradual increase in LV wall thickness, valve thickening and development of a "speckled" myocardium are evident. (Reproduced with permission from: Youn HJ, Chae JS, Lee KY, Hong SJ. Amyloidosis with cardiac involvement. Circulation 1998; 97: 2093–2094.)

Right ventricular hypertrophy (RVH) may be present with HCM and RV thickening present with restrictive cardiomyopathy. RVH is usually absent in hypertension. SAM of the mitral valve and mid-systolic closure of the aortic valve are associated with HCM, but may occasionally occur with hypertension.

Systolic function is preserved or increased in "early" stages of hypertension. In "late" stages of hypertension, hypertrophy may be inadequate to compensate for increased stress and systolic function may deteriorate with resultant LV dilatation (Fig. 11.30). Regression of mass is measurable within 3 months of treatment of hypertension. An increase in LV wall thickness can be noted within 4 weeks of cessation of hypertensive therapy. Whereas systolic function and LV dilatation may occur in "advanced" hypertension

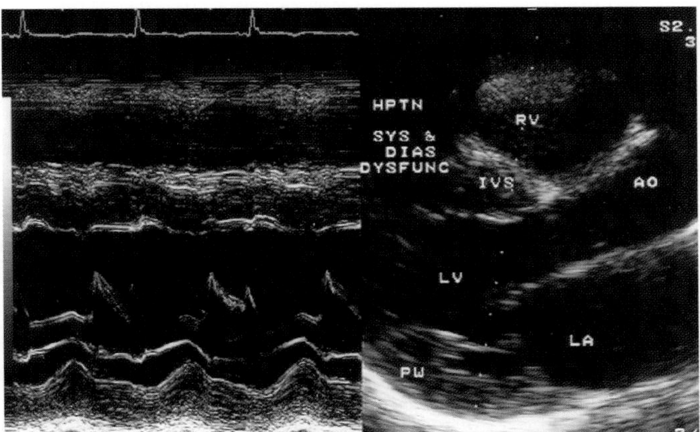

Fig. 11.30 M-mode and 2-D parasternal long axis image in a middle-aged patient with severe longstanding hypertension. The LA is dilated, aortic root (AO) generous, and both interventricular septum (IVS) and posterior LV wall (PW) are hypertrophied. The LV internal dimensions have increased as systolic dysfunction has developed.

and HCM, LV dilatation generally will not occur with systolic dysfunction in restrictive (infiltrative) disorders.

Echo clues for the diagnosis of hypertensive heart disease include:

- left atrial dilatation—secondary to increased LV diastolic pressure and/or MR
- aortic root dilatation
- mitral annular calcification
- aortic valve sclerosis.

Clues to help differentiate restrictive disorders from hypertensive heart or HCM include:

- absence of a history of hypertension
- RVH (may be present with HCM)
- moderate pulmonary hypertension
- generalized thickening of valves and atrial septum
- pericardial and pleural effusions may be present
- diffuse myocardial speckled appearance (localized usually to septum with HCM)
- presence of LVH on the electrocardiogram (LVH is usually present with hypertension or HCM, whereas with restrictive disorders relatively low voltage may be present).

The term hypertensive hypertrophic cardiomyopathy of the elderly is used for the following:

- elderly hypertensive patients
- normal or hyperdynamic LV systolic function
- LV hypertrophy
- evident diastolic abnormality
- LV cavity obliteration with a corresponding late systolic gradient may be present.

Differentiating *athlete heart* from *hypertensive heart* and *hypertrophic cardiomyopathy* may be difficult (Fig. 11.31). Whereas up to 46% of sudden deaths in

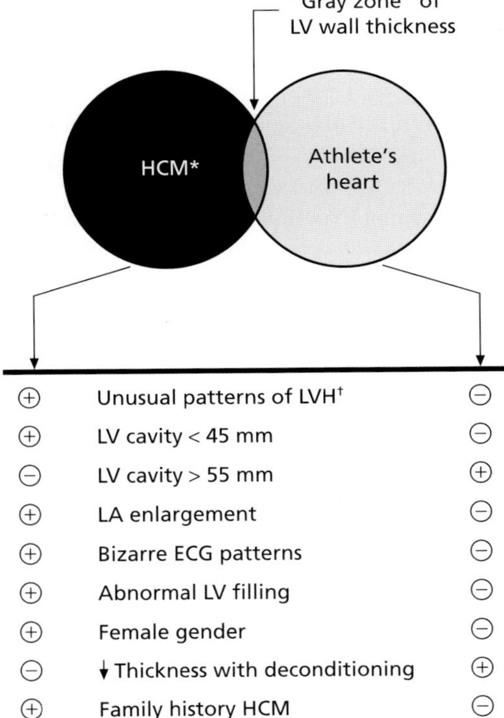

Fig. 11.31 Features that may help to distinguish between HCM and athlete's heart, in those patients with a pattern of LVH that overlap (gray zone). (Reproduced with permission from: Maron BJ, Pelliccia A, Spirito P. Cardiac disease in young trained athletes. Circulation 1995; 91(5): 1596–1601, figure 2.)

young athletes are due to HCM, it is important to differentiate athlete heart from HCM. Interventricular septal measurements greater than 11 mm are frequently noted in endurance athletes and increase as physical training progresses. The interventricular septal to posterior LV wall thickness ratio may become greater than 1.3, and approach 2.0. A method to distinguish physiologic septal hypertrophy in weight lifters (isometric exercise) from that of HCM is to divide the end-diastolic septal thickness by the end-systolic diameter. A value of 0.48 or more is consistent with HCM. The echocardiographic pattern of athlete heart hypertrophy (physiologic hypertrophy) differs from HCM by some of the following features:

- LV wall thickness is *homogeneous* as opposed to asymmetric (abrupt changes in wall thickness from one segment to another with HCM).
- LV wall contours are *smooth* as opposed to irregular.
- Maximum LV wall thickness usually will not exceed 16 mm.
- The LV cavity may be enlarged (LV end-diastolic dimension ≥55 mm) as opposed to normal or small.
- The LA size is normal as opposed to enlarged.
- Regression of LV wall thickness and mass into the normal range with deconditioning (<13 mm) is rapid in athlete heart (within 4 days of cessation of exercise changes may be noted) whereas within 3 months for treatment of hypertension.
- Highly trained endurance athletes (rowing sports or bicyclists—combination of isotonic and isometric exercise) often have generous LV diastolic cavity dimensions (55–63 mm) but rarely have substantial LV hypertrophy. In these endurance athletes, wall thickness is rarely ≥13 mm in men or ≥11 mm in women. Participants in other types of sports generally do not demonstrate substantial hypertrophy. Normal LV inflow patterns (mitral and pulmonary vein flow) are noted, whereas only a few patients with HCM (usually mild) have been noted to have normal diastolic filling.

With hypertension the pattern of symmetric hypertrophy may be similar to athlete heart, but the LV cavity (systolic and diastolic dimensions) will not be enlarged until systolic dysfunction ensues. Abnormal diastolic filling patterns are usually present with hypertensive cardiomyopathy.

A group of elite male triathletes were found to have mixed eccentric and concentric hypertrophy with "supernormal" LV diastolic function by transmitral flow (increased E/A ratio) and tissue Doppler echocardiography (increased peak early diastolic velocity and lower peak atrial systolic velocity).

CHAPTER 12

Pericardium and Effusions

The epicardium and pericardium (*visceral* and *parietal*) form a bright dense layer of echoes that cover the entire heart except for the posterior aspects of the left atrium. This normal appearance is changed by pericardial thickening or pericardial effusion.

Effusions

Echocardiography not only visualizes a *pericardial effusion* well, but also associated abnormalities (tumors, masses, and fibrin strands) are readily seen. Generally, as the cells and protein material increase within a pericardial effusion, its echogenicity increases. One cannot determine the exact composition, however, based upon echocardiography. Small effusions are usually only posterior (dependent position during echo study), whereas moderate and large effusions are both anterior and posterior. One may characterize a pericardial effusion as minimal, small, moderate, or large. A *minimal* effusion has less than 5 mm pericardial separation (50–100 ml), a *small* effusion 5–10 mm (100–250 ml), a *moderate* effusion 10–20 mm (250–500 ml), and a *large* effusion more than 20 mm (>500 ml) pericardial separation. The University of Maryland echocardiography laboratory uses the following criteria:

"small" (<100 ml)—<1.0 cm only posteriorly
"moderate" (100–500 ml)—<1.0 cm posteriorly but also an echo-free space anteriorly
"large" (>500 ml)—fluid both anteriorly and posteriorly >1.0 cm.

Usually pericardial fluid is not found behind the left atrium because the pericardial attachments are reflected onto the pulmonary veins. Occasionally fluid can be visualized in the oblique sinus, which is located behind the left atrium.

The following findings may help differentiate a *pericardial effusion* from a *left pleural effusion*:

- A pericardial effusion may "surround" the heart—it appears circular in the parasternal short axis and outlines the ventricles and atria in the apical views.
- A pericardial effusion lies anterior to the aorta and a left pleural effusion lies posterior to the aorta (Figs 12.1 & 12.2).
- A moderate to large pericardial effusion is often associated with "enhanced" cardiac motion.
- If a left pleural effusion and a pericardial effusion coexist, a parietal pericardium–pleural interface line will be present (Fig. 12.3).
- Imaging the patient in a semisitting position from the left posterior thorax may help identify a left-sided pleural effusion. The pleural effusion may allow

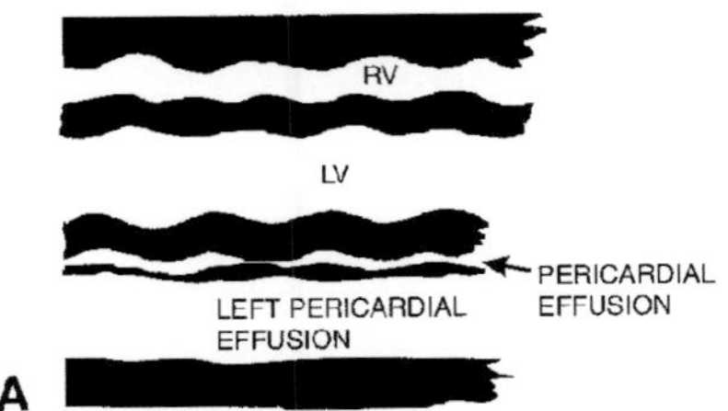

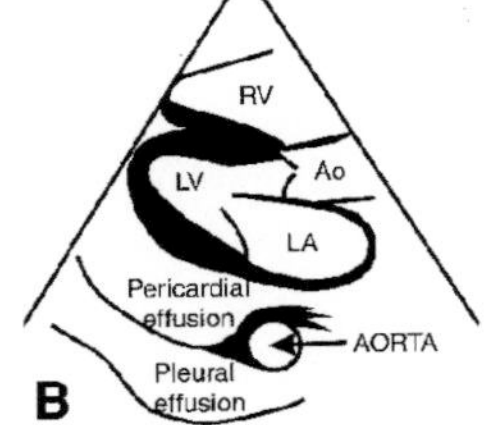

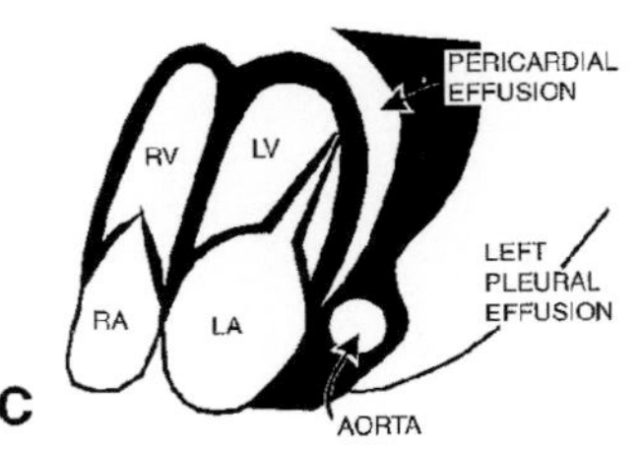

Fig. 12.1 Pericardial and left pleural effusion. (A) M-mode from a parasternal view at the LV level. (B) Parasternal long axis two-dimensional (2-D) image and (C) apical four-chamber view. In (B) and (C) note the position of the descending aorta (AORTA) as posterior to the pericardial effusion and anterior to the left pleural effusion.

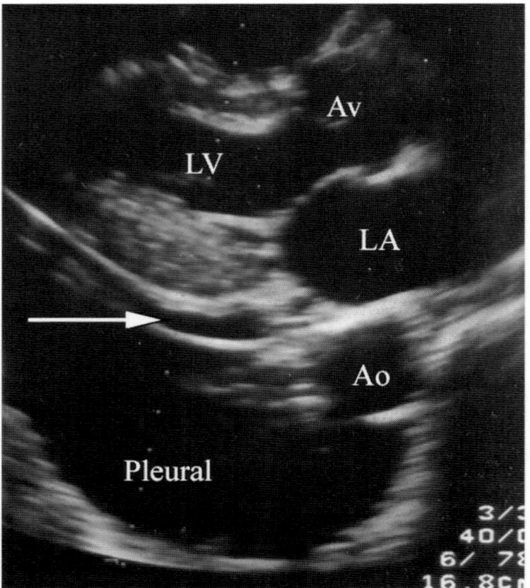

Fig. 12.2 Two-dimensional echocardiogram from a parasternal long axis view of a patient with a small pericardial effusion (arrow) and a left pleural effusion. Av, aortic valve; Ao, descending thoracic aorta.

excellent visualization of the heart through the fluid. (Fig. 12.4).

A *loculated pericardial effusion* is usually associated with cardiac surgery. In the first few days post surgery an effusion may be visualized anteriorly (along the right heart), and several months post surgery may be seen adjacent to the left heart as adhesions form anteriorly along the right heart border, not allowing the pericardial effusion to form in that location (Figs 12.5 & 12.6).

A *right pleural effusion* may be seen in the subcostal view with the transducer pointing toward the right shoulder. It will be seen posterior to the right atrium and superior to the liver (Fig. 12.7).

Ascites may be confused with a pericardial effusion. Subcostal imaging may view ascites anterior to the heart, simulating a loculated pericardial effusion. Low parasternal imaging, directing the transducer toward the abdomen, may view ascites posterior to the left ventricle, simulating a posterior pericardial effusion (Figs 12.8 & 12.9).

Congenital absence of the pericardium usually occurs on the left but rarely may involve the right side. With absence of the left side of the pericardium the heart shifts toward the left; therefore, the right heart will appear enlarged from the parasternal window and appear in the middle of the screen from the standard apical window. Exaggerated cardiac motion (especially the LV posterior wall) may also be noted. More common in males, absence of the pericardium is also associated with atrial septal defect and bicuspid aortic valve. Magnetic resonance imaging or computed tomography will help make the diagnosis.

Pericardial cyst is usually suspected by routine chest X-ray. A pericardial cyst is most often seen in the right costophrenic angle but may appear elsewhere. It appears as a fluid-filled echo-free structure by

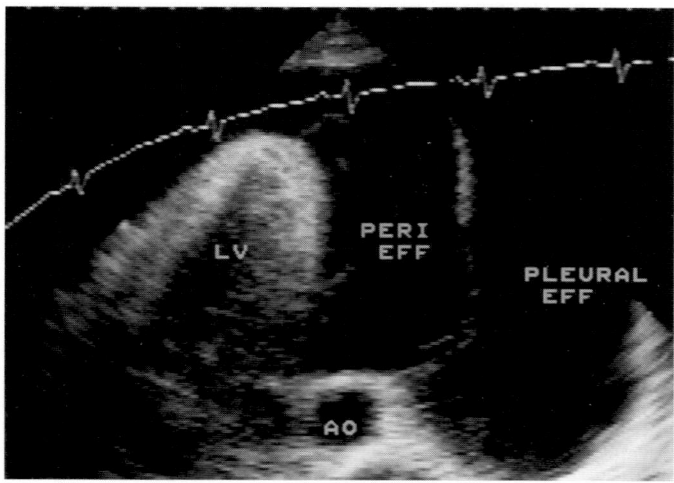

Fig. 12.3 Apical four-chamber view of a patient with a left pleural effusion and a large pericardial effusion. Note the pericardial–pleural line (arrow). PERI EFF, pericardial effusion; PLEURAL EFF, left pleural effusion; AO, descending thoracic aorta.

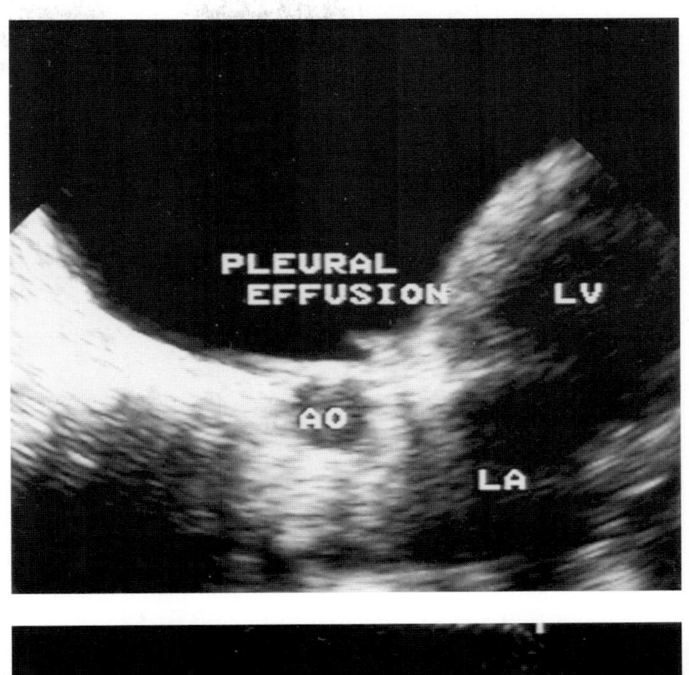

(a)

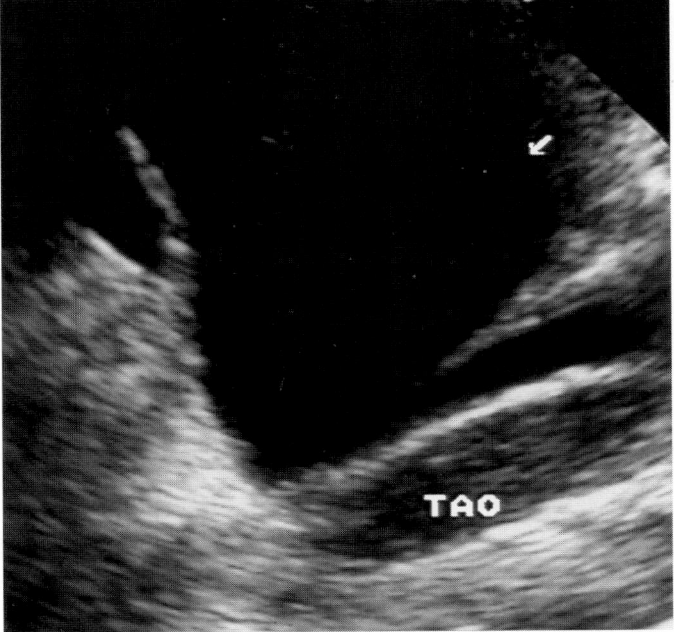

(b)

Fig. 12.4 Imaging of a left pleural effusion in a semierect patient from the left posterior thorax. (a) Transverse section of the descending aorta (AO). (b) Longitudinal section of the descending aorta (TAO). Note the position of the aorta in relation to the left pleural effusion. As the transducer is located on the posterior thorax and the pleural effusion is closest to the transducer, the pleural effusion is posterior to the descending aorta.

two-dimensional (2-D) echocardiography, usually located outside the true pericardial cavity.

A *teratoma* is located outside the heart in over 99% of cases, but often within the pericardial cavity. It receives its blood supply from the ascending aorta or main pulmonary artery, presumably from the vasa vasorum. Recurrent large pericardial effusions in children should suggest an intrapericardial teratoma.

Rarely a *large left atrium* may partially prolapse posterior to the LV. This may be falsely interpreted as a localized pericardial effusion (Fig. 12.10).

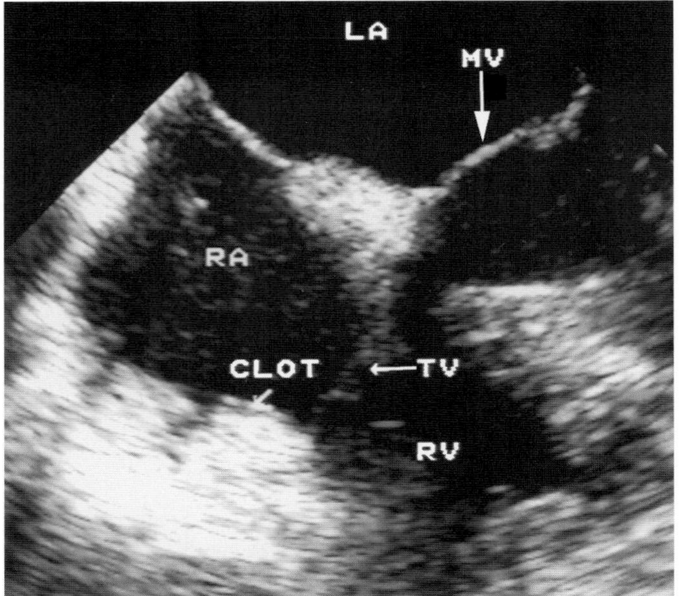

Fig. 12.5 A patient 6 h post coronary bypass surgery with unstable hemodynamics. The patient developed sudden hypotension with a drop in cardiac output. The pulmonary capillary wedge pressure (PCWP) was 12 mmHg, with a central venous pressure (CVP) of 24 mmHg. Transesophageal echocardiography (TEE) imaging revealed a localized pericardial clot (CLOT) causing a "localized" cardiac tamponade. Surgical evacuation resulted in resolution of the unstable hemodynamics. Note prominent spontaneous echo contrast within the RA. In each case of localized postoperative tamponade of the right heart, seen by the authors, there has been prominent RA spontaneous echo contrast observed by TEE. (Chuttani K, Pandian NG, Mohanty PK, *et al.* Left ventricular diastolic collapse: an echocardiographic sign of regional cardiac tamponade. Circulation 1991; 83: 1999–2006, p 2002, figure 1.)

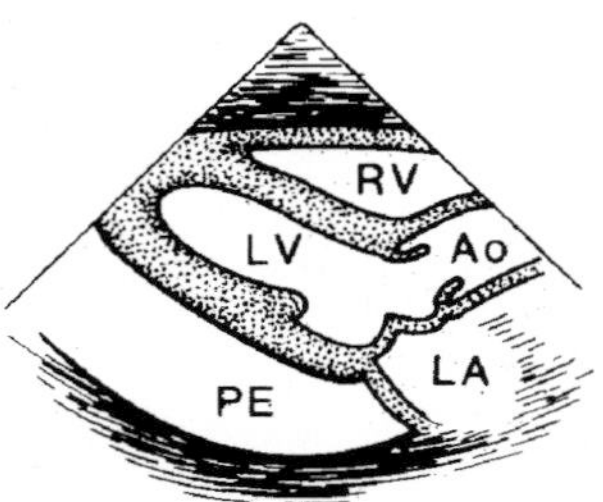

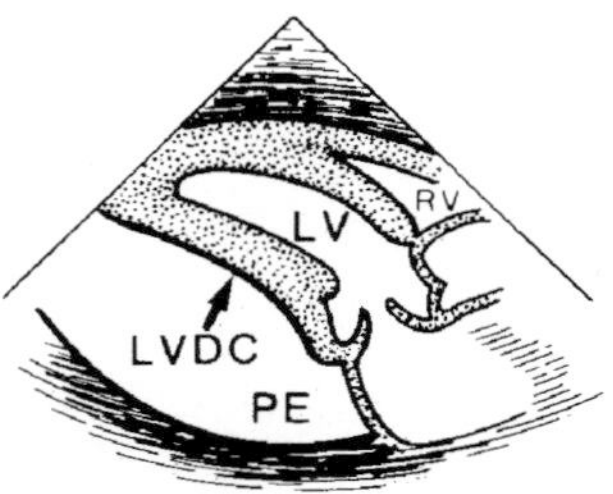

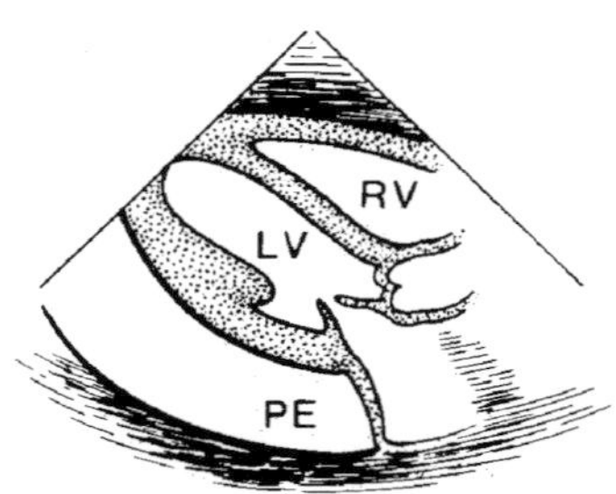

Fig. 12.6 Serial drawings of parasternal long axis images of a patient with localized cardiac tamponade with a large posterior pericardial effusion. The RV is adherent to the anterior chest wall, but in early diastole the LV bows inward (arrow), consistent with LV diastolic collapse. This LV diastolic collapse is only evident during early diastole. (Reproduced with permission from: Chuttani K, Pandian NG, Mohanty PK, *et al.* Left ventricular diastolic collapse: an echocardiographic sign of regional cardiac tamponade. Circulation 1991; 83: 1999–2006.)

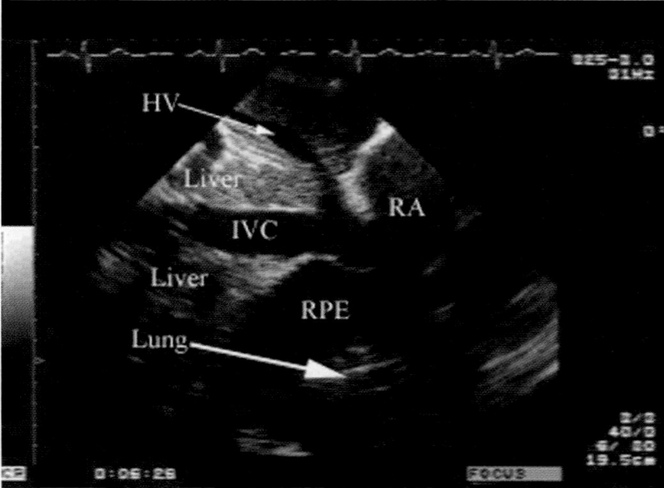

Fig. 12.7 Right pleural effusion (RPE) and right lung (LUNG) visualized from a subcostal view, with the transducer pointing toward the right shoulder. The RPE is posterior to the RA, and superior to the liver. Note the IVC and hepatic vein (HV).

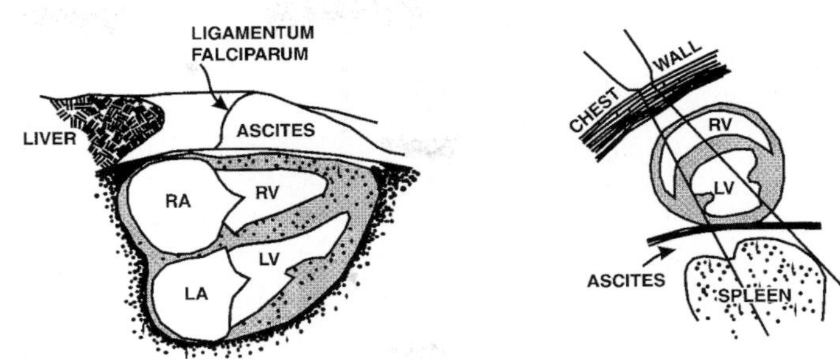

Fig. 12.8 Ascites visualized from the subcostal (left panel) and low parasternal (right panel) (pointing towards the abdomen) windows. The *ligamentum falciparum* may appear as a moving "flap" within the ascitic fluid.

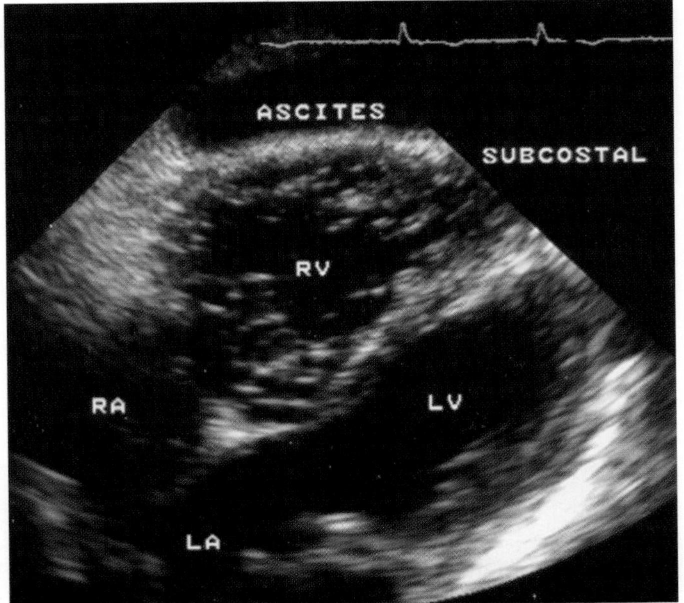

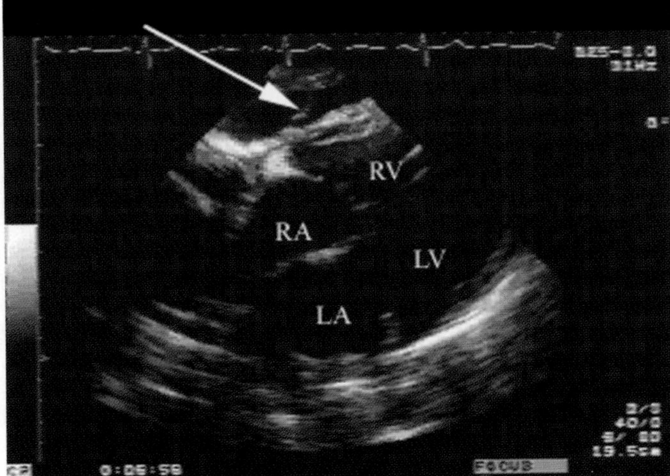

Fig. 12.9 Subcostal long axis view of ascites appearing anterior to the RV (a,b). The ligamentum falciparum (b) (arrow) is well seen.

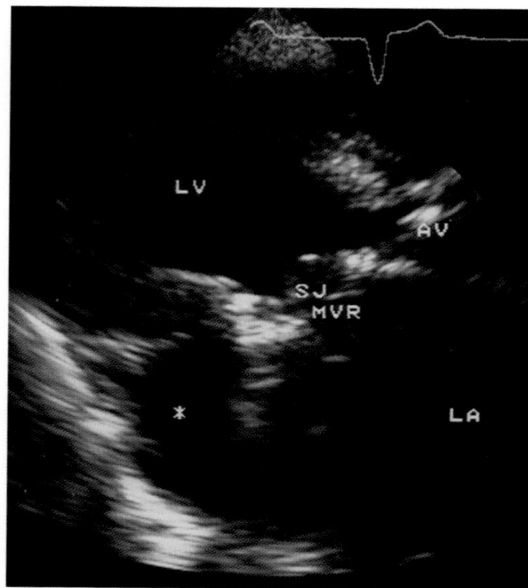

Fig. 12.10 Parasternal long axis view of a patient with a mechanical mitral valve prosthesis. The patient has a markedly enlarged left atrium with partial prolapse posterior to the LV (*). SJ MVR, St Jude mitral valve replacement; AV, aortic valve.

Cardiac tamponade

Cardiac tamponade represents a spectrum of hemodynamic changes. It is not an "all-or-none" phenomenon, but represents changes from mild to severe hemodynamic impairment. Echocardiographic (M-mode and 2-D) features of tamponade physiology include:

- *Early diastolic RV collapse*—specific but not sensitive for tamponade (Fig. 12.11). RV collapse may not be present when the RV is hypertrophied and stiff, as with pulmonary hypertension.
- *Late diastolic RA collapse (inversion)*—sensitive for tamponade, but not specific. It occurs with less severe hemodynamic compromise than RV collapse. The longer in late diastole that RA collapse is present and the longer it persists into early systole, the more useful it is as a sign of tamponade (Fig. 12.12). If RA inversion lasts longer than a third of an RR interval, it is suggestive of hemodynamically significant tamponade.
- *Late LA collapse*—late diastole and early systole (Fig. 12.13)
- *"Swinging" heart*—the heart will often "swing" with large effusions (the etiology of ECG *electrical alternans* with tamponade).

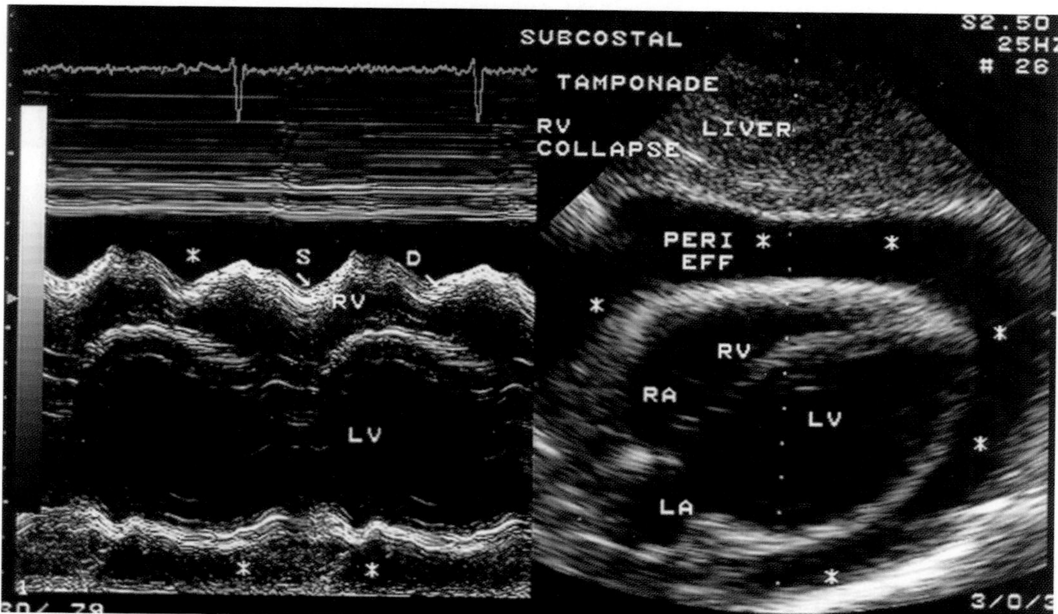

Fig. 12.11 Subcostal long axis image of a patient with a large pericardial effusion (*) and early right ventricular diastolic collapse (D) noted well by M-mode imaging.

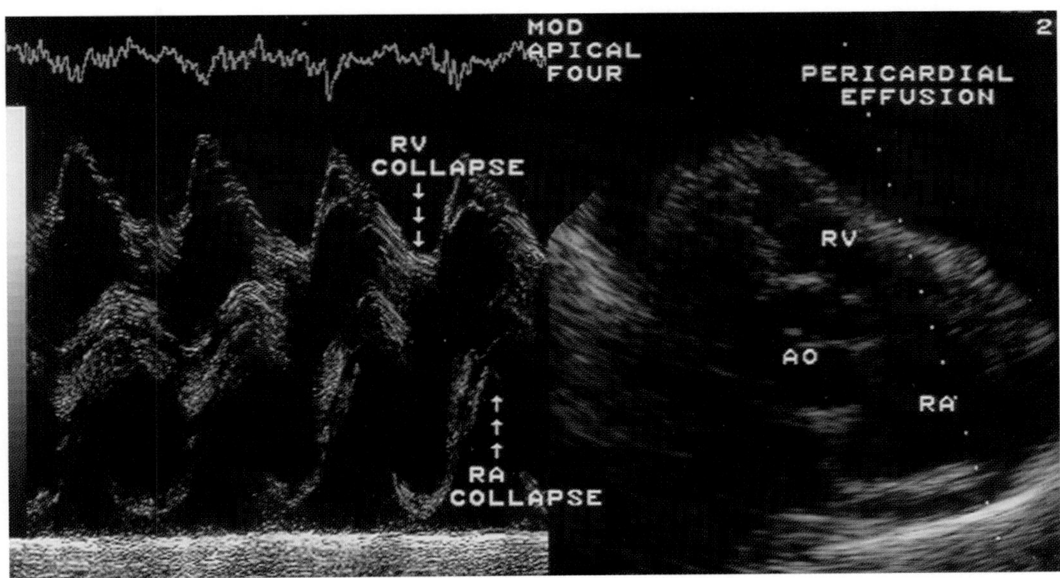

Fig. 12.12 Modified parasternal RV long axis demonstrates both early RV collapse and late RA collapse. M-mode is best for accurate timing of events.

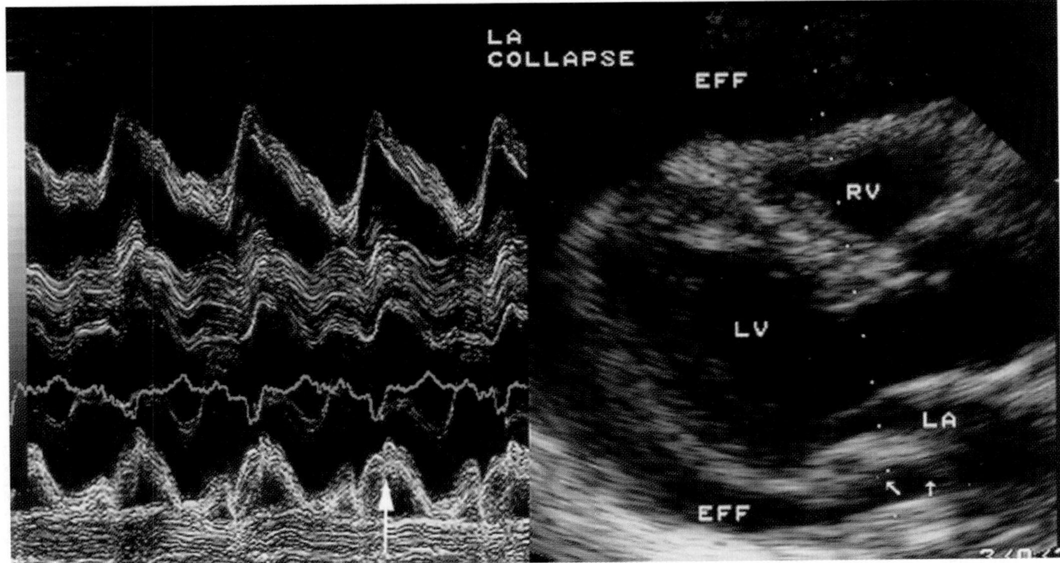

Fig. 12.13 Parasternal long axis view with an M-mode slice through the LA. Note late diastolic collapse of the LA, extending into systole (arrows).

• *IVC plethora without inspiratory collapse*—appears to be very sensitive but less specific for tamponade. With *low pressure tamponade* (RA <12 mmHg), however, patients often will not have IVC plethora. In this group of patients that are presumably volume depleted, tamponade physiology may become evident with volume loading.

• *Abnormal ventricular septal motion*—the septum moves toward the LV with inspiration and toward the RV upon expiration.

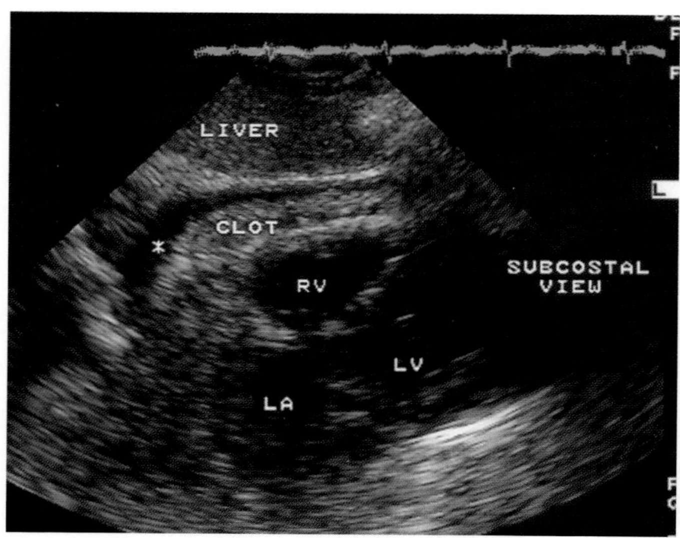

Fig. 12.14 Subcostal long axis view in a patient undergoing an electrophysiologic study using an electrode within the RV. The patient developed hypotension. Echocardiography demonstrates a pericardial effusion (*) with clot within the pericardial space.

• *Respiratory right and left ventricular chamber size variation*—with inspiration the RV chamber increases and the LV chamber decreases. The opposite occurs with expiration.

• *Clotted blood in the pericardium*—with myocardial infarction and rupture, Type I aortic dissection with dissection into the pericardial space or complications of cardiac procedures, clotted blood (hemopericardium) may be diagnosed by echocardiography. The effusion may not be very large as it develops rather quickly and tamponade physiology may occur with relatively little pericardial fluid (Fig. 12.14).

Doppler features appear to be more sensitive for diagnosis of tamponade than M-mode and 2-D findings. Normally there is a relatively small decrease in LV pressure and intrathoracic pressure to a similar degree (hence little change in transmitral gradient) with inspiration. With tamponade, however, since the "heart is separated from the chest by the effusion," intrathoracic pressure will fall more than intrapericardial pressure. The transmitral velocity gradient will diminish substantially during inspiration as the pulmonary wedge pressure (transthoracic pressure)–LV diastolic pressure gradient will be decreased. As the RV and LV are "coupled" during tamponade (relatively fixed heart volume), there will be a significant increase in transtricuspid gradient during inspiration.

Other Doppler features found may include an increase in hepatic and tricuspid flow velocities with inspiration (decrease in pulmonary vein diastolic and mitral E wave flow velocities), and a decrease in hepatic and tricuspid flow velocities with expiration (increase in pulmonary vein diastolic and mitral E wave flow velocities). Mitral and tricuspid E wave flow velocities will generally vary by 33% or more (Figs 12.15–12.17).

Other Doppler features of tamponade include:

• *Aortic and pulmonic valve flow velocity variation*—aortic valve flow velocity will vary corresponding with mitral flow velocity variations, and pulmonic valve flow velocity will vary corresponding with tricuspid valve flow velocity variations.

• *Superior vein flow velocity variation*—variation in flow velocity parallels that of the IVC.

One may falsely diagnose tamponade in the following situations: pericardial effusion with *hypovolemia*, *pleural effusion*, *pericardial constriction* with pericardial effusion, pericardial effusion with *lung disease* (chronic obstructive lung disease, asthma), or pericardial effusion and *obesity*. With tamponade, changes in transmitral and transtricuspid flow velocities occur with the first beat after initiation of a change in respiration, whereas with lung disease or obesity changes may begin with the second or third beat after initiation. This change in flow velocity with the first beat after initiation of inspiration or expiration is noted in constrictive pericarditis also. In RV infarction or pulmonary embolism, one may find variations in right-sided flow velocities as well.

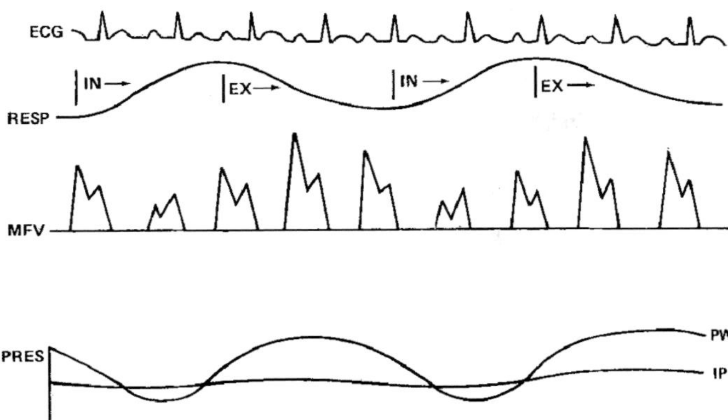

Fig. 12.15 A patient with cardiac tamponade. The upper panel depicts the ECG, and the second panel the respiratory phase by use of a *nasal thermistor* (RESP). Onset of inspiration (IN) and expiration (EX) are shown. The lowest panel (PRES) depicts pulmonary capillary wedge pressure (PW) and also intrapericardial pressure (IP). During inspiration there is a more pronounced reduction of PW compared to IP (approximates LV diastolic pressure). Therefore, a reduced PW–IP gradient results in reduced flow across the mitral valve. With the onset of expiration, the PW–IP gradient increases, and therefore mitral flow will increase. The third panel (MFV) illustrates this early mitral inflow (E wave) variation with the respiratory cycle. (Reproduced with permission from: Appleton CP, Hatle LK, Popp RL. Cardiac tamponade and pericardial effusion: respiratory variation in transvalvular flow velocities studied by Doppler echocardiography. Journal of the American College of Cardiology 1988; 11: 1020–1030, figure 6.)

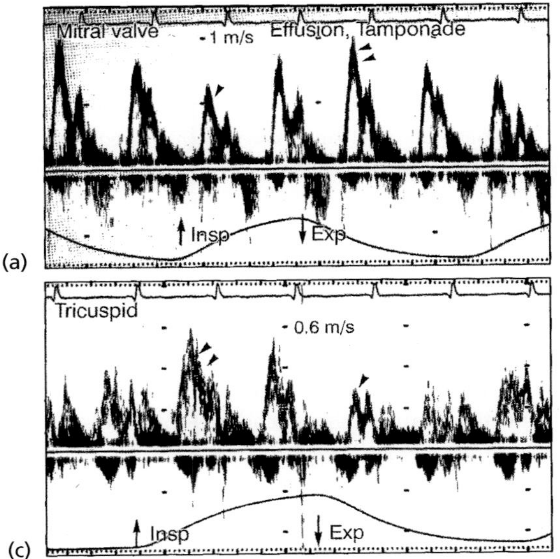

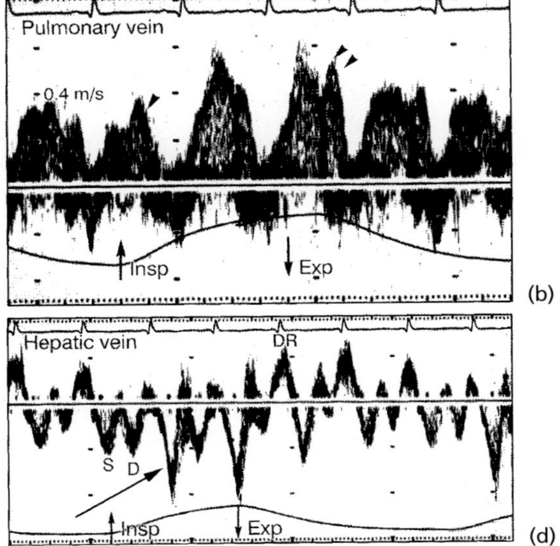

Fig. 12.16 Doppler patterns of cardiac tamponade. Note a nasal thermistor recording in each panel. With *inspiration*, mitral early inflow (E wave) decreases (single arrow in (a)) as does pulmonary vein diastolic (pulmonary vein D wave) forward flow (single arrow in (b)). Also, tricuspid early diastolic inflow (tricuspid E wave) increases (double arrow in (c)) and hepatic vein flow (arrow in (d)) demonstrates an increase in systolic and diastolic forward flow. With *expiration*, the opposite effect is noted. Note that hepatic flow (right lower panel) demonstrates a dramatic reduction in forward flow, and diastolic flow reversal (DR) is increased. (Reproduced with permission from: Oh JK, Hatle LK, Mulvagh SL, Tajik AJ. Transient constrictive pericarditis: diagnosis by two-dimensional Doppler echocardiography. Mayo Clinic Proceedings 1993; 68: 1158–1164.)

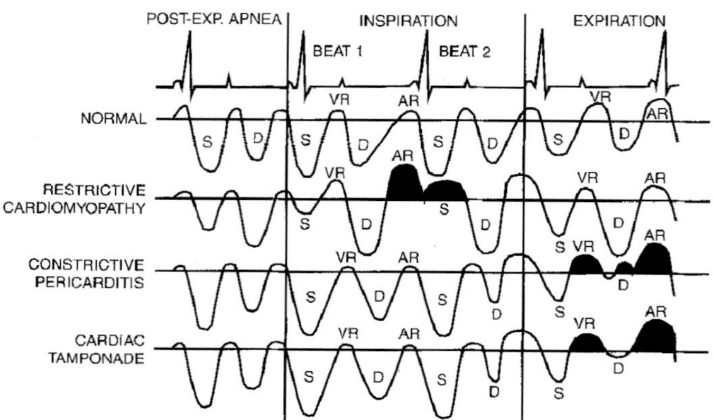

Fig. 12.17 Hepatic vein flow patterns with various disorders. With restrictive cardiomyopathy, an inspiratory decrease or flow reversal is noted (dark shaded) in systole and during atrial contraction (AR, atrial reversal). With constrictive pericarditis and cardiac tamponade an expiratory decrease of forward diastolic flow and marked reversal of flow is noted at AR. (Reproduced with permission from: Bansal RC, Chandrasekaran K. Role of echocardiography and Doppler techniques in the evaluation of pericardial diseases. Echocardiography 1989; 6: 293.)

One may miss the diagnosis of tamponade in the presence of *elevated right heart filling pressures*, *pulmonary hypertension*, *right ventricular hypertrophy*, *localized pericardial effusion*, or *pericardial clot*.

Echo-guided pericardiocentesis

Two-dimensional echocardiography (Fig. 12.18) helps locate the ideal site for puncture. One may determine the distance from the puncture site and note results of drainage. The following outline should be followed:

1 A full echo-Doppler study should be performed.

2 An entry site should be chosen, preferably the site should be closest to the fluid and where a large amount of fluid is located.

3 The patient should remain in the same position for the procedure.

Pericardial constriction

Uncomplicated viral pericarditis is associated with a normal echocardiogram. Pericardial effusion may be associated, and in myopericarditis one may see development of systolic or diastolic dysfunction.

With constrictive pericarditis, the pericardium thickens, and diastolic filling is then hindered by a given pericardial volume. Diastolic pressures in the four cardiac chambers are elevated and generally equal. Early diastolic filling is rapid as atrial pressures are high. Ventricular filling then abruptly stops, as the heart chamber volume is fixed. With inspiration, flow is reduced through the pulmonary vein and across the mitral valve. This reduction in flow prolongs the isovolumic relaxation time (IVRT) and the mitral deceleration time (DT), findings not seen with restrictive cardiomyopathy (the DT is generally shortened with constriction, but not with tamponade). Right heart filling will simultaneously increase.

Often, M-mode and 2-D findings of constrictive pericarditis are nonspecific. No single M-mode or 2-D finding is diagnostic. However, features include:

• *Pericardial thickening and calcification*—echo may have limited applicability, but computed tomography (CT) or magnetic resonance imaging (MRI) appears good for thickness measurement; however, pericardial thickness may not correlate well with hemodynamic compromise. Transesophageal echocardiography (TEE) may be helpful in identifying pericardial thickening.

• *Posterior LV wall early diastolic rapid posterior motion with sudden mid-diastolic cessation of motion with subsequent "flattening"*—this is seen in upwards of 85% of patients, but also 20% of normal subjects (Fig. 12.19).

• *Ventricular septal early diastolic notch (bounce) and end-diastolic notch followed by anterior septal motion*—an early diastolic septal bounce is an exaggeration of normal motion and the late diastolic bounce is followed by normal anterior motion (Fig. 12.19).

• *Rapid M-mode E to F slope.*

• *Early pulmonic valve opening*—best noted by M-mode through the pulmonic valve from a "high" parasternal short axis image. This is due to high RV diastolic pressure that is greater than pulmonary artery diastolic pressure toward mid-diastole, resulting in early valve opening.

• *IVC plethora with little respiratory variation*—with marked volume depletion, IVC plethora may not be prominent, and some respiratory variation may be noted.

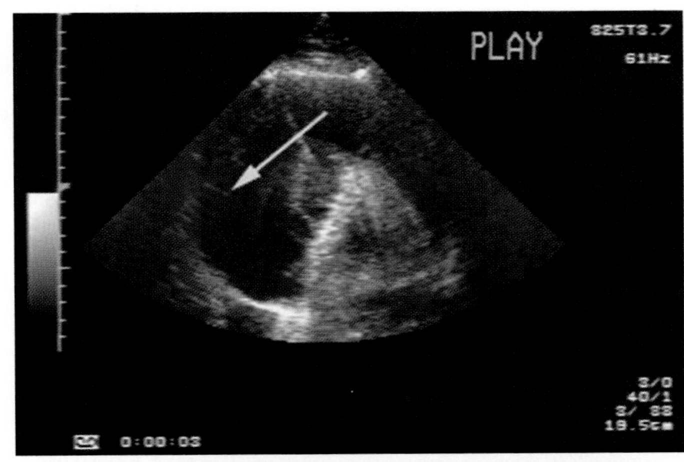

(a)

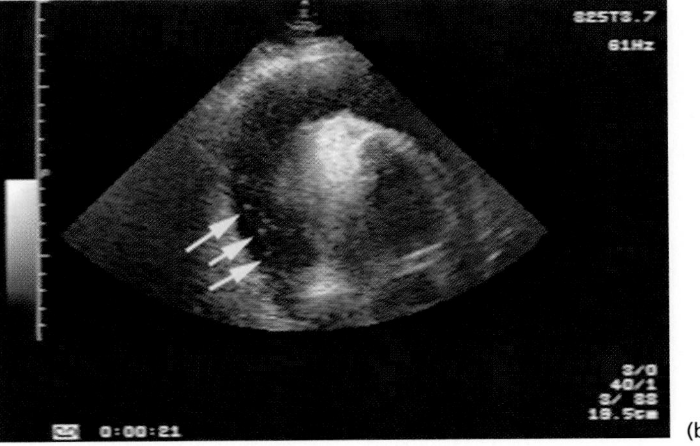

(b)

Fig. 12.18 A middle-aged patient presents with cardiac tamponade. He is several weeks post mechanical mitral valve replacement, and had an INR >6.0. The echocardiographic transducer is located at the cardiac apex with the needle entering from a subxiphoid approach. (a) The needle noted entering within the pericardial fluid (arrow). (b) The syringe "draws back" bloody appearing fluid, and then injection demonstrates bubbles (arrows) within the pericardial fluid, thus documenting needle position. (*Continued on p. 198.*)

When evaluating Doppler features of constriction, it is helpful to use a respirometer to help record Doppler flow as it relates to the respiratory cycle. Doppler features of pericardial constriction include:

1 Left heart:

(a) Reduction of mitral E wave velocity ≥25% with inspiration (increased velocity with expiration)—normally <10% respiratory variation is found.

(b) Prolongation of the mitral isovolumic relaxation time (IVRT) ≥25% with inspiration—the IVRT is usually but not always shortened (<160 ms).

(c) Decreased pulmonary vein systolic and diastolic flow velocities with a reduced systolic : diastolic flow ratio—this is a nonspecific finding consistent with elevated left heart filling pressures

(d) Inspiratory decrease in pulmonary vein flow—most prominently the diastolic flow component will vary ≥25% with respiration.

(e) Mild reduction in aortic systolic forward flow with inspiration

2 Right heart:

(a) Inspiratory increase in tricuspid E wave velocity (expiratory decrease).

(b) Mild increased tricuspid regurgitation (TR) velocity (and time velocity integral) with inspiration—increased filling increases RV preload and therefore TR during inspiration. Normally there is a small decrease in TR velocity with inspiration.

(c) Increased hepatic vein flow with inspiration and marked reduction and flow reversal with expiration—end-systolic and diastolic flow reversal with expiration may be noted. Expiratory diastolic flow reversal may be ≥25% of the forward diastolic flow velocity. Either predominant early diastolic forward flow or predominant systolic flow

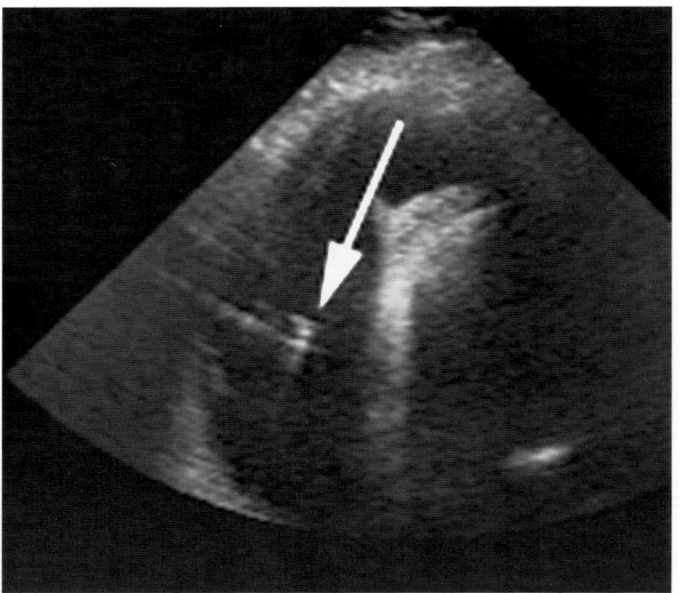

(c)

(d)

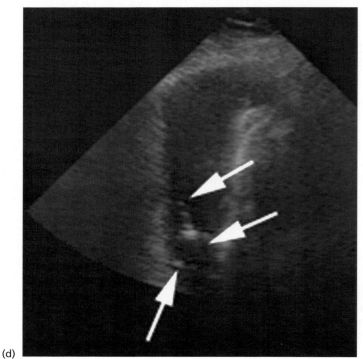

Fig. 12.18 (*cont'd*) (c) A guidewire (arrow) is noted with shadowing distally. (d) A pigtail catheter (arrows) is directed over the guidewire and then fluid is withdrawn. Echocardiography subsequently demonstrated a reduction in the pericardial effusion as fluid was removed.

may be seen, with most forward flow evident during inspiration.

(d) Mild increased pulmonary valve forward flow with inspiration.

Respiratory variation with constrictive pericarditis may not be present in the setting of markedly elevated filling pressures. Reduction of preload, by having the patient assume an upright position or with diuresis, will then reveal the expected Doppler respiratory changes.

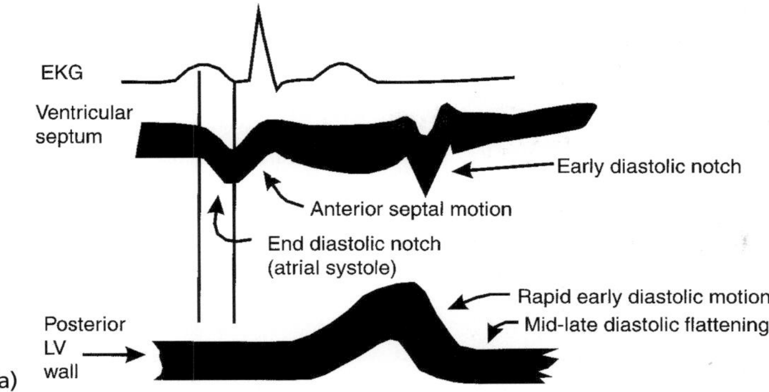

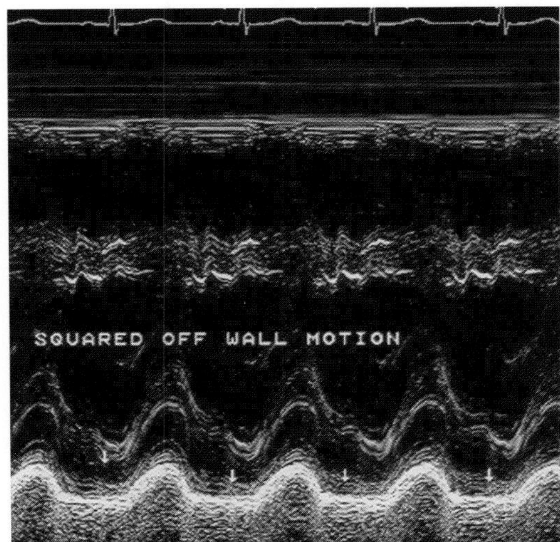

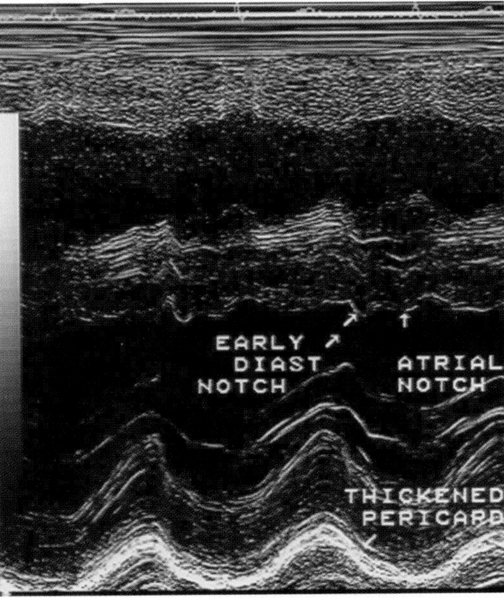

Fig. 12.19 Ventricular septal and posterior wall motion with pericardial constriction. (a) The LV posterior wall demonstrates rapid early diastolic posterior motion followed by an abrupt cessation of motion and a "flattened" posterior wall throughout the remainder of diastole. The ventricular septum demonstrates a *late diastolic notch* (posterior movement) before the normal anterior septal motion. This is due to a transient elevation in RV pressure above LV pressure with atrial systole onset. An *early diastolic notch* also occurs as an exaggerated normal posterior early diastolic motion. LV pressure decay is faster than RV pressure decay, resulting in this finding. (b) M-mode through the LV of a patient with constrictive pericarditis. There is rapid early diastolic posterior motion of the posterior wall with sudden mid-diastolic cessation of motion, with "flattening" (arrows) noted. (c) The interventricular septum demonstrates an early diastolic notch and a late diastolic notch (atrial notch; see text).

Constrictive pericarditis versus restrictive cardiomyopathy

Differentiation of restrictive cardiomyopathy from constrictive pericarditis may be difficult. Both restrictive and constrictive physiology may coexist. Generally respiratory variations in left heart and tricuspid Doppler flow velocity patterns are not present with restriction. Hepatic vein flow with restriction is predominantly forward during diastole, with increased systolic and diastolic flow reversal noted during *inspiration* (in distinction to prominent flow reversal in constriction during *expiration*). The mitral deceleration time (DT) is generally less than 160 ms

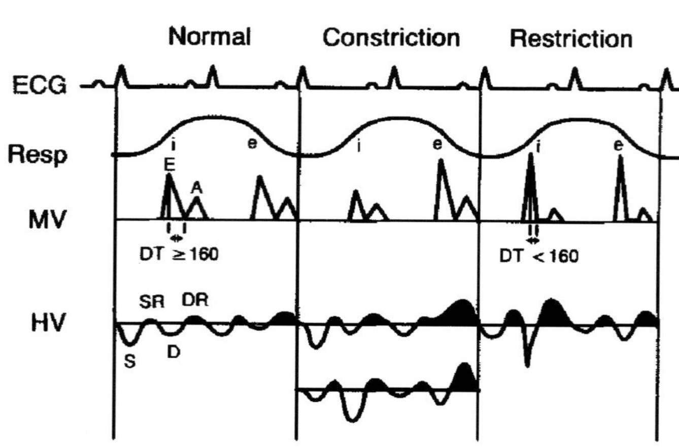

Fig. 12.20 Pulsed wave Doppler velocity patterns of mitral inflow (MV) and hepatic vein (HV) flow in normal, constriction and restriction. A respirometer (Resp) and ECG are also shown. A, mitral A wave; D, diastolic hepatic vein forward flow; DR, late diastolic hepatic vein reversed flow; DT, mitral deceleration time; E, mitral E wave; i, inspiration on the respirometer; e, expiration on the respirometer; S, systolic hepatic vein forward flow; SR, late systolic hepatic vein flow reversal. (Reproduced with permission from: Oh JK, Hatle LK, Seward JB, *et al.* Diagnostic role of Doppler echocardiography in constrictive pericarditis. Journal of the American College of Cardiology 1994; 23: 154–162, figure 1.)

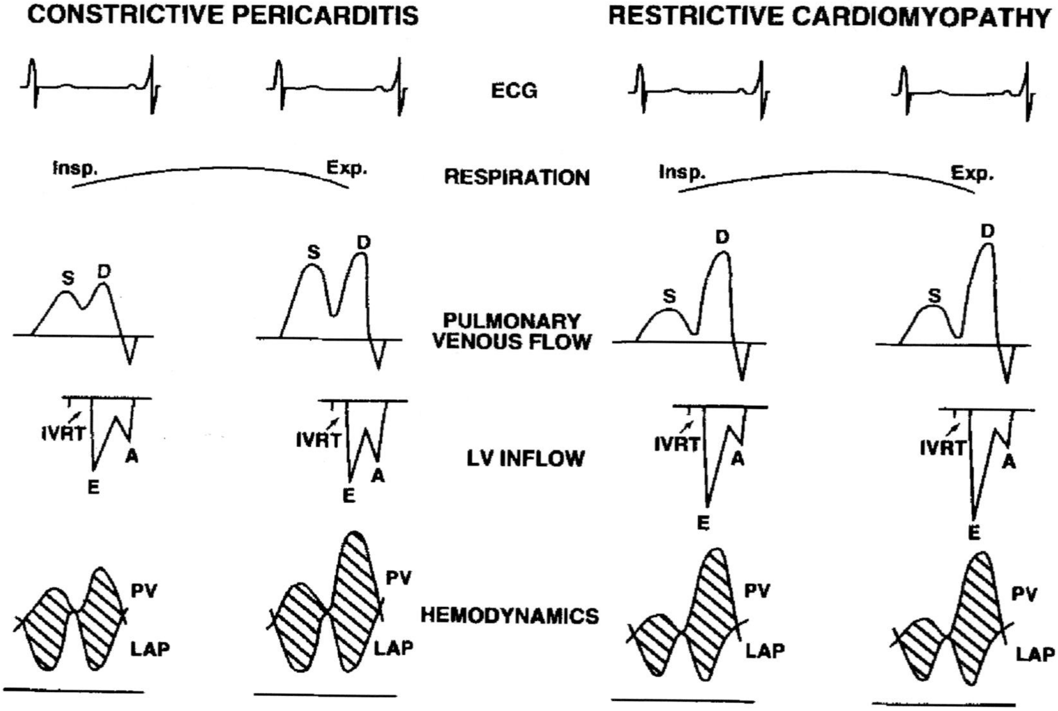

CONSTRICTIVE PERICARDITIS

RESTRICTIVE CARDIOMYOPATHY

ECG

Insp. Exp.

RESPIRATION

Insp. Exp.

S D

PULMONARY VENOUS FLOW

IVRT A E

LV INFLOW

PV LAP

HEMODYNAMICS

Fig. 12.21 Pulmonary venous flow and mitral flow along with hemodynamics in constrictive pericarditis and with restrictive cardiomyopathy. Patterns during inspiration (Insp) and expiration (Exp) are shown. Pulmonary venous patterns reveal marked blunting of systolic flow and a reduced systolic : diastolic flow ratio with restriction. Flow does not vary with respiration. With constriction there is a significant reduction in systolic and diastolic flow with inspiration, most notably variation noted with the diastolic flow component. Mitral inflow decreases with inspiration in constriction and the IVRT will also prolong. In restriction the mitral inflow pattern and IVRT will not change. (Reproduced with permission from: Klein AL, Cohen GI, Pietrolungo JF, *et al.* Differentiation of constrictive pericarditis from restrictive cardiomyopathy by Doppler transesophageal echocardiographic measurements of respiratory variations in pulmonary venous flow. Journal of the American College of Cardiology 1993; 22: 1935–1943, figure 4.)

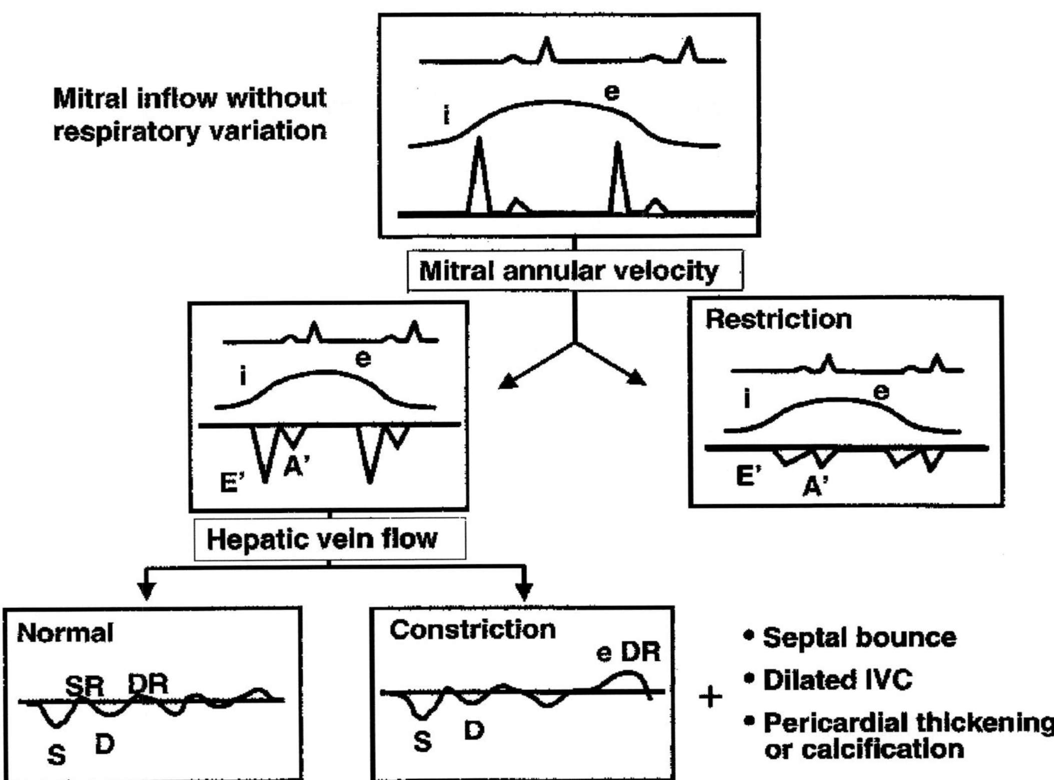

Fig. 12.22 When the mitral inflow patterns reveal a prominent E wave, short deceleration time, and lack of respiratory variation, three possibilities are present: normal, restriction, or constriction (constriction without respiratory variation). This flowchart shows that mitral annular velocity (*E′*) by TDI is low (usually <7 cm/s) with restriction, and preserved in normal individuals and with constriction. Two-dimensional features and hepatic vein flow should help differentiate between normal and constriction. *A′*, mitral annular velocity during atrial systole; e, expiration; *E′*, early diastolic mitral annular velocity; I, inspiration; S, systole; SR, systolic flow reversal. (Reproduced with permission from: Ha JW, Oh JK, Ommen SR, Ling LH, Tajik AJ. Diagnostic value of mitral annular velocity for constrictive pericarditis in the absence of respiratory variation in mitral inflow velocity. Journal of the American Society of Echocardiography 2002; 15: 1468–1471, figure 2.)

with constriction and restriction, but variation in the DT is not seen with restriction. Pulmonary vein flow may reveal systolic flow to be more prominent with constriction as opposed to restriction (Figs 12.17 & 12.21). Also, pulmonary artery systolic pressure tends to be higher in patients with restriction (≥60 mmHg) than in those with constriction (35–40 mmHg).

Tissue Doppler imaging (TDI) appears to be good in differentiating restriction from constriction. Normal volunteers and patients with constriction were found to have an early diastolic velocity (TDI of the lateral mitral annulus from the apical window) of ~14.5 ± 4.5 cm/s, whereas those with restriction had an early diastolic velocity of 5.1 ± 1.4 cm/s. When a patient without mitral inflow respiratory variation is thought to have constriction, use of TDI and hepatic vein flow parameters may help differentiate constriction and restriction from normal (Fig. 12.22). The utility TDI measures for combined restriction and constriction is unknown.

13

CHAPTER 13

Ischemic Heart Disease and Myocardial Infarction

Echocardiography may aid in the early diagnosis of acute myocardial infarction (MI), help diagnose complications of MI, and help with post-MI prognostication. The role of echocardiography in ischemic heart disease includes the following:

- detection of wall motion abnormalities in acute chest pain syndromes
- use of a left ventricular *wall motion score index* (WMSI) to predict infarction complications and survival
- determine myocardial *"area at risk"* during infarction
- assess effects of reperfusion therapy
- assess infarct *extension/expansion*
- assess for myocardial *viability*
- assess for left ventricular segment *"remote" dyssynergy*
- detection of right ventricular infarction
- detection of post-MI *mechanical complications*
- detection of other complications of MI—*aneurysm, thrombus.*

Myocardial segments

The American Heart Association Writing Group on Myocardial Segmentation and Registration for Cardiac Imaging (in association with the American Society of Echocardiography, American Society of Nuclear Cardiology, North American Society of Cardiac Imaging, Society for Cardiac Angiography and Interventions, and Society for Cardiovascular Magnetic Resonance) published standardized recommendations for orientation of the heart, names for cardiac planes, and number and nomenclature of myocardial segments, along with assignment of these segments to coronary artery territories (Figs 13.1–13.3). Originally in the past, the number of segments recommended to be used was 20, but this was subsequently reduced to 16 (Fig. 13.1). These segments were developed for systematic segmental wall motion analysis, but with the advent of myocardial perfusion agents, the 17-segment model was introduced (Fig. 13.2). In describing the segments, the terms *basal, mid-cavity* and *apical* are used. Both the basal and mid-cavity divide into six segments each (*anterior, anteroseptal, inferoseptal, inferior, inferolateral*, and *anterolateral*). Although the term *posterior* is used by some, the term *inferior* is recommended (Figs 13.4–13.6). The RV wall attachments to the LV identify the septum from the LV anterior and inferior free walls. The four apical segments are *apical anterior, apical septal, apical inferior*, and *apical lateral.* The 17th segment is the *apex* (apical cap), defined as that myocardium apically past the LV cavity (see Fig. 9.2 for an illustration of right ventricular segments). At times, the origin of coronary arteries may be visualized by transthoracic (TTE) and transesophageal (TEE) echocardiography (Fig. 13.7).

Acute ischemia, myocardial infarction, and the wall motion score index

Acute ischemia is initially manifested as abnormal diastolic function, followed by abnormal systolic function. These changes have been noted prior to acute ECG changes or the development of chest pain. Systolic dysfunction results in a decrease in systolic contractility. A normally functioning LV segment should have *systolic thickening* that is 40% or greater, whereas a segment with systolic thickening less than 30% is termed *hypokinetic*, and a segment with systolic thickening of less than 10% is considered *akinetic. Dyskinesis* is myocardial systolic motion of a segment outward. Myocardial necrosis (*subendocardial*) begins about 30 min after coronary occlusion, and proceeds

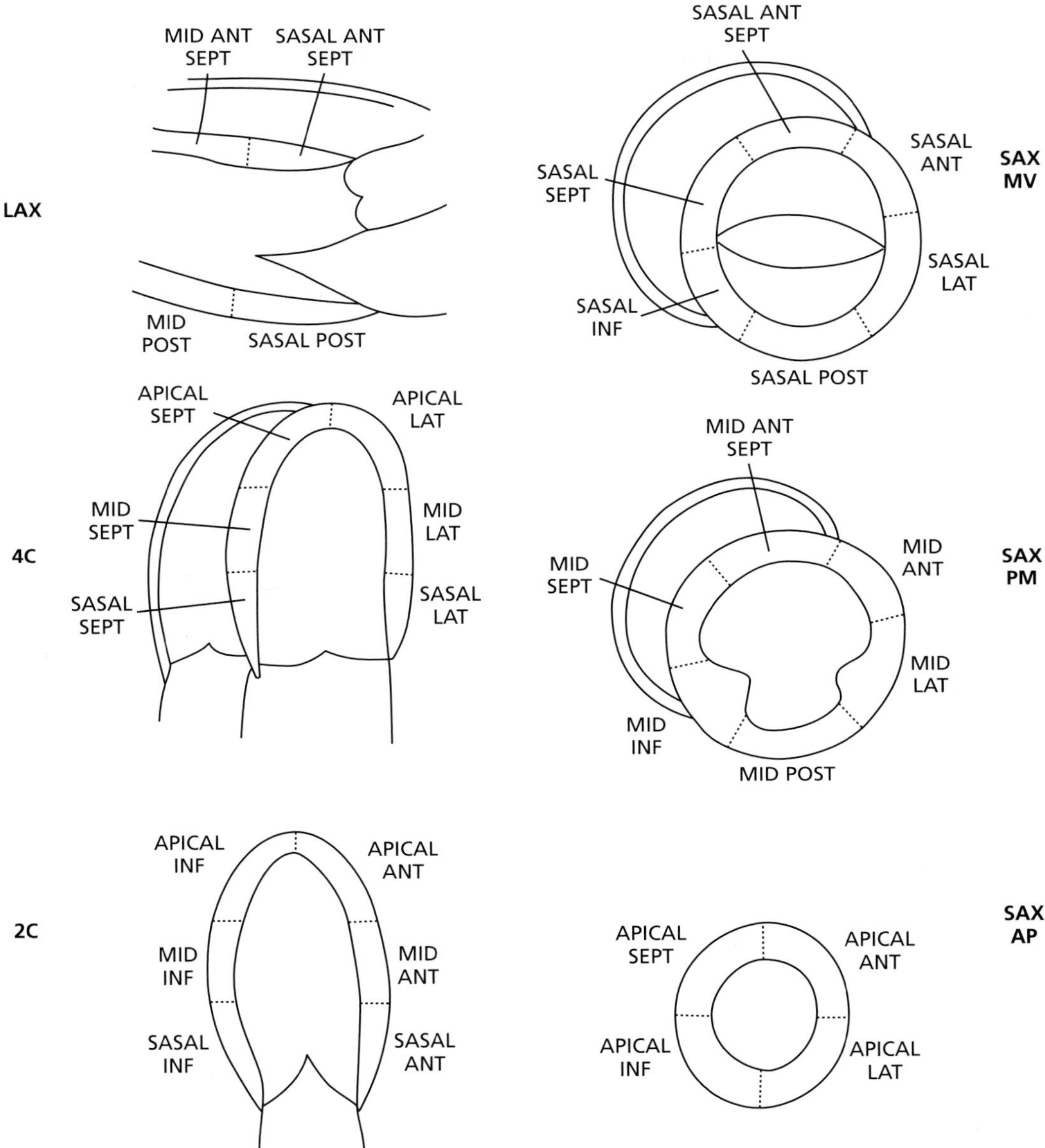

Fig. 13.1 The LV divided into 16 segments for 2-D (two-dimensional) echocardiography. LAX, long axis; 4C, four-chamber; 2C, two-chamber; SAX MV, short axis mitral valve level (basal); SAX PM, short axis papillary level (mid-cavity); SAX AP, short axis apex. (Reproduced with permission from: Standardized myocardial segmentation and nomenclature for tomographic imaging of the heart. Circulation 2002; 105: 539–549, figure 2.)

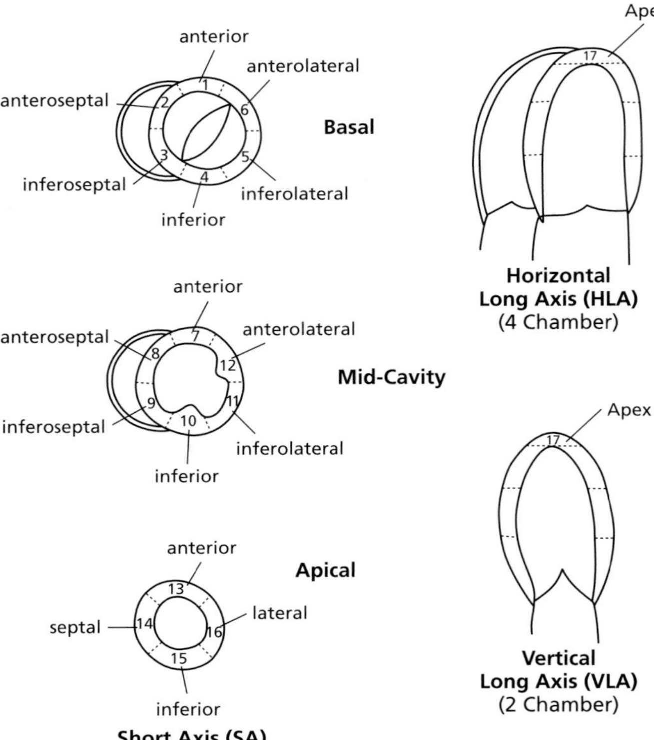

Fig. 13.2 The 17-segment model for assessment of the LV with echocardiography. In this model the apical cap beyond the LV cavity becomes the 17th segment. (Reproduced with permission from: Standardized myocardial segmentation and nomenclature for tomographic imaging of the heart. Circulation 2002; 105: 539–549, figure 3.)

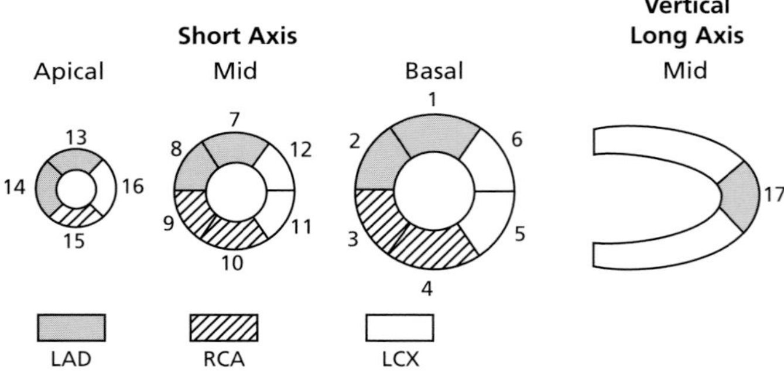

Fig. 13.3 Each of 17 segments has been assigned to a coronary artery, despite the known variability in coronary artery blood supply to the myocardial segments. Segment 17 may be supplied by either of the three major coronary vessels (LAD, RCA, or LCX). LAD, left anterior descending; RCA, right coronary artery; LCX, left circumflex. (Reproduced with permission from: Standardized myocardial segmentation and nomenclature for tomographic imaging of the heart. Circulation 2002; 105: 539–549, figure 5.)

from the endocardium to the epicardium. A *transmural infarction* may be evident with longer occlusion.

Acute coronary syndromes are syndromes that reflect acute myocardial ischemia. These syndromes have been divided into those with and without definite evidence of myocardial necrosis. Patients with necrosis, that is MI, have been subdivided into those with or without ST-segment elevation (ST-segment elevation MI or non-ST segment MI elevation, respectively). Although in the past ST-segment MIs have been labeled transmural or Q-wave MIs and non-ST segment MIs have been labeled subendocardial or-non-Q-wave MIs, there is much overlap and the former terms are preferred in clinical practice. Acute coronary syndrome without myocardial necrosis has been labeled "unstable angina."

Echocardiography is an excellent technique to assess the wall motion abnormality that occurs with

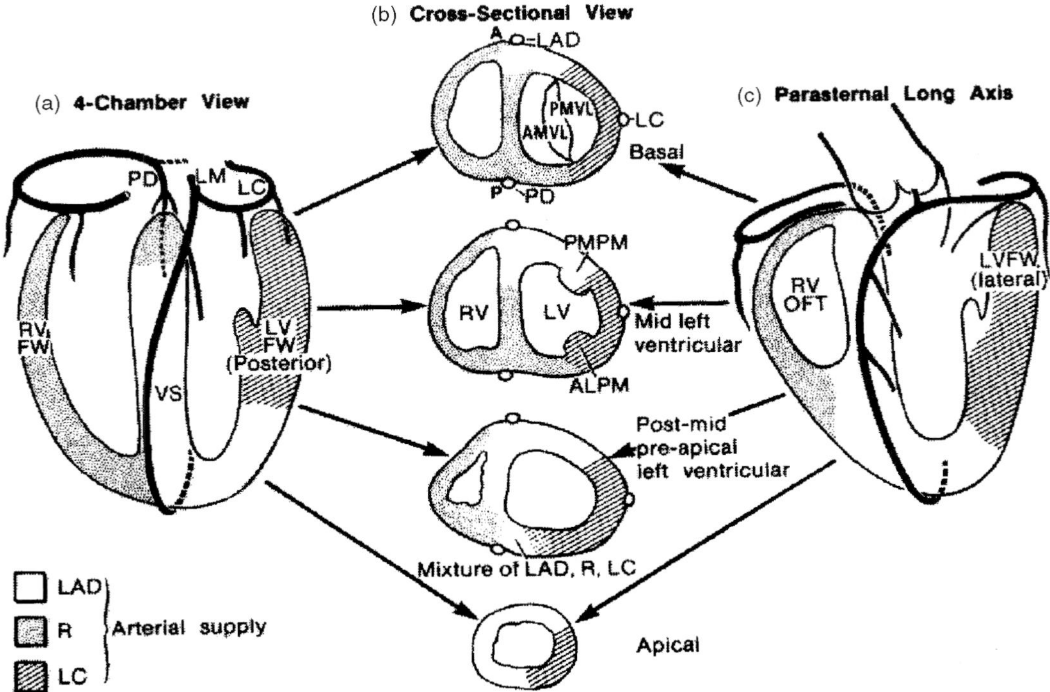

Fig. 13.4 The coronary arteries and respective myocardial segments perfused from the apical four-chamber (a), parasternal short axis (b), and parasternal long axis (c) views. A, anterior; ALPM, anterolateral papillary muscle; LC, left circumflex; LM, left main coronary artery; LVFW, left ventricular free wall; P, posterior; PMPM, posteromedial papillary muscle; RVFW, right ventricular free wall; RVOFT, right ventricular outflow tract. (Reproduced with permission from: Waller BF. Anatomy, histology, and pathology of the major epicardial coronary arteries relevant to echocardiographic imaging techniques. Journal of the American Society of Echocardiography 1989; 2: 232–252.)

the acute ischemic syndromes. Echocardiography may be particularly helpful in patients with acute ischemic syndromes who have ECG findings of left ventricular hypertrophy (LVH), paced rhythms, or bundle branch block. Echo may miss small nontransmural infarctions, however. The location and extent of LV dysfunction ("*area of risk*") may help in the decision process for reperfusion therapy, especially in patients at high risk for complications of reperfusion therapy.

Echocardiography helps localize the coronary vessel involved in acute infarction (Fig. 13.3). Infarction involving the inferior and inferoseptum segments suggests dominant right coronary artery (RCA) obstruction, whereas infarction involving the inferior and inferolateral segments suggests left circumflex coronary artery (LCX) involvement. Infarction of the anterior wall and anteroseptum denotes left anterior descending coronary artery infarction.

The WMSI may be used to semiquantitatively assess the degree of wall motion abnormalities. Most often the 16-segment model of the LV is used (Fig. 13.1). This method assigns a score to each segment: 0, hyperkinetic; 1, normal; 2, hypokinetic; 3, akinetic; 4, dyskinetic; 5, aneurysm. The score for each segment is added up and then divided by the number of segments (16 in the 16-segment model). The WMSI is a good predictor of complications of acute MI. It is better than the LV ejection fraction in this setting, as regional abnormalities rather than global function are assessed. Generally a WMSI of 1.7 (>20% LV myocardial damage) indicates an increased risk of postinfarction complications. A WMSI performed before hospital discharge is a good predictor of complications with 1 year.

Compensatory hyperkinesis in nonfarcted LV segments, over the first few days after MI, is often noted. This is probably related to an elevated catecholamine

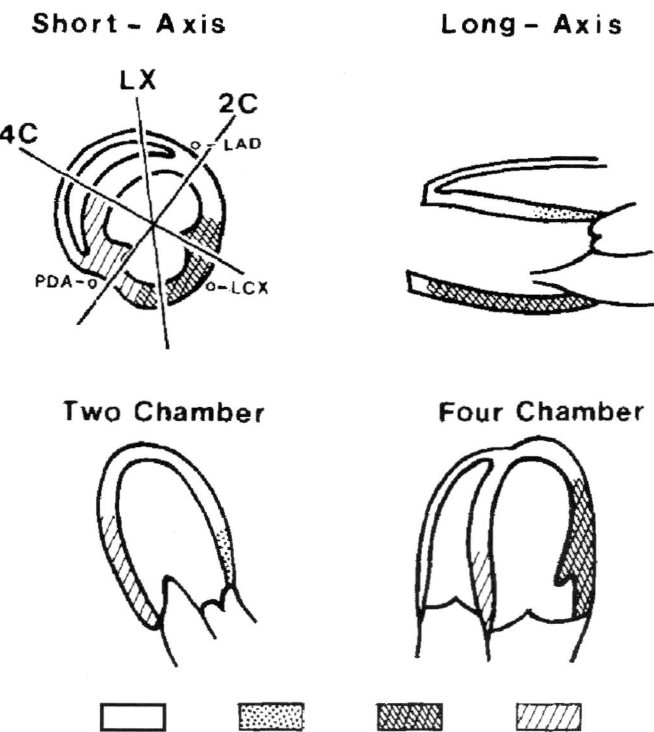

Fig. 13.5 2-D echocardiographic views and representative coronary artery territories. (Reproduced with permission from: Feigenbaum H. Echocardiography, 4th edn. Philadelphia: Lea & Febiger, 1986: p. 467, figure 8-8.)

state. Lack of this compensatory hyperkinesis may indicate significant coronary disease in those non-infarcted segments.

Ischemia at a distance is transient LV segmental wall dysfunction in a region outside the distribution of the infarct-related artery. It carries a poorer prognosis than ischemia localized only to the infarct zone, and indicates multivessel coronary disease. Ischemia at a distance may be due to: (i) a prior myocardial infarction; (ii) increased demand on these segments in which coronary disease is present and thus adequate oxygen cannot be supplied to those segments; (iii) sudden termination of collaterals to that territory in which the collateral circulation originated from the acutely occluded coronary vessel, or (iv) two ongoing acute myocardial infarctions (distinctly unlikely).

Echocardiography appears to be reliable for estimating infarct size after permanent coronary occlusion. After coronary occlusion with subsequent reperfusion, however, echocardiography is not reliable for about the first 10–14 days. Echocardiography will usually overestimate infarct size because of *myocardial stunning* and *myocardial tethering* (adjacent myocardial segments appear abnormal as endocardial motion may be affected, without any ischemia/injury evident).

Myocardial stunning is temporary myocardial segment dysfunction that subsequently improves following an acute ischemic insult. Intravenous dobutamine will improve contractility in stunned myocardium, hence detecting *myocardial viability*. *Myocardial contrast echocardiography* (MCE) will demonstrate flow into myocardium in stunned myocardium, whereas if permanent myocardial injury is present no flow will be noted in the myocardium despite a patent epicardial coronary vessel (*no reflow* phenomenon from microvascular occlusion).

Echocardiography may underestimate infarct size in subendocardial infarction in which less than 25% of the myocardial thickness is involved, as the remaining myocardial will provide normal segmental contractility. Also, in patients with myocardial infarction over

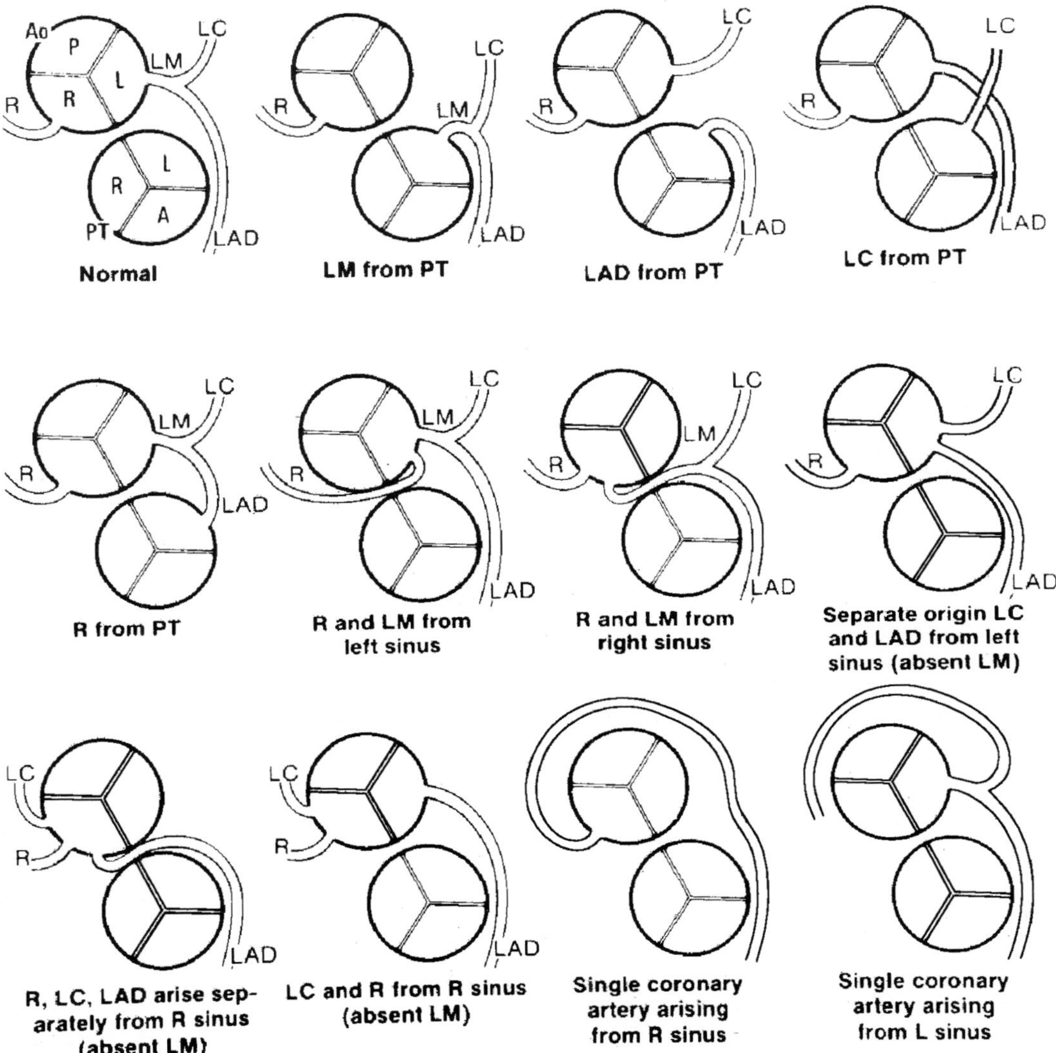

Fig. 13.6 Anomalies of the coronary arteries as would be noted by transesophageal echocardiography (TEE). Ao, aorta; PT, pulmonary trunk; R, right. (Reproduced with permission from: Waller BF. Anatomy, histology, and pathology of the major epicardial coronary arteries relevant to echocardiographic imaging techniques. Journal of the American Society of Echocardiography 1989; 2: 232–252, figure 29.)

6 months prior, echocardiography will tend to underestimate the number of infarcted segments.

Some patients with *end-stage liver disease* may demonstrate a flattening or inward anterior displacement of the inferior-posterior wall in diastole. In early systole there is then an outward posterior expansion (LV resumes a rounded shape) followed by thickening and appropriate anterior motion in mid to late systole. Then, in early diastole a paradoxical rapid anterior movement is noted. These patients have elevated intra-abdominal pressures from either organomegaly or ascites, with an elevated diaphragm likely causing external compression of the inferoposterior LV wall. This (a recognizable finding in patients undergoing evaluation for liver transplantation) should not be confused with ischemia, and may alert the unsuspecting sonographer to the possibility of elevated intra-abdominal pressures.

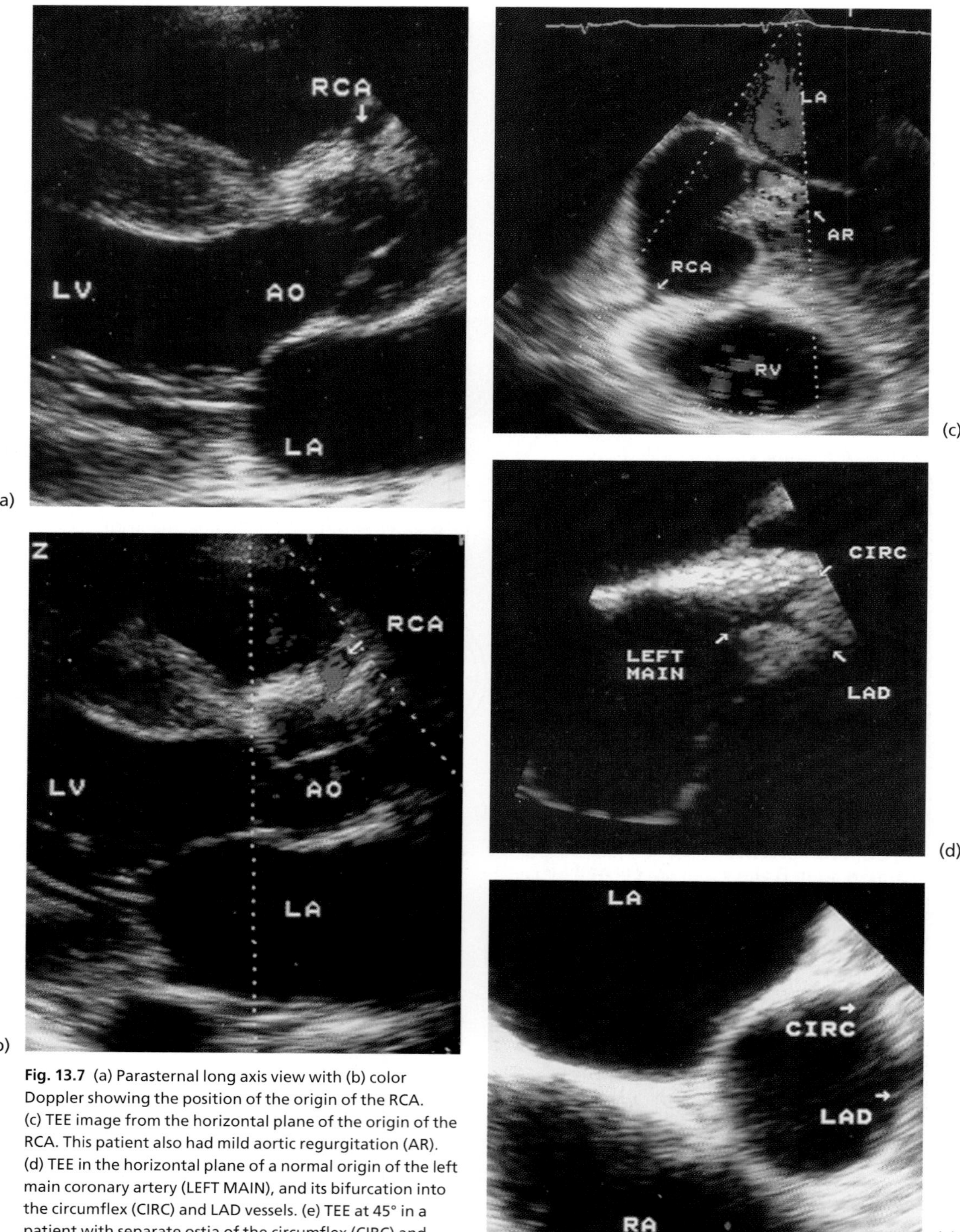

Fig. 13.7 (a) Parasternal long axis view with (b) color Doppler showing the position of the origin of the RCA. (c) TEE image from the horizontal plane of the origin of the RCA. This patient also had mild aortic regurgitation (AR). (d) TEE in the horizontal plane of a normal origin of the left main coronary artery (LEFT MAIN), and its bifurcation into the circumflex (CIRC) and LAD vessels. (e) TEE at 45° in a patient with separate ostia of the circumflex (CIRC) and LAD vessels. (*Cont'd.*)

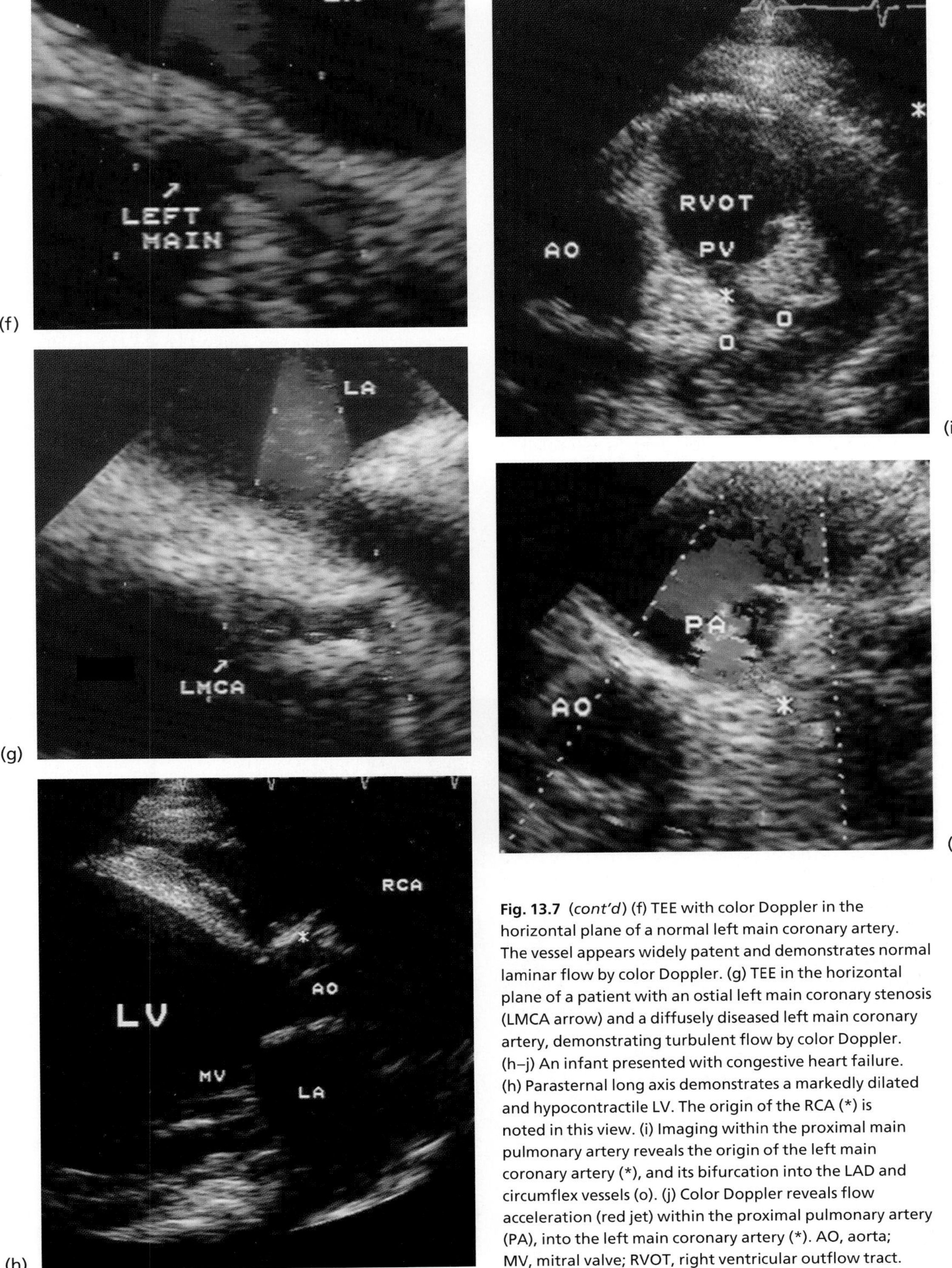

Fig. 13.7 (*cont'd*) (f) TEE with color Doppler in the horizontal plane of a normal left main coronary artery. The vessel appears widely patent and demonstrates normal laminar flow by color Doppler. (g) TEE in the horizontal plane of a patient with an ostial left main coronary stenosis (LMCA arrow) and a diffusely diseased left main coronary artery, demonstrating turbulent flow by color Doppler. (h–j) An infant presented with congestive heart failure. (h) Parasternal long axis demonstrates a markedly dilated and hypocontractile LV. The origin of the RCA (*) is noted in this view. (i) Imaging within the proximal main pulmonary artery reveals the origin of the left main coronary artery (*), and its bifurcation into the LAD and circumflex vessels (o). (j) Color Doppler reveals flow acceleration (red jet) within the proximal pulmonary artery (PA), into the left main coronary artery (*). AO, aorta; MV, mitral valve; RVOT, right ventricular outflow tract.

Infarct extension, expansion and remodeling

Infarct extension is further infarction of the same affected coronary area, with further myocardial segments becoming involved with necrosis.

Infarct expansion involves acute stretching and thinning of the infarcted segment. Significant expansion may occur within the first 3 h following an acute MI, increase within 3–5 days of the injury, and progress over weeks to months. Myocardial expansion almost always occurs following an anterior infarction. Infarct expansion is associated with a poorer prognosis but can be reduced by the use of cardiac medications (e.g. angiotensin converting enzyme inhibitors—ACEi). This reduction in infarct expansion is manifest as a reduction in LV enlargement. Infarct expansion may result in *aneurysm* formation and rarely *myocardial rupture*.

Remodeling of the left ventricle is related to infarct expansion. Whereas infarct expansion involves stretching and thinning of the infarcted segments only, remodeling involves adjacent and remote non-ischemic segments, with LV dilatation and subsequent altered LV geometry. The LV will subsequently assume a spherical shape, as a pattern of volume-overload hypertrophy is seen. Remodeling may begin soon after myocardial infarction and continue well past the hospital course. Risk factors for remodeling include infarction size, early infarct expansion, a persistently occluded infarct-related coronary artery, and myocardial dysfunction secondary to coronary ischemia. ACEi drugs attenuate remodeling. Development of clinical heart failure is related to both infarct expansion and remodeling.

Left ventricular aneurysm and thrombus formation

Left ventricular aneurysm (Figs 13.8–13.11) results from infarct expansion and is found in 10–20% of transmural infarcts. An aneurysm is a deformity or bulging of a thinned infarcted segment during both diastole and systole. An aneurysm can be differentiated from a dyskinetic segment by its abnormal shape in diastole. A myocardial *dyskinetic segment* is defined as deformation during systole only, but does not display a diastolic bulging or deformity and usually does not appear thinned. An aneurysm will display myocardial segment scarring (thinned walls <7 mm) with increased segment echogenicity (increased collagen formation). With time, the aneurysm may calcify.

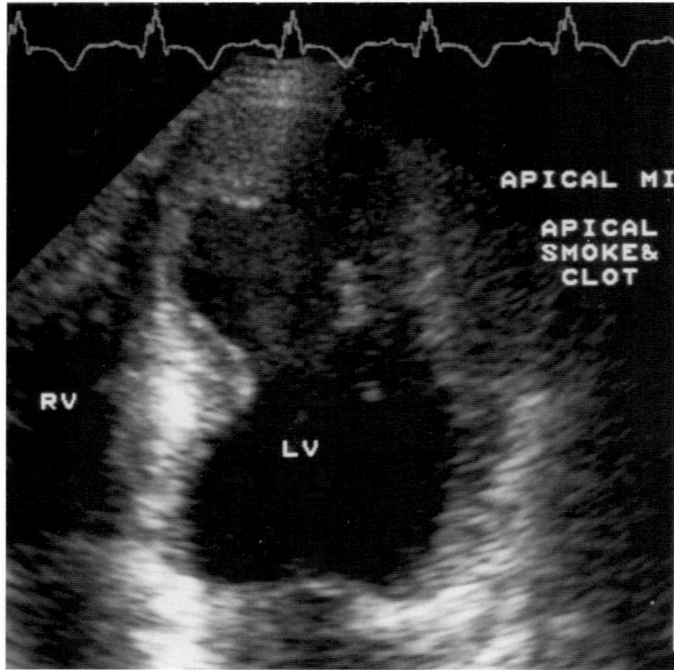

Fig. 13.8 Apical four-chamber view in a patient with a LV apical aneurysm. Note spontaneous echo contrast and thrombus within the apex.

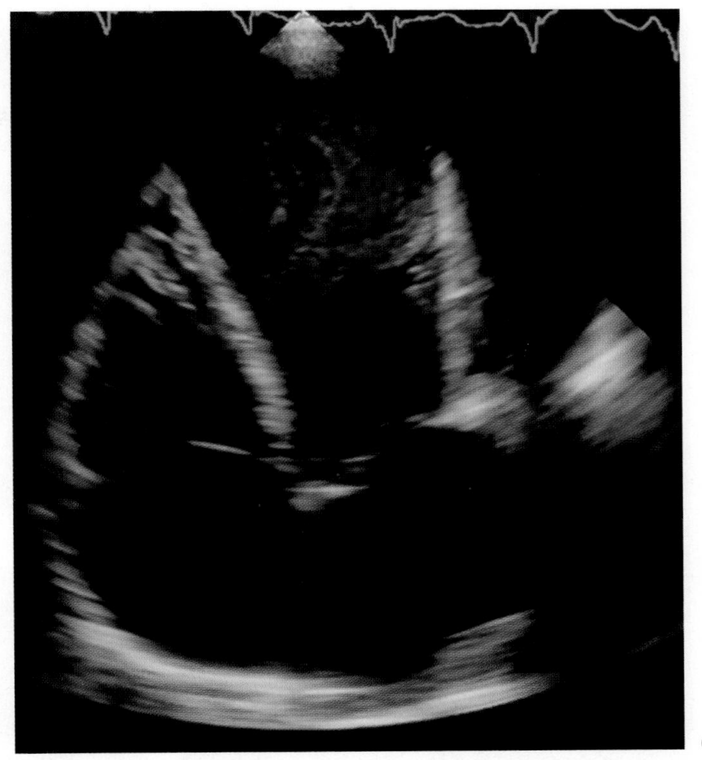

(a)

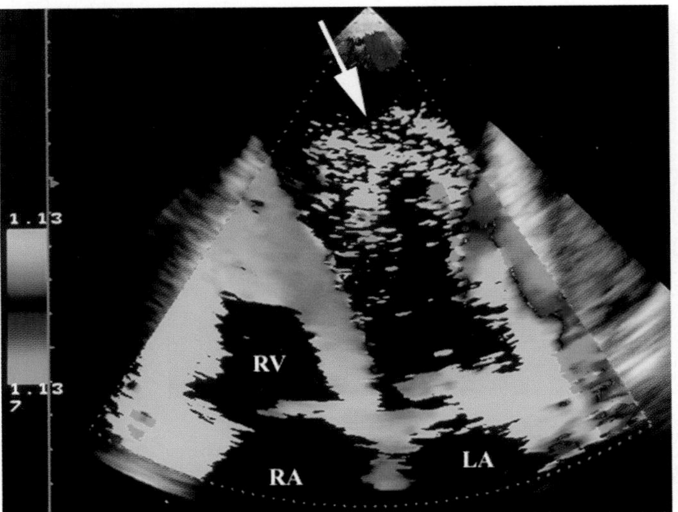

(b)

Fig. 13.9 (a) A patient with an apical myocardial infarction (MI) and noted heavy spontaneous echo contrast. (b) Another patient with an apical aneurysm with spontaneous echo contrast (arrow) noted by tissue Doppler imaging. With real-time imaging, a characteristic gentle swirling motion is noted.

An aneurysm is most commonly found at the LV apex (90%), but may involve any other segment. Posterobasal aneurysms must be carefully differentiated from a pseudoaneurysm.

LV thrombus (Figs 13.12–13.14) forms most commonly in a LV aneurysm. Thrombi that are pedunculated embolize more frequently than those that are laminated. It may be difficult to identify a laminated thrombus. To improve visualization of a thrombus, one should angle the ultrasound transducer from the LV apex to obtain an apical short axis view (so called "bread-loaf" section of the LV apex). Peripheral

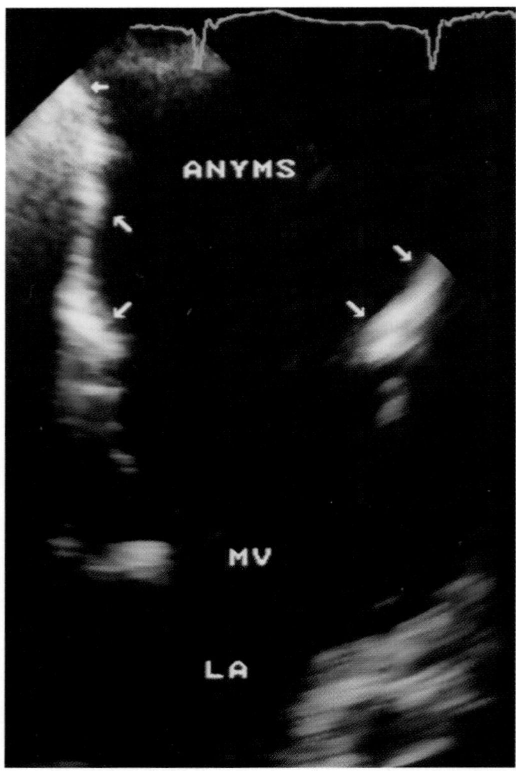

(a)

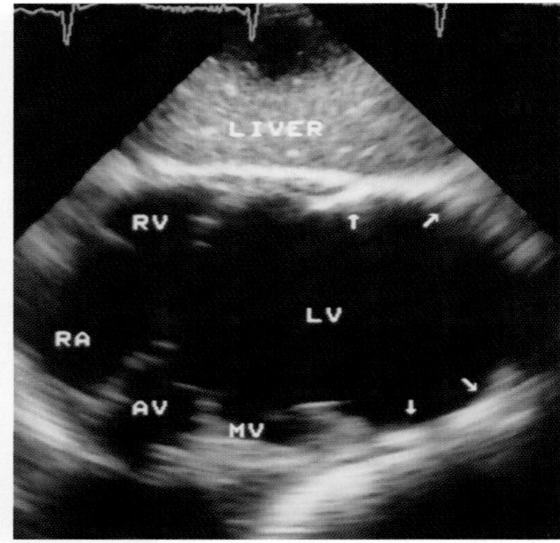

(b)

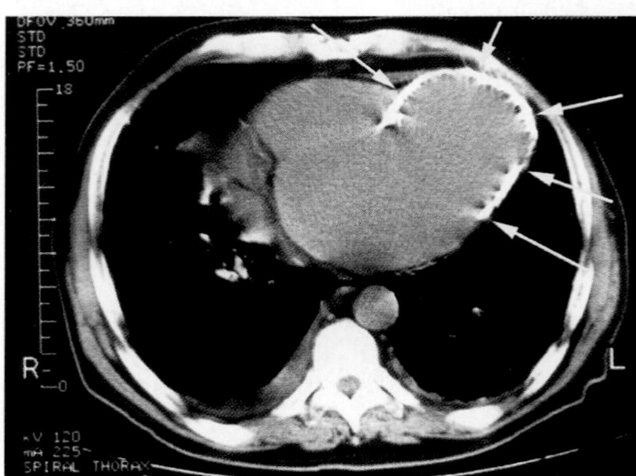

(c)

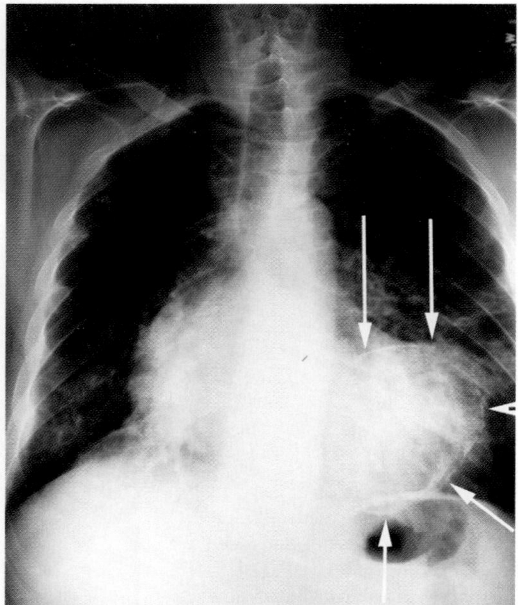

(d)

Fig. 13.10 An elderly patient with a history of a heart attack some 15 years earlier. (a) A large calcified (arrows) LV aneurysm (ANYMS) is noted. (b) Subcostal long axis imaging demonstrates the large calcified LV aneurysm (arrows). (c) Computed tomography with transverse imaging through the LV, and (d) an upright posterior-anterior chest X-ray also demonstrates the large calcified LV apical aneurysm. Calcification location by chest X-ray may help distinguish this from pericardial calcium, as pericardial calcification is mostly located over the right heart and atrioventricular groove. Isolated calcification over the LV apex or posterior wall is suggestive of a calcified LV aneurysm.

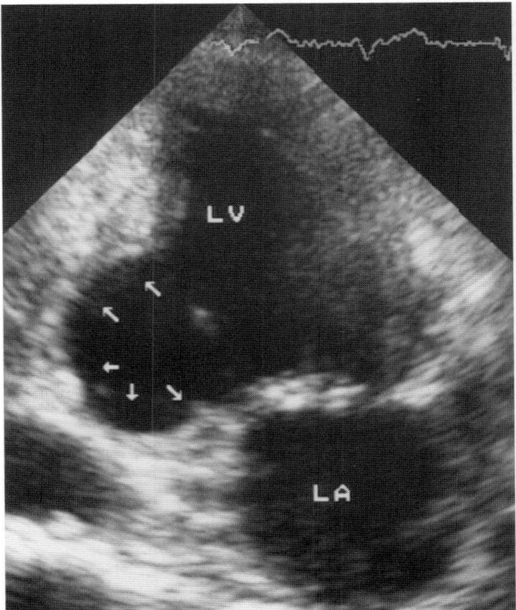

Fig. 13.11 Apical two-chamber view in a patient with a posterobasal aneurysm (arrows). It is important to differentiate this from a pseudoaneurysm.

injection of contrast agents with LV opacification may also help identify a thrombus by the observation of a filling defect.

Echo features of LV thrombus include:

- LV wall motion abnormality—usually akinetic/dyskinetic
- LV apex most common site
- thrombus border "disrupts" the endocardial appearance
- apparent "increase in LV wall thickness" due to the thrombus
- occasional pedunculated appearance—the thrombus may change from being mobile and pedunculated to sessile relatively quickly
- echo/texture appearance may be different from the LV wall—a chronic thrombus may appear layered with areas of calcification (*lines of Zahn*)
- pedunculated thrombus with sonolucent center—a higher incidence of embolism than a flat, layered thrombus.

When using low frequency transducers, one may mistakenly misdiagnose LV trabeculations, a false tendon or near-field artifact as a LV thrombus.

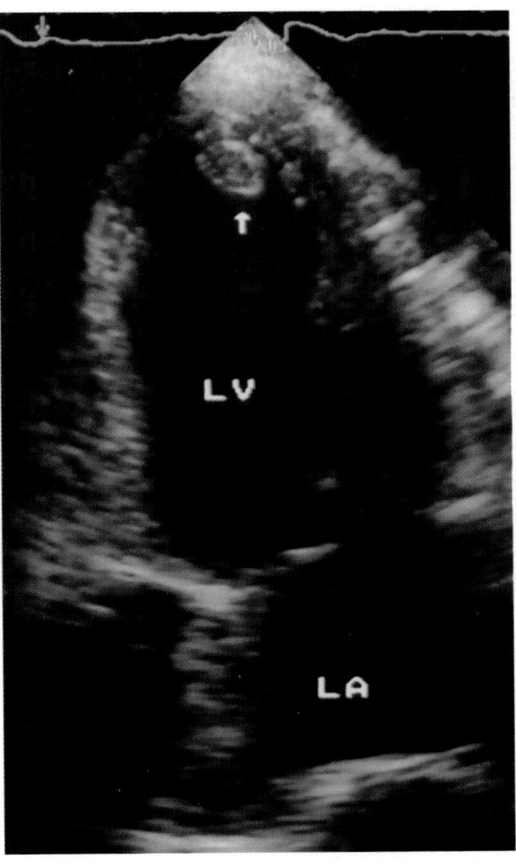

Fig. 13.12 Apical four-chamber view demonstrating an apical LV clot. There appears to be some calcification, suggesting a chronic clot.

Pseudoaneurysm

LV pseudoaneurysm occurs with rupture of the LV free wall and formation of a localized hemopericardium (Fig. 13.15). A true aneurysm located in the inferobasilar area may mimic a pseudoaneurysm because both may have a narrow neck. Echo features of a pseudoaneurysm include:

- sharp discontinuity of the endocardial edge
- a globular contour of the pseudoaneurysm
- a relatively narrow neck compared to that of an aneurysm
- displacement of the other cardiac chambers or compression of the right ventricle anteriorly against the chest wall
- expansion of a pseudoaneurysm during systole, whereas the LV cavity gets smaller during systole

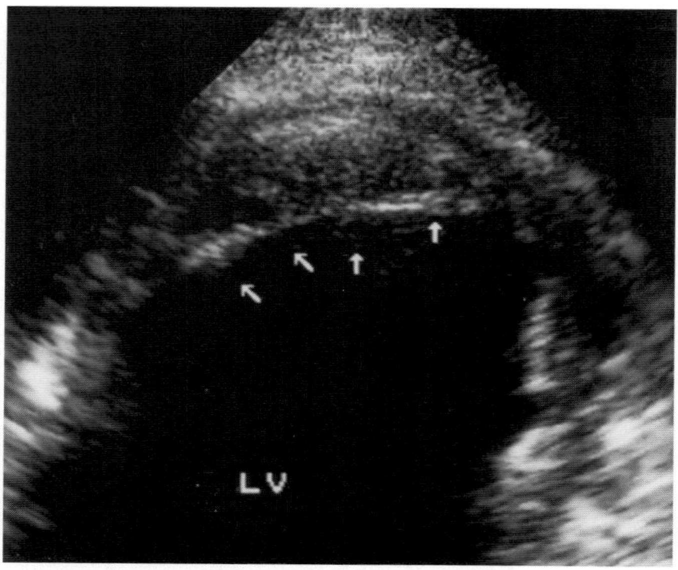

Fig. 13.13 Apical transducer position in a patient with an apical infarction. A high frequency probe and close evaluation reveals a laminated apical thrombus (arrows). Note an apparent increase in LV wall thickness, and a "disruption" in the endocardial border.

- demonstration of Doppler flow between the LV cavity and pseudoaneurysm (Fig. 13.16)—generally, flow occurs into the pseudoaneurysm beginning in late diastole and flows back into the left ventricle beginning in late systole and ending in early to mid diastole
- thrombus usually lining the pseudoaneurysm.

Occasionally a posterobasal pseudoaneurysm will develop as a result of perforation of the LV with a valve strut during implantation of a high profile bioprosthesis. This complication may not become immediately apparent, and may even be found years later.

If large, a *LV diverticulum* may resemble a pseudoaneurysm. A LV diverticulum is a congenital defect that may be associated with embolic events, cardiac rupture, mitral regurgitation, or arrhythmias. Doppler flow may help differentiate the two. With a diverticulum, systolic flow occurs from the diverticulum into the LV and diastolic flow occurs from the LV into the diverticulum.

Subepicardial aneurysm and left ventricular free wall rupture

A rare but important complication of MI is *subepicardial aneurysm*, demonstrating partial rupture of the LV wall. Epicardium prevents rupture and forms the wall of the aneurysm (hematoma). These tend to rupture, forming a pseudoaneurysm. Echo features of a subepicardial aneurysm include:

- abrupt interruption of myocardium at the aneurysm neck
- narrow neck of the aneurysm
- systolic expansion of the aneurysm wall.

LV free wall rupture usually leads to immediate death, with sudden cardiovascular collapse and electromechanical dissociation. Forty per cent of ruptures occur within 24 h of the onset of symptoms of myocardial infarction, and 85% occur within the first week. Characteristics of patients most likely to rupture include:

- older
- female
- no prior history of MI
- no evidence of LV hypertrophy
- no evidence of mural thrombus
- less angina
- presence of an acute transmural MI.

A pattern of free wall rupture with a subacute course from hours to days may occur, termed *subacute LV free wall rupture* (Fig. 13.17). Nearly all patients with subacute rupture will have a pericardial effusion of 5 mm or larger and intrapericardial echos suggestive of clot. Pericardial fat may be confused with

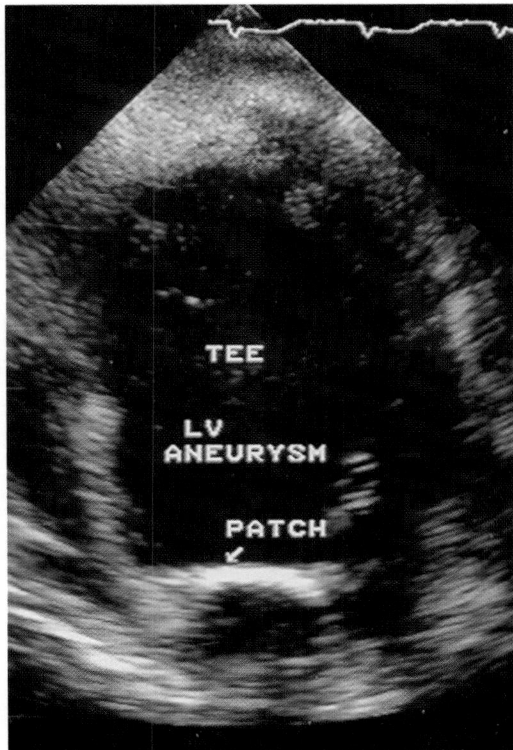

Fig. 13.14 Mid-esophageal TEE image of a patient 10 years after surgical placement of an intraventricular patch (PATCH) for a discrete LV apical aneurysm. The foreshortened LV apex is most distant from the transducer.

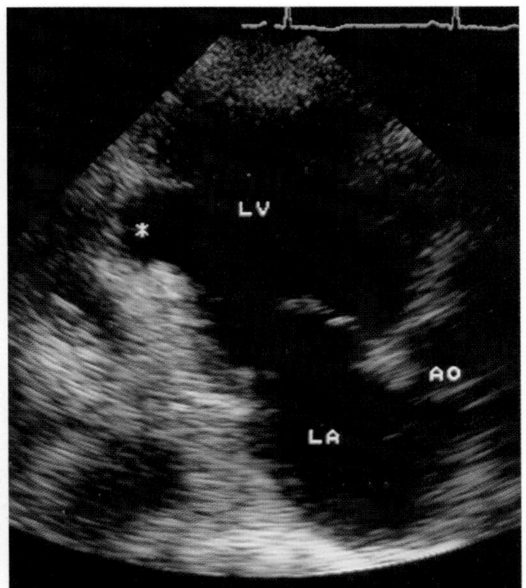

(a)

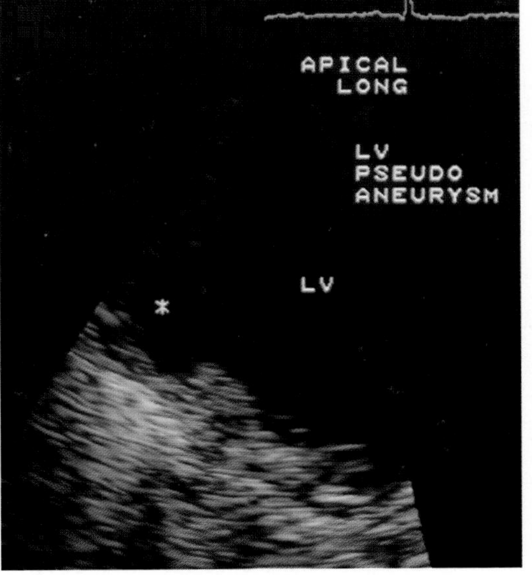

(b)

Fig. 13.15 (a,b) Apical long axis imaging demonstrates a relatively small LV pseudoaneurysm (*). (b) Close-up view of the pseudoaneurysm. The patient underwent successful multivessel coronary artery bypass surgery with resection of the pseudoaneurysm.

thrombus. However, thrombus may have a higher echodensity and may appear layered compared to fat.

Ventricular septal rupture

Ventricular septal rupture (Fig. 13.18) may occur in the setting of either anterior or inferior MI. Echo features of a ventricular septal defect include evidence of right ventricular volume overload and visualization of an irregular discontinuity of the ventricular septum. The defect is commonly associated with development of a ventricular septal aneurysm and is usually at the "hinge point" between normal and abnormal tissue. Color Doppler is helpful in demonstrating turbulent flow on the RV side of the defect (Fig. 13.19). Off-angle imaging is often necessary to best image these defects. Associated RV infarction manifested by RV segmental contraction abnormalities indicates a poor prognosis. TEE monitoring during surgical repair is helpful in assessing anatomy and evaluating for a postoperative residual shunt. A small amount of residual flow is usually present, but a large amount of flow indicates a need for reoperation.

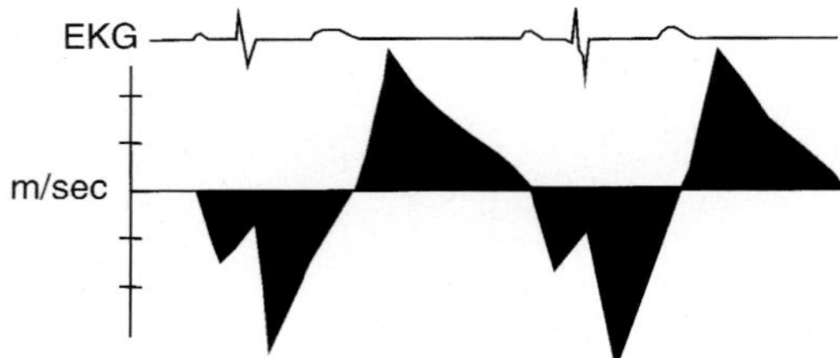

Fig. 13.16 Biphasic Doppler flow between a pseudoaneurysm and the LV. Blood flow from the LV to pseudoaneurysm occurs in presystole (atrial systole) and in early to mid systole. Pseudoaneurysm to LV flow then occurs in late systole through diastole.

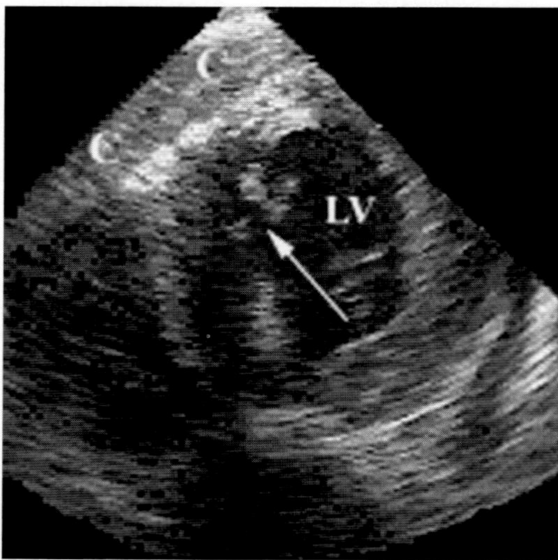

Fig. 13.17 Subacute LV free wall rupture in an elderly female. TEE near the gastro-esophageal junction, reveals rupture in the basal infero-septum (arrow). Clot (C) is noted in the pericardial space.

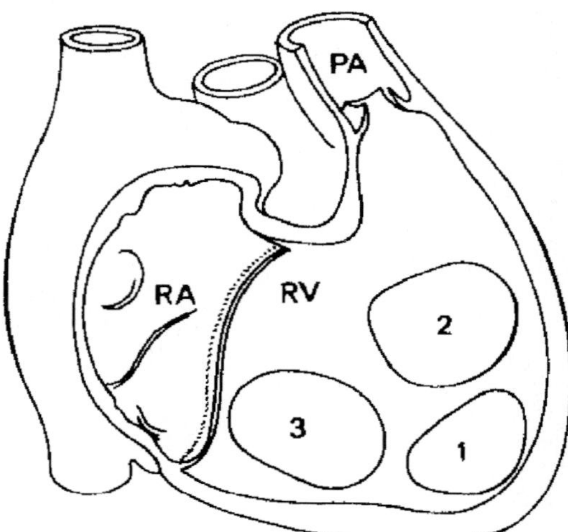

Fig. 13.18 Diagrammatic representation of the RV side of the interventricular septum. Postinfarction sites are: (1) apical defects—confined to the apical septum; (2) anterior trabecular defects—anterior and central septum; (3) posterior defects—posterior septum. PA, pulmonary artery. (Reproduced with permission from: Smyllie JH, Sutherland GR, Geuskens R, *et al.* Doppler color flow mapping in the diagnosis of ventricular septal rupture and acute mitral regurgitation after myocardial infarction. Journal of the American College of Cardiology 1990; 15: 1449–1455, figure 3.)

Acute mitral regurgitation

Acute mitral regurgitation may be due to:

• papillary dysfunction—ischemia or infarction of papillary muscles and the contiguous portion of the LV wall

• papillary tip rupture

• rupture of the trunk of the papillary muscle—less common

• rupture of chordae tendinae—rare in the setting of acute MI

• mitral annulus dilatation due to severe LV dysfunction—central regurgitant jet from abnormal coaptation

• ischemic mitral regurgitation/dynamic mitral regurgitation.

Posteromedial papillary muscle dysfunction or *rupture* (Fig. 13.20) is more common than that from the anterolateral papillary muscle, in that the former has a single blood supply and the latter has a dual arterial supply. With papillary tip or trunk rupture, a mobile mass may be seen attached to the tips of the mitral leaflets. Mitral regurgitation (see also Chapter 8) due to papillary muscle ischemia is usually associated with hypokinesis or akinesis of the adjoining segment of LV myocardium.

Ischemic mitral regurgitation results from development of LV dilatation from infarcted myocardium. The LV will assume a spherical shape (normally elliptical) and subsequently papillary muscles become apically displaced with mitral chordae "stretching." With this change in geometry, abnormal mitral leaflet apposition occurs and the coaptation point is displaced below the plane of the annulus toward the LV apex. Thus, mitral regurgitation ensues.

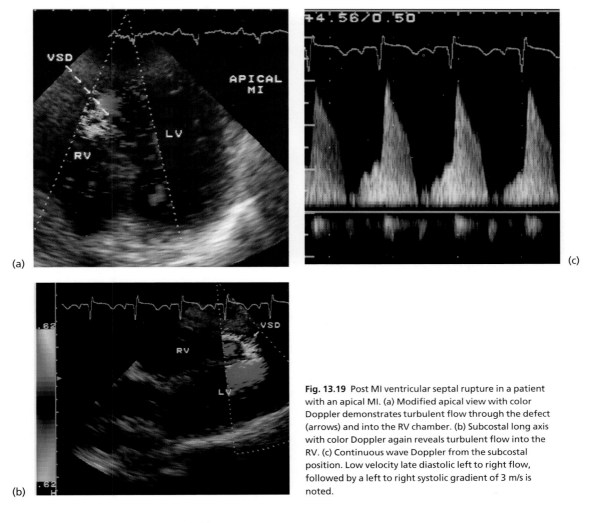

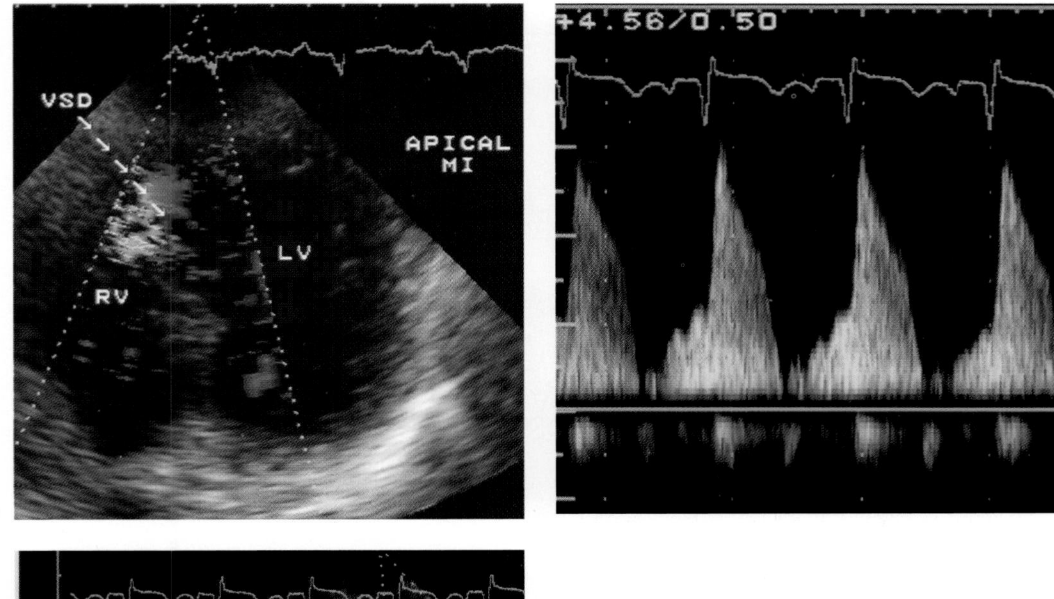

Fig. 13.19 Post MI ventricular septal rupture in a patient with an apical MI. (a) Modified apical view with color Doppler demonstrates turbulent flow through the defect (arrows) and into the RV chamber. (b) Subcostal long axis with color Doppler again reveals turbulent flow into the RV. (c) Continuous wave Doppler from the subcostal position. Low velocity late diastolic left to right flow, followed by a left to right systolic gradient of 3 m/s is noted.

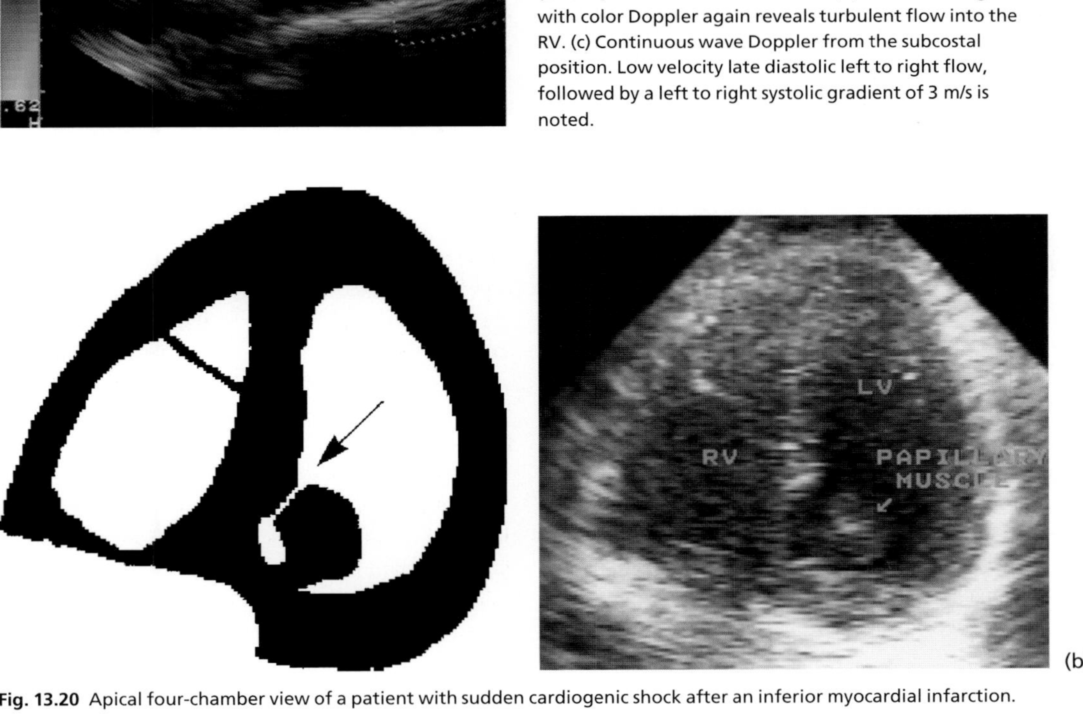

Fig. 13.20 Apical four-chamber view of a patient with sudden cardiogenic shock after an inferior myocardial infarction. Rupture of the papillary muscle trunk is evident (arrow).

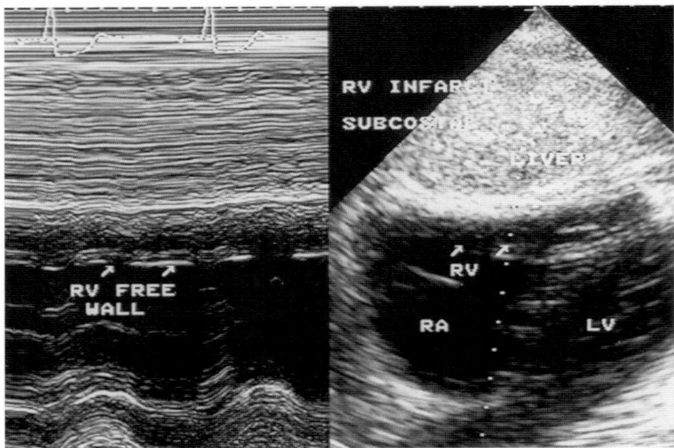

Fig. 13.21 A patient with an inferior myocardial infarction and RV involvement. Subcostal image with M-mode demonstrating an akinetic RV free wall (arrows). Note that the RV in this patient is not dilated.

Dynamic mitral regurgitation occurs when acute transient ischemia develops at "distant" segments resulting in subsequent acute LV geometry dilatation. As with ischemic MR, the papillary muscles are relatively apically displaced with subsequent stretched chordae. The mitral coaptation point is then displaced toward the apex resulting in regurgitation. The larger the LV is at rest, the more likely dynamic MR will occur with ischemia. Patients with dynamic MR with acute ischemic events tend to describe more dyspnea that chest pain.

Right ventricular infarction

When *right ventricular infarction* occurs, it is most commonly associated with an inferior myocardial infarction (IMI) and involvement of the inferior septum. The extent of RV wall motion contraction abnormalities (see Fig. 9.2) correlates with hemodynamic abnormalities. Echocardiographic features (Fig. 13.21) of RV infarction include:

- RV segmental wall motion abnormalities
- RV dilatation—not always found
- tricuspid papillary muscle dysfunction with resultant tricuspid regurgitation (TR)
- paradoxical ventricular septal motion—may occur with significant TR
- RV thrombus formation—easy to miss unless multiple RV echo views are used
- ventricular septal rupture—poor prognosis when RV infarction coincides
- abnormal IVC hemodynamics indicating an elevated RV end-diastolic pressure.

CHAPTER 14

Critical Care

Transesophageal echocardiogarphy (TEE) may be extremely helpful in the critical care situation (see also Chapter 4). Common indications for performing TEE in this setting include evaluation of the following:

- aortic dissection or transection (see Chapter 19)
- hemodynamic instability
- unexplained shock
- unexplained hypoxemia
- "ruling out" cardiac contusion—with unstable hemodynamics, donor heart
- possible tamponade, particularly "localized" tamponade following surgery (see Chapter 12)
- myocardial infarction complications (see Chapter 13)
- source of embolism (see Chapter 17)
- endocarditis complications (see Chapter 18)
- identifying complications of procedures (Figs 14.1 & 12.14)
- documenting placement of devices (Fig. 14.2).

Unexplained hemodynamics/hypotension

Unexplained unstable hemodynamics are a common indication for TEE in the critical care situation. Often the transthoracic echo is limited due to a poor acoustic window, especially in patients on mechanical ventilators. Both transthoracic echo and TEE may be used to obtain the following hemodynamic information:

- estimation of RA pressures—hepatic veins, IVC
- calculation of PA pressures
- evaluation of LV systolic function
- assessment of ventricular preload
- assessment of tamponade physiology
- evaluation of valvular function.

With positive pressure ventilation (PEEP) the jugular venous pressure may be increased even with normal intravascular volumes. LV preload may be reduced secondary to a reduced RV venous return.

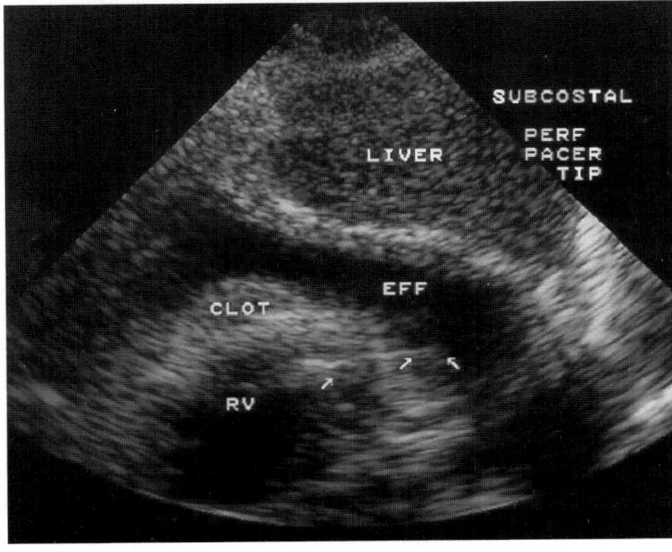

(a)

Fig. 14.1 Subcostal imaging of a patient who developed sudden hypotension during placement of a pacemaker. In these three views a pericardial effusion with clot is noted. The pacer tip appears to be within the pericardial space. (*Continued on p. 220.*)

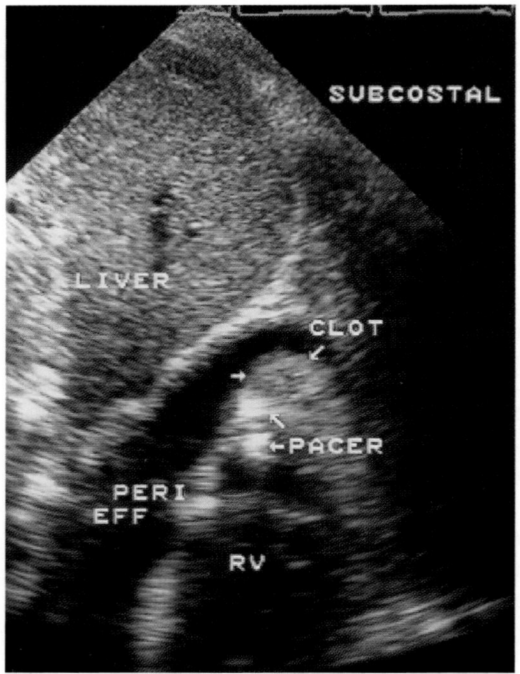

(b)

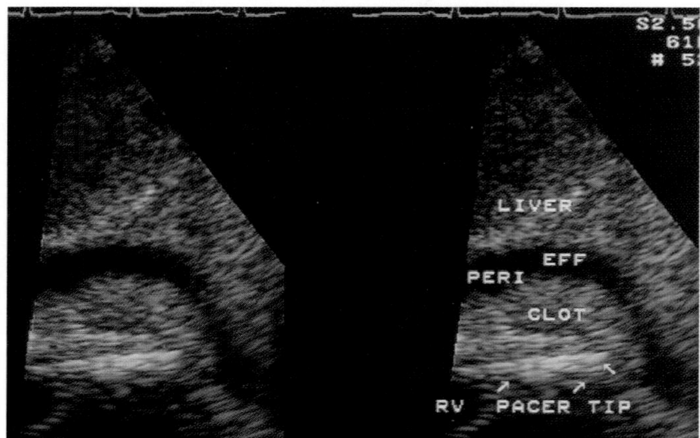

(c)

Fig. 14.1 (*cont'd*)

Right-to-left shunting and the platypnea–orthodeoxia syndrome

The *platypnea–orthodeoxia syndrome* describes both dyspnea (platypnea) and arterial desaturation in the upright position with improvement in the supine position (orthodeoxia). This occurs with an intracardiac or intrapulmonary shunt and often with some form of lung disease. The postpneumonectomy patient (particularly having the right lung removed) may develop symptoms many months after the surgical procedure. A ventilation-perfusion lung scan may reveal systemic uptake of isotope. Patent foramen ovale (PFO) diagnosis has been made with a tilt table and saline contrast using both transthoracic echocardiography (TTE) and TEE. A typical history with a significant drop in oxygen saturations while in the upright position, along with a large PFO found as the only source of a shunt, has been considered diagnostic.

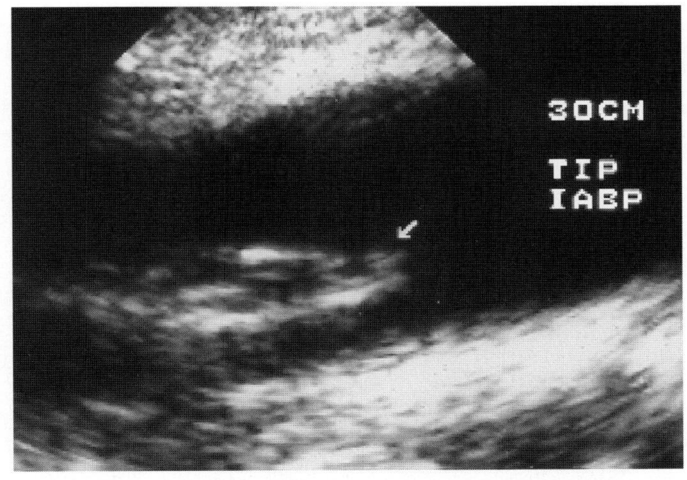

(a)

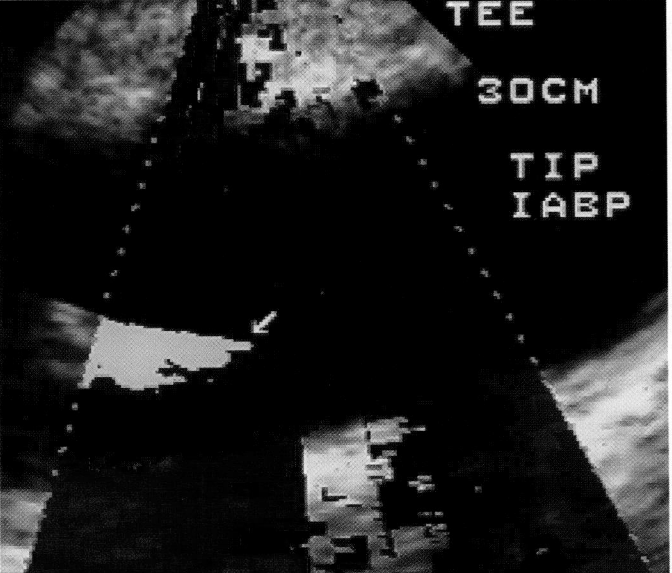

(b)

Fig. 14.2 Transesophageal echocardiography (TEE) (a) in the longitudinal view and (b) with tissue Doppler imaging documenting placement of an intra-aortic balloon pump just distal to the left subclavian artery. TEE was being performed to help characterize a patient's unstable hemodynamics.

Shunting from right to left may also occur at the pulmonary level. When associated with liver disease (seen in up of cases 30% in hepatic cirrhosis), it is termed the *hepatopulmonary syndrome.* Agitated saline contrast will appear in the left atrium (LA) when injected in a peripheral vein. Appearance of contrast within the LA will usually occur after at least three cardiac cycles from its appearance in the right atrium (RA).

Pulmonary arteriovenous shunts associated with certain congenital disorders and/or their therapies have been detected. Multiple pulmonary arteriovenous shunts may develop in patients in whom flow from the liver bypasses a segment of lung. An interesting example of this is when there is placement of a surgical shunt from the SVC directly into the right pulmonary artery with proximal ligation of the right pulmonary artery. The left pulmonary artery receives mixed venous blood from the right ventricle. It has been postulated that the absence of IVC (e.g. liver) flow into the right pulmonary artery territory may be causally related to the subsequent development of the multiple pulmonary venous shunts detectable by saline contrast imaging.

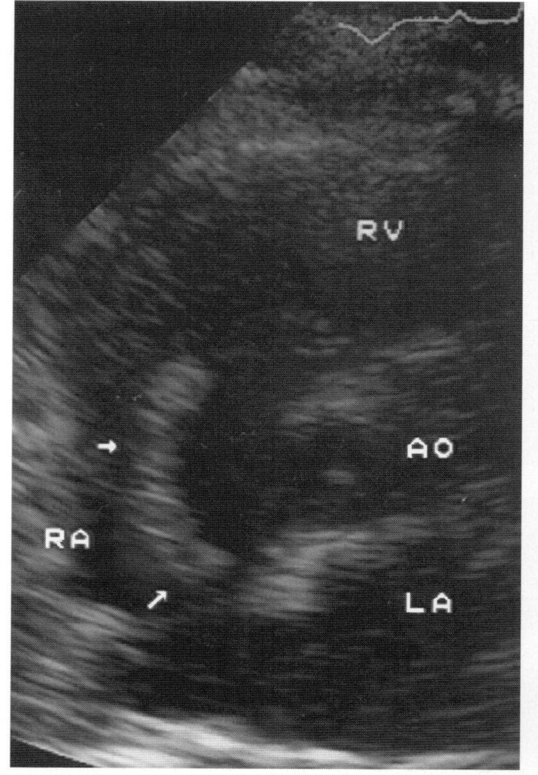

(a)

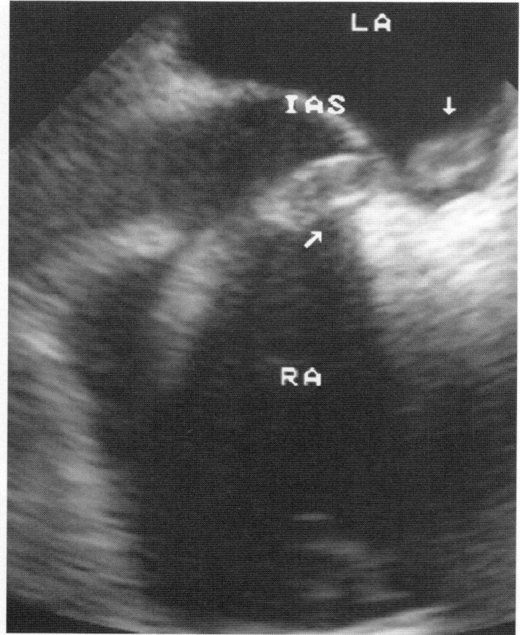

(b)

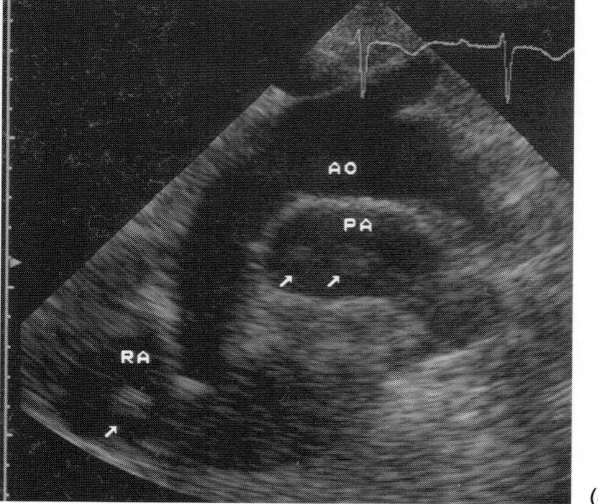

(c)

Fig. 14.3 Venous embolism from the lower extremities. (a) Parasternal short axis demonstrating a long thrombus "cast" of a lower extremity vein within the RA (arrows) extending into the RV. In real time it appeared "fixed" to the atrial septum and (b) TEE imaging at 75° demonstrates the clot to be "jammed" in a PFO (arrows). (c) Suprasternal thoracic imaging demonstrates a faint clot in the right pulmonary artery (PA, arrows). The RA clot was again seen in this view (single arrow).

Pulmonary embolism

Thrombi within the right heart or proximal pulmonary arterial vessels (main pulmonary artery and most of right pulmonary artery but rarely past 2 cm of proximal left pulmonary artery) may be directly visualized by TTE or TEE (Fig. 14.3). *Right heart thrombi* originating in the lower extremities usually appear as mobile "casts" of the veins swirling with the heart chambers. These "emboli in transit" have a characteristic serpentiginous motion (note that *intravenous leiomyomatosis* may have a similar mobile serpentiginous appearance within the right atrium). Thrombi originating in the lower extremities are the presumed etiology of *paradoxical arterial embolism* in patients with arterial embolic events and a PFO (see Chapter 17). In patients with a major pulmonary embolism, detection of a PFO may be a predictor of arterial embolic events and of an increased risk of death.

If right ventricular hypertrophy (RVH) and high pulmonary artery pressures are present in a patient with an *acute pulmonary embolism*, a coexistent pulmonary problem should be considered. If right-sided chamber dilatation, RV systolic dysfunction, and a small LV chamber size (due to diminished LV preload) are present, one should suspect acute pulmonary embolism.

The hemodynamic severity of pulmonary emboli may be detected by the Doppler findings:

- "minor"—normal mean pulmonary artery (PA) pressures
- acute massive—≥20 mmHg mean PA pressure
- subacute massive—≥40 mmHg mean PA pressure, >70 mmHg systolic PA pressure.

RV dilatation and RV wall motion abnormalities have been found in most patients with acute and subacute massive pulmonary emboli, but generally not in those with a minor embolic event (Figs 14.4 & 14.5).

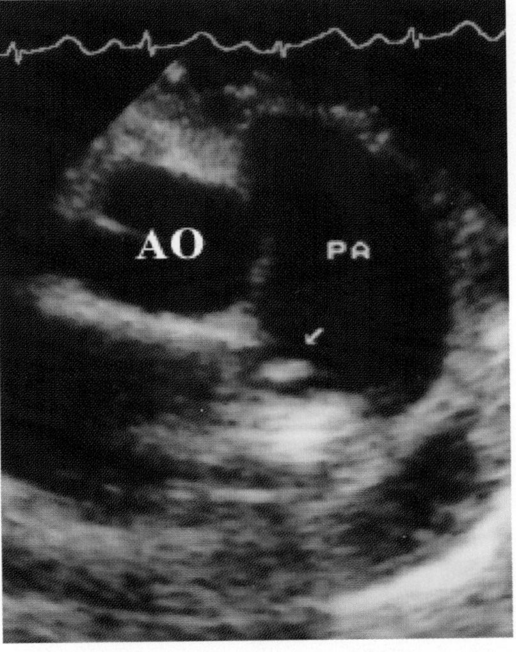

(a)

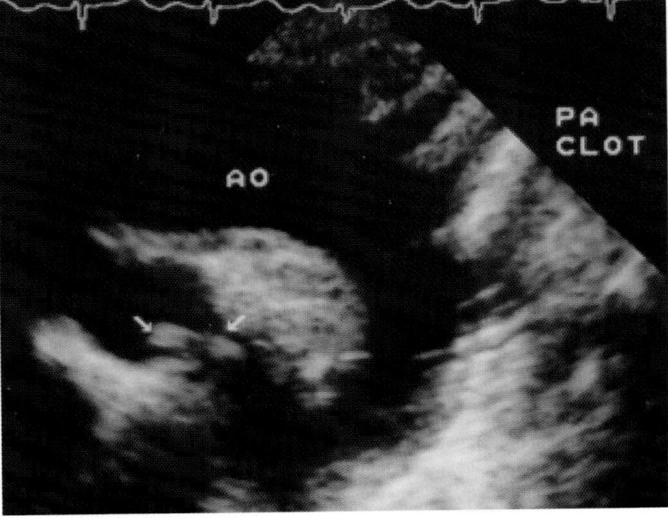

(b)

Fig. 14.4 A 20-year-old-female who at 2 days after a caesarean section developed unstable hemodynamics. By transthoracic echocardiography, a mobile clot was noted attached near the origin of the right pulmonary artery. (a) High parasternal short axis view demonstrates the clot (arrow). The proximal ascending aorta (AO) is noted. (b) (c) Suprasternal imaging with tissue Doppler imaging highlights the mobility of the clot. (*Continued on p. 223.*)

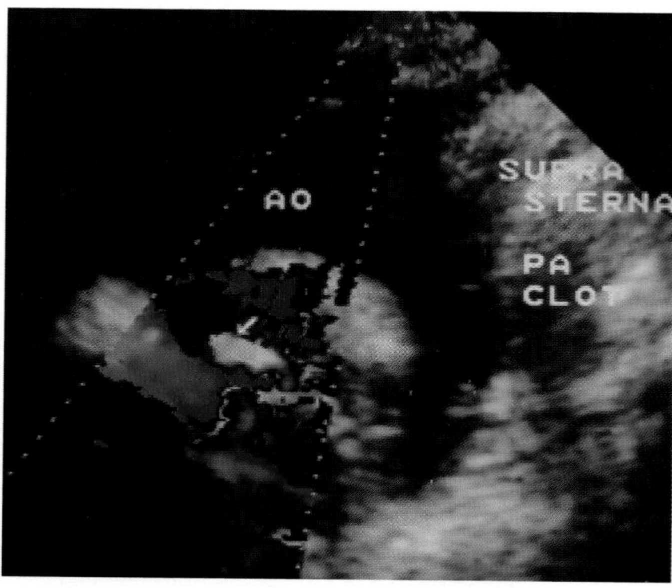

(c) Fig. 14.4 (*cont'd*)

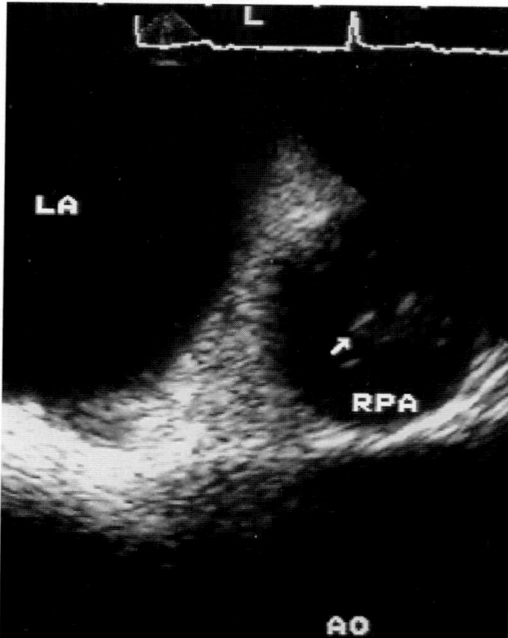

Fig. 14.5 A TEE was performed as part of a work up to look for the etiology of a patient's progressive exertional dyspnea and dilated right heart. The purpose of the TEE was to look for a suspected atrial septal defect. During evaluation an "echo-soft" mass (arrow) was noted within the right pulmonary artery (RPA). Subsequent evaluation documented chronic pulmonary emboli.

Blunt trauma to the heart and great vessels

Blunt chest injury (often from a steering wheel injury or from a fall from a height) may commonly result in:

- myocardial contusion
- traumatic ventricular septal defect (VSD)
- tricuspid/mitral valve trauma
- aorta—hematoma, intimal tear, transection (Fig. 14.6).

Deceleration may result in an injured thoracic artery despite lack of external evidence of chest trauma. If a patient has first or second rib fractures, thoracic spine fractures, or an abnormal chest X-ray manifesting an abnormal mediastinum or blurred aortic knob, aortic trauma should be considered. *Traumatic disruption of the thoracic aorta* (*TDA*) may generally occur *anywhere the aorta is "attached."* It is located in the *aortic isthmus* in ~90% of cases (2–3 cm past the left subclavian artery origin). The aortic arch is connected to the thorax by the ligamentum arteriosum at that location. The second most common location of aortic tear is the *ascending aorta*. Disruption of the middle of the descending thoracic aorta is rarely found, but may be associated with marked hyperextension of the thoracic vertebra. The *diaphragm level* may also be a site of injury.

Patients may be subgrouped by type of traumatic

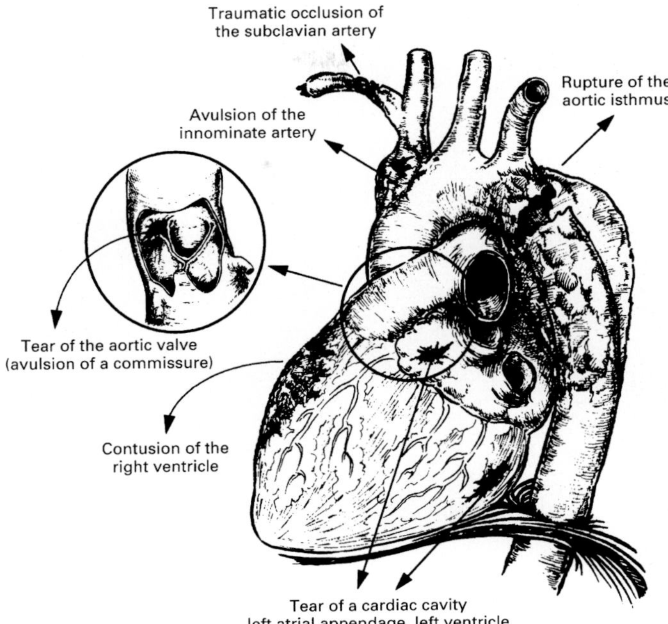

Fig. 14.6 Blunt chest trauma most commonly will affect the heart and great vessels, as illustrated. (Reproduced with permission from: Pretre R, Chilcott M. Blunt trauma to the heart and great vessels. New England Journal of Medicine 1997; 336(9): 626–632.)

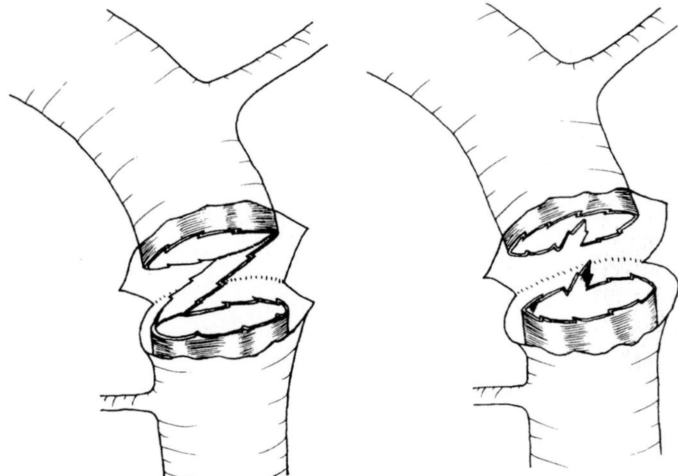

Fig. 14.7 An image of a subtotal disruption of the aortic isthmus in a spiral tear pattern (left) and a complete disruption (right). (Reproduced with permission from: Vignon P, Gueret P, Vedrinne JM, *et al.* Role of transesophageal echocardiography in the diagnosis and management of traumatic aortic disruption. Circulation 1995; 92: 2959–2969.)

aortic injury: (i) *subadventitial TDA* and (ii) *traumatic intimal tears*. Patients with subadventitial TDA should have immediate surgical repair, whereas many of these patients with intimal tears are treated conservatively. *Mediastinal hematoma* may be found in conjunction with aortic trauma (see Chapter 19).

Subadventitial TDA involves the aortic intima and medial layers, thus there is a risk of adventitial rupture. They may be clinically subcategorized as:

1a *Subtotal subadventitial aortic disruption*—disruption of more than two thirds of the aortic circumference, usually in a spiral pattern in the posterior aorta (Fig. 14.7 left).

1b *Complete subadventitial aortic disruption*—disruption of the entire aortic circumference (Fig. 14.7 right).

1c *Partial subadventitial aortic disruption*—limited discontinuity of both the intimal and medial layers, either with or without pseudoaneurysm development.

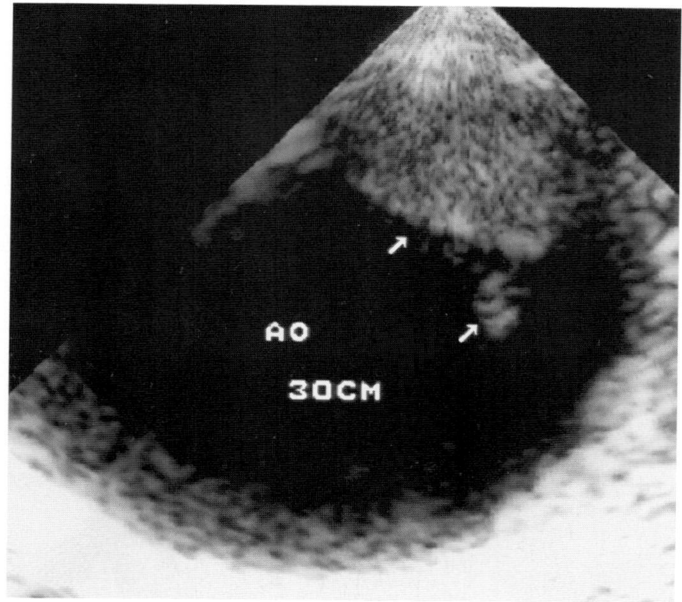

(a)

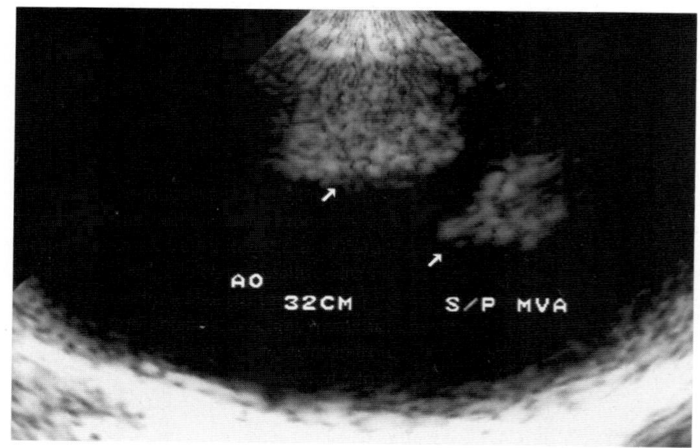

(b)

Fig. 14.8 (a,b) A 24-year-old male was an unrestrained driver and drove his vehicle into a ditch. The steering wheel was bent. Intimal tears are noted in the proximal descending aorta by TEE (arrows). The membrane was noted to be "thin" in real time, and there was no turbulence by color flow Doppler. Aortography and CT of the chest were "normal." A repeat study 1 week later was unchanged, but 5 weeks after the initial study revealed intimal healing.

A *traumatic intimal tear* by definition involves only the intima. It appears as a *thin, mobile* structure, usually near the aortic isthmus (Figs 14.8 & 14.11B). Color flow Doppler will generally *not show any flow turbulence*. Often, aortography will be normal.

With subadventitial TDA, color Doppler appears to be the same on both sides of the media, and usually has an area of flow turbulence (with aortic dissection there are two distinct flow channels). A *subtotal subadventitial aortic disruption* reveals a *thick* membrane (termed "medial flap") across the aorta lumen (as opposed to a thin mobile membrane usually nearly perpendicular to the isthmus wall seen in traumatic intimal tears and acute aortic dissection). *Color flow turbulence* will probably be seen (Fig. 14.9).

A *complete subadventitial aortic disruption* will appear as a thick "open circle" within the aortic lumen. The medial flap will move with each cardiac cycle, and color turbulence will be noted on both sides of the medial flap (Fig. 14.10). In distinction to this, with aortic dissection, the "open circle" is a thin intimal membrane, not very mobile, and has most flow noted only in the true lumen.

Partial subadventitial disruption appears as a discontinuity of the intimal and medial layers with no intraluminal medial flap evident (Fig. 14.11 left).

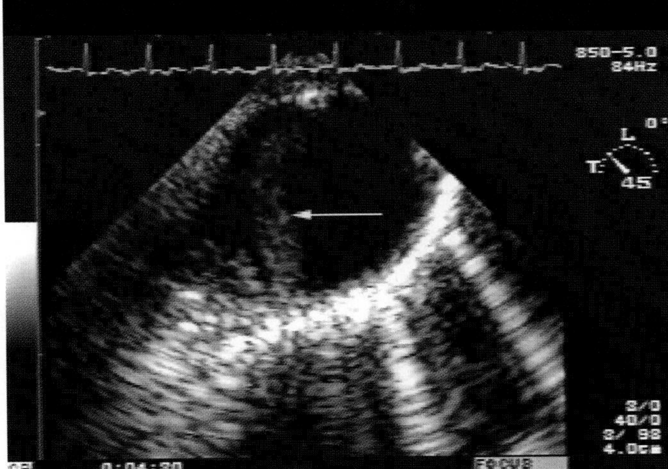

Fig. 14.9 A young man fell from a height of 15 feet (4.5 m) onto his head, upon a barge on the Mississippi River. TEE revealed a "thick" medial flap, localized to the area of the aortic isthmus. In addition, color flow Doppler revealed localized turbulent flow. At surgery a localized pseudoaneurysm was also found.

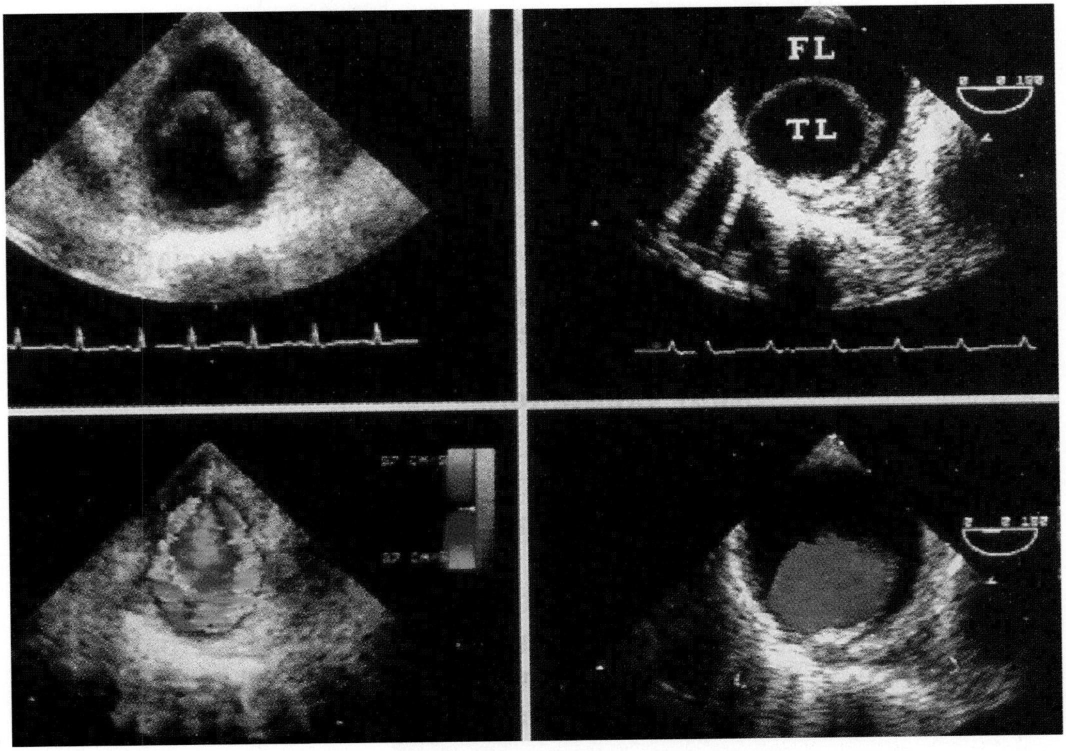

Fig. 14.10 (a) Complete subadventitial aortic disruption is manifested by a thick, mobile circular medial flap, with (c) color flow/turbulence on both sides of the flap. In distinction, an acute aortic dissection (b) will have a thin, immobile flap, with (d) different flow patterns in each lumen. (Reproduced with permission from: Vignon P, Gueret P, Vedrinne JM, *et al*. Role of transesophageal echocardiography in the diagnosis and management of traumatic aortic disruption. Circulation 1995; 92: 2959–2969.)

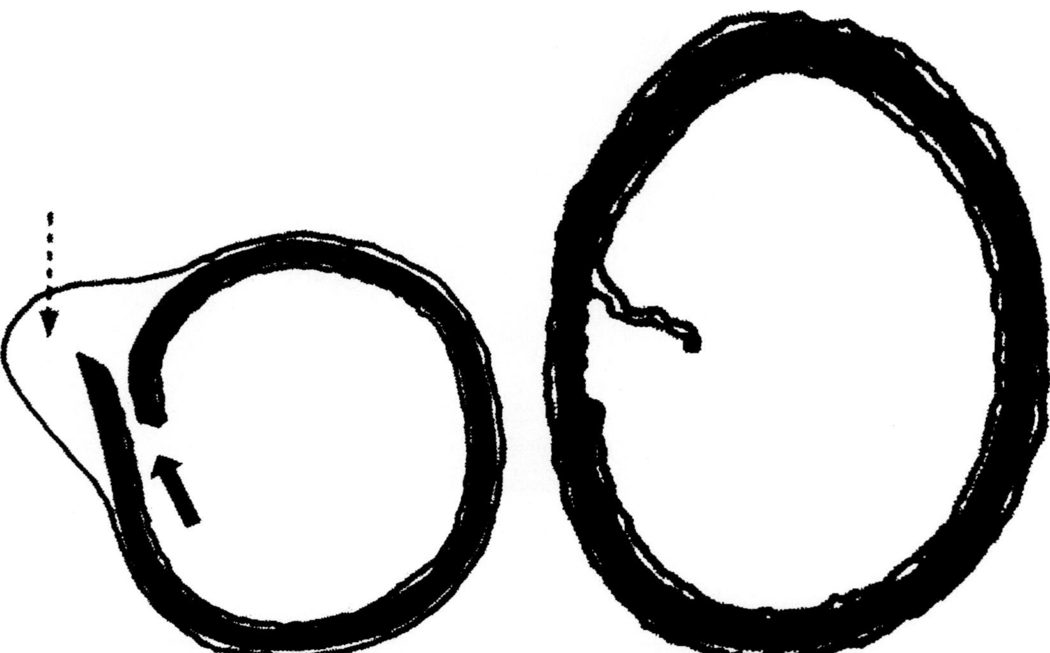

Fig. 14.11 (Left) Partial subadventitial disruption of the aortic isthmus. The entire intima and media are involved. If a pseudoaneurysm is formed, color flow Doppler may reveal turbulent flow at that site. (Right) Traumatic intimal tear. The media remains intact. Usually there is *no turbulent flow* noted by color flow Doppler. (Reproduced with permission from: Vignon P, Gueret P, Vedrinne JM, *et al*. Role of transesophageal echocardiography in the diagnosis and management of traumatic aortic disruption. Circulation 1995; 92: 2959–2969, figure 6.8.)

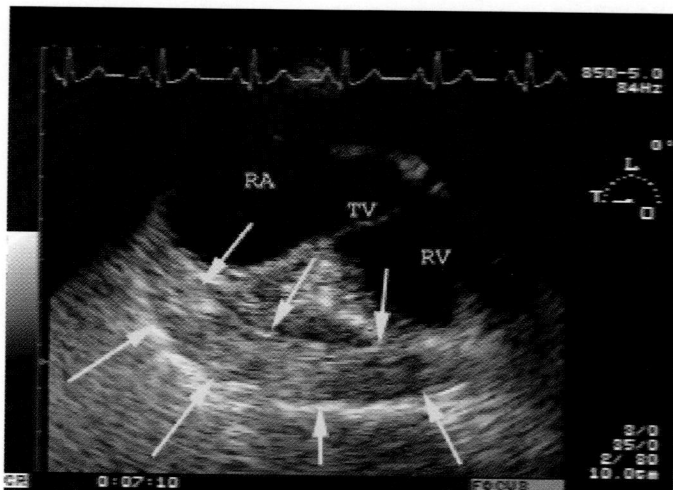

Fig. 14.12 A 32-year-old male fell out of a helicopter from 25 feet (7.5 m) above a platform on an oilrig, landing upon his chest. TEE and CT scan of the chest revealed a hematoma between the sternum and anterior portion of the pericardium. With real-time imaging the hematoma remained motionless, independent of cardiac motion. The patient's hemodynamics remained stable, and the next day he left the hospital against medical advice.

Table 14.1 Differential findings by TEE to distinguish traumatic subadventitial aortic disruption from that of aortic dissection. (Reproduced with permission from: Vignon P, Lang RM. Use of transesophageal echocardiography for the assessment of traumatic aortic injuries. Echocardiography 1999: 16(2): 211).

	Aortic disruption: presence of a disrupted wall traversing the aortic lumen	*Aortic dissection: presence of two distinct aortic channels separated by a flap*
2-D echocardiography		
Transverse view	Thick and mobile "medial flap"	Thin and less mobile "intimal flap"
	Abnormal aortic contour (false aneurysm formation)	Normal aortic contour
	Normal/increased aortic size	Enlarged aorta
	Presence of hemomediastinum	Absence of hemomediastinum
	No entry/re-entry tear or thrombus	Entry/re-entry tear, thrombus in the false channel
Longitudinal view	"Medial flap" traversing the aortic lumen perpendicular to isthmus wall	"Intimal flap" parallel to the aortic wall
Color Doppler mapping	Similar blood flow velocities on both sides of the "medial flap"	Different blood flow velocities (slower velocities in the false lumen)
	Mosaic of colors surrounding the disrupted wall (blood flow turbulence)	No mosaic of colors at the vicinity of the "intimal flap" (near laminar flow)
Location of TEE signs	Confined to the aortic isthmus (25–35 cm from incisors)	More extended, according to anatomic type

Color flow Doppler may reveal turbulent flow entering a pseudoaneurysm. Small disruptions may be missed using ultrasound techniques.

The differential of TEE diagnostic criteria to distinguish aortic disruption from acute aortic dissection is given in Table 14.1.

With deceleration injury one should also consider trauma to the cardiac structures (Figs 14.6 & 14.12), including the tricuspid and mitral valves, ventricular septum, pulmonary veins, and left atrial appendage.

15

CHAPTER 15

Operating Room

Intraoperative transesophageal echocardiography (TEE) serves mostly as a monitoring device for the anesthesiologist and as a diagnostic tool for the surgeon and cardiologist. As the anesthesiologist is responsible for hemodynamic monitoring and the airway, the TEE probe is usually placed by the anesthesiologist. TEE is used during both noncardiac and cardiac surgical procedures.

Noncardiac surgery

Generally, for *noncardiac surgery* TEE has been used to assess for:

- LV ischemia
- LV function (systolic and diastolic)
- hemodynamics
- air embolism.

The LV chamber has been divided into a 16-segment model by the ASE/SCA Guidelines (Fig. 15.1). Typical coronary territories of the LV are illustrated (Figs 15.2 & 15.3). With development of ischemia, abnormalities of wall motion and thickening will appear. Systolic wall thickening is generally related to hypokinesis, as shown in Table 15.1.

These changes occur before the onset of ECG changes. A *transgastric transverse view at the papillary level* is often used to monitor all three coronary territories during surgical procedures. Often hemodynamics will not change with the development of intraoperative ischemia. Patients undergoing vascular operations or other high risk procedures are typically monitored during surgery for the development of intraoperative ischemia.

Global LV function may be estimated using the end-diastolic volume (area) for preload and the end-systolic volume (area) for afterload. The measure that seems to be of high clinical value to the anesthesiologist is the ejection fraction estimation based upon a transgastric horizontal plane view (mid short axis view in Fig. 15.2). Hemodynamics routinely obtained include mitral and pulmonary vein flow (see Chapter 6). *Stroke volume* may be obtained using the mitral or pulmonary artery time velocity integral (see Chapters 3 & 5). When measuring the mitral orifice, one should measure the diameter in both the four- and two-chamber views. The equation for area (Ar) will then be:

$$Ar = \pi\left(\frac{D_a}{2}\right)\left(\frac{D_b}{2}\right)$$

where D_a is the diameter in the four-chamber view and D_b is the diameter in the two-chamber view. A high esophageal horizontal plane will generally provide a good position to obtain pulmonary artery flow and diameter measurements.

Air embolism may be problematic during neurosurgical and craniofacial procedures performed in the sitting position. Air becomes entrapped in noncollapsible cerebral venous sinuses and will travel from the SVC to the RA. From the RA, air may pass through a patent foramen ovale (PFO) or other shunt (cardiac or pulmonary), leading to air cerebral embolism. Significant air embolism into the right ventricular outflow tract (RVOT) may cause obstruction with an increase in RA pressure and marked right-to-left

Table 15.1 Relationship of systolic wall thickening to systolic motion.

Systolic motion	*Systolic thickening*
Normal	30–50%
Mild hypokinesis	10–30%
Severe hypokinesis	<10%
Akinesis	None
Dyskinesis	Thinning or bulging

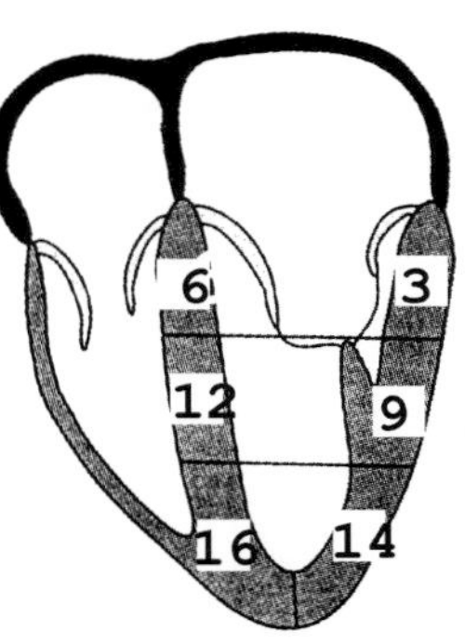

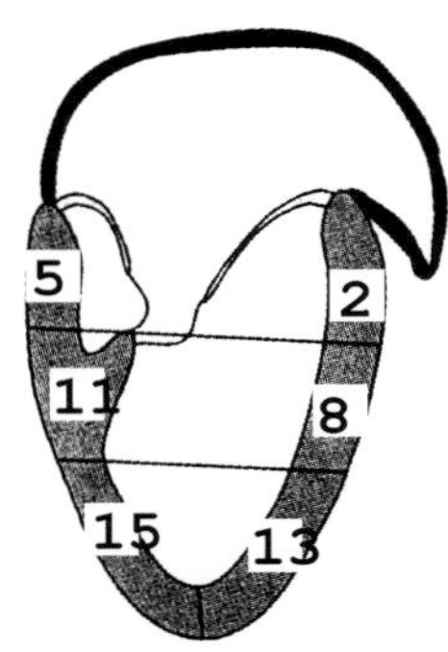

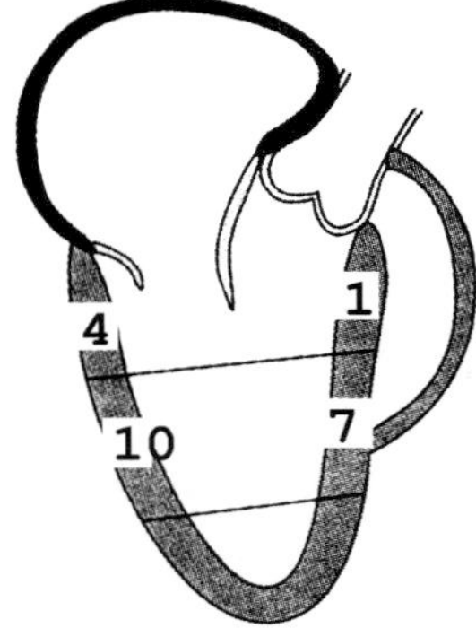

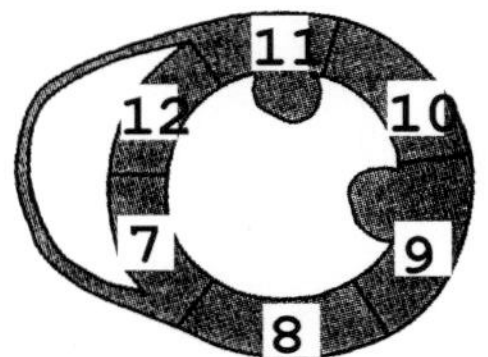

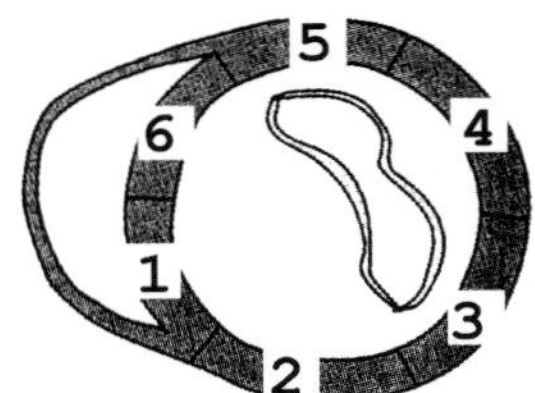

Fig. 15.1 Sixteen LV segments by transesophageal echocardiography (TEE), as recommended by the ASE/SCA Guidelines. Basal segments: 1, anteroseptal; 2, anterior; 3, lateral; 4, posterior; 5, inferior; 6, septal. Mid segments; 7, anteroseptal; 8, anterior; 9, lateral; 10, posterior; 11, inferior; 12, septal. Apical segments: 13, anterior; 14, lateral; 15, inferior; 16, septal. (Modified with permission from: ASE/SCA Guidelines for Performing a Comprehensive Intraoperative Multiplane Transesophageal Echocardiography Examination. Recommendations of the American Society of Echocardiography Council for Intraoperative Echocardiography and the Society of Cardiovascular Anesthesiologists Task Force for Certification in Perioperative Transesophageal Echocardiography. Journal of the American Society of Echocardiography 1999; 12(10): 884–900, figure 4.)

shunting through a PFO. It seems advisable to avoid this type of surgery if possible in a patient found preoperatively to have a significant PFO.

Cardiac surgery

There are several applications for intraoperative echocardiography (mostly TEE) during cardiac surgery, in addition to assessment of hemodynamics and for ischemia. The advantage of TEE over epicardial echocardiography is that the probe is located away from the operative field and may be left in place during the entire surgical procedure. *Epicardial echocardiography*, however, has been used in certain intraoperative settings, including:

- evaluation of the RVOT and anterior heart
- evaluation of hypertrophic cardiomyopathy
- assessment of atherosclerotic plaque in the ascending aorta for cross-clamping the aorta and/or for placement of vein grafts (TEE may have a blind spot in the upper ascending aorta).

Mitral valve repair

The mitral valve (see also Chapters 4 & 8) is evaluated from the mid-esophagus and from the transgastric views (Fig. 15.4). The anterior leaflet is composed of the lateral, mid and medial segments and the posterior leaflet is composed of the lateral, middle and medial scallops.

Functional surgical echocardiographic criteria (as described by Carpentier) classify regurgitation (MR) by leaflet mobility—normal, excessive, or restrictive (Fig. 15.5). Normally, the coaptation point of the valve leaflets is on the ventricular side of the mitral annulus.

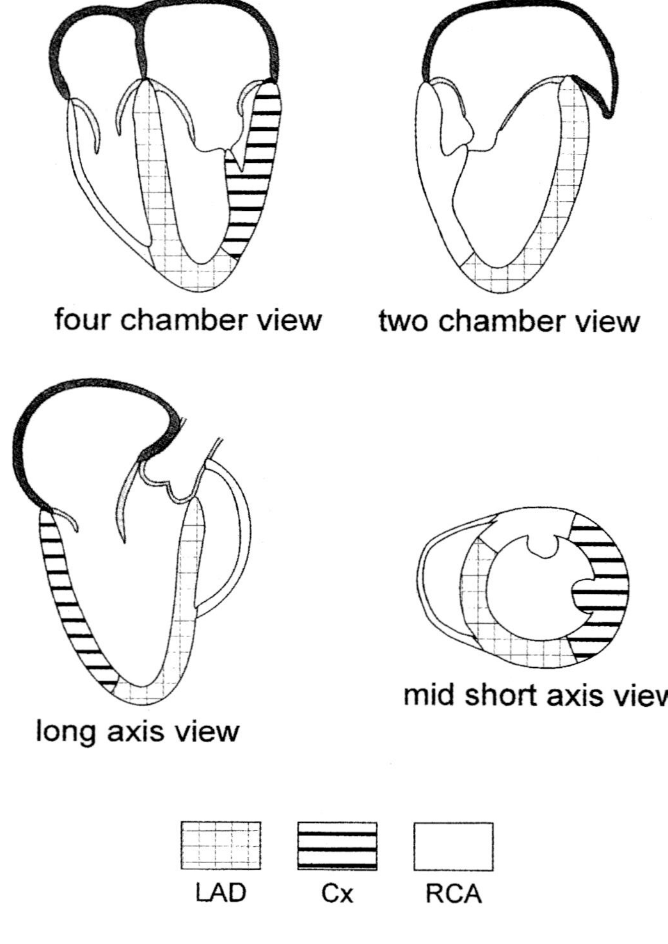

Fig. 15.2 Regions of myocardium perfused by the LV major coronary arteries. LAD, left anterior descending; Cx, circumflex; RCA, right coronary artery. (Reproduced with permission from: ASE/SCA Guidelines for Performing a Comprehensive Intraoperative Multiplane Transesophageal Echocardiography Examination. Recommendations of the American Society of Echocardiography Council for Intraoperative Echocardiography and the Society of Cardiovascular Anesthesiologists Task Force for Certification in Perioperative Transesophageal Echocardiography. Journal of the American Society of Echocardiography 1999; 12(10): 884–900 figure 5.)

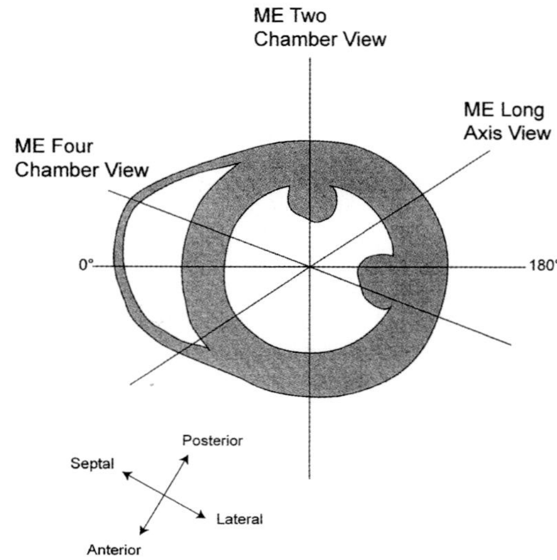

Fig. 15.3 Short axis of the LV (mid short axis view in Fig. 15.2) demonstrates the transection of the LV from the mid-esophageal (ME) TEE views. (Reproduced with permission from: ASE/SCA Guidelines for Performing a Comprehensive Intraoperative Multiplane Transesophageal Echocardiography Examination. Recommendations of the American Society of Echocardiography Council for Intraoperative Echocardiography and the Society of Cardiovascular Anesthesiologists Task Force for Certification in Perioperative Transesophageal Echocardiography. Journal of the American Society of Echocardiography 1999; 12(10): 884–900, figure 6.)

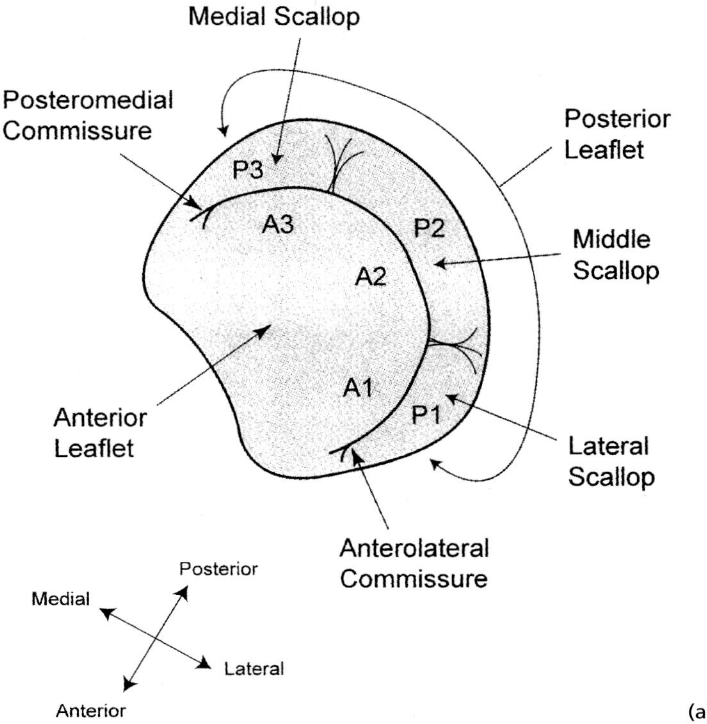

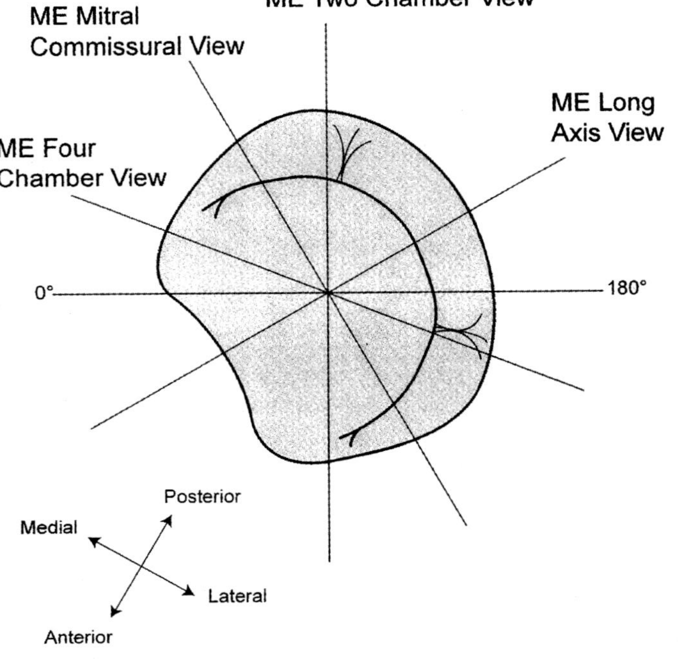

Fig. 15.4 (a) Anatomy of the mitral valve as viewed from the horizontal plane at the gastro-esophageal junction. (b) Transections through the mitral valve as viewed from the mid-esophageal (ME) views. A1, lateral third of the anterior leaflet; A2, middle third of the anterior leaflet; A3, medial third of the anterior leaflet; P1, lateral scallop of the posterior leaflet; P2, middle scallop of the posterior leaflet; P3, medial scallop of the posterior leaflet. (Reproduced with permission from: ASE/SCA Guidelines for Performing a Comprehensive Intraoperative Multiplane Transesophageal Echocardiography Examination. Recommendations of the American Society of Echocardiography Council for Intraoperative Echocardiography and the Society of Cardiovascular Anesthesiologists Task Force for Certification in Perioperative Transesophageal Echocardiography. Journal of the American Society of Echocardiography 1999; 12(10): 884–900, figure 7.8.)

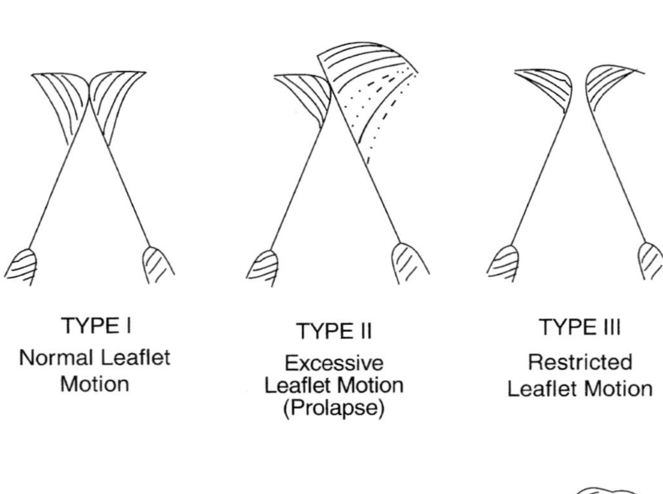

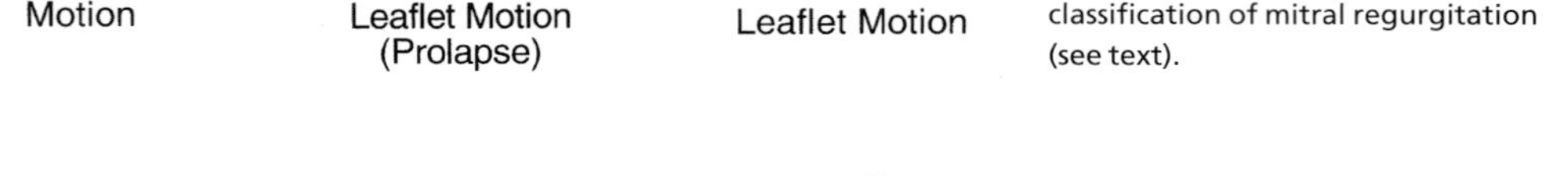

Fig. 15.5 Carpentier functional surgical classification of mitral regurgitation (see text).

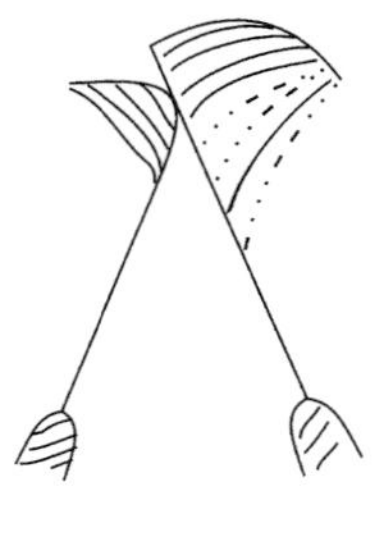

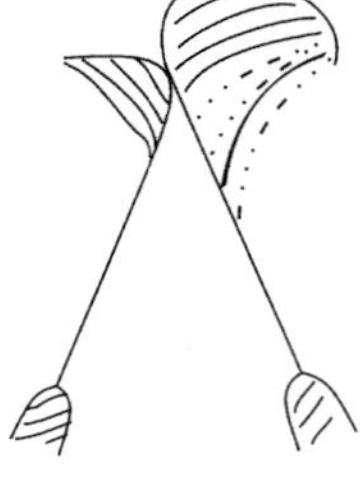

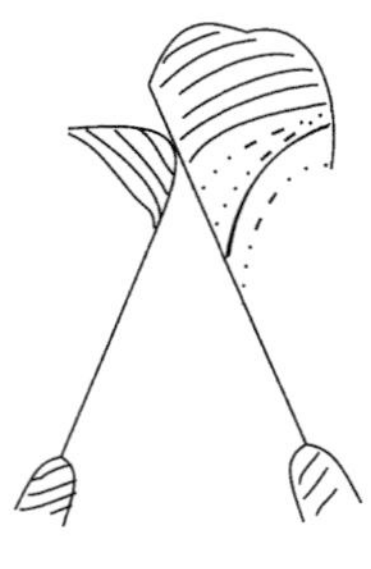

Fig. 15.6 Barlow's description of *prolapse* (one leaflet overrides another) and *billowing* (protrusion of tissue into the LA but free edges are in apposition).

Type I—normal leaflet motion:
- mitral annular dilatation (most common)
- leaflet perforation
- cleft valve.

Type II—excessive leaflet motion:
- rupture or elongation of chordae or papillary muscle.

Type III—restricted leaflet motion:
- fusion of leaflets or subvalvular structures
- congenital parachute valve.

The Carpentier surgical definition of leaflet prolapse (Type II) is present when one leaflet overrides the edge of the other above the mitral annulus plane. The "*billowing valve*" (Fig. 15.6) describes excessive systolic leaflet tissue protruding into the left atrium. The free edges of the leaflets remain in apposition below the mitral valve plane.

Functional echocardiographic classification is necessary when evaluating the mitral valve preoperatively for a mitral valve repair procedure. Preoperative TEE is important to determine the etiology of MR for the proper surgical repair procedure to be performed (Fig. 15.7).

It is important to identify which sections of leaflets are involved (Fig. 15.4). The middle scallop of the posterior leaflet is involved in about 75% of posterior leaflet repairs. From the *horizontal plane in the mid-esophagus*, the left ventricular outflow tract (LVOT) view (visualize the LA, LV, and LVOT) will generally view A1/A2 and P1/P2, whereas the four-chamber view will view A2/A3 and P2/P3. A *long axis view* (120–135°) will image A2 and P2 (this is an excellent view of the posterior middle scallop) (Fig. 15.8). A short axis view of the mitral valve (Fig. 15.4) may be obtained in the horizontal plane near the gastro-esophageal junction. This view is useful not only to identify the part of the leaflet that is abnormal, but also with color flow Doppler it will help to localize the site of origin of MR.

The "easiest" valve for repair is a flail posterior leaflet with ruptured chordae to one of its scallops (Fig. 15.9). A flail anterior leaflet is more difficult (Fig. 15.10), and a rheumatic valve even more difficult. Heavy calcification within the posterior mitral annulus is a contraindication to repair.

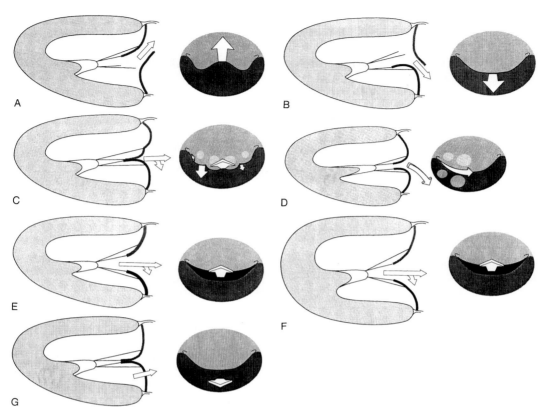

Fig. 15.7 Mitral regurgitation as determined by transthoracic echocardiography and color flow Doppler. The left side of each pair of images represents a parasternal long axis view, and the right side of each pair a parasternal short axis view. Arrows indicate flow direction. (A) Posterior leaflet flail or prolapsing with an anteriorly directed jet (B) Anterior leaflet flail or prolapse with a posteriorly directed jet (C) Chordal elongation, flail or prolapse of both leaflets with a central or posteriorly directed jet (D) Posteromedial papillary muscle infarction with elongation or disruption of the support of both leaflets at the commissure, with a jet from the medial commissure posterolaterally directed. (E) Restriction of leaflet motion (posterior leaflet) with a central or posteriorly directed jet. (F) Dilatation of the mitral annulus with resultant apically displaced papillary muscles and a central or posteriorly directed jet. (G) Perforation of a leaflet with an eccentric jet origin and flow away from the line of coaptation. (Reproduced with permission from: Stewart WJ, Currie PJ, Salcedo EE, *et al*. Evaluation of mitral leaflet motion by echocardiography and jet direction by Doppler color flow mapping to determine the mechanism of mitral regurgitation. Journal of the American College of Cardiology 1992; 20: 1353–1361, figure 1.)

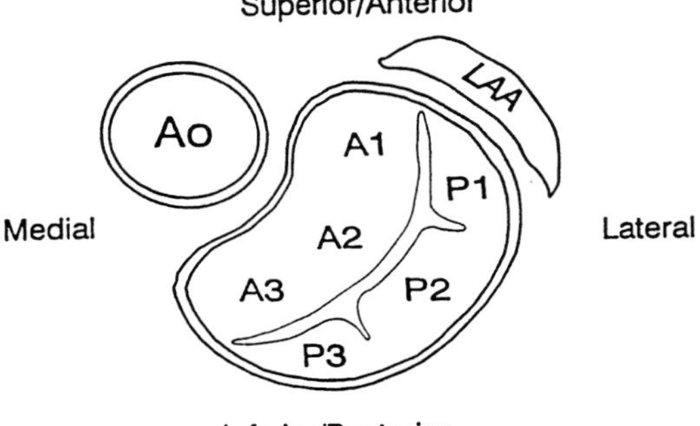

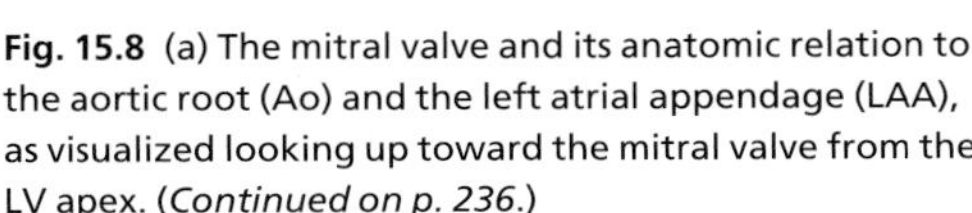
Fig. 15.8 (a) The mitral valve and its anatomic relation to the aortic root (Ao) and the left atrial appendage (LAA), as visualized looking up toward the mitral valve from the LV apex. (*Continued on p. 236.*)

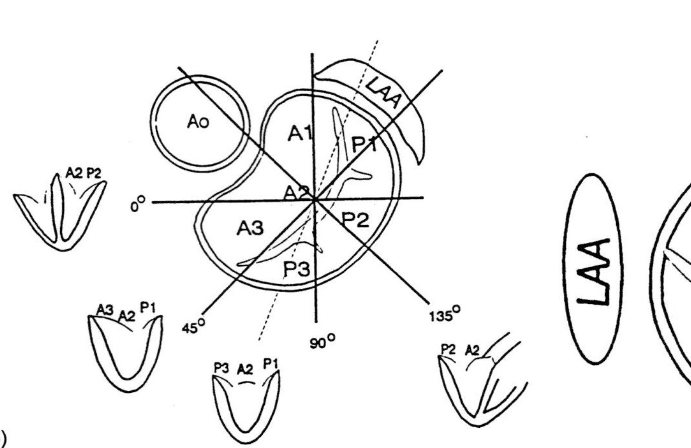

(b)

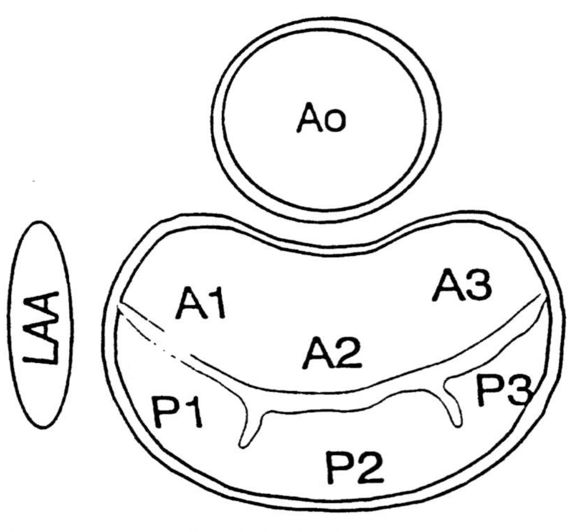

(c)

Fig. 15.8 *(cont'd)* (b) Reference image illustrating the relation of the TEE mitral imaging planes with the probe in the mid-esophagus. (c) View of mitral structures as seen by the surgeon. (Reproduced with permission from: Foster GP, Isselbacher EM, Rose GA, *et al*. Accurate localization of mitral regurgitant defects using multiplane transesophageal echocardiography. Ann Thorac Surg 1998; 65: 1025–1031, figure 1.)

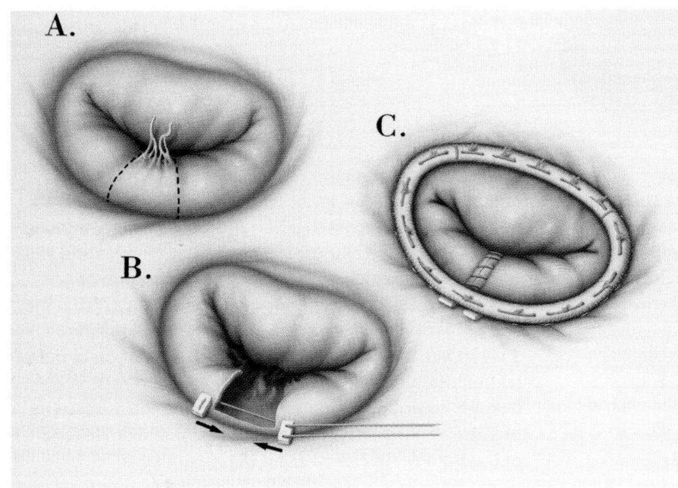

Fig. 15.9 Method for repair of ruptured chordae of the middle scallop of the posterior mitral leaflet. A quadrangular (trapezoidal) area (A) is identified and resected (B). The resected leaflet is repaired and an annuloplasty ring (C) is sutured in place. (Reproduced with permission from: Mitral Valve Reconstruction: Tampa II, Laboratory Manual. Dennis F Pupello, MD, Chief, Cardiac Surgery, St Joseph's Heart Institute, Tampa, Florida, figure 5.)

Postoperatively, the structure and valve motion are examined (Fig. 15.11). Potential complications of MV repair include: (i) significant *residual MR*; (ii) an excessively narrowed MV orifice with *resultant mitral stenosis* or *ring dehiscence*; and (iii) *systolic anterior motion* (SAM) of the MV apparatus with dynamic outflow tract obstruction.

Postoperatively, one should assess coaptation of resected MV leaflets. The LA should be evaluated with color flow Doppler and the pulmonic veins interrogated with pulsed wave (PW) Doppler. Significant residual MR is often corrected with another "pump run." Postoperatively, MR may be underestimated due to preload/afterload reduction or arrhythmias; therefore, one should assess the postvalve repair for residual MR by simulating physiologic conditions. Preload should be adjusted (using volume loading) and afterload may be manipulated (e.g. using an alpha-agonist such as phenylephrine) to help decide if the repair was adequate.

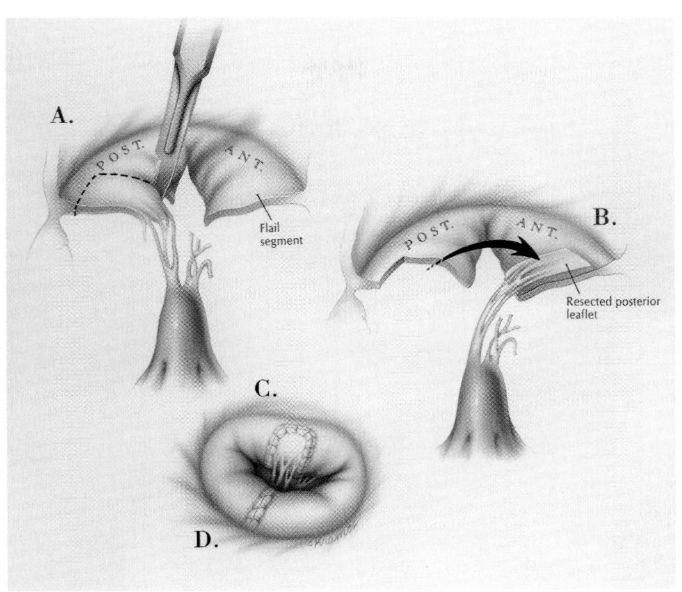

Fig. 15.10 Method for repair of the anterior mitral leaflet by resection (A) of the posterior leaflet with primary chordae, opposite the flail segment of anterior leaflet. The posterior leaflet segment is then (B) "flipped over" to the atrial side of the anterior leaflet, and (C) sutured into position. The posterior leaflet quadrangular defect (D) is then sutured. (Reproduced with permission from: Mitral Valve Reconstruction: Tampa II, Laboratory Manual. Dennis F Pupello, MD, Chief, Cardiac Surgery, St Joseph's Heart Institute, Tampa, Florida, figure 8.)

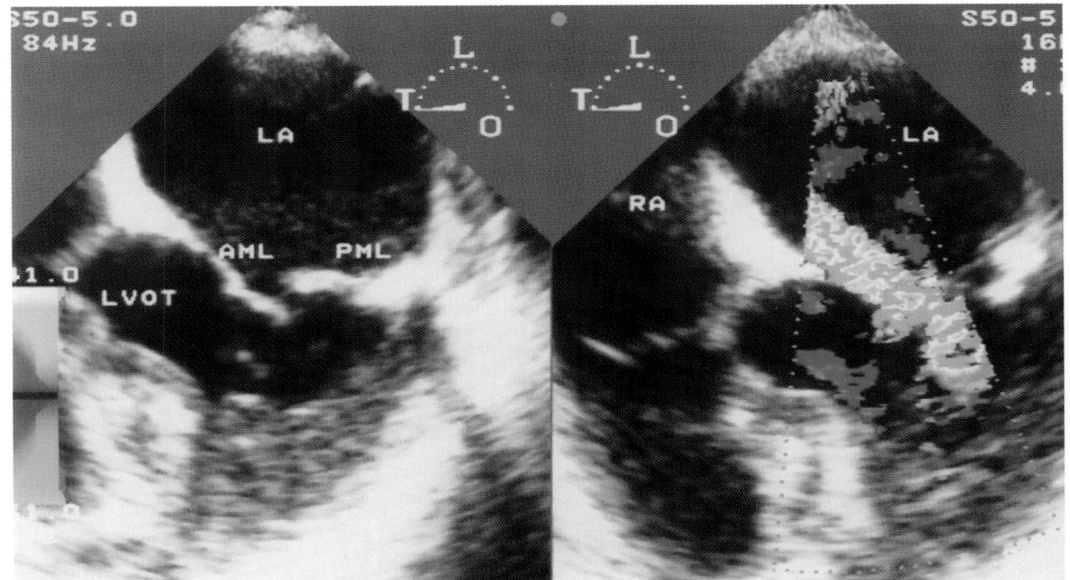

Fig. 15.11 Preoperative TEE (a,b) of a patient with a flail posterior mitral leaflet. Color (b) demonstrates marked coexistent MR. Postoperatively (c,d) color Doppler reveals no evident residual MR in systole (c) and good valve excursion in diastole (d). (*Continued on p. 238.*)

Post repair the mean MV gradient should be measured across the orifice. If the mean gradient is ≥6 mmHg, one should consider a repeat pump-run. Valve dehiscence may occur rarely (Fig. 15.12).

About 2–3% of patients may develop SAM with *dynamic LV outflow tract obstruction*. This will occur almost exclusively with a stiff valve ring (Carpentier) as opposed to a flexible (Duran) ring. SAM should be

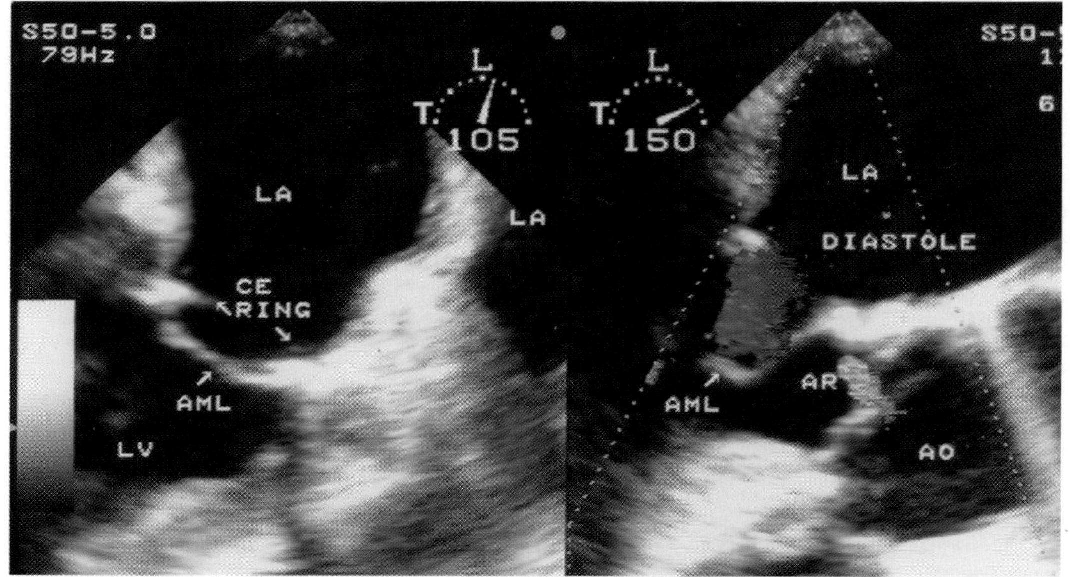

(c) (d)

Fig. 15.11 *(cont'd)*

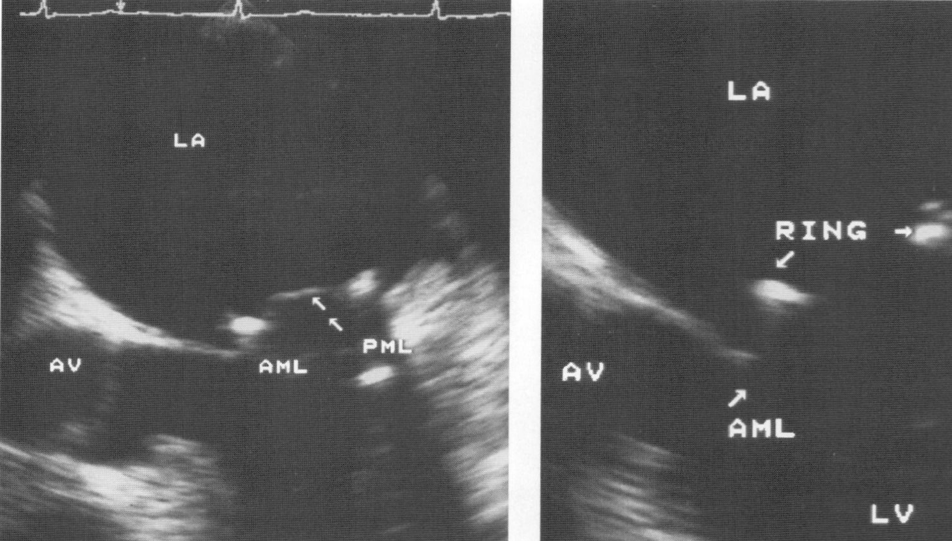

(a) (b)

Fig. 15.12 TEE images in (a) systole and (b) diastole in a patient several weeks post mitral valve (MV) repair, who was referred for progressive exertional dyspnea and noted to have a systolic murmur. Mitral ring dehiscence is evident.

identified in the operating room and may resolve with fluids (especially if it occurs with a flexible ring). "Risk factors" for SAM post ring insertion include:

- myxomatous mitral degeneration
- small LVOT
- hyperkinetic heart
- excessive posterior leaflet resection
- large anterior leaflet
- extensive mitral annulus narrowing
- catecholamines/hypovolemia.

It has been found that those at risk for postoperative SAM have a low anterior leaflet length to posterior leaflet length ratio (AL/PL). Measurements of leaflet lengths are performed during valve coaptation preoperatively. If this ratio is 1.3 or less, then posterior leaflet height reduction seems to be indicated. If the distance from the mitral coaptation point to the septum is 2.5 cm or less with a AL/PL ratio less than 1.3, then the patient appears to have the greatest risk of postoperative SAM.

Patients with ischemic and dynamic mitral regurgitation (see Chapters 8 & 13), particularly those with a dilated annulus, may require a valve ring, and those with a *posterobasal infarction* may require valve replacement.

Tricuspid valve repair

The tricuspid valve is usually evaluated for possible annular ring insertion in cases of tricuspid annulus dilatation with marked tricuspid regurgitation. The tricuspid annulus along the septum (about one third of the annulus circumference and part of the fibrous skeleton) does not dilate. Most dilatation occurs at the base of the posterior and anterior tricuspid leaflets. The decision for repair should be made preoperatively and assessment can usually be done adequately by transthoracic echo. Hemodynamic shifts in the operating room will affect the degree of tricuspid regurgitation (TR) seen intraoperatively and should not affect the preoperative decision for a tricuspid annuloplasty ring.

Aortic valve repair

The aortic valve repair procedure is more difficult than mitral valve repair. Patients with aortic regurgitation (AR) are categorized in a similar way to the mitral valve system (excessive, restricted or normal leaflet motion). The aortic valve pathology most amenable to repair is a prolapsing valve in a patient with a bicuspid valve. When prolapse occurs in a patient with a tricuspid valve, most often the right coronary cusp is involved. Central jet AR due to aortic root dilatation can also be repaired (see also Chapter 7).

CHAPTER 16

Congenital Heart Disease*

Most congenital defects encountered by the adult cardiologist will be discussed.

Congenital heart disease occurs in approximately 0.5–0.8% of live births. This does not include mitral valve prolapse (~5% of the population) or bicuspid aortic valve (1–2% of the population). About 50% of all cardiac congenital defects are simple shunts (atrial septal defect (ASD), ventricular septal defect (VSD), or patent ductus arteriosus (PDA)). Another 20% are simple obstruction lesions (congenital aortic stenosis, pulmonic stenosis, coarctation of the aorta), and approximately 30% are complex lesions (including tetralogy of Fallot).

Identification of cardiac anatomy

Identification of cardiac anatomy involves the "sequential" approach, which includes determination of situs, concordance of connections, and positional relationship of cardiac structures. Some points to remember include:

Atria:

right—usually systemic veins connected to the RA

right atrial appendage (RAA)—triangular shape, trabeculated

left—pulmonary veins attached

left atrial appendage (LAA)—narrow, "fingerlike," near AV groove

foramen ovale—usually "flap" on the left side.

Atrioventricular connection:

right—tricuspid valve attachment is apical relative to mitral attachment

left—mitral valve is "septal-phobic" except with primum ASD.

Ventricles:

right—tricuspid valve almost always associated with the RV trabeculae, conus, moderator band

left—mitral valve almost always associated with the LV.

Great vessels:

aorta—coronary arteries arise

pulmonary artery—pulmonary branches.

Viscera:

atria and abdominal situs is usually the same.

Pulmonary:

lungs may be reversed.

Overview of surgical repair of congenital defects

Over the past several years there has been a trend for early *corrective* (goal of achieving normal anatomy or hemodynamics) surgical procedures (improved infant intraoperative management) for complex congenital defects, whereas mostly *palliative* procedures (temporary surgical procedure for a severe derangement) were performed in the past. Palliative surgical procedures may be performed when a corrective procedure is not possible. Those palliative procedures include:

- *Blalock–Taussig shunt*—subclavian artery to pulmonary artery
- *modified Blalock–Taussig shunt*—GoreTex graft between subclavian artery and pulmonary artery
- *Waterston shunt*—ascending aorta to right pulmonary artery
- *Pott's shunt*—descending aorta to left pulmonary artery
- *central shunt*—ascending aorta to pulmonary artery GoreTex graft
- *Glenn shunt*—superior vena cava (SVC) to right pulmonary artery
- *pulmonary artery band*—band around the main pulmonary artery.

* Dynamic LV and RV outflow obstruction (hypertrophic cardiomyopathy, Chapter 11), congenital aortic valvular stenosis (Chapter 7), and pulmonic stenosis (Chapter 9) are discussed elsewhere in this text.

Complications of the Blalock–Taussig shunts, Waterston shunt, Pott's shunt (less so with the central shunt), and pulmonary artery band include distorted pulmonary arteries. The Glenn shunt is associated with development of *pulmonary AV fistulas* (that part of the pulmonary circulation not receiving IVC flow—flow from the liver—will develop fistulas).

The *Fontan procedure* combines the IVC and SVC using a tunnel through the right atrium, with subsequent direct connection to the pulmonary arteries (*total cavopulmonary anastomosis*). The pulmonary artery is also ligated. This procedure allows for one ventricle to pump to the systemic circulation. There is no ventricular chamber pumping into the pulmonary circulation. The Fontan procedure may be used for single ventricle, hypoplastic left or right heart, and tricuspid valve atresia amongst others.

Atrial septal defect

Atrial septal defects (ASD) are classified by the location within the atrial septum. An ASD is an abnormal opening between the atria through the atrial septum. A patent foramen ovale (PFO) is not classified as an ASD (see Chapter 17). A hemodynamically significant left-to-right shunt results in echocardiographic findings of right ventricular diastolic volume overload and increased pulmonary flow. Left-to-right shunting occurs primarily because the right ventricle is more compliant than the thicker walled LV and fills easier. The pulmonary artery resistance is also lower than systemic resistance, thus facilitating left-to-right shunting. Whenever RV enlargement is noted, an ASD should be excluded.

Occasionally caval flow may be confused with ASD flow. Color Doppler can help differentiate these two by evaluating the response to respiration. Caval flow increases with inspiration whereas shunt flow through an ASD decreases with inspiration and has much less peak velocity variability over the respiratory cycle. With a hemodynamically substantial shunt, the mean flow velocity across the shunt measured with pulsed wave Doppler is usually 0.3–0.9 m/s with peak velocities up to 2 m/s. Flow begins in early systole, continuing nearly through the entire cardiac cycle. A broad peak is noted in late systole, ending in early diastole.

Saline contrast injections may reveal a small right-to-left shunt that is accentuated by the Valsalva maneuver, and a "negative" contrast effect within the right atrium. A PFO demonstrating a right-to-left shunt can be discerned from a secundum type ASD with transesophageal echocardiography (TEE) by its consistent location (Figs 7.25 & 7.29).

If a hemodynamically substantial ASD is suspected, tricuspid valve diastolic flow will be increased. Likewise, increased flow noted across the tricuspid valve should warrant further investigation for an ASD. The ratio of transtricuspid to transmitral maximum flow velocities is normally less than 0.75. Measurements should be made from an apical four-chamber view at the level of the valve annulus. Pulmonic valve flow velocity will also be increased up to 1.0–1.5 m/s with a significant shunt. This may be up to 1.5 times as high as the aortic velocity. With the development of pulmonary hypertension and right ventricular hypertrophy (RVH), however, the amount of left-to-right shunting and increased tricuspid and pulmonic flow will diminish. It is important to calculate the ASD shunt ratio (QP/PS) (see Chapter 3).

Types of ASDs (Fig. 16.1) include secundum, primum, sinus venosus, and the coronary sinus types.

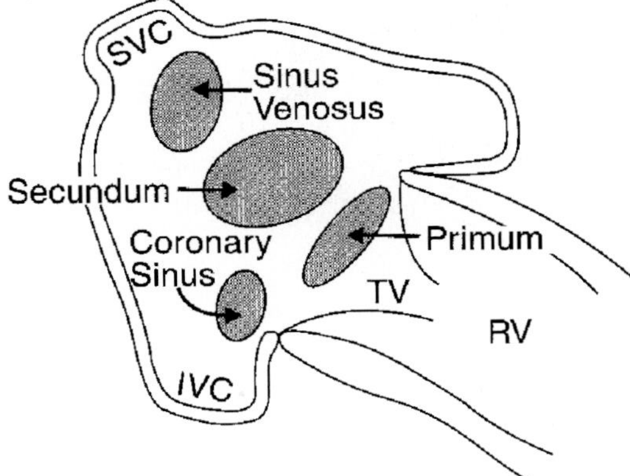

Fig. 16.1 Types of atrial septal defects (ASDs) as viewed from the right atrium. The *primum ASD* lies anteroinferior to the fossa ovalis and is often associated with a cleft anterior leaflet of the mitral valve. It may also be associated with a cleft septal leaflet of the tricuspid valve. The *sinus venosus ASD* lies posterior to the fossa ovalis and is most often associated with anomalous drainage of the right upper pulmonary vein—drains near the superior junction of the SVC–RA–LA. Rarely anomalous drainage of the left upper pulmonary vein (into the innominate vein) will also be found. The *coronary sinus ASD* lies at the site of the coronary ostium. If present, the coronary sinus will straddle the defect. A very rare form of defect involves an *"unroofed" coronary sinus*, in which LA shunting occurs into the coronary sinus and then into the RA.

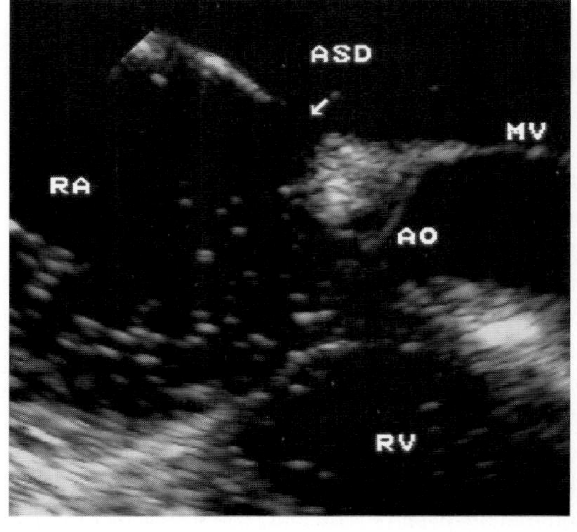

(a)

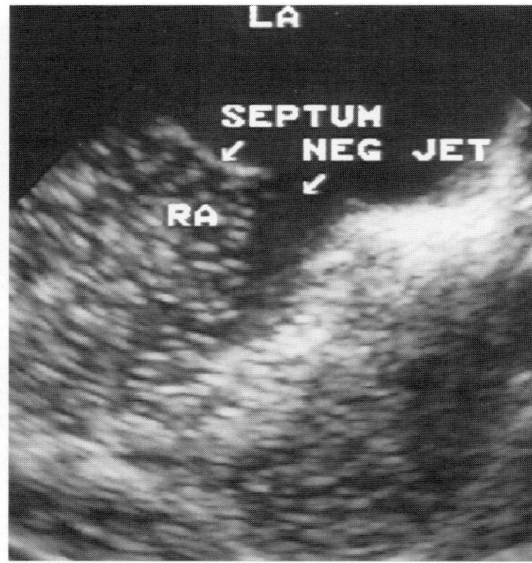

(c)

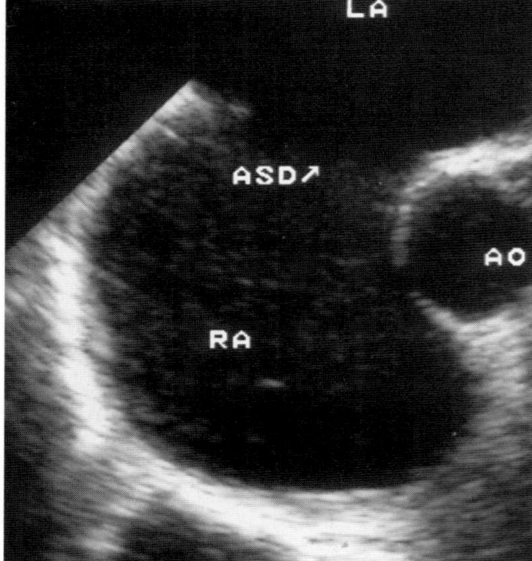

(b)

Fig. 16.2 Examples of secundum ASDs. (a) Transesophageal echocardiography (TEE) of a "medium" sized secundum ASD, (b) large secundum ASD, and (c) agitated peripheral venous saline injection performed to illustrate a negative contrast effect (NEG JET) in the right atrium (RA). The septum primum (SEPTUM) has a defect with a resultant secundum type ASD. (*Cont'd.*)

The most common is the secundum type, followed by primum, sinus venosus, and coronary sinus defects. The *secundum defect* (Fig. 16.2) lies in the region of the fossa ovalis. A secundum defect (defect in the septum primum) may be multiple or fenestrated (Fig. 16.3).

A *primum defect* (a form of atrioventricular (AV) canal) is in contact with the AV valve ring (Figs 16.4 & 16.5) and may be associated with complex AV junction and AV valvular abnormalities. A cleft anterior leaflet of the mitral valve is almost always present. A cleft septal leaflet of the tricuspid valve with coexistent significant tricuspid regurgitation may also be present. From an apical four-chamber view, the normal apical displacement of the tricuspid annulus in relation to the mitral annulus is not found. Both the tricuspid and mitral annulus are in the same plane.

The sinus venosus defect (*superior sinus venosus defect*) is best visualized by TEE in the esophageal longitudinal view (Fig. 16.6). It may be seen also, especially in the pediatric population, from a subcostal view highlighting the SVC–RA junction. The defect involves the posterosuperior atrial septum and is immediately inferior to the RA–SVC junction. As

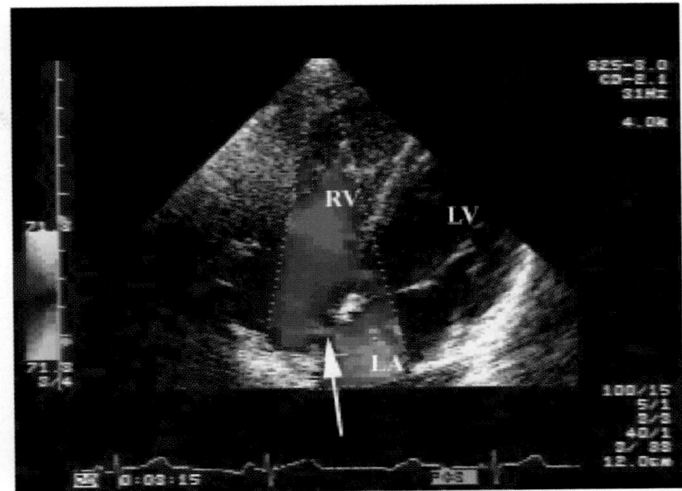

(d)

Fig. 16.2 (*cont'd*) (d) Transthoracic modified apical view with color Doppler demonstrates flow (arrow) through a secundum ASD, from the LA to right atrium. One must be careful not to confuse caval flow and flow through an ASD. A small restrictive secundum ASD is illustrated in Fig. 17.29.

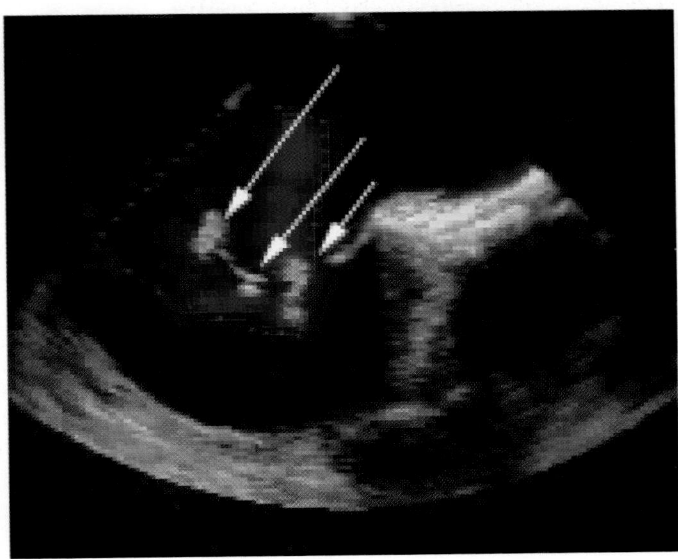

Fig. 16.3 TEE at 90° in a 23-year-old-commercial diver with unexplained decompression sickness. The diver was referred for evaluation for percutaneous closure. By TEE multiple fenestrations (arrows) were found, along with an atrial septal aneurysm.

mentioned, it is usually associated with anomalous right upper pulmonary vein insertion into the SVC, and sometimes anomalous left upper pulmonary vein drainage (into the innominate vein). A very rare form of sinus venosus defect is the *inferior sinus venosus defect*. This is located near the junction of the IVC and RA.

A *coronary sinus defect* lies at the site of the coronary sinus orifice, in the posteroinferior septum. It is usually associated with a persistent left SVC, which drains into the coronary sinus. The coronary sinus defect may also be associated with a secundum type ASD, persistent left SVC, and rarely an unroofed coronary sinus.

During echocardiographic evaluation of patients with an ASD, one should:

- identify all four pulmonary veins—the suprasternal "crab" view is often helpful
- evaluate for RV enlargement
- identify the defect structurally and measure its size
- document flow by color and PW Doppler

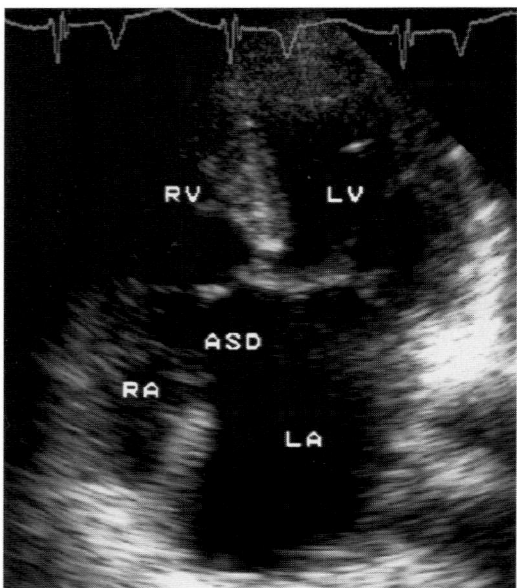

Fig. 16.4 Apical four-chamber view of a patient with a septum primum type ASD. Note that the tricuspid septal leaflet and mitral anterior leaflet lie in the same plane.

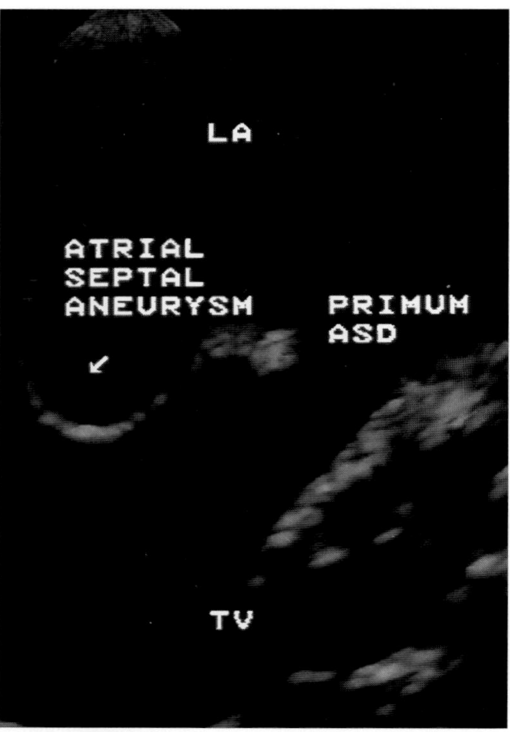

Fig. 16.5 TEE in the horizontal plane of a patient with a septum primum ASD. The defect is in contact with the atrioventricular valve ring.

• evaluate the mitral and tricuspid valves (anatomy and for regurgitation)
• calculate pulmonary artery pressures
• calculate pulmonary flow/systemic flow (Q_P/Q_S).

Percutaneous closure of atrial level shunts

Transesophageal echocardiography (TEE) plays an important role in selection of patients for *percutaneous closure of an ASD or PFO* (Fig. 16.7). First described in 1974 by Drs Terry King and Noel Mills, the procedure has gained momentum. Features to be evaluated include the defect size, length of the interatrial septum, amount of remaining rim around the defect, and mobility or aneurysm of the septum primum (fossa ovalis). As the percutaneous closure procedure is performed with continuous TEE monitoring, we perform most procedures with the patient under general anesthesia.

Before introduction of the device, TEE evaluation should be performed to look for other abnormalities. The defect morphology, size and location should then be measured using horizontal and vertical planes. The distance from the edge of the defect to the mitral annulus, right pulmonary vein orifice, SVC, posterior wall of the ascending aorta, and coronary sinus should all be measured. Using the Amplatzer septal occluder, a 5-mm margin is needed around the entire rim. A common area for insufficient "rim" to be present is between the edge of the defect and the aortic root, which can be well seen in a short axis view of the aortic valve.

Sizing of the defect is important as this determines the size of Amplatzer device to be used. The "stretch diameter" measured uses a balloon deployed across the defect and inflated. A balloon (spherical or cylindrical) should be inflated across the defect (partly in the LA and partly in the RA) causing a waist in the central portion of the balloon, as the defect will indent the balloon. This indentation should be measured by fluoroscopy and TEE. One must be careful to measure the largest diameter, as the defect may be oval in shape. Also, the tissue rim may be pliable and may be pushed aside during device deployment. In this case, the diameter should be measured to a margin that is thicker and essentially nonmobile. In a few cases, the measured defect size will still be underestimated.

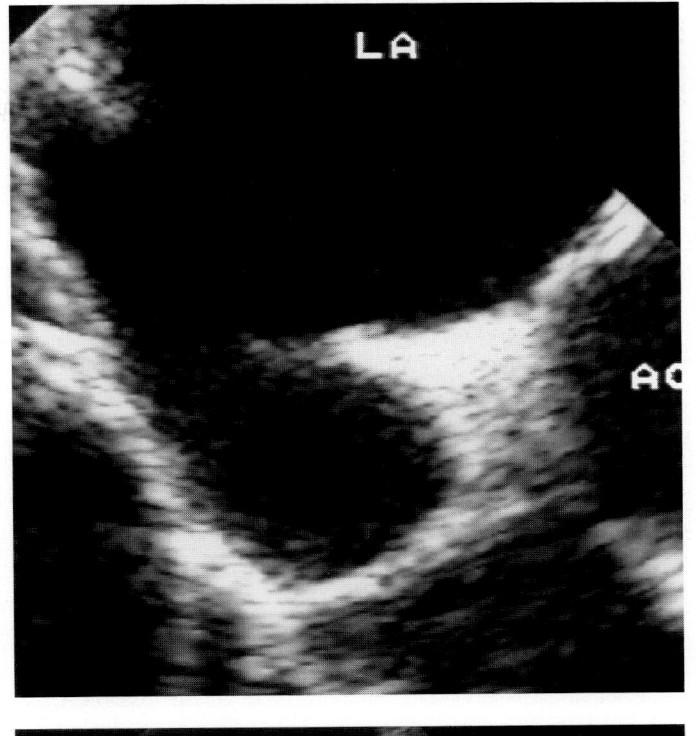

(a)

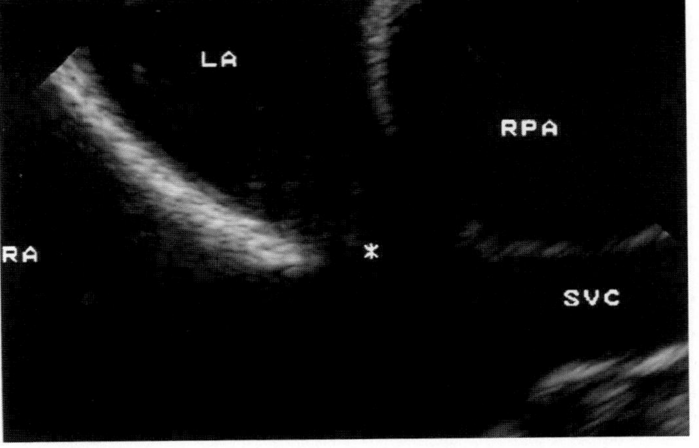

(b)

Fig. 16.6 TEE images of a superior sinus venosus type ASD. (a) Transverse view illustrating the SVC–LA communication, and (b) longitudinal view illustrating the defect (*). SVC, superior vena cava; RPA, right pulmonary artery.

A delivery catheter is then passed over a guidewire, and into the LA. The catheter tip needs to be visualized free in the body of the LA, away from the left atrial appendage (LAA), mitral valve orifice, and pulmonary veins. Also, the tip of the catheter may become entangled in the Chiari network when passing through the right atrium. If multiple defects are present, the catheter should go across the largest defect.

The LA disk is then deployed in the left atrium, and positioned against the interatrial septum. If the catheter tip is too close to the distal LA wall or LAA, the left atrial disk may assume a twisted shape, as part of it will be ensnared (*cobrahead shape*) by the LA or LAA. Also, the deployed disk should not (partially) prolapse into the right atrium. If the LA disk is not against the septum, when the right atrial disk is deployed, it will prolapse into the left atrium. TEE confirms both disks on either side of the septum. The right atrial disk will not flatten completely until the device is released. The atrial septum may be distorted

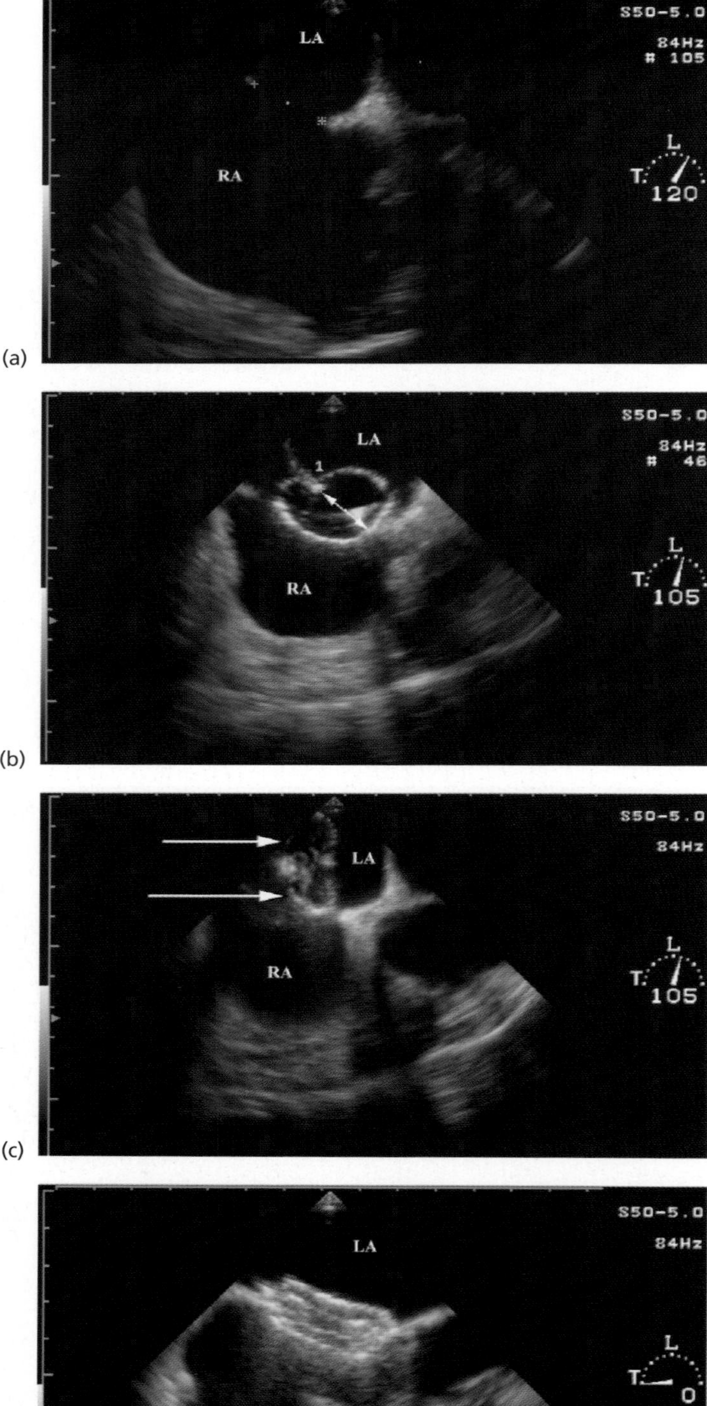

Fig. 16.7 A 43-year-old-female was referred for percutaneous closure of a secundum type ASD. An Amplatzer device was used. (a) Measurement of the ASD size is performed from multiple views. The view shown is from 120°. (b) Sizing the defect with a balloon (double-headed arrow) at 105°. (c) The left-sided occluder (arrows) has been deployed and is being pulled toward the atrial septum. (d) Both devices are deployed and appear well seated against the atrial septum. Imaging is from the horizontal plane. (*Cont'd.*)

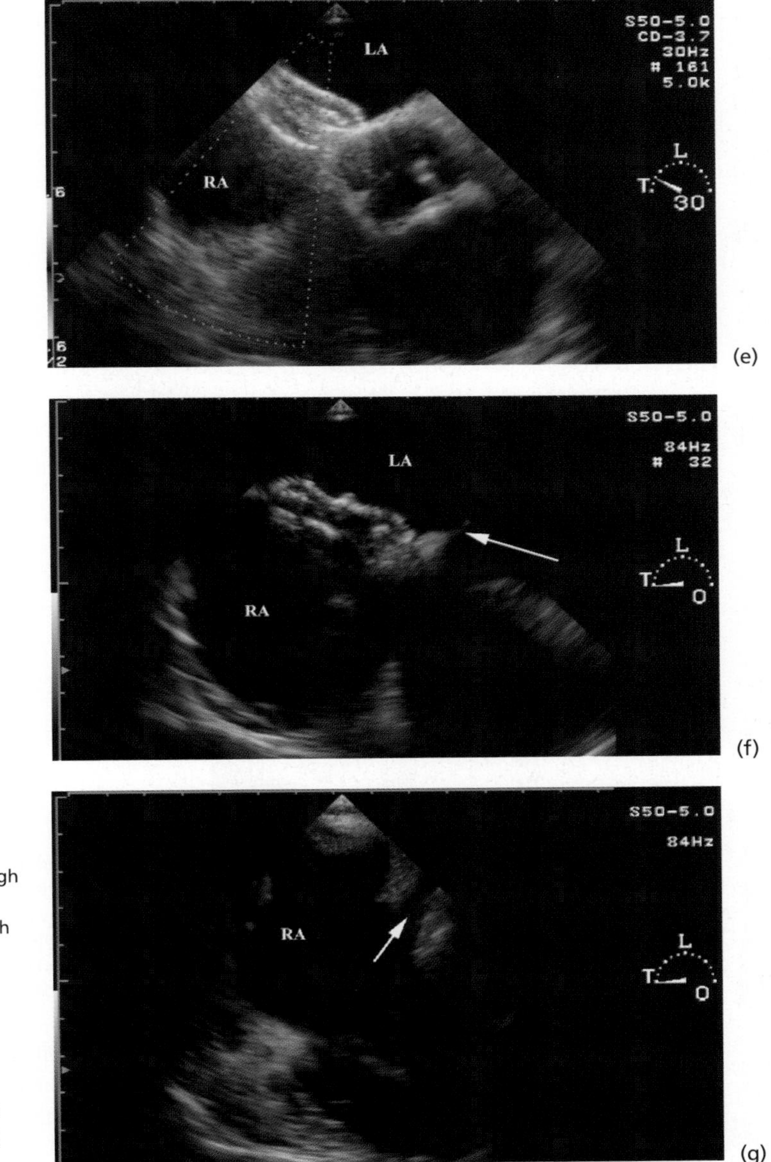

Fig. 16.7 (*cont'd*) (e) "Foaming" through the Amplatzer device (see text) is manifested as color turbulence through the device. Imaging is from 30°. (f) Documentation of the Amplatzer device seated away from the mitral apparatus (arrow, anterior leaflet mitral valve) in the horizontal plane. (g) Documentation that the occluder device is not in proximity to the orifice of the coronary sinus (arrow). Imaging was in the horizontal plane.

up to 60° before release from the catheter. The angle of distortion will generally resolve upon release of the catheter. Excessive distortion, however, may increase the risk for device embolization, when the catheter is released.

The shunt is then evaluated by color Doppler before release from the catheter. A small amount of flow through the device (termed *foaming*) and some small amount of color around the device may be seen. Trivial color flow around the device generally resolves when the device is released. If more significant flow around the device is noted, it may be necessary to withdraw the device and insert a larger Amplatzer occluder.

Before the device is released, one should evaluate the device to make sure it is not obstructing the mitral valve, coronary sinus, and right upper pulmonary vein orifice. A gentle tugging on the attached catheter (*Minnesota wiggle*) will document a stable device

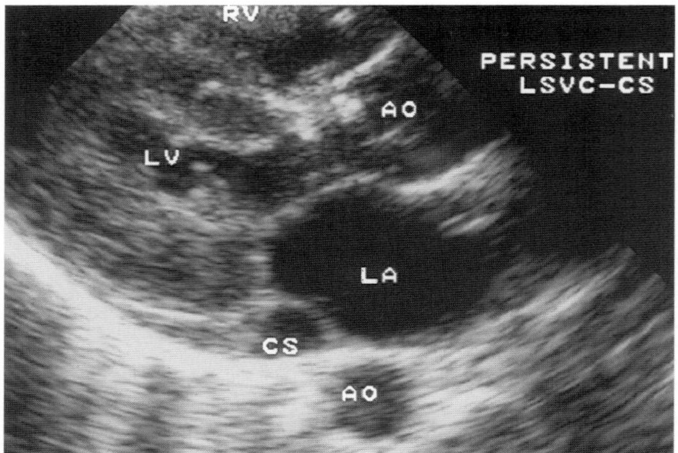

(a)

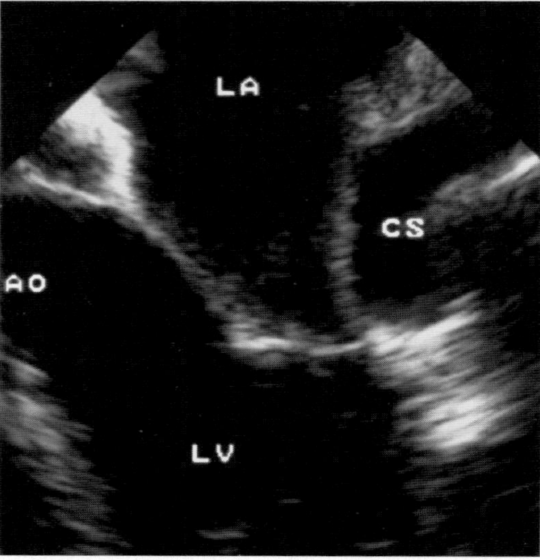

(b)

Fig. 16.8 Dilated coronary sinus (a) Parasternal long axis view of a patient with a persistent left SVC and resultant dilated coronary sinus (CS). The CS will "move" with the cardiac cycle, whereas the descending aorta (AO) remains relatively stationary. (b) TEE in the transverse plane of a patient with a dilated CS.

position. After catheter release from the device, re-evaluation for residual shunt should be performed.

Follow-up transthoracic echocardiography should be performed at day 1, and at 1, 3, and 6 months. One should document device position (particularly in relation to the mitral valve), any residual shunting, device appearance, right heart size and function, and pulmonary artery pressures.

Coronary sinus and persistent left superior vena cava

When dilated, the *coronary sinus* is prominently noted by echocardiography. Dilatation of the coronary sinus is associated with:

- persistent left SVC
- total anomalous pulmonary venous drainage and drainage into the coronary sinus
- coronary AV fistula with coronary sinus drainage
- anomalous hepatic vein drainage into the coronary sinus
- right heart failure with elevated RA pressure
- severe tricuspid regurgitation
- surgical complication of tricuspid valve replacement.

A dilated coronary sinus (Fig. 16.8) may appear as a mass in the left atrium but actually lies in the posterior AV groove and collapses during ventricular systole. Knowing this characteristic position, following its "drainage" into the RA and demonstrating flow by Doppler allows one to make the diagnosis. The cor-

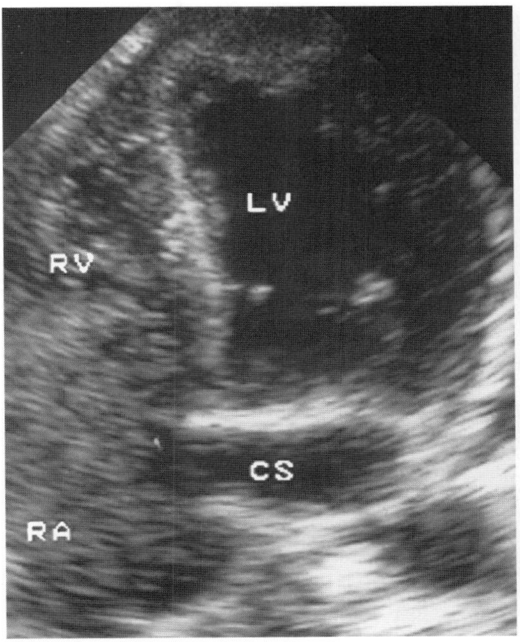

(a)

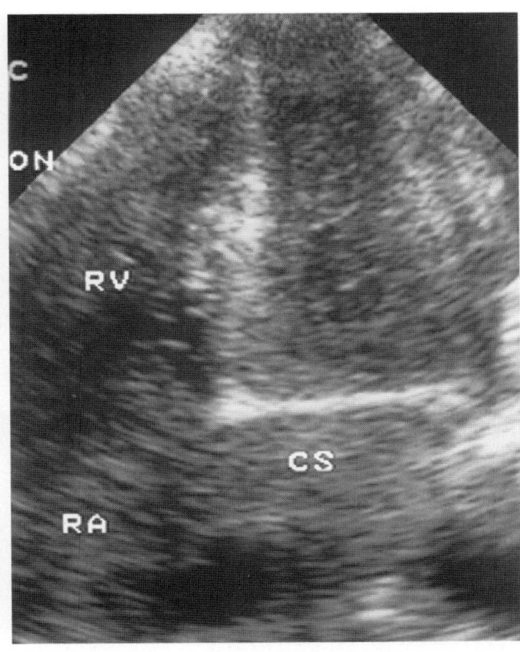

(b)

Fig. 16.9 Persistent left SVC. (a) Agitated saline contrast injected into the right antecubital vein reveals no contrast in the CS, whereas in (b) injection into the left antecubital vein reveals contrast entering the right heart via the CS.

onary sinus can be differentiated from the descending thoracic aorta in that the latter usually will not "move" with the cardiac cycle.

Persistent left SVC occurs occasionally (~0.5%) in the general population, and in 3–10% of patients with an ASD (Figs 16.9 & 16.10). It drains into the coronary sinus; hence the coronary sinus will be dilated. Diagnosis is made by seeing the appearance of saline contrast in the coronary sinus before it appears in the RA following injection of the sonocated saline in the left antecubital vein. When saline contrast is injected via the right antecubital vein, contrast will appear first in the normal right SVC, followed by the RA. Some reflux of agitated saline may occur into the orifice of the coronary sinus.

Ventricular septal defect

Classification of VSDs is made according to location, size (restrictive or nonrestrictive), type (muscular or nonmuscular), and alignment (alignment or malalignment). VSDs are the most common form of congenital heart disease (~25% of congenital defects), and may be isolated (only 25–30% are isolated) or

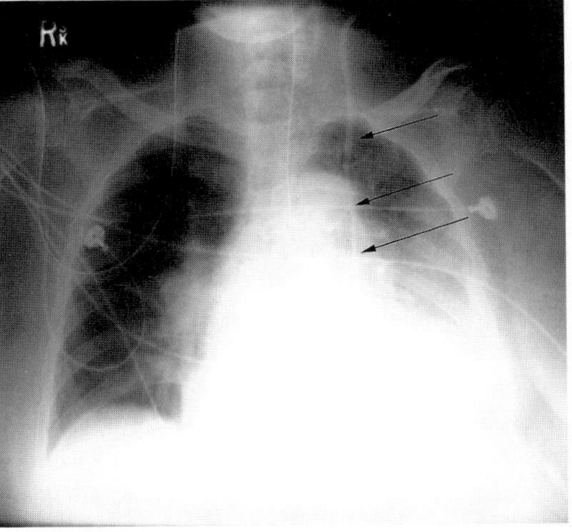
(a)

Fig. 16.10 A patient received a central venous line catheter via the left jugular vein. (a) Chest X-ray was performed to document position, and revealed an unusual course (arrows), suggesting the possibility of a persistent left SVC. Transthoracic echocardiography with imaging from the parasternal right ventricular inflow view was then performed. (*Continued on p. 250.*)

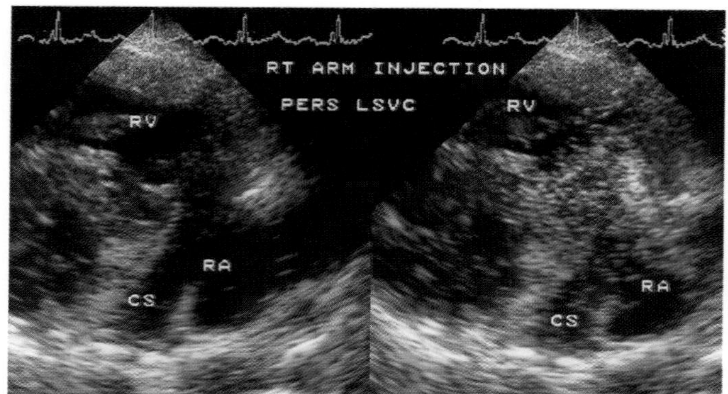

(b)

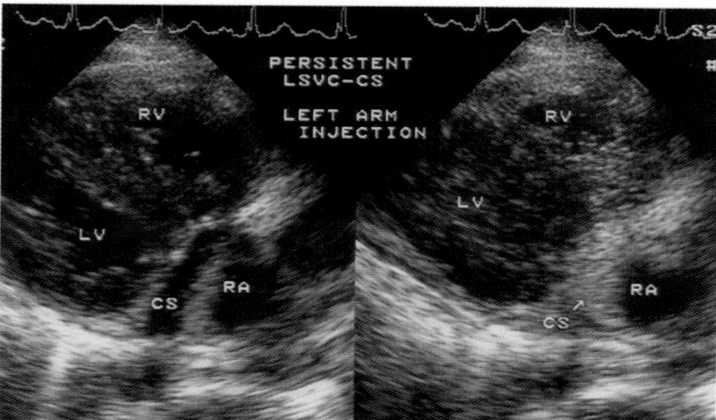

(c)

Fig. 16.10 (*cont'd*) (b) Injection of saline contrast into the right antecubital vein documented contrast entering the RA via the normal right SVC. (c) Injection of saline contrast into the left antecubital vein resulted in contrast first appearing in the CS, followed by the RA. (Reproduced with permission from: Dearstine M, Taylor W, Kerut EK. Persistent left superior vena cava: chest X-ray and echocardiographic findings. Echocardiography 2000; 17(5): 453–455.)

associated with other abnormalities such as with tetralogy of Fallot. The ventricular septum (Fig. 16.11) is divided into membranous and muscular portions. The muscular septum is further divided into inlet (posterior), trabecular, and outlet (anterior) portions (Fig. 16.12).

Perimembranous VSDs are the most common form of VSD in the adult (Fig. 16.13) and lie under the aortic valve ring. These defects may extend posteriorly to involve the RV inlet muscular septum (*perimembranous inlet VSD*), anteriorly to involve the RV outlet muscular septum (*perimembranous outlet VSD*), or apically to involve the RV trabecular septum. Most (50–80%) small perimembranous VSDs will close spontaneously.

A *ventricular septal aneurysm* (Fig. 16.14) usually is formed from the septal leaflet of the tricuspid valve. It will cover a perimembranous defect, and may decrease the amount of left-to-right shunting. Aneurysms may become large, causing flow turbulence by color Doppler, and may even cause RV outflow tract obstruction. If the tricuspid septal leaflet becomes distorted, flow may occur from the LV outflow tract into the RA (*Gerbode defect*). A Gerbode defect may lead to RV volume overload, increased RA size, and subsequent atrial arrhythmias. *Prolapse of the aortic valve right coronary cusp,* secondary to a perimembranous defect, may lead to progressive aortic regurgitation. Also, associated with a perimembranous VSD, a *subaortic discrete membrane* may develop in youth or early adulthood, leading to fixed subaortic stenosis.

Muscular VSDs are the second most common defect. Most small defects close spontaneously. These defects may be multiple. If hypertrophy of the RV outflow tract develops, this may protect the pulmonary vasculature and pulmonary hypertension may be avoided (*Gasul phenomenon*). If an apical muscular VSD is present, moderator band hypertrophy may restrict shunt flow. The LV apex and RV apex essentially becomes one chamber, having a cardiac apical aneurysmal configuration.

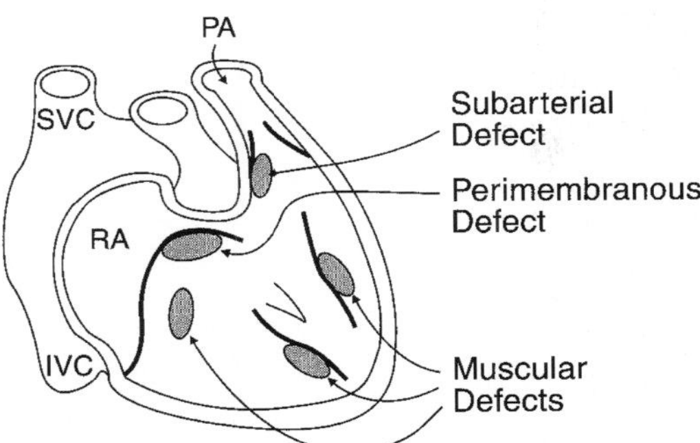

Fig. 16.11 Classification of ventricular septal defects (VSDs) as viewed from the RV.

Supracristal or *subarterial defects* (most common in patients of Asian descent) are associated with aortic valve right or left coronary cusp prolapse into the VSD, and development of aortic regurgitation.

Inlet septal defects are usually associated with abnormalities of the AV septum. A primum ASD is often associated, as are clefts in the anterior leaflet of the mitral valve or septal leaflet of the tricuspid valve. Tricuspid chordae may cross the VSD to insert into the LV. This type of VSD is most often found in patients with *Down's syndrome*.

Echocardiographic evaluation in a patient with a VSD should include the following:

- size the defect (systolic dimension) in several views
- document flow with color and CW Doppler
- measure the CW Doppler gradient—one may estimate RV pressure ($RV_{systolic}$) using the modified Bernoulli equation, as $RV_{systolic}$ = (Cuff systolic BP) – $4(Vel)^2$, where (Vel) is the peak velocity across the VSD
- calculate pulmonary artery pressure
- measure aortic annulus size in systole
- evaluate LA size (a significant VSD will increase the LA size)
- evaluate LV size and function—chronic volume overload of the LV may develop with LV enlargement of failure
- evaluate for the presence of aortic regurgitation (supracristal and some perimembranous defects)
- calculate Q_P/Q_S if the shunt is relatively small.

In the clinical setting of *endocarditis*, vegetations may develop on a membranous septal aneurysm, tricuspid septal leaflet, aortic valve, or at the site the color jet strikes the RV or RV outflow tract.

Shunting is determined by the size of the defect and by the outflow resistance. A *restrictive VSD* maintains

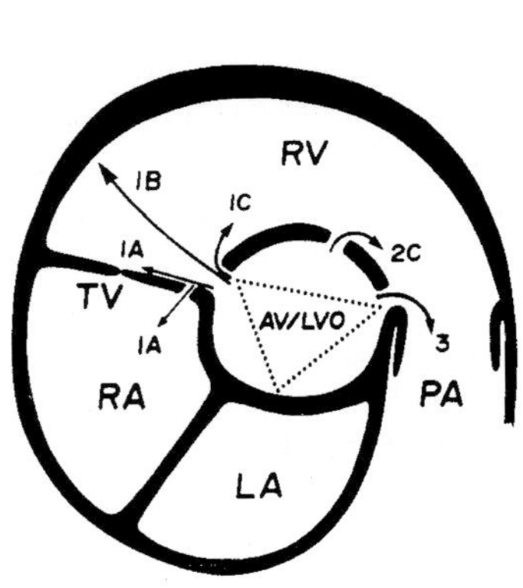

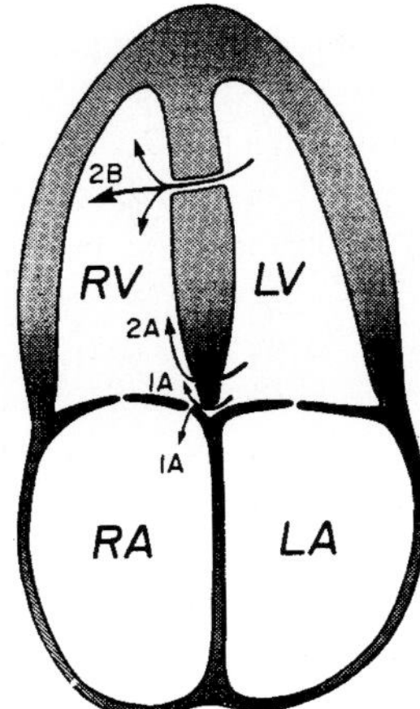

Fig. 16.12 Representation of the relative positions by echocardiography of various types of VSDs. Group 1 (*perimembranous defects*) may be identified as *inlet extension* (1A) when flow is directed toward the tricuspid valve, *trabecular extension* (1B) when flow is directed toward the RV free wall, and *outflow extension* (1C) when directed toward the RV outflow tract. Group 2 (*muscular defects*) may be divided into *muscular inlet* (2A), *muscular trabecular* (2B), or as a *high muscular defect* (2C) with flow directed toward the RV outflow tract. Group 3 is the *juxtaarterial doubly committed defect* which is continuous with the pulmonic valve. (Reproduced with permission from: Helmcke F, *et al*. Two-dimensional and color Doppler assessment of ventricular septal defect of congenital origin. American Journal of Cardiology 1989; 63: 1112.)

(a)

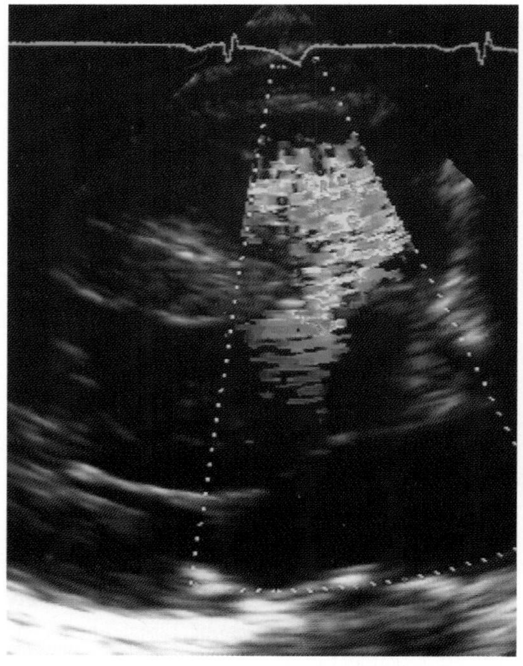

(b)

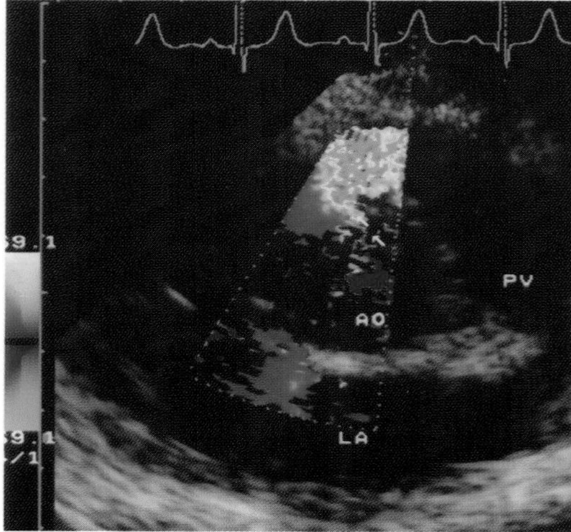

Fig. 16.13 Parasternal (a) long axis and (b) short axis images of an adult with a rather large perimembranous VSD.

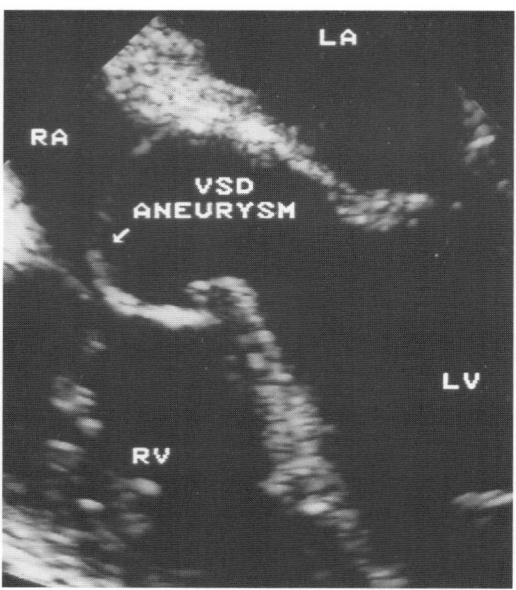

Fig. 16.14 TEE transverse plane image of a VSD covered by the septal leaflet of the tricuspid valve to form an aneurysm.

a systolic gradient between the LV and RV (Fig. 16.15), whereas in a *nonrestrictive defect* the LV and RV systolic pressures become equal. Bidirectional shunting will occur in patients with increased RV outflow resistance, as with elevated pulmonary vascular resistance (*Eisenmenger's syndrome*) or RV outflow obstruction (tetralogy of Fallot).

Sinus of Valsalva aneurysm

A *sinus of Valsalva aneurysm* probably results from a defect within the aortic media at the annulus. A diverticulum (finger-like or windsock appearance) will arise most commonly from the right (~70%) or noncoronary (~25%) cusp, or from the left coronary cusp (~5%). The sinus from which the aneurysm originates may be mildly enlarged whereas the aortic root and valve are usually nearly normal. A right coronary cusp aneurysm will end usually within the RA or RV, and a noncoronary cusp aneurysm will usually end in the RA. A sinus of Valsalva aneurysm may also dissect into the interventricular septum or back into the LV, which may be confused with aortic regurgitation (AR) if not carefully imaged. Some degree of AR may be noted with a sinus of Valsalva aneurysm, but marked AR should be an alert to look for rupture back into the LV, or for aortic valve endocarditis.

Color Doppler of a ruptured sinus of Valsalva aneurysm will demonstrate flow turbulence extending into the receiving chamber. LA and LV enlargement may develop secondary to left heart volume overload.

Echocardiography will help distinguish this entity from other abnormalities. When evaluating a patient

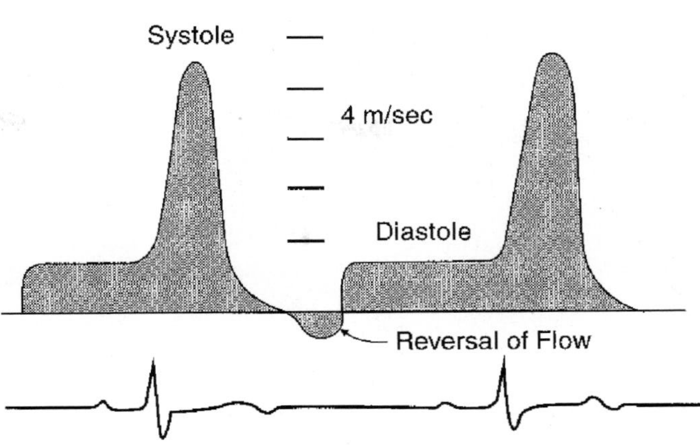

Fig. 16.15 Diagram of continuous wave (CW) Doppler of a restrictive VSD. Early systolic left-to-right shunting (isovolumic contraction phase) with a minimal amount of right-to-left reversal of flow in late systole and early diastole (isovolumic relaxation—RV pressure decay is slower than LV pressure decay) is noted. Mid-to-late diastolic left-to-right shunting occurs if the RV is more compliant than the LV (indicative of normal pulmonary vascular resistance). Note that predominant shunting occurs during early systole.

with a continuous murmur (patent ductus arteriosus and a coronary artery fistula will also have a continuous murmur), echo will readily identify the etiology. Echo evaluation of the origin of the aneurysm will also distinguish sinus of Valsalva aneurysm from the more common aneurysm of the membranous interventricular septum. Doppler flow is different from a VSD, in that there will be high flow from left to right during both systole and diastole (continuous murmur), as a significant pressure gradient exists between the aorta and right heart throughout the cardiac cycle. Aneurysms secondary to healed endocarditis do not have a windsock appearance. An *aortico-left ventricular tunnel* (presents as severe AR in infancy) forms a communication between the aorta and LV. The origin lies in the anterior aortic wall, superior to the right coronary artery. It lies adjacent but outside the right coronary cusp aspect of the aortic annulus, and terminates in the LV, just below the right and left aortic coronary cusps. This may be distinguished from a ruptured sinus of Valsalva aneurysm, in that the origin of the aneurysm of the sinus of Valsalva is inferior to the coronary arteries.

Patent ductus arteriosus

Patent ductus arteriosus is most often an isolated defect, but may occur associated with other cardiac abnormalities. The ductus originates within the lesser curvature of the aorta just distal to the left subclavian artery and connects to the pulmonary artery bifurcation near the left pulmonary artery. Infective endocarditis involving the pulmonary artery side may occur, usually in early adulthood. A *PDA aneurysm* or a closed *ductus diverticulum* (off the aorta) may rupture. A patient with a substantial shunt will usually develop an enlarged LA and an enlarged LV, secondary to left heart volume overload. With development of pulmonary hypertension, the right heart will develop right heart pressure overload with RVH. The shunt will diminish and a right-to-left shunt may ensue, with cyanosis evident in the lower extremities (not the upper extremities). The PDA shunt ratio may be calculated (see Chapter 3), keeping in mind that the value in the numerator is flow through the aortic valve and the value in the denominator is flow through the pulmonary valve.

A PDA may be short and wide, or long, tortuous and narrow, making direct two-dimensional (2-D) imaging difficult. TEE may help visualize and characterize Doppler flow. Imaging from a high left parasternal short axis window and the suprasternal notch may help visualize a PDA (Fig. 16.16). If color flow is seen within the ductus itself, a continuous color Doppler flow signal should be seen. Imaging of the main pulmonary artery, however, may reveal color flow from the PDA toward the pulmonary valve in diastole only, as the systolic portion will proceed toward the distal pulmonary artery branches, along with flow ejected into the main pulmonary artery from the RV.

With the development of pulmonary hypertension, ductal flow velocities will decrease. It may become difficult to distinguish ductal flow from low velocity *late systole* retrograde flow in the main pulmonary artery in patients with a dilated pulmonary artery (idiopathic dilated pulmonary artery, pulmonary hypertension). Flow from the ductus into the main

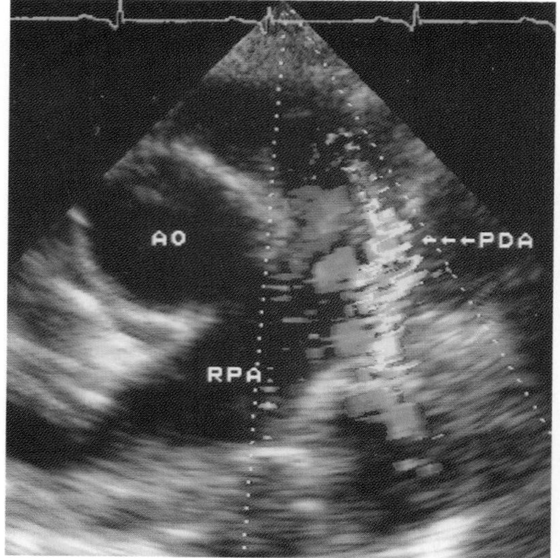

(a)

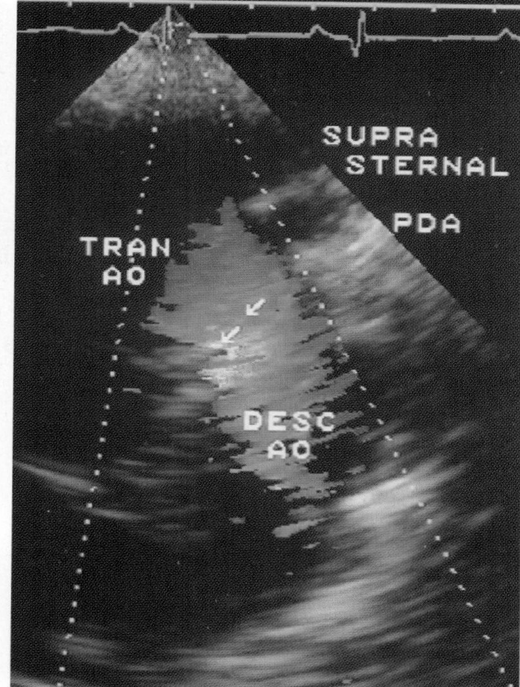

(b)

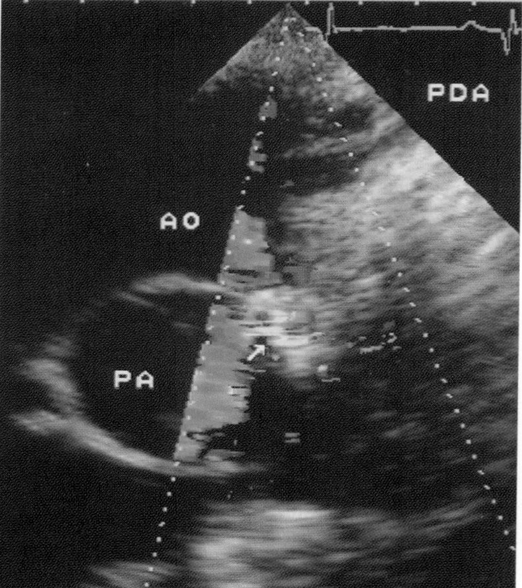

(c)

Fig. 16.16 Echocardiography in a 42-year-old female with a continuous murmur, found to have a patent ductus arteriosus (PDA). (a) High parasternal short axis view reveals turbulent color flow emanating from the main pulmonary artery, near the origin of the left pulmonary artery. Suprasternal imaging in (b) reveals color flow beginning from the lesser curvature of the proximal descending thoracic aorta (DESC AO). (c) By following the path of the calcified short (and wide) PDA, its entrance into the pulmonary artery (PA) is visualized. TRAN AO, transverse aorta.

pulmonary artery, however, occurs in *diastole*. One may distinguish flow from other systemic–pulmonary connections (coronary artery fistula, aortopulmonary window) by noting that color flow originates in the proximal descending aorta and ends in the main pulmonary artery near the origin of the left pulmonary artery.

Continuous wave Doppler will reveal continuous flow from the aorta into the pulmonary artery (Fig. 16.17). Peak velocity will occur in late systole. One may use the modified Bernoulli equation to calculate the pulmonary artery pressure by subtracting the PDA gradient from the arm cuff blood pressure. However, if the PDA is a long narrow structure, the pressure may be underestimated using the simplified Bernoulli equation. Also, with a left-to-right shunt, the CW

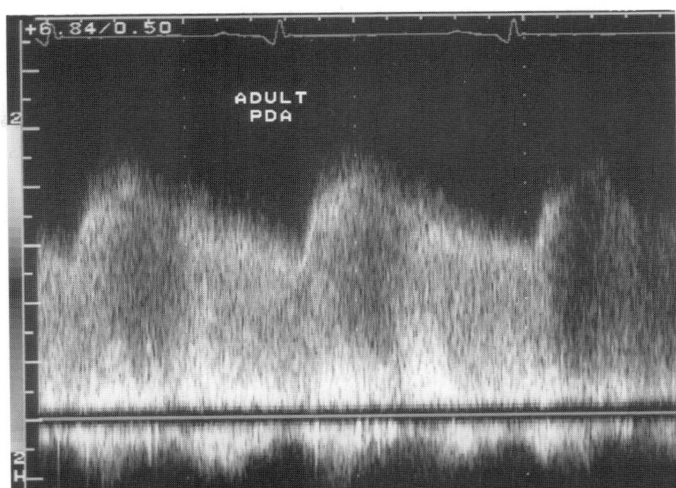

Fig. 16.17 Continuous wave Doppler of the same patient in Fig. 16.16. The high velocity continuous flow travels from the thoracic aorta into the pulmonary artery. Peak velocity occurs in late systole and is ~4.5 m/s.

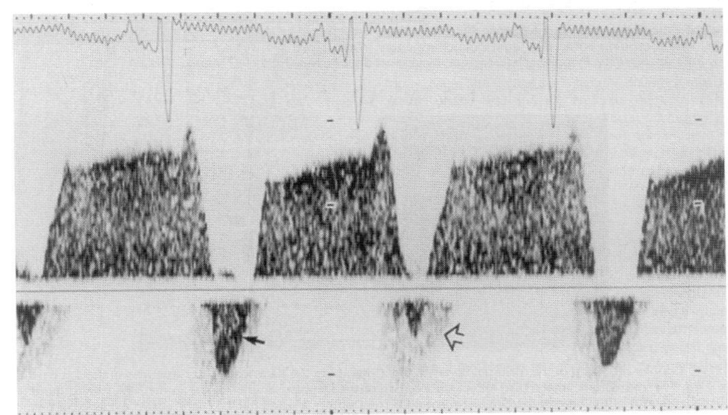

Fig. 16.18 Continuous wave Doppler in an infant with a PDA and pulmonary hypertension. Bidirectional shunting is evident with systolic flow (peaking in mid-to-late systole indicative of an oxygen saturation difference in the pulmonary artery proximal and distal to the ductus of 5–30%) away from the transducer (solid arrow). Late systolic flow extending through diastole (toward the transducer) represents left-to-right ductal flow. Flow from the left pulmonary artery (open arrow) may be confused with ductal flow. (Reproduced with permission from: Snider AR, Serwer GA, Ritter SB. Echocardiography in Pediatric Heart Disease, 2nd edn. St Louis, MO: Mosby, 1997: p 457, figure 11.7.)

beam should be near the pulmonary side of the ductus, and with a right-to-left shunt, the CW beam should be near the aortic side of the ductus.

Bidirectional flow may be noted in patients with marked pulmonary hypertension. Right-to-left flow will occur in systole (away from the transducer in a high parasternal window), and left-to-right flow from late systole through diastole (Fig. 16.18). Those patients with no oxygen saturation difference in the pulmonary artery proximal and distal to the ductus will have right-to-left flow peaking in early systole. Patients with an oxygen saturation change of from 5% to 30% will have peaking in mid to late systole. Echocardiography helps document positioning and success of placement of a PDA closure device (Fig. 16.19).

Coronary fistula

A *coronary fistula* (usually an incidental finding in ~0.2% of coronary arteriograms) is a rare defect involving the connection of a coronary artery with a cardiac chamber, great vessel, or other vascular structure without passing first through the myocardial capillaries. Over 90%, however, connect to the right heart (RA, RV, pulmonary artery (PA), coronary sinus, and SVC) (Fig. 16.20). Connection to the RV and PA are the most common. Most originate from the right coronary artery (RCA), but may arise from the left anterior descending (LAD) or circumflex coronary artery. The murmur of a coronary fistula is continuous, differing from that of a PDA only by its location.

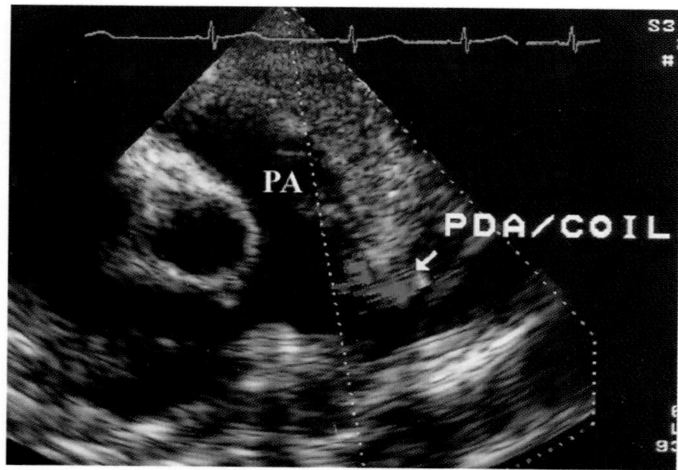

Fig. 16.19 High parasternal short axis image of an adolescent after closure of a PDA with an occluder device. Color Doppler reveals a small residual left-to-right shunt through the device.

(a)

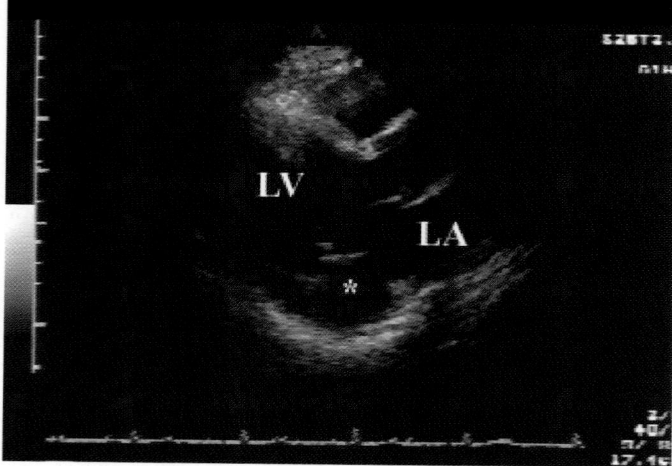

(b)

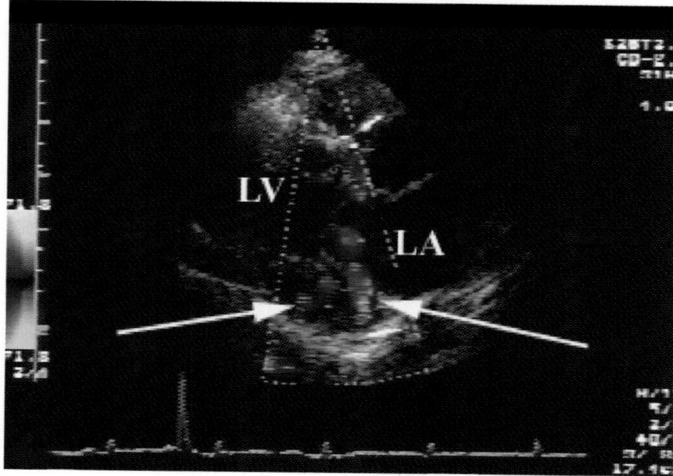

Fig. 16.20 A middle-aged male underwent echocardiography for a continuous murmur. He was found to have a circumflex artery to coronary sinus connection, with drainage into the RA. Real-time imaging demonstrated a dilated tortuous circumflex artery connecting to the coronary sinus. (a) Parasternal long axis imaging demonstrates an echo free space (*) posterior to the LA and LV, within the atrioventricular groove. (b) Color Doppler imaging reveals two distinct jets of flow (arrows) from the circumflex artery and the coronary sinus. (*Cont'd.*)

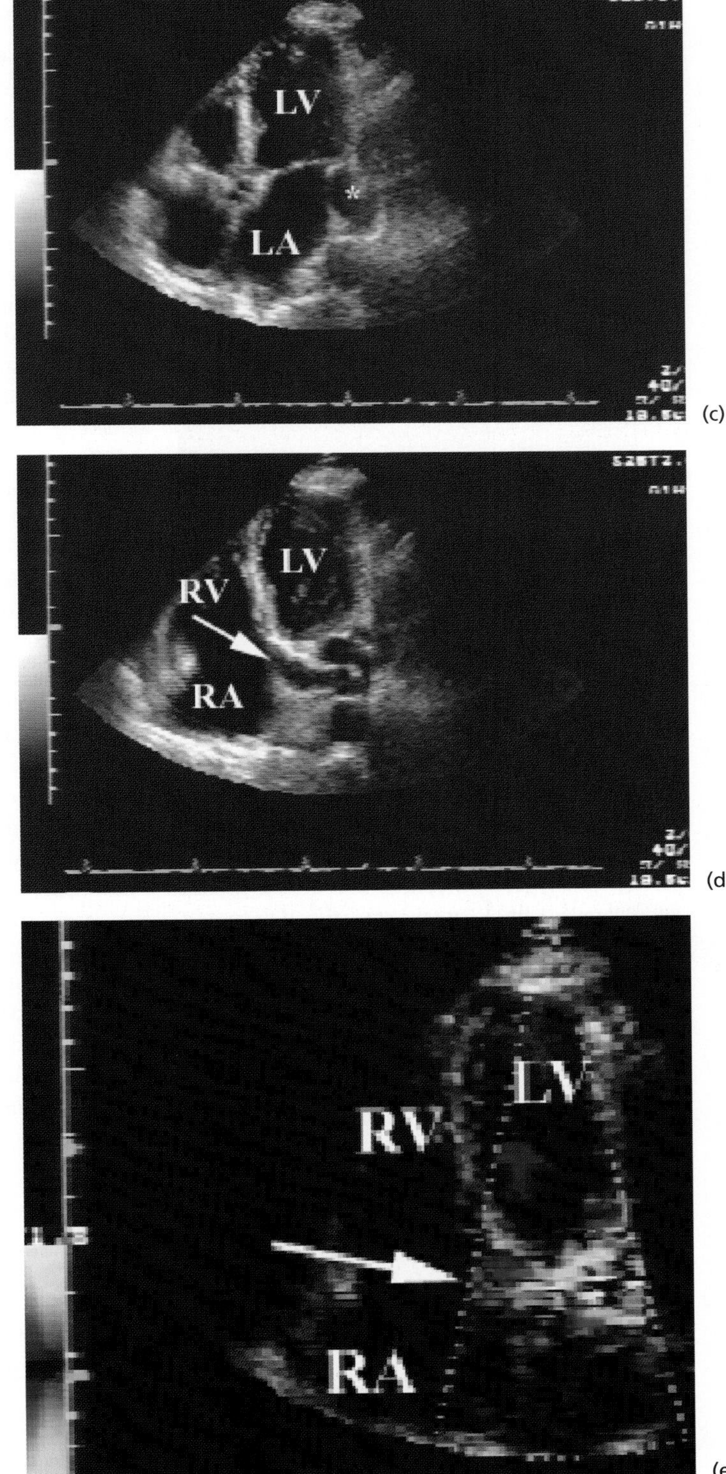

Fig. 16.20 (*cont'd*) (c) Apical four-chamber view again reveals an echo free space (*). One could follow its drainage (d) into the coronary sinus and subsequently the RA (arrow). (e) By color Doppler imaging, continuous flow was documented to enter the RA, via the coronary sinus (arrow).

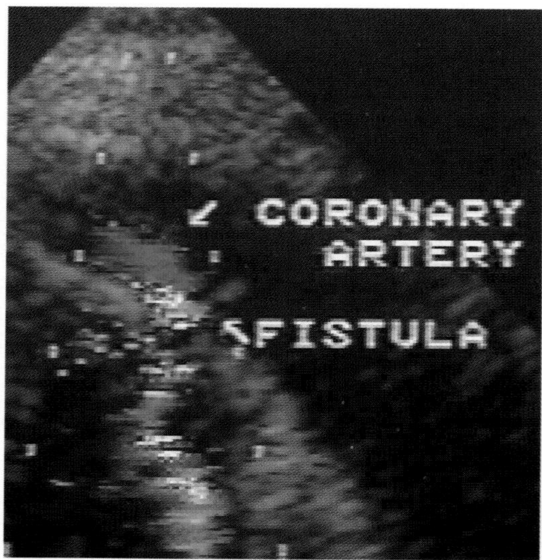

Fig. 16.21 Apical imaging of an 18-year-old female with a soft apical continuous murmur. The patient had a coronary artery (red) to RV fistula. Continuous turbulent flow at the RV apex was a feature that helped make the diagnosis.

When the fistula connects to the left ventricle, the murmur will be heard only in diastole.

The involved coronary will be dilated from its origin throughout its length. Its origin may be imaged best from a high parasternal short axis view. The uninvolved coronary artery should remain normal in size. Color Doppler helps locate the entry site. If the fistula enters the right heart there will be continuous color turbulence (Fig. 16.21), and if the fistula enters the left ventricle there will be color turbulence in diastole. If a LAD branch enters the main pulmonary artery, a small turbulent continuous color flow jet will be noted to enter the proximal main PA.

Coarctation of the aorta

Coarctation of the aorta may present in infants, adolescents, and adults. Infants will generally have a severe form—*aortic isthmal hypoplasia*—and may have other associated defects. Adolescents and adults often will be asymptomatic. These patients will usually have a discrete "shelf" at the junction of the transverse and descending aorta, which projects from the posterior aortic wall (an anterior shelf proximal to the ductus may be a normal finding). It is nearly always opposite the prenatal ductus arteriosus (*ligamentum arteriosum*), just distal to the left subclavian artery in the aorta (Fig. 16.22). Proximal to the coarctation, the transverse aorta is often somewhat small, and post-stenotic enlargement of the descending thoracic aorta is usually found (Fig. 16.23). Patients with the "infant" aortic isthmal hypoplasia form or even a complete aortic interruption may rarely present in adulthood.

An *abdominal coarctation* may rarely be found, and when present is usually associated with Turner's syndrome, neurofibromatosis, Takayasu's arteritis, or William's syndrome. This should be suspected in patients with any one of the above diagnoses or in patients with a substantial difference in arm and leg blood pressures.

Coarctation is an isolated finding in about 50% of cases. Associated congenital abnormalities include bicuspid aortic valve (50%) and occasionally a VSD or PDA. Coarctation of the aorta is the most common associated cardiac anomaly in patients with *Turner's syndrome*. The *Shone complex* involves left heart obstructive lesions at multiple levels which could include coarctation of the aorta, parachute mitral valve, bicuspid aortic valve, discrete or fibromuscular subaortic stenosis, or supravalvular mitral ring. An elongated *redundant mitral chordal apparatus* may be

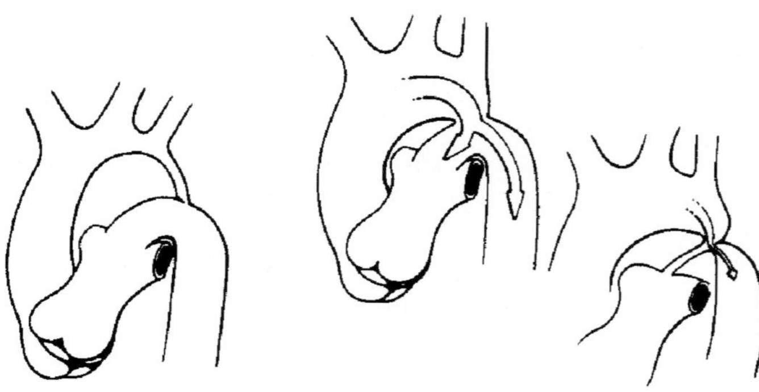

Fig. 16.22 Anatomic findings of coarctation of the aorta. (Left) Aortic isthmal hypoplasia most often found in infants. (Middle, right) Juxtaductal aortic ridge most often seen in older children and adults. (Reproduced with permission from: Cyran SE. Coarctation of the aorta in the adolescent and adult: echocardiographic evaluation prior to and following surgical repair. Echocardiography 1993; 10(5): 553.)

(a)

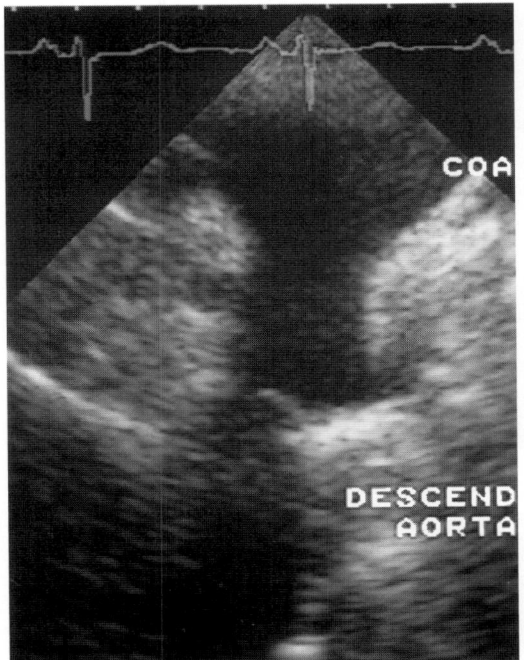

(b)

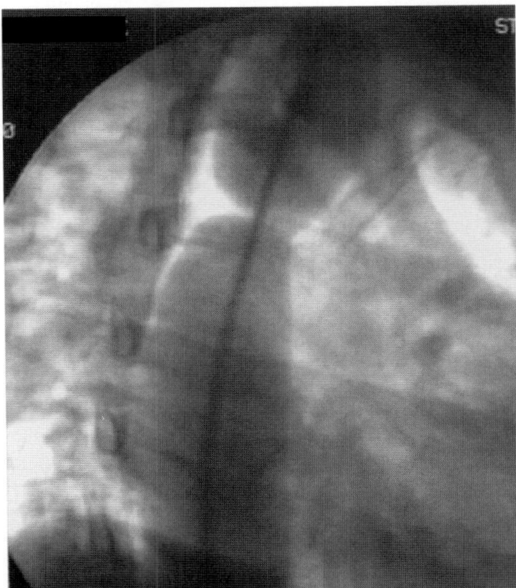

Fig. 16.23 "Adult" form of coarctation of the aorta with a "ridge" located opposite the ductus arteriosus (ligamentum arteriosum). (a) Suprasternal notch imaging of the descending thoracic aorta, and (b) corresponding aortogram.

associated with coarctation of the aorta. The chordae may be dramatically elongated and "prolapse" into the left ventricular outflow tract (LVOT) during systole. If this is noted, one should look for an associated coarctation.

It is important to search for associated congenital defects by echocardiography. TEE is better than transthoracic echocardiography (TTE) for identifying and characterizing the coarctation. Surface imaging of the aortic arch is usually performed from the suprasternal notch, but occasionally a better image is obtained from the medial right or left supra- (or sub-) clavicular areas. The area of coarctation may be best visualized from the suprasternal or right parasternal windows. For suprasternal imaging, the patient should be in the supine position. A towel can be placed under the shoulders, to allow the neck to be slightly hyperextended. Sometimes a better image can be obtained if the patient is sitting up with the neck extended. In patients with coarctation, one should use 2-D echo to:

- evaluate for associated defects, such as bicuspid aortic valve
- assess the ascending aorta
- assess the transverse aorta and great vessels for excessive narrowing
- assess the descending aorta—visualize the "shelf" and measure the distance of the shelf from the left subclavian artery
- evaluate LV and LV hypertrophy.

Color flow Doppler will help localize the site of coarctation by identifying the area of the development of flow turbulence. With color guidance, one can use continuous wave (CW) Doppler to obtain a velocity profile. Typically, a high systolic velocity with extension of a forward flow pattern into diastole will be found (Fig. 16.24). Collateral blood flow around the coarctation will result in a reduction of the Doppler-derived systolic gradient. The pressure difference across the coarctation will be reduced as the pressure in the aorta distal to the coarctation will not drop as much as would be expected secondary to collateral flow, but importantly, the diastolic forward gradient will persist, helping to make the diagnosis. The classic pattern may not be found in patients with diminished cardiac output or patients with a large patent ductus arteriosus in whom the gradient will be diminished. At times, the peak Doppler gradient across the coarctation may overestimate the true gradient if the

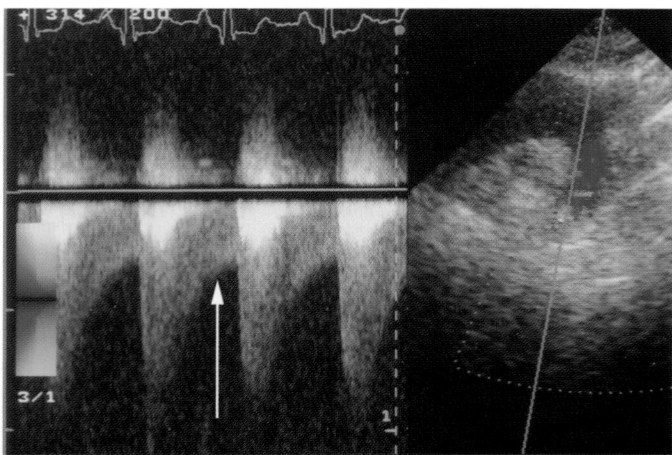

Fig. 16.24 Coarctation of the aorta. (Left panel) CW Doppler of the descending thoracic aorta demonstrates a high systolic gradient and diastolic persistence (arrow). (Right panel) Suprasternal imaging of the descending aorta with color Doppler to help "line up" the CW probe.

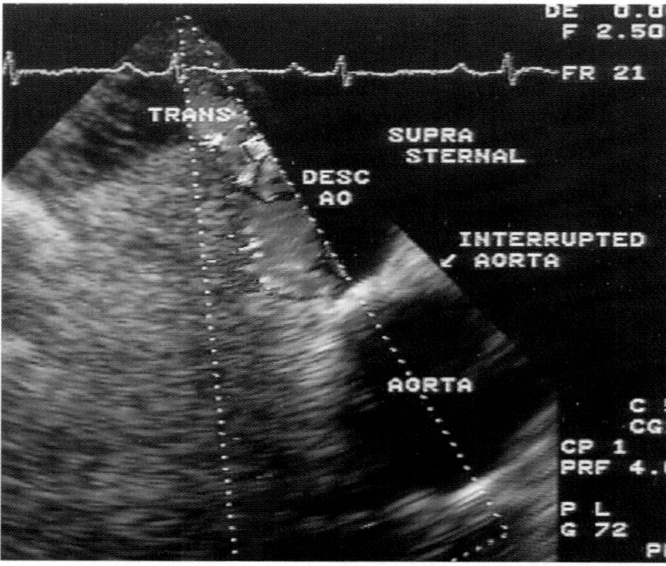

Fig. 16.25 A 40-year-old-male presented with congestive heart failure. He was found to have severe aortic regurgitation and LV dysfunction. Cardiac catheterization was attempted via the femoral arterial route, but a catheter could not be passed into the aortic arch. The procedure was then performed via the right antecubital artery. Aortography revealed an interrupted aorta with excellent collateral circulation distal to the aortic obstruction. Transthoracic suprasternal imaging with color Doppler documents an enlarged transverse aorta (TRANS) and proximal descending aorta (DESC AO) with subsequent complete interruption. The aorta distal to the obstruction (AORTA) is also visualized.

velocity proximal to the narrowing is elevated. The proximal velocity term must be included in calculating the gradient when using the Bernoulli equation (see Chapter: 3) as:

$$\text{Pressure gradient} = 4(V_2^2 - V_1^2)$$

where V_2 is the CW Doppler-derived peak velocity across the obstruction and V_1 is the velocity proximal to the obstruction.

Interrupted aorta is a severe form of coarctation. Rarely will it present in adulthood. Extensive collateral flow is necessary (Fig. 16.25). Repair of coarctation of the aorta may be accomplished by balloon catheter dilatation in children. It is also often used for recurrence of residual stenosis postoperatively. TEE is helpful for the diagnosis of dilatation-associated dissection.

Surgical repair includes an end-to-end anastomosis, patch aortoplasty with a prosthetic patch, or subclavian flap aortoplasty (Fig. 16.26). One should evaluate a postoperative patient in a manner similar to that of an uncorrected patient. Several anatomic variations may be found postoperatively:

- normal patent aorta
- mild narrowing or arch

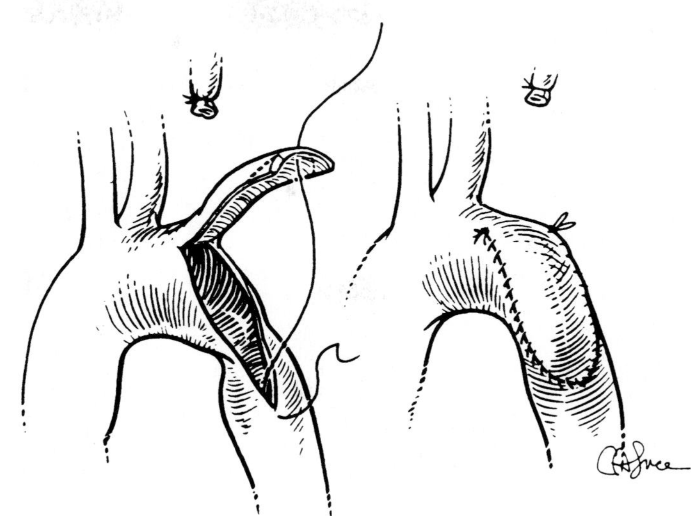

Fig. 16.26 Subclavian flap aortoplasty repair of aortic intimal hypoplasia. (Reproduced with permission from: Dron IL, *et al*. Incidence and risk after coarctation repair. Annals of Thoracic Surgery 1990; 49: 910–926.)

- inverted "V" configuration of the transverse arch
- small nonobstructed arch shelf
- mild tortuosity of the arch and descending aorta.

Continuous wave Doppler evaluation of the postoperative descending aorta helps evaluate for postoperative residual narrowing. A peak velocity of more than 2.5 m/s correlates with narrowing of more than 25%. Persistent antegrade diastolic flow suggests restenosis or aneurysmal dilatation of the aorta. Some patients have no Doppler gradient at rest, but manifest a significant systolic gradient with exercise. Patients in the immediate postoperative period do not need stress testing, but later on postoperative patients should be evaluated with exercise stress testing for exercise-associated hypertension. A Pedoff CW transducer may be placed in the suprasternal notch for velocity measurements in each stage of the Bruce protocol, during peak exercise (standing), and then serially in the recovery phase (supine position).

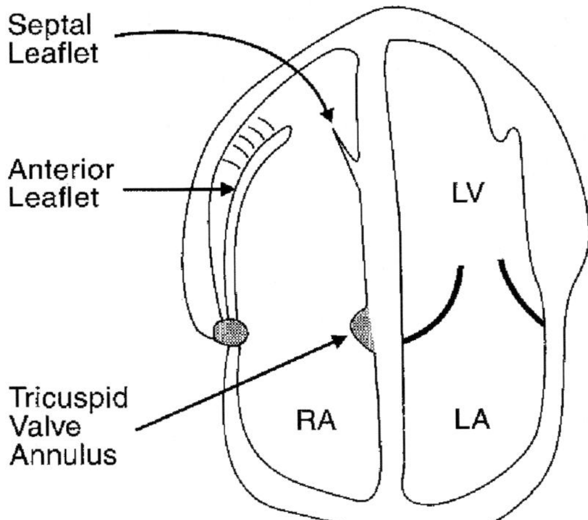

Fig. 16.27 Representation of Ebstein's anomaly. The septal and posterior leaflets are apically displaced, and may be hypoplastic. The anterior leaflet inserts into the tricuspid annulus, but is often redundant and thickened, and is attached to the wall of the right ventricle.

Ebstein's anomaly

Ebstein's anomaly involves a malformation of the septal and posterior leaflets of the tricuspid valve with apical displacement (the septal leaflet may be absent or rudimentary). These leaflets may be dysplastic. The anterior leaflet is enlarged and elongated. Its origin is from the normal position of the tricuspid annulus (Fig. 16.27), and is attached to the trabecular and outflow portions of the RV. Tethering of the anterior leaflet is defined as three or more accessory attachments of the leaflet to the RV wall, causing restricted valve leaflet motion.

Often present, an associated ASD is of the secundum type (40–60% of patients) but a PFO or sinus venosus ASD with partial anomalous pulmonary venous return may be seen. Because of substantial tricuspid regurgitation (TR) and RV dysfunction, a right-to-left shunt may be present. Patients with an ASD may demonstrate significant right-to-left

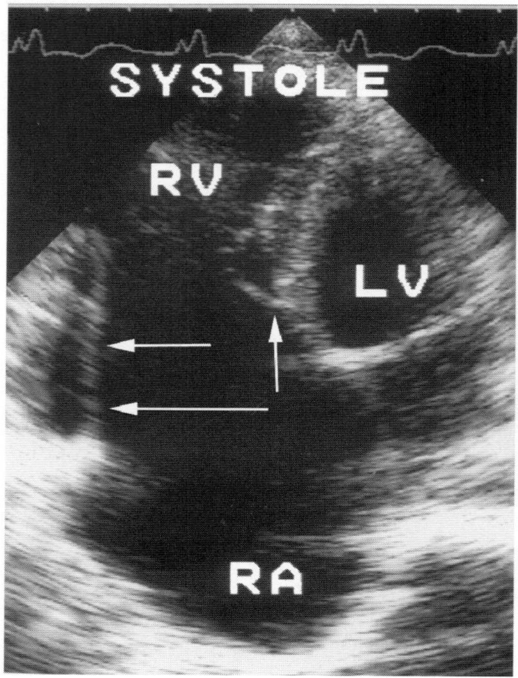

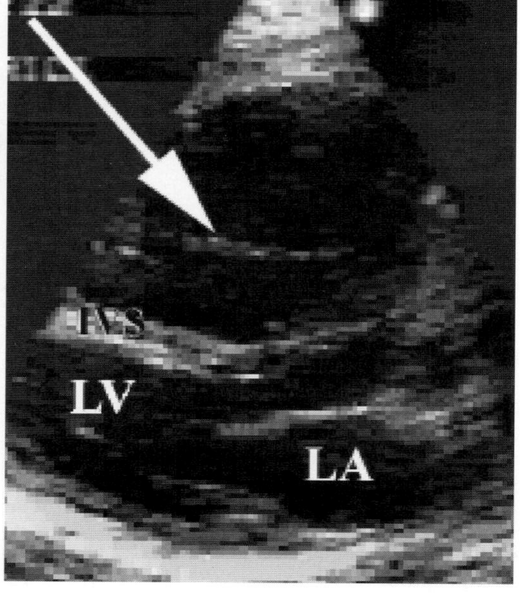

Fig. 16.28 (a) Apical four-chamber view of an adult patient with Ebstein's anomaly. The anterior leaflet (horizontal arrows) has the tricuspid valve (TV) annulus as its origin. It is elongated and tethered to the RV wall. The septal leaflet (vertical arrow) is apically displaced. (b) Parasternal long axis view of a patient with Ebstein's anomaly. The long anterior leaflet of the tricuspid valve (arrow) appears serpentine during real-time imaging. IVS, interventricular septum.

shunting in early adulthood. Wolff–Parkinson–White syndrome may be found in 10–15% of patients. Some degree of obstruction to RV inflow and also RV outflow (anterior leaflet redundancy causing obstruction) may also be found. Tricuspid regurgitation is a hallmark, with TR emanating from the RV cavity at the site of valve tips. Because of apically displaced septal and posterior leaflets, the RA is enlarged with an "atrialized" portion of the RV found. The anatomic RV is often small and dysfunctional.

Septal leaflet insertion displacement should be measured. A displacement of 20 mm beyond the level of the mitral valve annulus is definitely abnormal, but a more accurate criterion is 8-mm/m^2 body surface area. Also delayed closure of the tricuspid valve, as compared with the mitral valve, of more than 80 ms may be found by M-mode echocardiography.

The apical four-chamber view is best to find the origin of the septal leaflet, the attachments of the anterior leaflet, and the true right ventricle (Fig. 16.28). From the parasternal long axis view during real-time imaging, the elongated anterior leaflet within the body of RV may have a serpentine-like undulating appearance.

By echocardiography, one should be sure to assess TV septal leaflet displacement, evaluate the anterior leaflet for tethering and mobility, evaluate for an atrial level shunt (and shunt direction), and evaluate both right and left ventricular function.

Marfan's syndrome

Marfan's syndrome (see Chapter 19) is a generalized disorder of connective tissue occurring in 1 in 15 000 persons. Around 60–70% of patients have an affected parent. It is characterized by musculoskeletal abnormalities, including tall stature, arachnodactyly, scoliosis, pectus deformities, and laxity of ligaments. Other abnormalities include lens dislocation and myopia. The mitral and aortic valves are characterized by

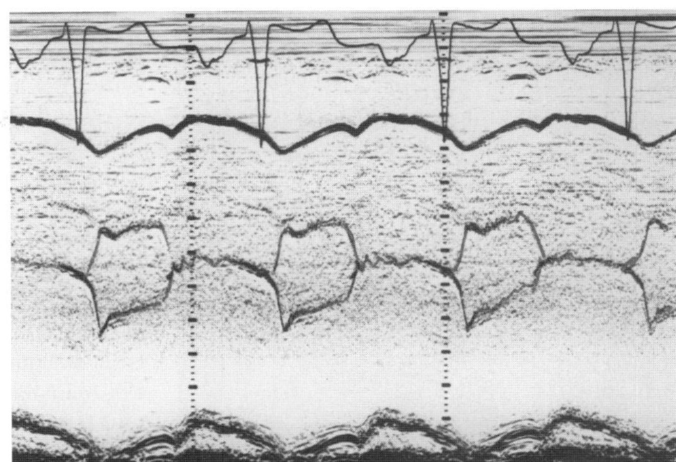

Fig. 16.29 Annuloaortic ectasia in a patient with Marfan's syndrome. M-mode at the level of the aortic valve reveals a profoundly dilated aortic root.

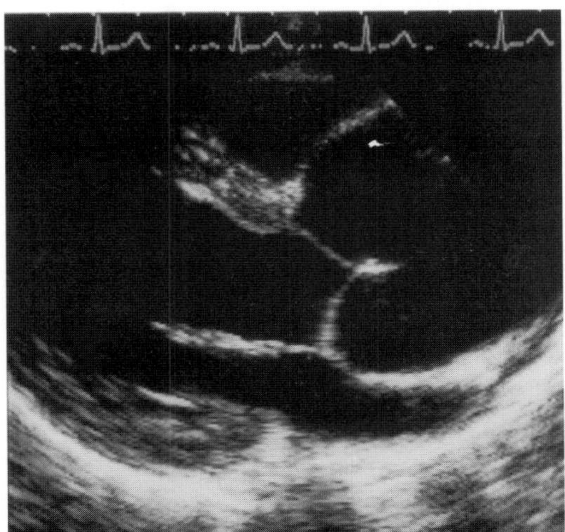

Fig. 16.30 Two-dimensional parasternal long axis image in a patient with Marfan's syndrome and annuloaortic ectasia.

myxomatous degeneration with material separating the normal cells of the valves.

Annuloaortic ectasia is common in patients with *Marfan's syndrome* and probably is a result of an abnormality of the media (sometimes termed *cystic medial necrosis*). The proximal ascending aorta is symmetrically dilated (Figs 16.29 & 16.30), often with dilatation of the sinuses of Valsalva and aortic annulus. The sinuses of Valsalva are often dilated at birth. Aortic regurgitation is due to annular dilatation with inadequate leaflet coaptation. Because of the dilated aortic root, the left atrium may be reduced in dimension. Annuloaortic ectasia may also occur with Ehlers–Danlos syndrome, osteogenesis imperfecta, autosomal dominant polycystic kidney disease, or may be idiopathic. Aortic dissection typically starts in the ascending aorta. It may propagate retrograde into the pericardium, and also antegrade to involve the thoracic and abdominal aorta.

In 60–80% of patients with Marfan's syndrome, *mitral valve prolapse* (MVP) has been found by echocardiography. The mitral valve leaflets may appear elongated and redundant. The mitral annulus may dilate, adding to the mitral regurgitation. Ruptured chordae have been reported.

Fixed "discrete" subaortic outflow tract obstruction

Subaortic obstruction should be considered whenever the LVOT region is narrower than the aortic annulus. Fixed obstructive lesions of the LVOT are generally categorized into one of three groups: *discrete fibrous membrane*, *thick fibrous ring*, or *fibromuscular tunnel*. With each type, *early systolic closure* of the aortic valve leaflets (Fig. 16.31) may be noted by M-mode echocardiography (mid-systolic closure is generally noted with hypertrophic cardiomyopathy).

It is important to properly classify the discrete fibrous membrane, since surgical resection of a membrane will usually improve the gradient (Fig. 16.32). With the other two forms a more extensive surgical

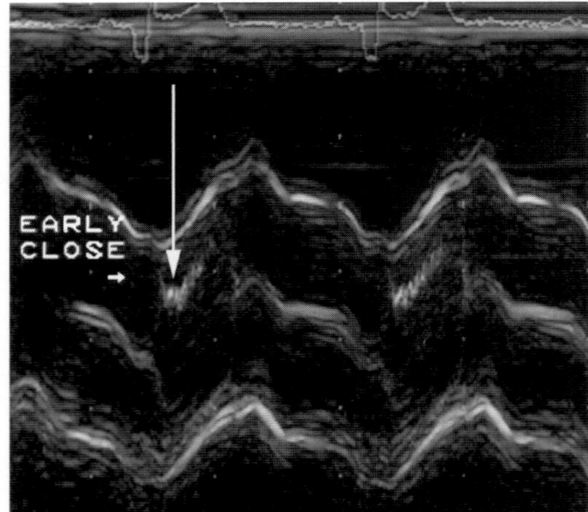

Fig. 16.31 Discrete subaortic stenosis. M-mode of the aortic valve reveals early closure (vertical arrow) followed by coarse systolic leaflet fluttering. Early systolic closure may be absent if there is coexistent aortic valve thickening or a bicuspid valve.

resection is usually required. With a discrete fibrous membrane, the edges usually appear brighter than the membrane itself. During systole, the membrane may appear to move toward the aortic valve, and then move back toward the LV in diastole.

Defects associated with a discrete fibrous membrane include a perimembranous VSD, bicuspid aortic valve, and coarctation of the aorta.

A *thick fibrous ring* produces a more diffuse area of LVOT obstruction. It may involve the anterior leaflet of the mitral valve. The *fibromuscular tunnel* involves both borders of the LVOT. Obstructive LVOT lesions will involve the anterior leaflet of the mitral valve (Fig. 16.33).

The CW Doppler pattern of a discrete fibrous membrane is similar to that of a fixed obstruction (such as found with valvular aortic stenosis) and differs from the concave shape found with dynamic LVOT (such as found with hypertrophic obstructive cardiomyopathy). The CW velocity envelope is generally representative of the pressure gradient across the membrane. With a LVOT tunnel, however, the modified Bernoulli equation may not be accurate, and the Doppler gradient may overestimate the gradient measured by catheterization.

Supravalvular aortic stenosis

Supravalvular aortic stenosis may present in young adults but is rare. Obstruction may present as an "hour-glass" narrowing of the aortic sinotubular

(a)

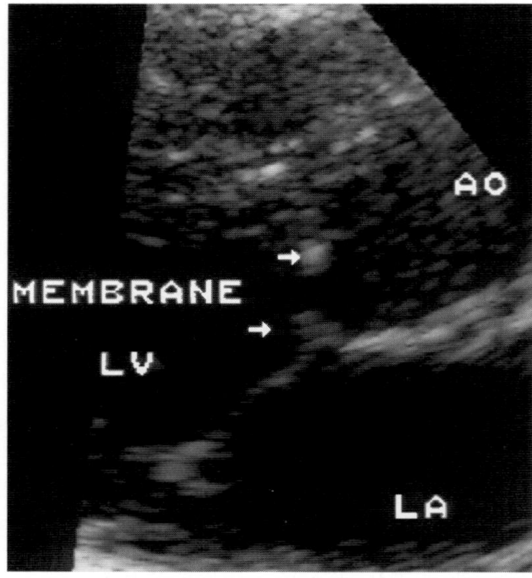

(b)

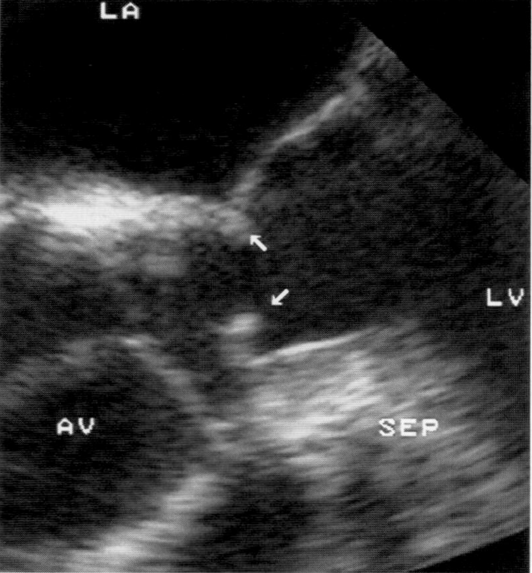

Fig. 16.32 A patient with exertional dyspnea and a murmur was found to have discrete subaortic stenosis. Fifteen years earlier the patient had a perimembranous VSD surgically closed. (a) Parasternal long axis and (b) TEE transverse image demonstrate the subaortic membrane (arrows). AO, ascending aorta; AV, aortic valve; SEP, ventricular septum.

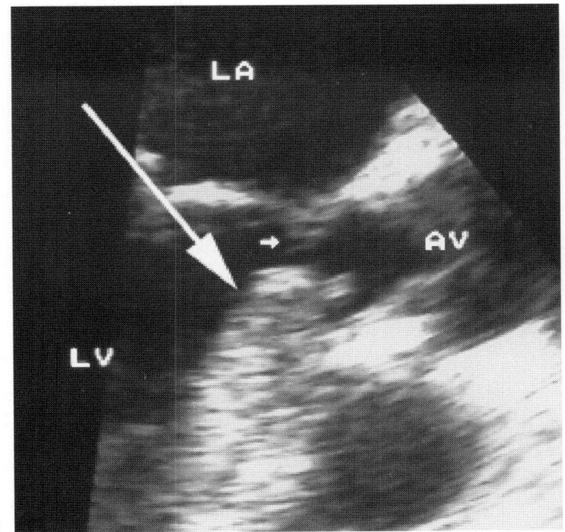

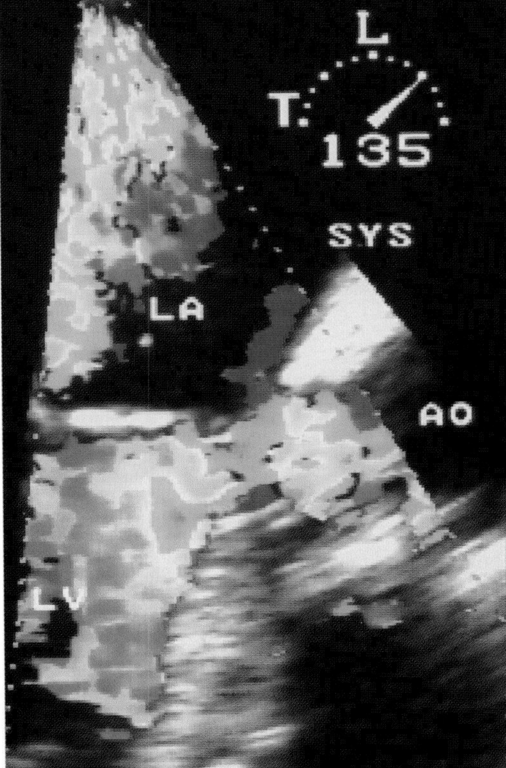

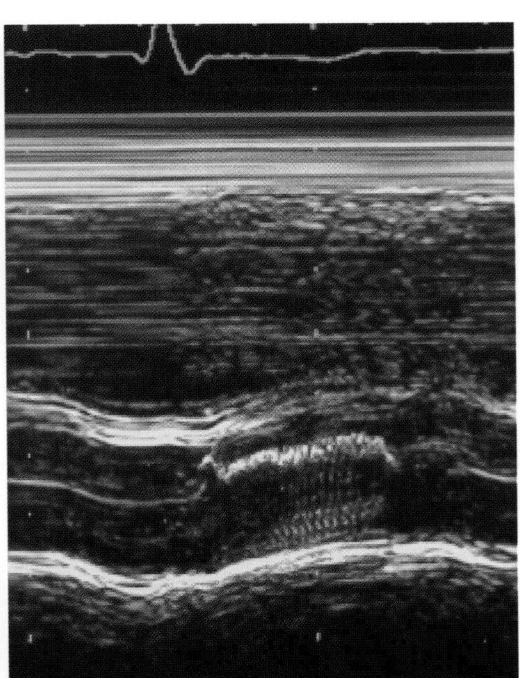

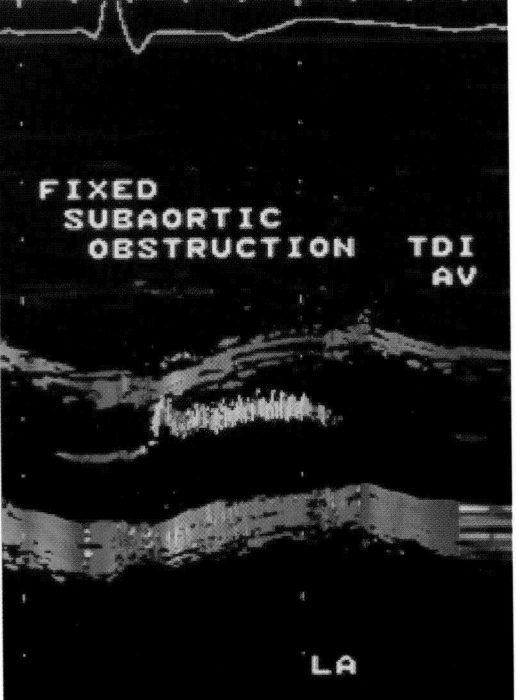

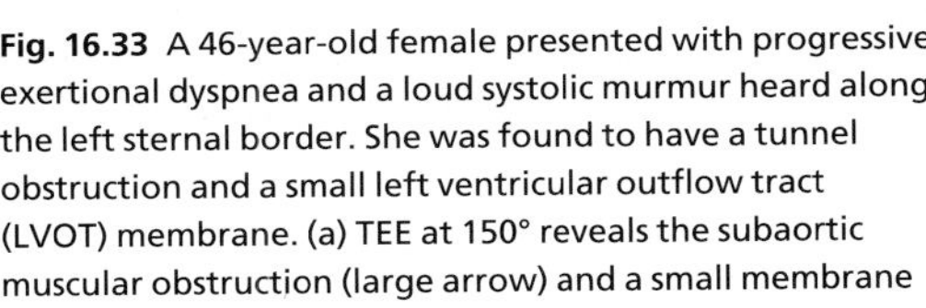

Fig. 16.33 A 46-year-old female presented with progressive exertional dyspnea and a loud systolic murmur heard along the left sternal border. She was found to have a tunnel obstruction and a small left ventricular outflow tract (LVOT) membrane. (a) TEE at 150° reveals the subaortic muscular obstruction (large arrow) and a small membrane (small arrow). (b) Corresponding color Doppler (at 135°) image reveals that turbulent flow begins within the LVOT. (c,d) An M-mode tracing through the aortic valve. (d) Tissue Doppler imaging (TDI) highlights the observed early systolic notching followed by aortic leaflet vibratory motion. (*Continued on p. 266.*)

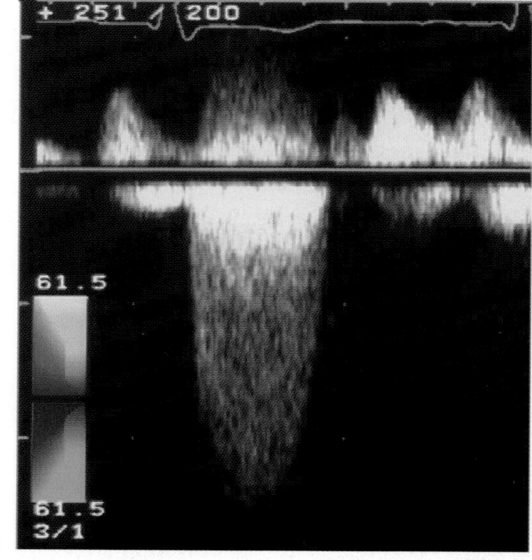

(e)

(f)

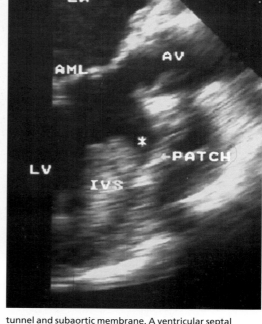

Fig. 16.33 (*cont'd*) (e) Continuous wave Doppler of the LVOT from an apical five-chamber view reveals a fixed obstruction pattern, with a peak velocity of 5 m/s. (f) TEE at 135° after the patient underwent resection of the muscular tunnel and subaortic membrane. A ventricular septal defect (*) was created, with a patch (PATCH) placed on the right ventricular side of the defect.

junction (two thirds of cases), discrete membranous or weblike obstruction at the sinotubular junction (10% of cases), or as a diffuse hypoplasia of the ascending aorta (20% of cases). *Normally, the sinotubular junction will not be smaller than the aortic annulus* (if so it is abnormally diminished in diameter). If one notes an increased turbulent flow across an anatomically normal aortic valve, one should look for supravalvular aortic stenosis. This is often best recorded from the right parasternal window in the right supine position, or from the suprasternal window.

Congenitally corrected transposition of the great arteries (l-transposition)

Transposition describes a discordant connection between the ventricles and great vessels (aorta arises from the morphologic RV and pulmonary artery arises from the morphologic LV). *Congenitally corrected transposition of the great arteries* will often present in adulthood. There is *atrioventricular discordance* (proper positioned RA connected to morphologic LV, and proper positioned LA connected to morphologic RV) and also *ventriculoarterial discordance* (morphologic LV connected to pulmonary artery, and morphologic RV connected to the aorta). The "l" describes the position of the aortic valve to that of the pulmonic valve. As the aortic valve is most often to the left of the pulmonic valve, this is termed an *l-transposition* (*d-transposition* describes the aortic valve to the right of the pulmonic valve).

With congenitally corrected transposition there are two disconcordant levels (basically the ventricles have "exchanged positions"); therefore the circulation is hemodynamically correct (hence the term "congenitally corrected transposition"). The tricuspid valve will be on the systemic side, and the mitral valve on the venous side of the circulation. The ventricular outflow tracts and the great vessels are parallel in orientation (Fig. 16.34).

Patients often lead a normal life, unless other

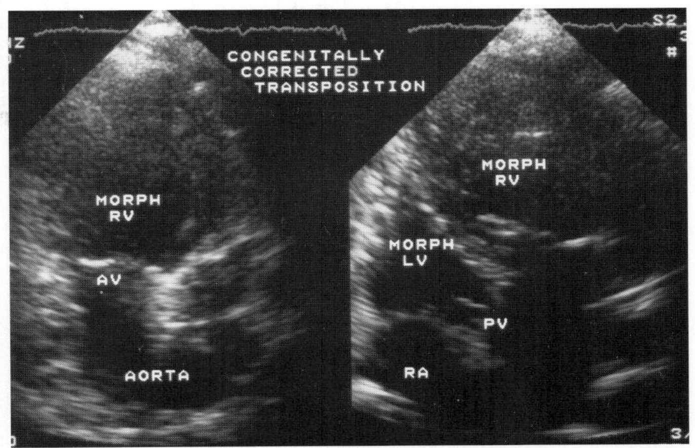

(a)

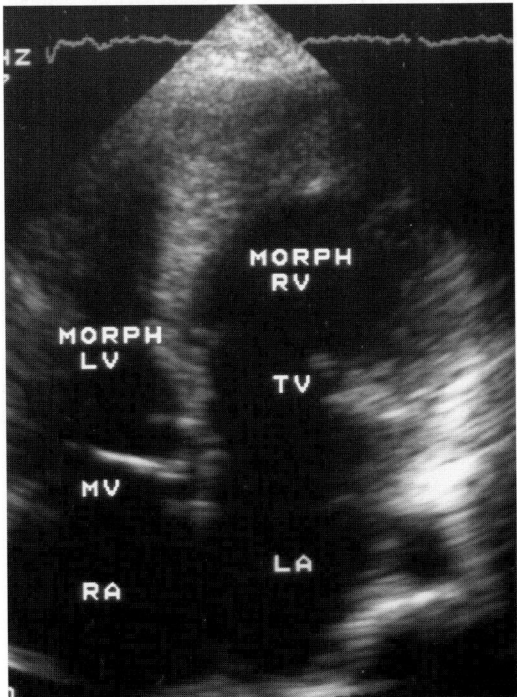

(b)

Fig. 16.34 A middle-aged male was referred for progressive exertional dyspnea and a systolic murmur at the cardiac apex. Echocardiography revealed congenitally corrected transposition of the great vessels, with significant regurgitation of the tricuspid valve (systemic AV valve connecting the left atrium and morphologic right ventricle). (a) Apical images of the ventriculo-arterial connections—(right panel) The RA and mitral valve connect to the morphologic LV (MORPH LV). This connects to the pulmonic valve (PV) and pulmonary artery. (Left panel) Anterior transducer angulation reveals the morphologic right ventricle (MORPH RV), which functions as the systemic ventricle, connected to the aortic valve (AV) and aorta. (b) Apical image demonstrates that the tricuspid valve maintains its relative apical displacement, as compared to the mitral valve. (*Continued on p. 268.*)

associated defects coexist. These defects include a VSD (70%—perimembranous), pulmonary outflow obstruction (40%—subvalvular), and an abnormal left-sided tricuspid valve (Ebstein-like valve). Complete heart block is also common. The left-sided tricuspid valve is abnormal in 90% of patients, with regurgitation often requiring surgical intervention. Symptoms related to left-sided atrio-ventricular valvular regurgitation is a relatively common presentation in the adult patient, who may have previously been asymptomatic and undiagnosed with this disorder.

Tetralogy of Fallot

Tetralogy of Fallot is defined as a large VSD, an overriding aorta, pulmonary stenosis, and RV hypertrophy. About 25% will have a right-sided aortic arch, and 15% an ASD (*pentalogy of Fallot*). Upwards

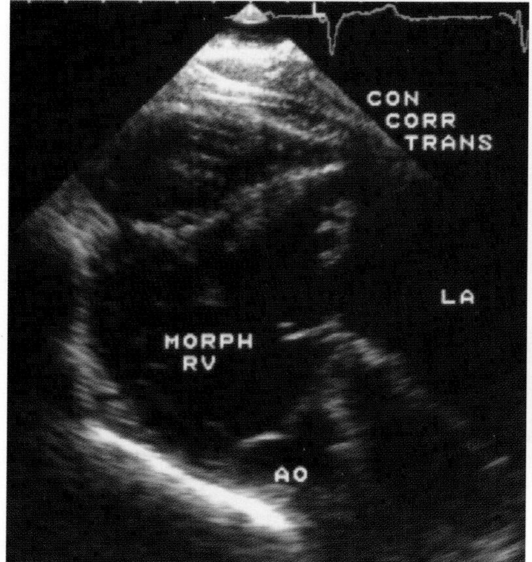

(c)

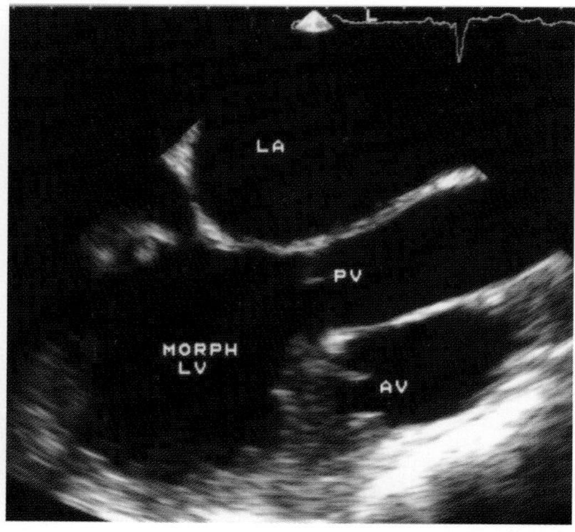

(d)

Fig. 16.34 (*cont'd*) (c) TEE in the longitudinal view reveals the properly positioned LA connected to the morphologic TV and RV (MORPH RV), which subsequently is connected to the aortic valve and aorta (AO). (d) TEE in the longitudinal view demonstrates the connection of the morphologic LV (MORPH LV) with the PV and pulmonary artery.

of 10% will have a left anterior descending coronary artery (LAD) that arises from the right coronary artery, or there will be bilateral LAD vessels.

The overriding aorta is best noted in the parasternal long axis view. The aorta and mitral valve remain in normal continuity, but the ventricular septum and anterior aortic annulus are discontinuous. From a high parasternal short axis view, an anteriorly deviated conal septum, resulting in narrowing of the right ventricular outflow tract (RVOT), is noted. The most common form of VSD is a large perimembranous outlet defect. The pulmonary valve is bicuspid in ~50% and tricuspid in ~40%. Stenosis is common. In addition, the valve may be atretic.

Postoperatively, one should evaluate the right heart for pulmonic stenosis (infundibular dynamic obstruction, pulmonic valve level, pulmonary artery branches, and distal suture line of patch), pulmonary regurgitation, and tricuspid regurgitation. Calculation of RV pressure using the tricuspid regurgitant velocity will assist in determining the degree of obstruction to RV outflow. Other abnormalities to assess include aortic regurgitation (which may result from placement of the ventricular patch), residual VSDs (which are usually insignificant), and a coronary artery to RV fistula. The latter may become manifest in the postoperative period as the high RV pressures drop toward normal levels.

17

CHAPTER 17

Source of Embolism

Of 500 000 strokes yearly in the United States, about 100 000 are of cardiac origin. Another 100 000–200 000 strokes are of undetermined cause (*cryptogenic stroke*). In this group, an increasing number of echocardiographic abnormal findings have been noted. Potential etiologies of a cardiac source of embolism include the following:

Left atrial/left atrial appendage (LAA) thrombus:
- atrial fibrillation
- atrial flutter.

Left ventricular (LV) thrombus:
- LV aneurysm
- myocardial infarction
- dilated (congestive) cardiomyopathy.

Valvular heart disease:
- rheumatic valvular disease
- prosthetic heart valves
- endocarditis (infective, marantic, Libman–Sacks)
- mitral annulus calcification (MAC).

Cardiac tumors:
- atrial myxoma
- papillary fibroelastoma.

Aorta:
- protruding or ulcerative atheroma.

Intracardiac shunt:
- patent foramen ovale (PFO)/atrial septal aneurysm (ASA)
- atrial septal defect (ASD)
- pulmonary AV shunt.

Fibrinous valve strands:
- prosthetic strands
- Lambl's excrescences.

Conditions classified as "high risk" for an association with cardioembolism include: LA/LAA thrombus, LV thrombus, prosthetic valve thrombus, endocarditis, intracardiac tumors, and protruding and/or mobile aortic atherosclerotic debris. Conditions classified as less of an association include PFO, ASA, and spontaneous echo contrast. Conditions classified as "low risk" of association with cardioembolism include mitral valve prolapse, fibrous strands, and MAC.

When performing transthoracic echocardiography (TTE) for source of embolism, specific attention should be paid to evaluation of *LA size* and LV function. Transesophageal echocardiography (TEE) has an advantage over TTE in better imaging of several sources of emboli including LA and LAA thrombus, PFO, and complex atheroma in the aorta.

Left atrium, left atrial appendage, and atrial fibrillation

Atrial fibrillation is clearly the most common cause of cardiac source of emboli. The likelihood of thrombus formation is highest in those with a dilated atrium. LA size can be measured by M-mode but is better quantified in the apical four- and two-chamber views. Calculation of atrial volumes is more accurate for identifying an enlarged LA (see Chapter 6). The LAA can occasionally be viewed by TTE, especially when enlarged. The best views to image the LAA by TTE are the high parasternal short axis or apical views (Fig. 17.1). TEE, however, consistently images the LAA and has a much greater chance of imaging a LAA thrombus. Chronic atrial fibrillation is associated with progressively enlarging atria. Resumption of sinus rhythm may reverse this process.

TEE is also better than TTE for detection of thrombus within the body of the LA, especially the upper atrial wall near the pulmonary veins, which is not well seen by TTE. As a rule of thumb, masses adjacent to the atrial septum are tumors, those laterally usually are thrombi, and on the roof of the LA either thrombi or tumors. There are exceptions to this rule, however (Fig. 17.2).

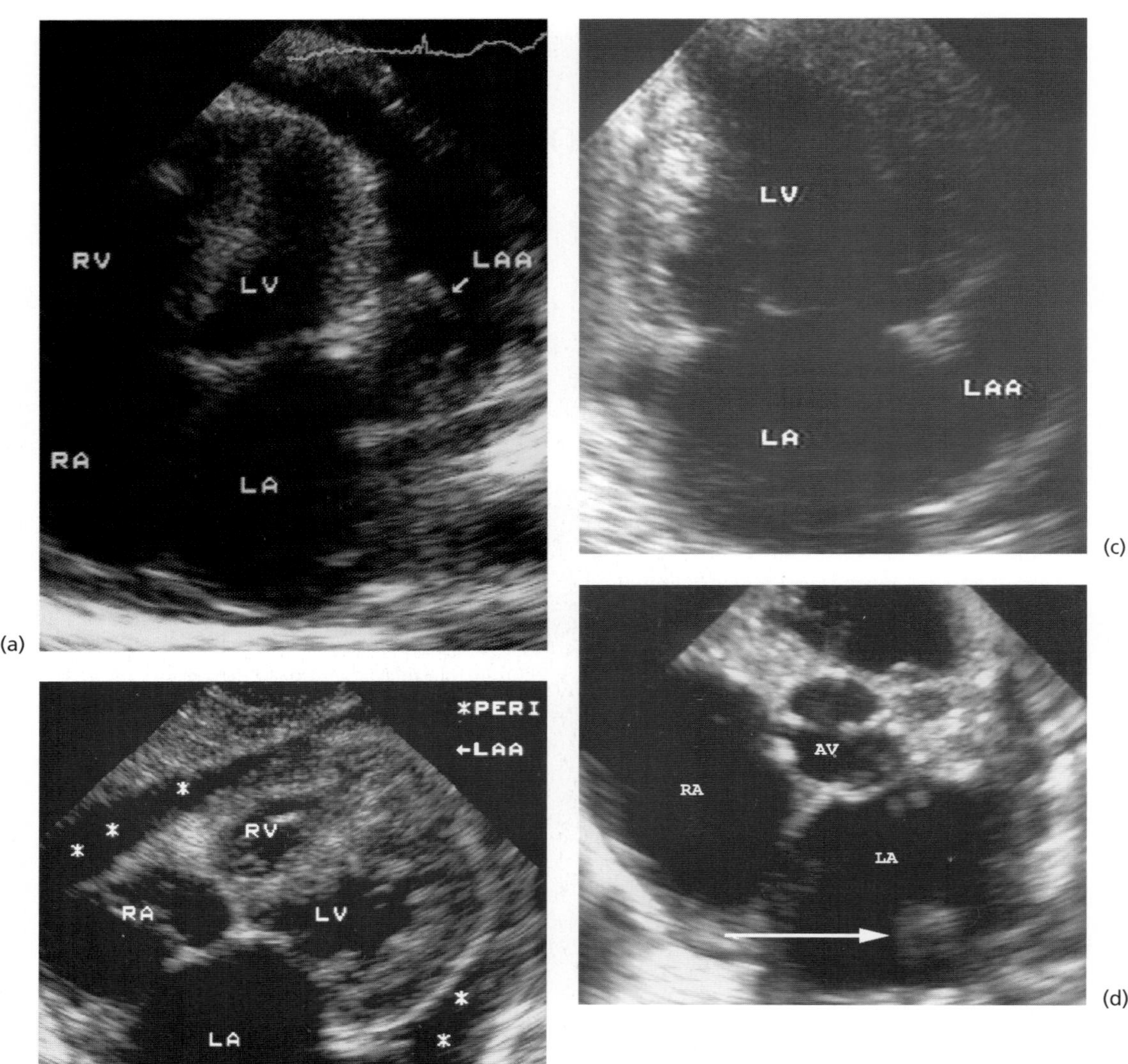

(a) (b) (c) (d)

Fig. 17.1 Transthoracic echocardiographic (TTE) imaging of the left atrial appendage (LAA). A patient with a pericardial effusion is imaged in (a) four-chamber view and (b) subcostal image. Another patient (c) is imaged in an apical two-chamber view, and in (d) parasternal short axis at the level of the aortic valve reveals not only the LAA, but a posterior LA thrombus (arrow).

The size of the LA alone is generally not a predictor of a successful cardioversion of atrial fibrillation to normal sinus. However, patients with *longstanding atrial fibrillation*, a *LA dimension greater than >60 mm*, or *rheumatic mitral valve disease* are not likely to remain in sinus rhythm.

It should be kept in mind that the LAA is a complex structure (Fig. 17.3), frequently having more than one "apex," and may be multilobed; therefore, several TEE positions should be used, with multiple imaging planes (often transverse and longitudinal).

It is important not to confuse LAA thrombus with normal findings, namely the normal *pectinate muscles*, noting that they remain continuous within the ridge of

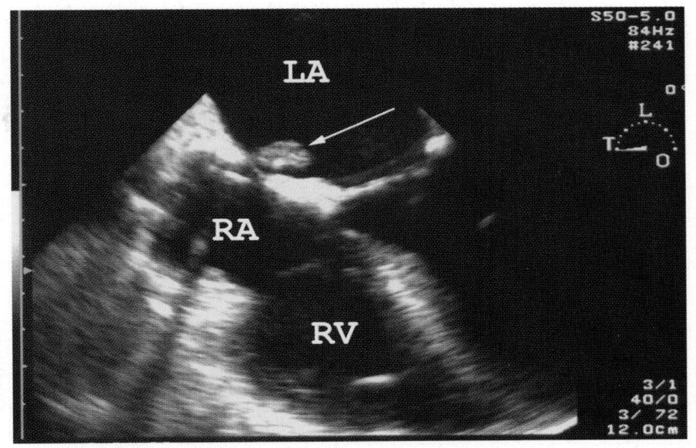

(a)

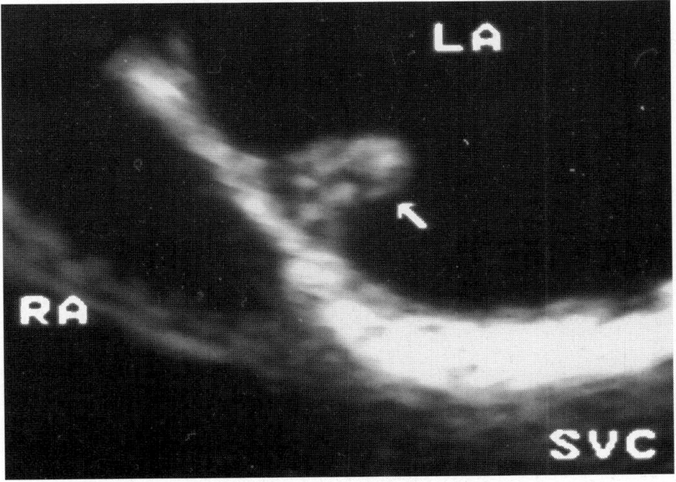

(b)

Fig. 17.2 Intraoperative TEE of a patient during aortic valve replacement for aortic stenosis. The patient was in normal sinus rhythm. The mass was attached to the interatrial septum as noted in (a) the horizontal plane and (b) the vertical plane. Histologic examination revealed the mass to be thrombus. (Reproduced with permission from: Kerut EK, Dearstine M, Everson CT, Giles TD. Left atrial septum thrombus masquerading as a myxoma in a patient with aortic stenosis in sinus rhythm. Echocardiography 2001; 18: 709–10.)

the LAA (Fig. 17.4). The *transverse sinus* may be evident on occasion and may have adipose tissue within it. This may be easily misinterpreted as thrombus in the LAA. To help differentiate the transverse sinus from LAA clot, rotation of the TEE probe may help confirm that the structure containing the presumed thrombus is not connected to the LA (Fig. 17.5). In addition, color and pulsed wave Doppler should reveal no "flow" within the structure.

When assessing the LAA for thrombus (Fig. 17.6), the following features should be evaluated to assess for LAA thrombus potential:

- LAA size
- LAA pulse wave Doppler flow patterns
- LAA/LA spontaneous echo contrast.

The presence of these features helps increase the likelihood that a potential abnormality is in fact a thrombus. Sometimes attempting to differentiate a thrombus from a normal structure is extremely difficult. As a rule of thumb, the smaller the size of the LAA, the less likely it is to harbor thrombus.

TEE has allowed for characterization of LA and LAA flow using pulsed wave Doppler. Patients with normal flow patterns within the LAA (normal 46 ± 18 cm/s) have a low likelihood of thrombus formation, whereas, those with reduced flow tend to have a higher likelihood. Some investigators have demonstrated that patients with atrial arrhythmia (atrial fibrillation, atrial flutter) may be risk stratified by the flow velocities found within the LAA. If flows remain high in patients with these arrhythmias, there is thought to be a relatively low likelihood of embolism or thrombus formation (Figs 17.7 & 17.8).

Low velocities (<15 cm/s) within the posterior LA, as detected by TEE, appear to be just as predictive of stroke as low velocities within the LAA proper.

(a)

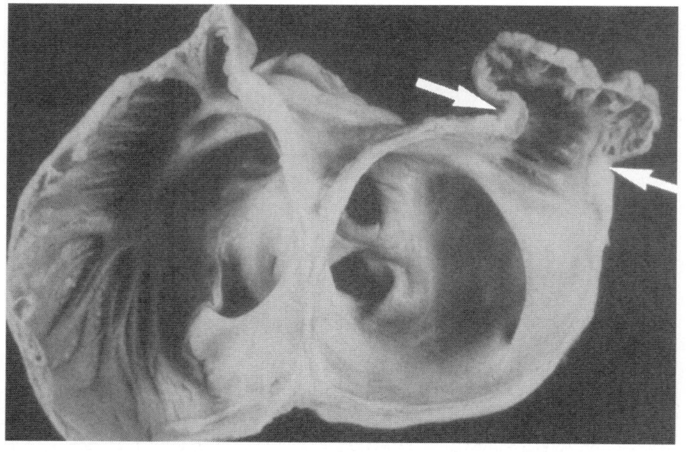

(b)

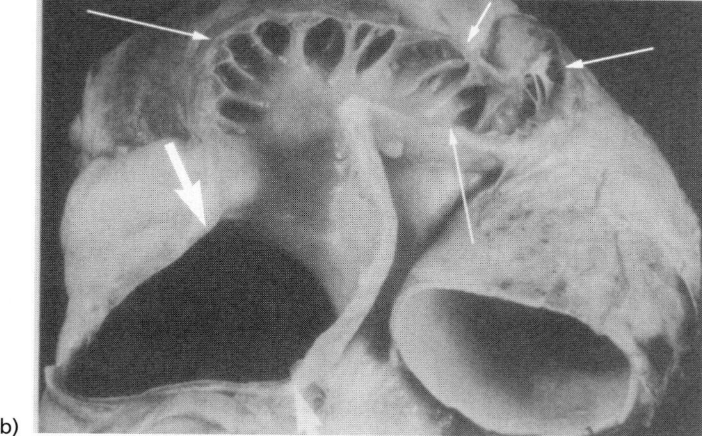

(c)

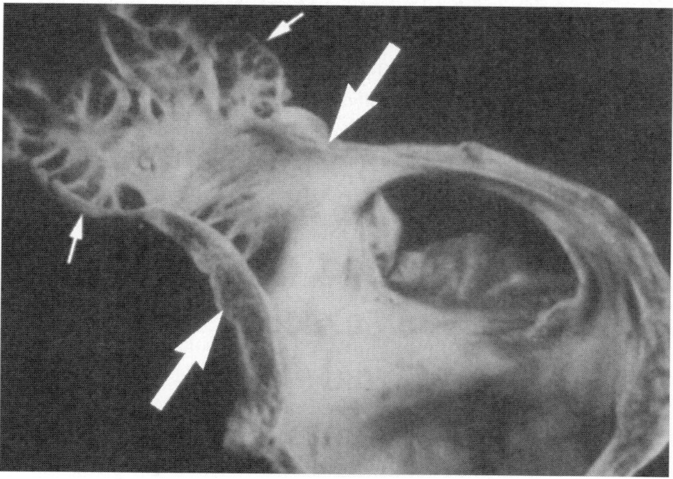

Fig. 17.3 Pathologic examples of the LAA demonstrate its complex and variable three-dimensional shape. In (a), the LAA is bilobed, In (b) it has a single long lobe, and (c) multiple small lobes. (Modified with permission from: Agmon Y, Khandheria BK, Gentile F, Seward JB. Echocardiographic assessment of the left atrial appendage. Journal of the American College of Cardiology 1999; 34: 1867–1877.)

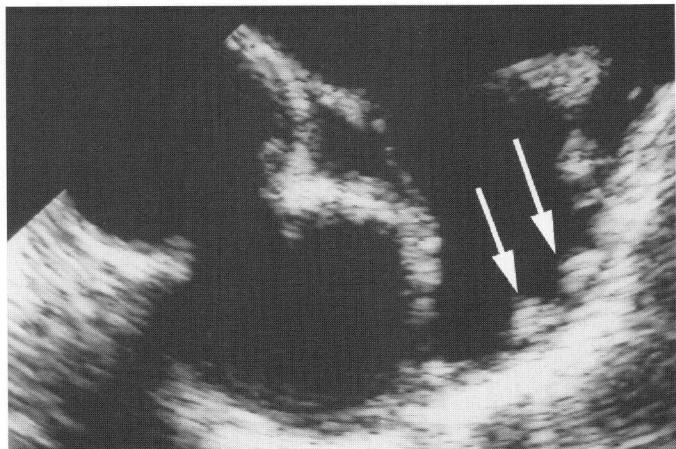

Fig. 17.4 TEE in the transverse view demonstrates a normal LAA with prominent pectinate muscles (arrows). The pectinate muscles are not to be confused with clot.

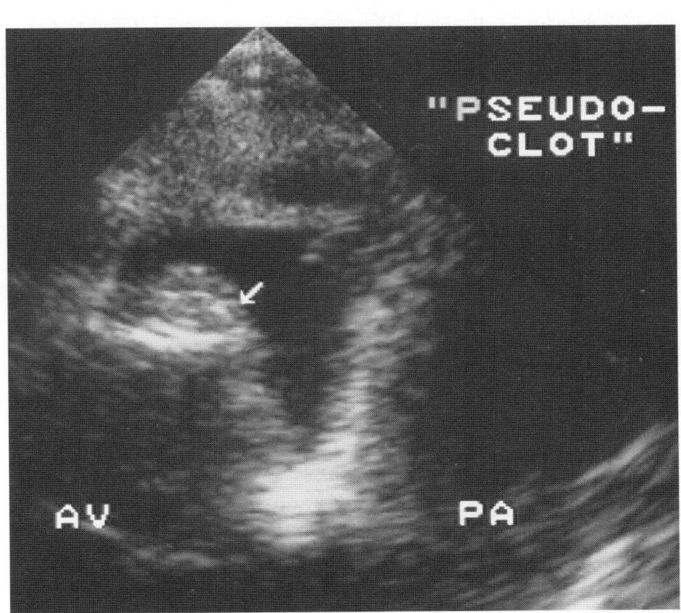

Fig. 17.5 TEE of the oblique sinus with material (fat) within the space, simulating a LAA clot. By rotating the transducer, and "following" the echo-free space, one notes that this space is not "attached" to the LA (see text).

There is risk of clot formation with other atrial arrhythmias, such as atrial flutter. Although the risk of forming LA thrombi in patients with atrial flutter does not appear as great as that of patients with atrial fibrillation, anticoagulation is still recommended.

Spontaneous echo contrast (SEC), or *smoke*, is defined as the presence of dynamic smoke-like swirling echoes within a cavity. A high frequency transducer should be used and the machine gain set high to best detect smoke (Figs 17.9 & 17.10). White noise may be confused as SEC, but SEC may be identified by its characteristic "swirling" motion. Probes higher than 5 MHz can sometimes reveal low intensity swirling echoes in normal subjects.

SEC can be found essentially anywhere there is a low flow state (LA, LAA, RA, LV, and descending aorta). It is felt to represent aggregation of blood cells at low shear rates. Severe mitral regurgitation tends to protect against the development of SEC within the LA, presumptively due to the rapid swirling and turbulent motion induced by the mitral regurgitant jet. However, SEC can be seen on occasion with mitral

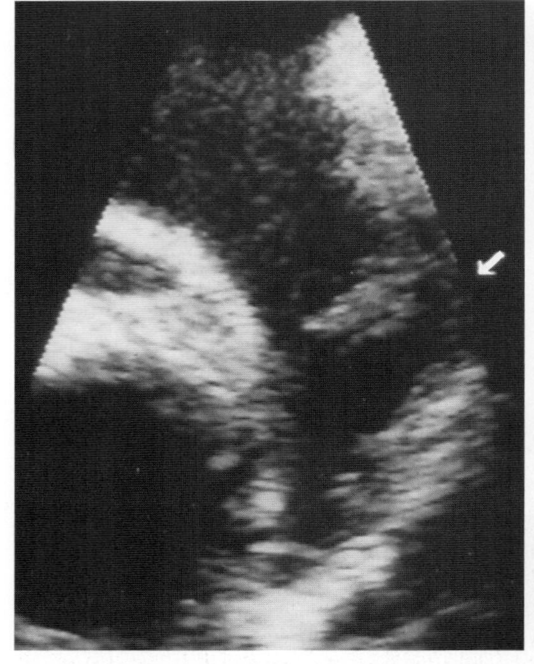
(a)

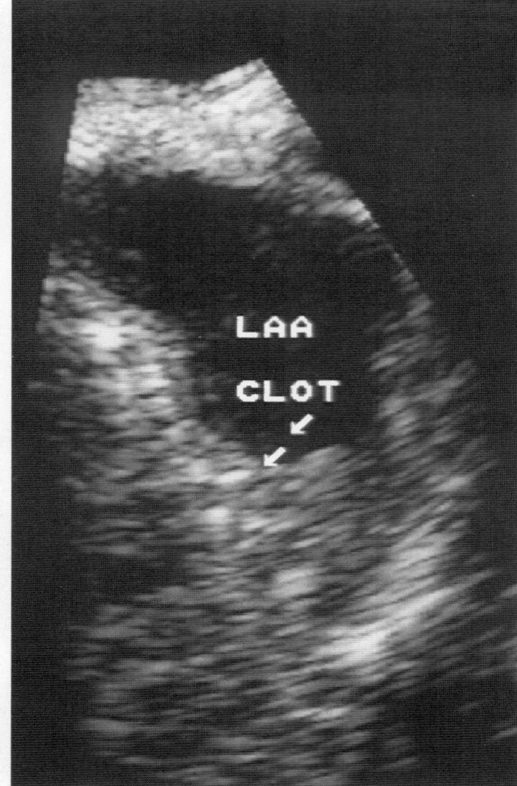

(c)

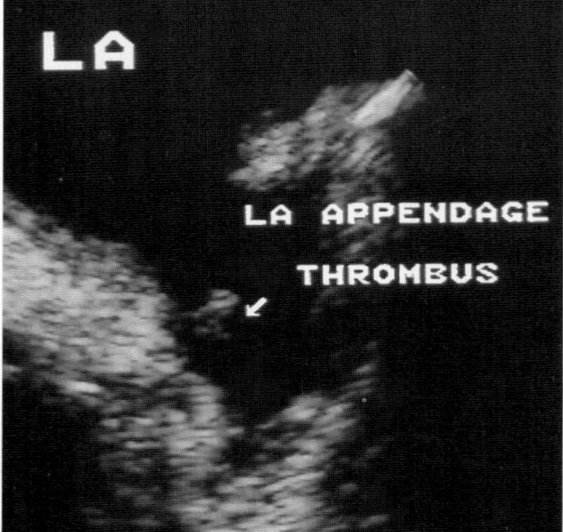

(b)

Fig. 17.6 LAA thrombus by TEE (horizontal plane) in three different patients. In (a) and (b) the thrombus was pedunculated and mobile, whereas in (c) the thrombus was layered.

regurgitation (MR) in patients with very large left atria. SEC is a predictor of embolism and of thrombus formation within the LA and LAA.

Upon conversion of atrial fibrillation or flutter to normal sinus rhythm (NSR), LAA "stunning" with low flow Doppler velocities, SEC, and thrombus formation may occur (Fig. 17.11). It is therefore recommended that full anticoagulation be in effect at the time of cardioversion (even if no thrombus is seen preconversion by TEE) and continued for at least 3 or 4 weeks after conversion to sinus rhythm. The need for lifelong anticoagulation has recently been recommended by some experts. Recovery of mechanical function of the LAA is generally delayed for anywhere

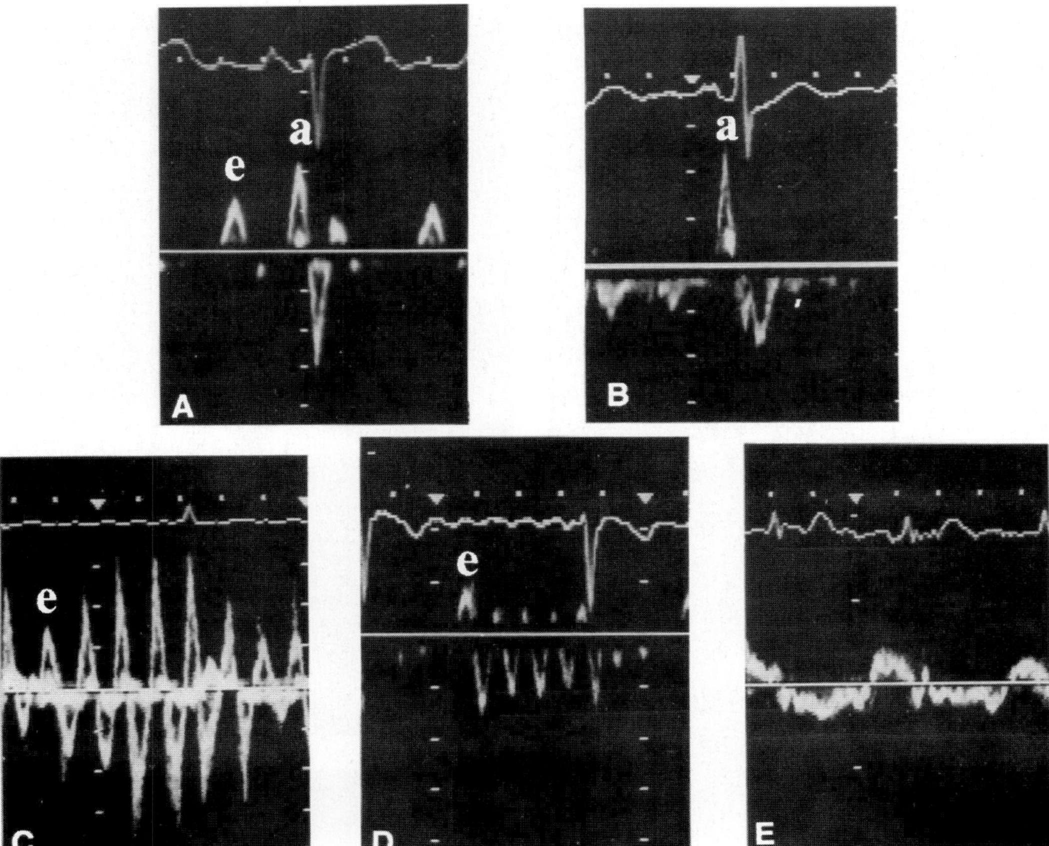

Fig. 17.7 Characterization of LAA flow types. Patterns were identified as Types I to V (A to E, respectively). Increasing spontaneous echo contrast severity was noted with diminishing LAA flow velocities (none with Type I, and increasing from II to V). Type I flow (normal) evidenced a small *e* wave and larger *a* wave, whereas Type II flow lacked an *e* wave. Three patterns were noted with atrial fibrillation. In Type III, an *e* wave was accompanied by relatively high velocity fibrillatory waves. The most common waveform noted was Type IV, where the *e* wave was associated with little or no fibrillatory velocities. Type V consisted of prolonged minimal LAA velocities. In this report, thromboembolic event prevalence was not progressively associated with decreasing velocities, as has been suggested by several others. (Reproduced with permission from: Fatkin D, Kelly RP, Feneley MP. Relations between left atrial appendage blood flow velocity, spontaneous echocardiographic contrast and thromboembolic risk in vivo. Journal of the American College of Cardiology 1994; 23(4): 961–969.)

from days to weeks after cardioversion, as is well documented by TEE. Electrical cardioversion of atrial fibrillation, as compared to chemical cardioversion, may be associated with a longer period of atrial mechanical inactivity. Thrombus in the LA may be found in patients with atrial fibrillation of a relatively brief duration (<48 h). One study demonstrated that LAA clot was present in ~14% of patients with atrial fibrillation for up to 3 days duration, and ~25% of patients with atrial fibrillation over 3 days. Predictors of atrial thrombus include SEC, decreased LV systolic function, and initial presentation with a thromboembolic event.

LAA ligation is often performed during mitral valve surgery to decrease the potential for an embolic source (Fig. 17.12). The LAA may be completely obliterated by clot and hence not "seen" by TEE. If the LAA is incompletely ligated, the cavity may be visualized

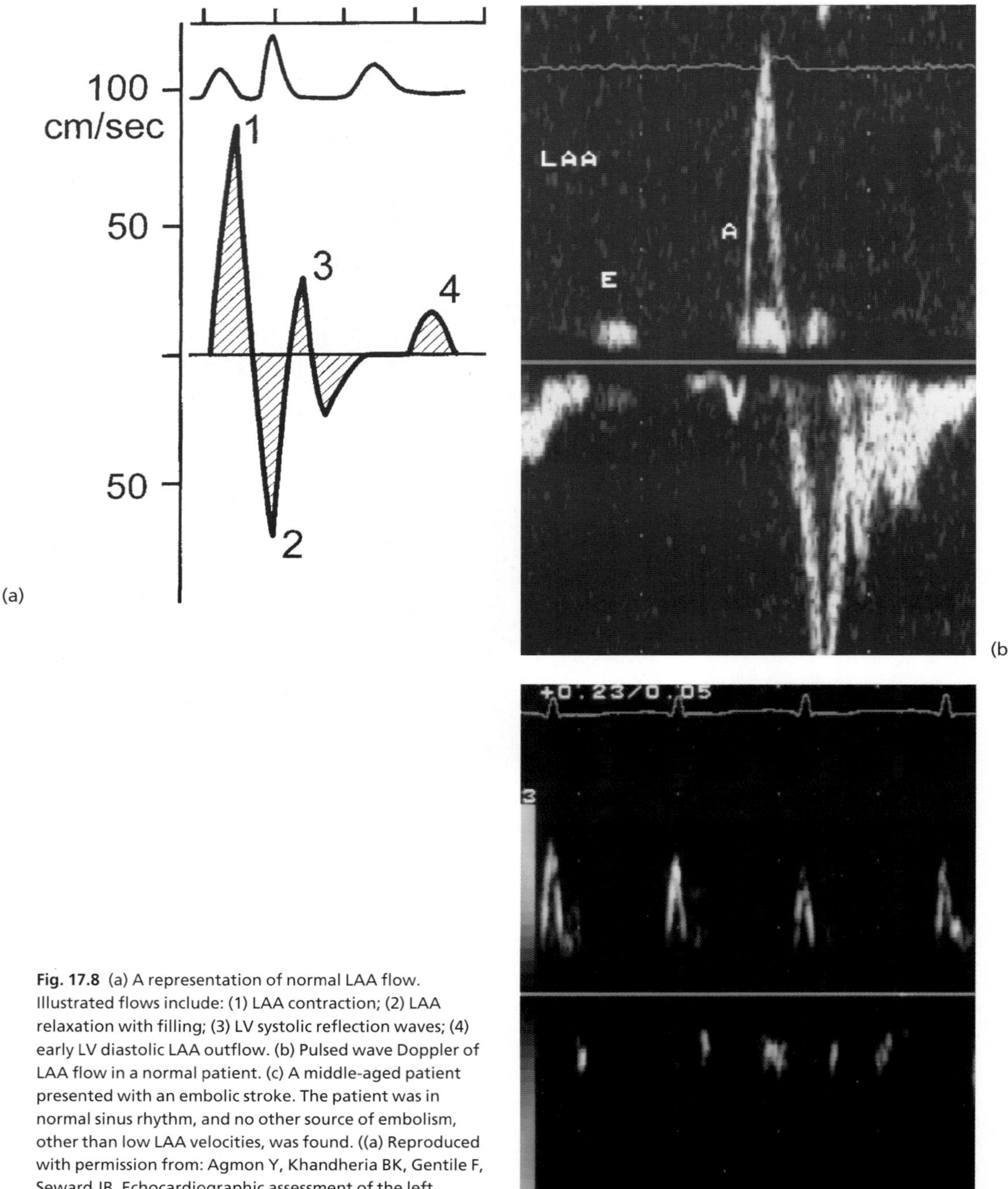

Fig. 17.8 (a) A representation of normal LAA flow. Illustrated flows include: (1) LAA contraction; (2) LAA relaxation with filling; (3) LV systolic reflection waves; (4) early LV diastolic LAA outflow. (b) Pulsed wave Doppler of LAA flow in a normal patient. (c) A middle-aged patient presented with an embolic stroke. The patient was in normal sinus rhythm, and no other source of embolism, other than low LAA velocities, was found. ((a) Reproduced with permission from: Agmon Y, Khandheria BK, Gentile F, Seward JB. Echocardiographic assessment of the left atrial appendage. J Am Coll Cardiol 1999; 34: 1867–1877, figure 17.4a.)

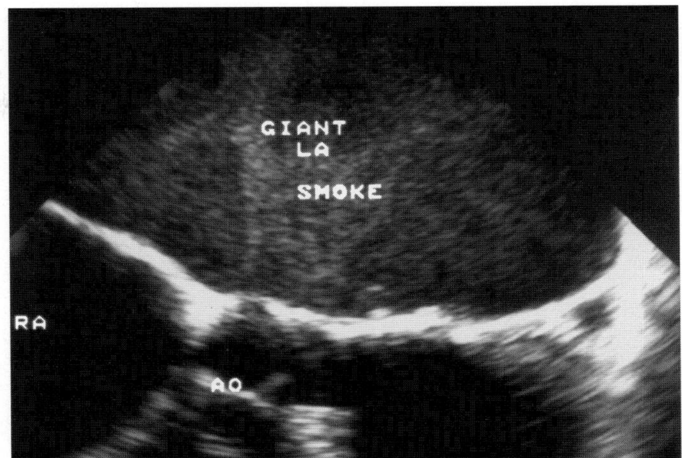

Fig. 17.9 A patient with mitral stenosis and giant LA by TEE in the horizontal plane. Prominent spontaneous echo contrast (SEC) is noted.

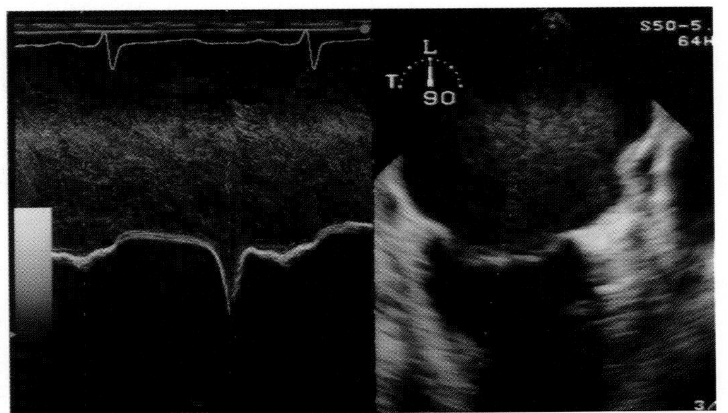

(a)

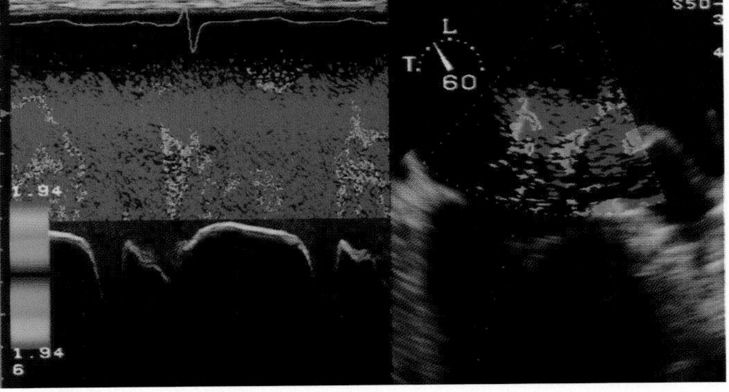

(b)

Fig. 17.10 TEE in a middle-aged patient with hypertension who presented with an embolic stroke. The patient had left ventricular hypertrophy (LVH) with preserved systolic function, but evidence of an elevated LV preload by mitral and pulmonary vein flow patterns. TEE M-mode and two-dimensional (2-D) imaging (a) revealed SEC within the LA. (b) Using M-mode and 2-D with TDI (low PRF of 1.94 cm/s in this example), the SEC is prominently noted. The M-mode recording highlights the "swirling" SEC motion.

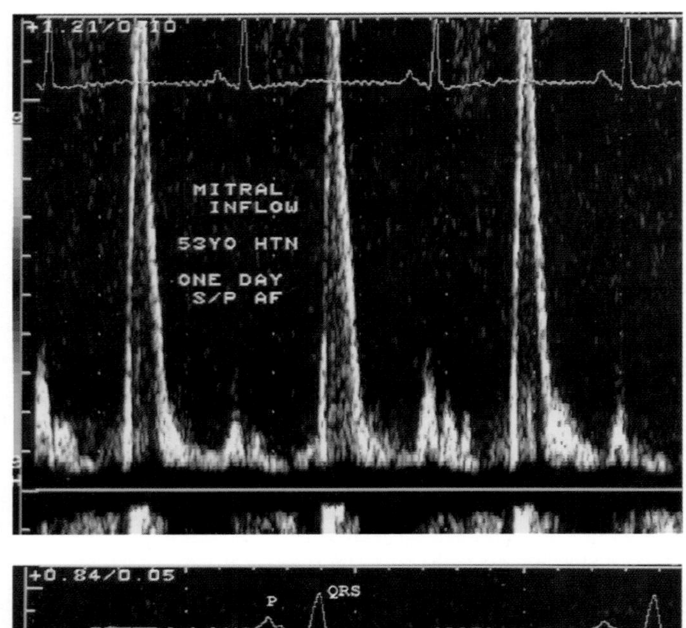

(a)

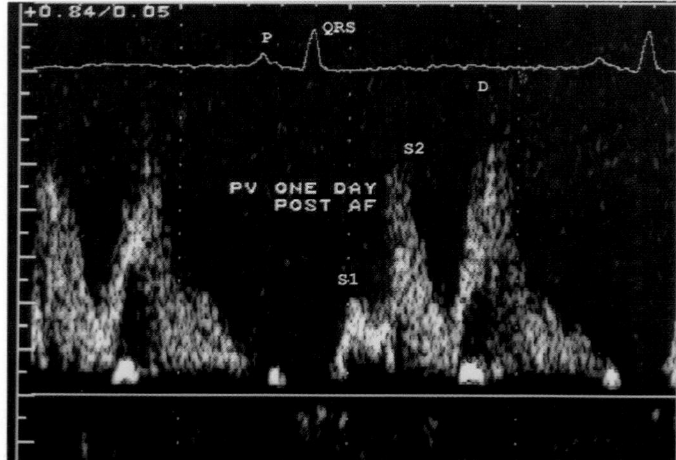

(b)

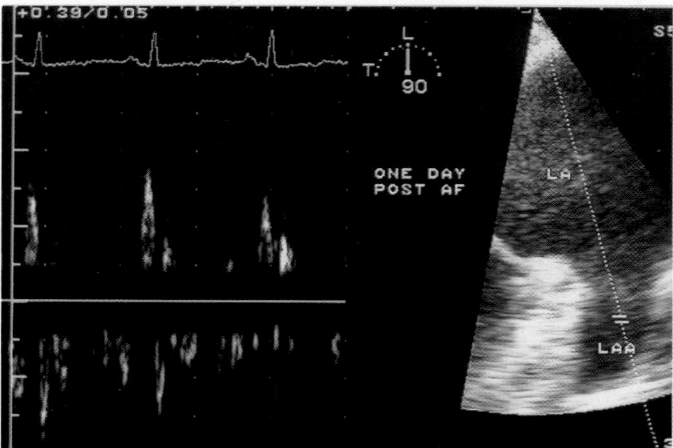

(c)

Fig. 17.11 Doppler findings of a patient who spontaneously converted from atrial fibrillation of unknown duration to normal sinus rhythm. (a) The mitral valve pulsed wave (PW) Doppler inflow pattern reveals essentially no A wave component, consistent with atrial "stunning". (b) The pulmonary vein flow pattern reveals essentially no atrial reversal wave, and S1 (due to atrial relaxation) is low. (c) Imaging reveals SEC within the LAA and LA. The LAA was noted to be essentially noncontractile, and PW Doppler flow patterns revealed low velocities (<20 cm/s).

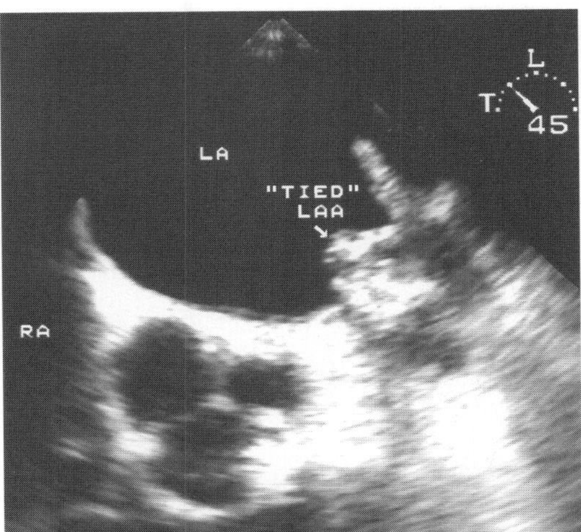

Fig. 17.12 Intraoperative visualization of a ligated LAA (see text).

and flow may be seen within the LAA cavity (and occasionally through an opening in the suture line) (Fig. 17.13).

The Stroke Prevention in Atrial Fibrillation (SPAF) study compared low dose coumadin with aspirin vesus full dose coumadin for long term therapy in chronic atrial fibrillation. A subset of 382 patients identified as high risk (females over 75 year, any aged person with hypertension, LV dysfunction or history of embolic events) underwent TEE as part of the initial evaluation. Fourteen per cent had LA clot and 18% had dense smoke. The patients were followed for 1.1 years. TEE predictors of embolism were LA clot, dense smoke, low LAA Doppler flow, and complex plaque in the descending thoracic aorta. Patients with an abnormality in the LA or with aortic complex plaques were at very high risk (21% per year) of embolism, whereas those with none of the above findings were at very low risk (1.3% per year) regardless of treatment.

The Assessment of Cardioversion Using Transesophageal Echocardiography (ACUTE) study compared TEE-guided cardioversion with the conventional approach in 1222 patients. Patients with atrial fibrillation of unknown duration for 2 days or longer were randomized to either:

1 "Conventional strategy" ($n = 603$)—3 weeks of warfarin, electrical cardioversion, and then 4 weeks of warfarin; or

2 "TEE-guided strategy" ($n = 619$)—TEE was performed. If no clot was found, patients received intravenous heparin and electrical cardioversion followed by 4 weeks of warfarin. If a clot was found by TEE, patients received 3 weeks of warfarin followed by a repeat TEE. If no clot was then visualized, the patient underwent electrical cardioversion followed by 4 weeks of warfarin.

Clot was initially found in 79/583 (13.6%) of patients. Of these, clots were found in the following chambers: LA, 5%; LAA, 85%; both LA/LAA, 2%; RA or RAA, 8%. In patients with thrombi, LAA velocity was 26.5 + 19.6 cm/s and in patients without

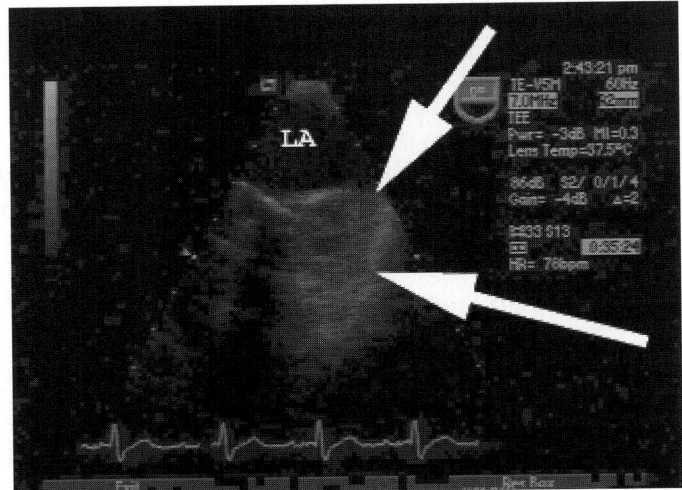

Fig. 17.13 TEE image of an incompletely ligated LAA several months after mitral valve replacement. Thrombus was noted within the LAA cavity (see text).

thrombi it was 37.1 + 21.7 cm/s. LA size by TTE was somewhat larger in the thrombus group (28.3 + 9.3 cm^2) than in the no thrombus group (25.8 + 9.8). Embolic events were 5/619 (0.81%) in the TEE-guided strategy group and 3/603 (0.50%) in the conventional strategy group. There was no difference between the groups in the 8-week maintenance of normal sinus rhythm. Hemorrhagic events were lower in the TEE group (2.9%) compared to the conventional group (5.5%).

Based on the above, some advocate use of TEE-guided early cardioversion with intravenous heparin or warfarin, especially if there is a relative contraindication to prolonged use of anticoagulation. The LA and LAA should be well visualized and clot carefully excluded. Patients should either be on full dose intravenous heparin or fully anticoagulated on warfarin. Anticoagulation is then continued for 3–4 weeks to prevent clots from forming in the postcardioversion period. If TEE reveals a thrombus, marked atrial or LAA smoke or LAA trabeculations that preclude exclusion of thrombus, the patient should first be treated with 4 weeks of warfarin. Many recommend a follow-up TEE to document the resolution of clot at that time prior to cardioversion. If the clot has not resolved, generally serial TEEs are of little benefit and cardioversion is not performed.

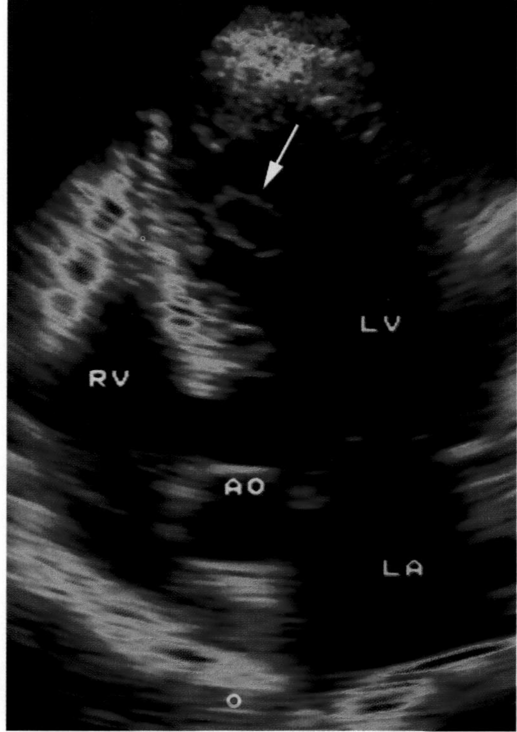

Fig. 17.14 Apical imaging (B-mode color image) of a mobile thrombus within the LV (arrow) noted several days after transmural myocardial infarction.

Left ventricular thrombus

Left ventricular thrombi may form in a patient with an acute myocardial infarction (during the first 2 weeks), a LV aneurysm, or a dilated cardiomyopathy (ischemic or nonischemic). The most common site for LV thrombus is in the LV apex. LV thrombus may be well visualized by TTE (see also Chapter 13). To decrease the likelihood of a false positive interpretation, the thrombus should be visualized throughout the cardiac cycle using at least two different echo views. LV thrombus forms in an area of LV wall motion abnormality, most often within an aneurysm (Figs 17.14–17.17). Occasionally a thrombus may form in the setting of transient LV ischemia with later visualization revealing preserved LV motion. TTE evaluates LV thrombus well, especially at the cardiac apex. Use of higher frequency transducers (3.75, 5 or even 7 MHz) and obtaining apical short axis images ("bread-loafing" the apex) will increase the diagnostic yield (Fig. 17.18). TEE may help in patients with difficult acoustic transthoracic windows.

Endocarditis (see also Chapter 18)

Endocarditis is associated with embolism. Large vegetations (>10 mm) attached to the mitral valve (especially the anterior leaflet) and involvement of multiple valves are associated with an increased incidence of embolism. In addition, one study found *Staphylococcus* infection, right-sided valve endocarditis and/or highly mobile vegetations (>15 mm) were associated with a very high risk of embolism.

Mitral annular calcification

There may be an association of mitral annular calcification (MAC) with stroke (see also Chapter 20), although this association is not strong. Presumptively,

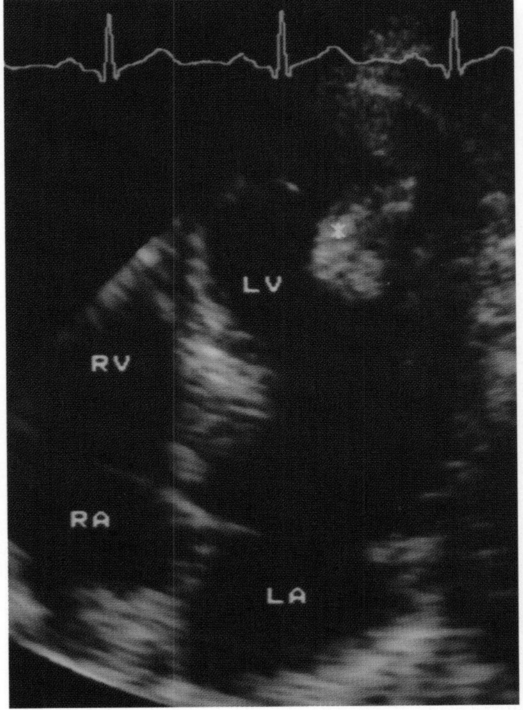

(a)

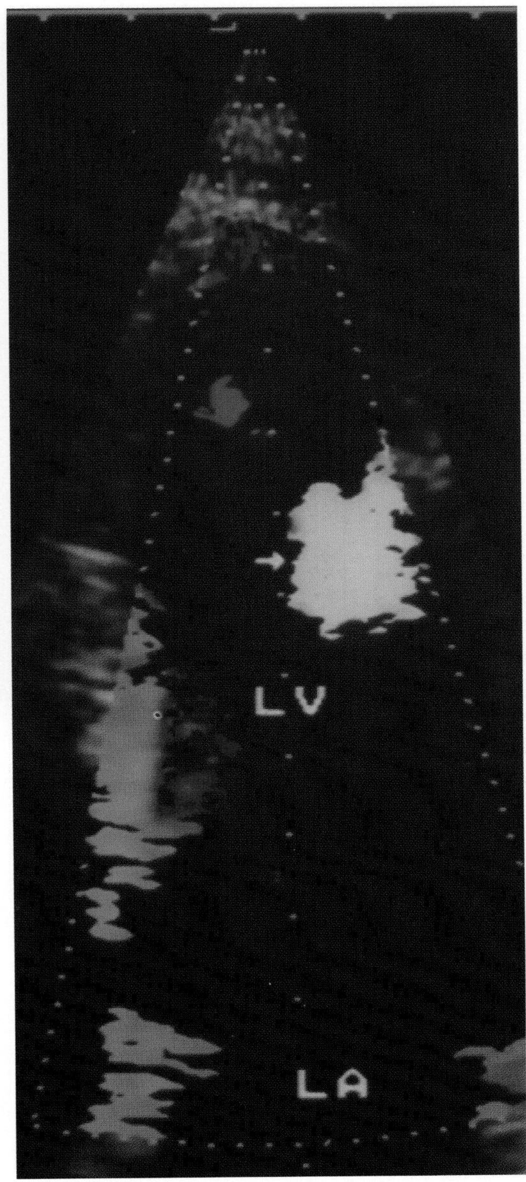

(b)

Fig. 17.15 Apical imaging of (a) LV thrombus and (b,c) with tissue Doppler imaging (TDI). In (b) the 2-D image reveals the clot as yellow in this still frame, and (c) by M-mode TDI through the clot, the clot is seen to "oscillate" throughout the cardiac cycle, demonstrating its mobility. (*Continued on p. 282.*)

the mechanism of stroke with MAC is either calcific emboli from the calcified annulus or thrombus formation (Fig. 17.19). Some contend that MAC is just a marker for increased aortic debris. MAC appears part of the aging process but is found particularly in elderly females, in patients on renal dialysis, or in patients with obesity, hypertension, aortic stenosis, or hypertrophic cardiomyopathy.

Tumors (see also Chapter 20)

Tumors may be associated with embolism. A small LA myxoma (which is usually attached to the foramen ovale) is more likely to embolize than a larger one. Those that are "polypoid" and prolapsing, as opposed to "round" and nonprolapsing, are also more likely to embolize (Fig. 17.20).

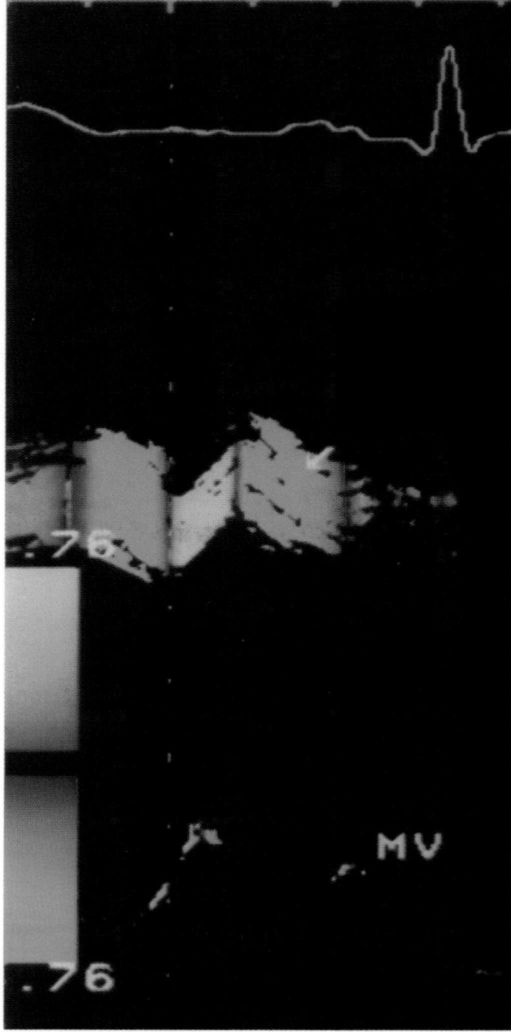

(c)

Fig. 17.15 *(cont'd)*

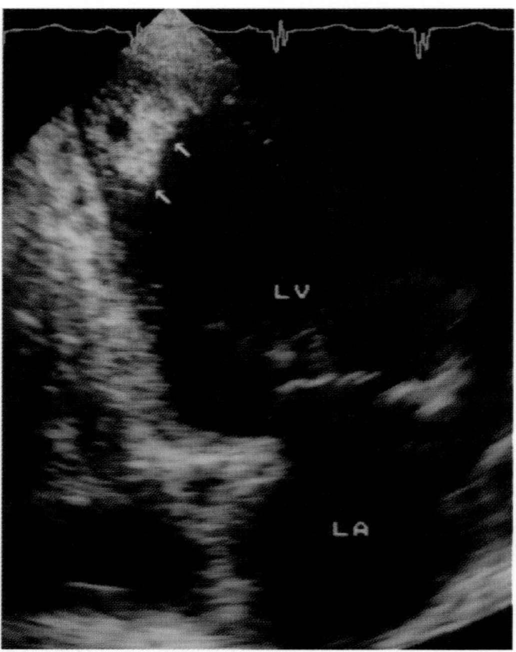

Fig. 17.16 Apical imaging of a patient with a myocardial infarction in the recent past. An area of sonolucency is noted within this thrombus.

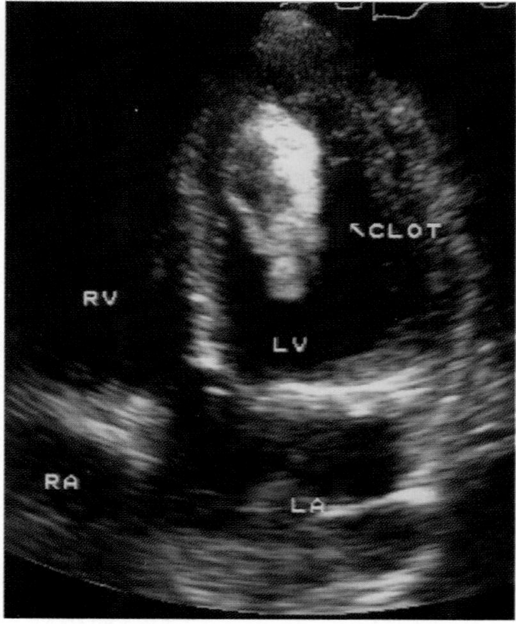

Fig. 17.17 A large partially calcified thrombus is noted in a patient with a remote small apical myocardial infarction.

A papillary fibroelastoma (Figs 17.21 & 17.22) may be associated with arterial embolism but the vast majority of patients with this tumor are found at autopsy and were asymptomatic. Echocardiographic characteristics of a papillary fibroelastoma include:

- usually solitary
- usually less than 1 cm in diameter
- usually arises from the midportion of valve leaflets (away from the line of closure in distinction to fibrous strands)
- typically pedunculated (occasionally sessile) and demonstrate a high frequency oscillation

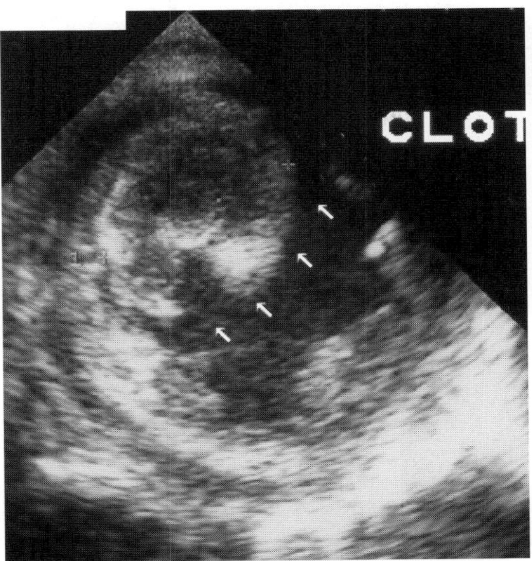

Fig. 17.18 By imaging the LV apex in a short axis view, apical thrombi may be detected that might be otherwise missed by apical four- or two-chamber imaging. This is a 22-year-old-male with a dilated cardiomyopathy and heart failure. Imaging in a short axis ("bread-loaf") view with a 3.75-MHz transducer revealed this apical thrombus (arrows).

Table 17.1 Comparisons between papillary fibroelastoma and Lambl's excrescences. (Reproduced with permission from: McAllister *et al*. Tumors of the heart and pericardium. Current Problems in Cardiology 1999; 24(2))

Papillary fibroelastoma	*Lambl's excrescences*
Usually arterial side semilunar valves or mural endocardium	Not usually arterial side semilunar valves or mural endocardium
Midpart or body of valve away from contacting surfaces	Along line of closure of valve
Rare	70–80% adult heart valves
Seldom multiple	Multiple in >90% affected hearts
No fibrin deposits	Fibrin deposits
Abundant acid mucopolysaccharide matrix	No abundant acid mucopolysaccharide matrix
Smooth muscle cells are significant	No smooth muscle cells as a significant component

• "fronds" appear on the mass (sometimes said to appear like a "cluster of grapes" or a "sea anemone").

Papillary fibroelastomas have been found on all four cardiac valves but are most commonly found on the aortic valve, originating from either its arterial or ventricular side. They are occasionally on the subvalvular apparatus of the mitral or tricuspid valve and very rarely are attached to the free wall of a ventricular chamber. A papillary fibroelastoma may serve as a nidus for platelet and fibrin aggregation, leading to embolic events. Some investigators recommend anticoagulation once a papillary fibroelastoma is visualized by echocardiography followed by surgical removal, even if the patient is asymptomatic.

Table 17.1 contrasts papillary fibroelastoma and Lambl's excrescences.

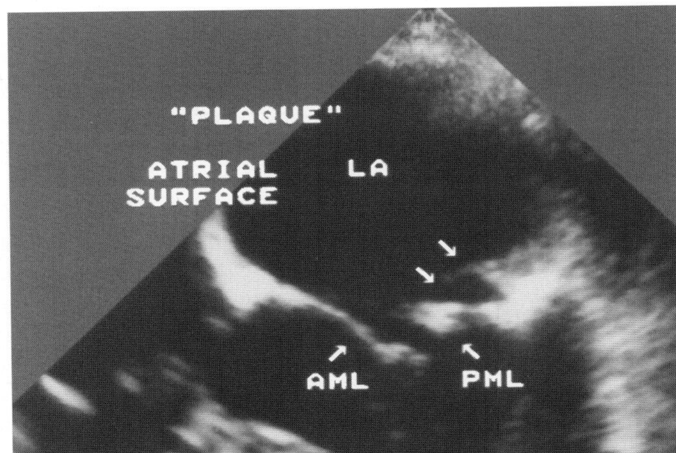

Fig. 17.19 Intraoperative TEE in the horizontal plane. Posteriorly within the atrial side of the mitral annulus was "extruded" calcium and also thrombus, documented histologically.

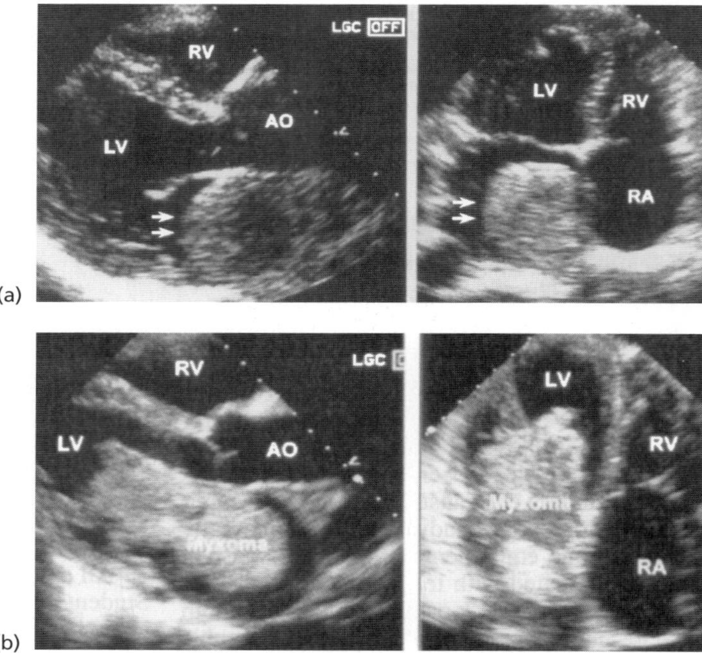

Fig. 17.20 TTE images of myxomas. In (a) the tumor is "smooth" and nonprolapsing, and in (b) it is "polypoid" and prolapsing. (Reproduced with permission from: Ha JW, Kang WC, Namsik C, *et al*. Echocardiographic and morphologic characteristics of left atrial myxoma and their relation to systemic embolism. American Journal of Cardiology 1999; 83: 1579–1582.)

Aortic atheroma

Aortic atheroma has been found at autopsy in the past but was not generally recognized as a source of embolism until the advent of TEE. The atherosclerotic process tends to be diffuse, involving the entire thoracic aorta (although there are exceptions). Atheromas at highest risk of embolization are those noncalcified plaques that protrude more than 4 mm into the aortic lumen, are ulcerated, pedunculated, and/or have mobile components (Fig. 17.23). Tissue Doppler imaging of the aorta may help locate small mobile atheroma (Fig. 17.24). Patients presenting with systemic embolic events and found to have mobile aortic atheromas on TEE have a high incidence of recurrent systemic events. Warfarin may reduce the recurrence rate. There may also be a role for statin drug therapy in these patients.

Patent foramen ovale and associated structures

Patent foramen ovale (PFO) is a remnant from embryology existing in about 25–30% of the general population. It has been associated with otherwise unexplained strokes in young patients (see also Chapter 14) as well as with the platypnea–orthodeoxia syndrome (dyspnea upon assuming an upright position) and decompression illness in divers, in high altitude aviators, and possibly in astronauts. Paradoxical embolism through a PFO has been postulated as a cause of stroke, particularly in patients in whom no other cause can be detected. Direct TEE visualization is considered the gold standard for PFO diagnosis (Fig. 17.25), but peripheral injection of agitated saline with TTE (Fig. 17.26) and/or transcranial Doppler (TCD) of a middle cerebral artery have also been used to detect a right-to-left shunt. During saline contrast injection, a Valsalva maneuver (with TTE, TCD, or TEE) should be used to increase the diagnostic yield. The patient should be asked to release the Valsalva as the right atrium is seen to begin to opacify with contrast (Fig. 17.27). If the patient is unable to perform the Valsalva maneuver, repetitive cough may be done with saline injection (but a well performed Valsalva probably has a higher yield).

From embryology, flow returning from the IVC is preferentially directed toward the interatrial septum (IAS) (Fig. 17.28) and flow from the SVC is directed laterally. Agitated saline injection via a femoral vein

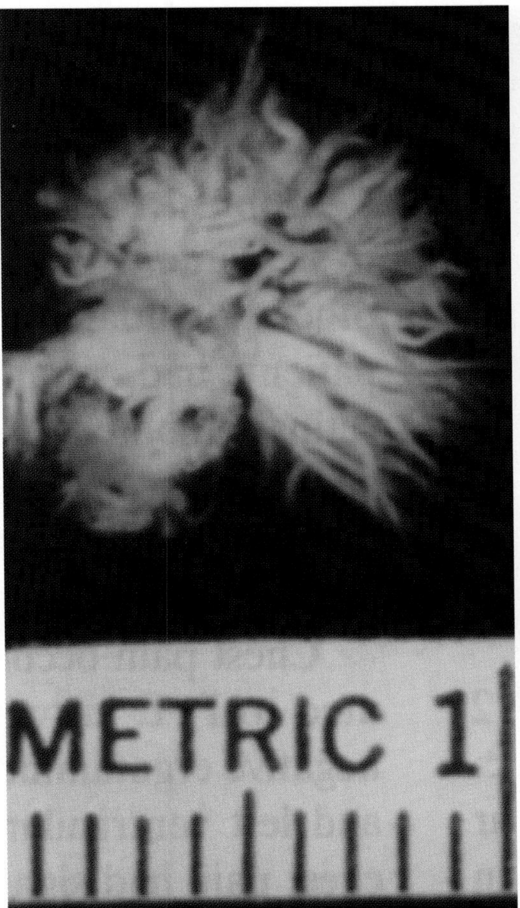

Fig. 17.21 Pathologic specimen of a mitral papillary fibroelastoma. The appearance of its frond-like structures is described as that of a sea anemone. (Reproduced with permission from: Klarich KW, Enriquez-Sarano M, Gura GM, *et al.* Papillary fibroelastoma: echocardiographic characteristics for diagnosis and pathologic correlation. Journal of the American College of Cardiology 1997; 30: 785, figure 1.)

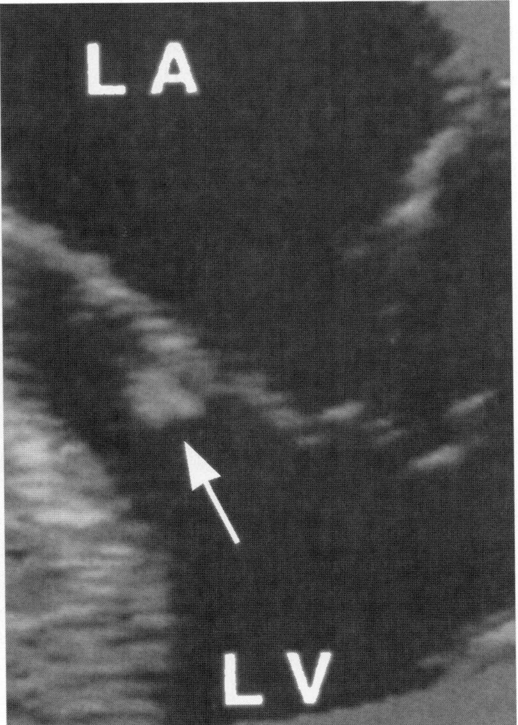

Fig. 17.22 TEE in the horizontal plane demonstrating a pathologically documented papillary fibroelastoma. (Reproduced with permission from: Moraes D, Philippides GJ, Shapira OM. Papillary fibroelastoma of the mitral valve with systemic embolization. Circulation 1998; 98: 1252.)

may yield a right-to-left shunt when antecubital injection has not demonstrated contrast in the left heart.

When imaging for PFO, the use of the longitudinal plane is more sensitive than the transverse plane for identification of the right-to-left shunt and to identify the exact location of the shunt (that is, to differentiate a PFO from a small secundum ASD) (Fig. 17.29).

That PFO is a common cause of stroke remains somewhat controversial. There may be a higher likelihood of stroke among patients with larger size PFOs or evidence of a larger amount of shunting (i.e. >20 bubbles seen in the left heart in any single frame following opacification of the right heart). The strongest association, however, appears to be in patients who also have an ASA.

The autopsy incidence of ASA is 1%. It is associated with PFO about 80% of the time. An ASA is a redundant and mobile membranous portion of the atrial septum defined as an excursion of more than 15 mm with a base width of 15 mm (Fig. 17.30; and see Chapter 20). Some suggest platelet aggregation with thrombus formation within the ASA as a source of embolism, but more often the associated PFO with paradoxical embolism is thought causal.

The Chiari network, a remnant from embryology, extends from the inferior part of the RA to the atrial septum in the region of the lower portion of the limbus of the fossa ovalis (see also Chapter 20). It has a

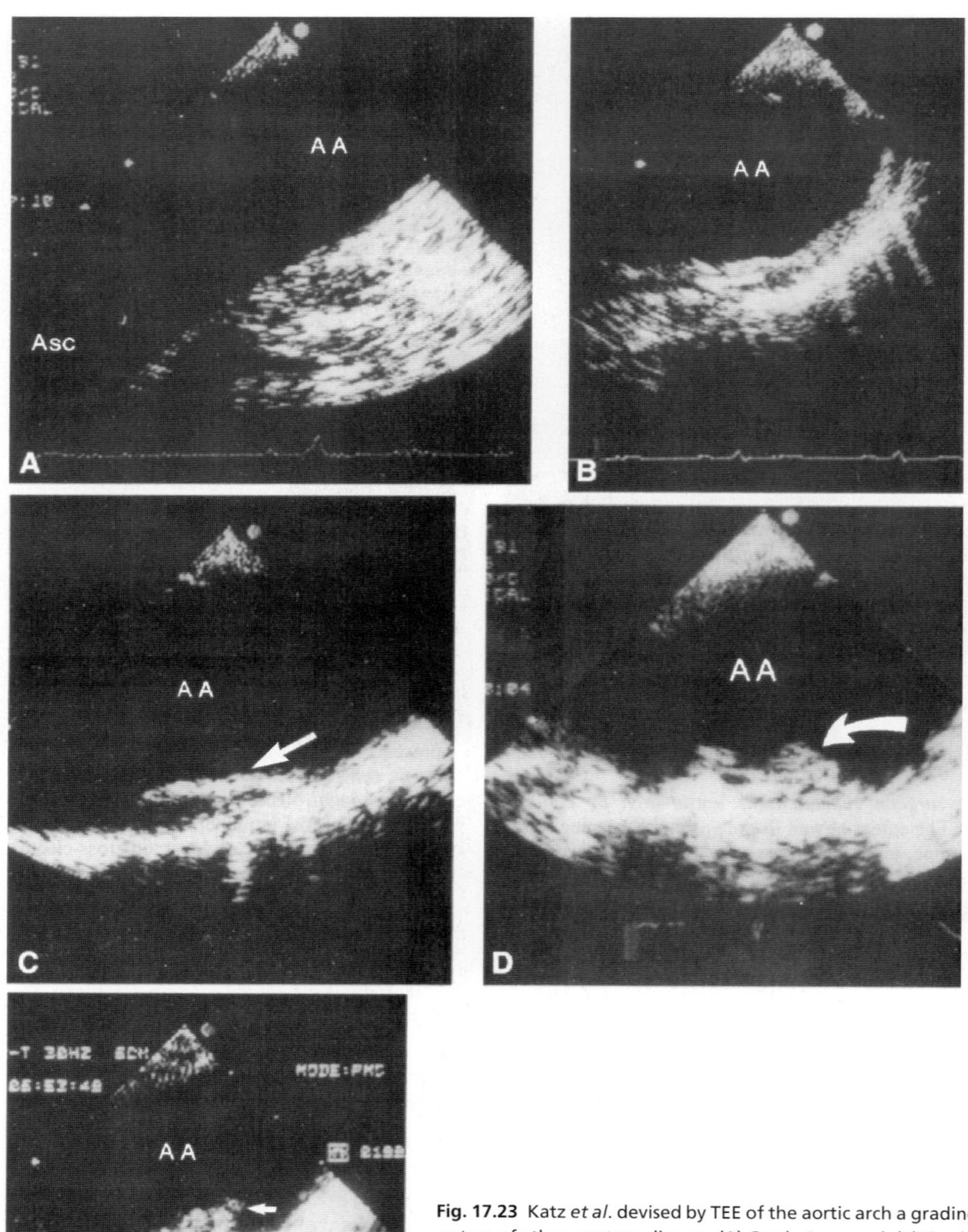

Fig. 17.23 Katz *et al.* devised by TEE of the aortic arch a grading system of atheromatous disease. (A) Grade 1: normal. (B) Grade 2: intimal thickening. (C) Grade 3: sessile atheroma <5 mm into the aorta. (D) Grade 4: atheroma >5 mm. (E) Grade 5: mobile atheroma. Sessile atheroma >5 mm or mobile atheromas are at highest risk of embolization. (Reproduced with permission from: Katz ES, Tunick PA, Rusinek H, *et al.* Protruding aortic atheromas predict stroke in elderly patients undergoing cardiopulmonary bypass: experience with intraoperative transesophageal echocardiography. Journal of the American College of Cardiology 1992; 20: 70–77, figure 1.)

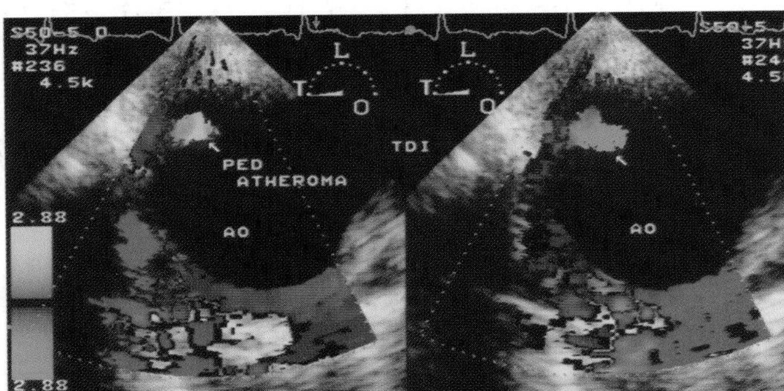

Fig. 17.24 TEE of the descending aorta in the horizontal plane. Sequential frames with tissue Doppler imaging (TDI) highlight the independent motion of a pedunculated atheroma (arrows).

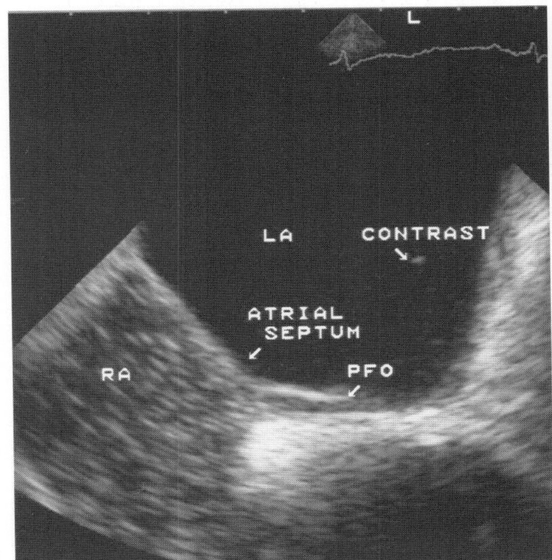

(a)

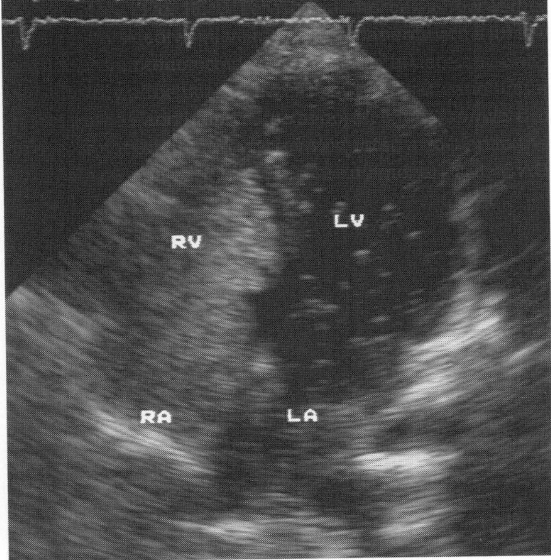

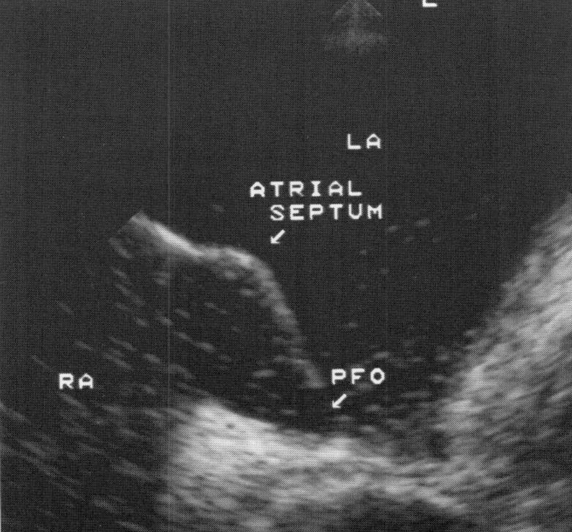

(b)

Fig. 17.26 (*above*) Apical four-chamber view of a patient with a PFO. Direct visualization or shunting of a PFO is usually not possible by TTE, but venous agitated saline injection revealed contrast appearance within the left heart. Often shunting at the atrial level is noted, but it is difficult to differentiate shunting from an ASD versus a PFO.

Fig. 17.25 (*left*) TEE images in the longitudinal plane of a patient noted to shunt agitated saline contrast from the RA to the LA through a PFO. Shunting was (a) minimal during normal resting respiration, but (b) dramatically increased when agitated saline was injected in conjunction with the Valsalva maneuver.

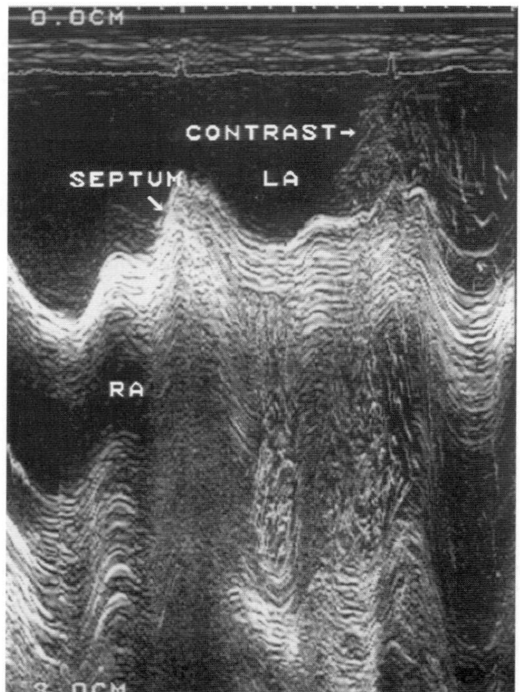

Fig. 17.27 TEE M-mode study in the transverse plane demonstrates appearance of agitated saline first in the RA and then in the LA. If contrast is seen in the LA within three cardiac cycles of appearance in the RA, it may be attributed to an atrial level shunt, whereas a pulmonary shunt should require five or more cardiac cycles before appearing in the LA.

typical undulating movement (some have described the motion as "seaweed"). It should not be confused with the Eustachian valve or a clot within the right heart. The Chiari network may facilitate IVC flow across a PFO (as in the fetus), and may contribute to an increased likelihood of paradoxical embolism.

Mitral valve prolapse

Earlier studies using TTE found a correlation of unexplained cerebrovascular accident (CVA) with mitral valve prolapse (MVP). However, using present-day guidelines for MVP diagnosis, this correlation has not been found. Rarely, platelet and fibrin deposits located on the atrial side of the posterior leaflet insertion site have been found at autopsy.

Fibrous strands

Fibrous strands identified by TEE appear as fine thread-like material arising on the line of closure ("contact surface") of the mitral valve (most often) and occasionally on the aortic valve line of closure. They have been described on prosthetic valves (Fig. 17.31), but are uncommonly found on the tricuspid or pulmonic valves. Fibrous strands are highly mobile with motion independent of the valve and may prolapse during valve closure. They are more likely to be multiple. These small fibrous strands

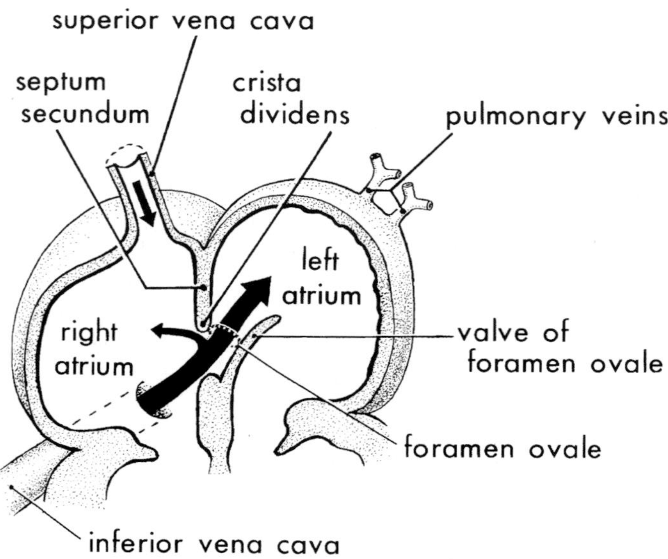

Fig. 17.28 How IVC blood flow *in utero* (oxygenated from the placenta) is preferentially directed toward and across the foramen ovale. Deoxygenated SVC flow is directed away from the atrial septum. This flow pattern of venous return into the RA often remains after birth. (Reproduced with permission from: Moore KL. The Developing Human, 2nd edn. Philadelphia: WB Saunders, 1977: p. 282, figure 14.24.)

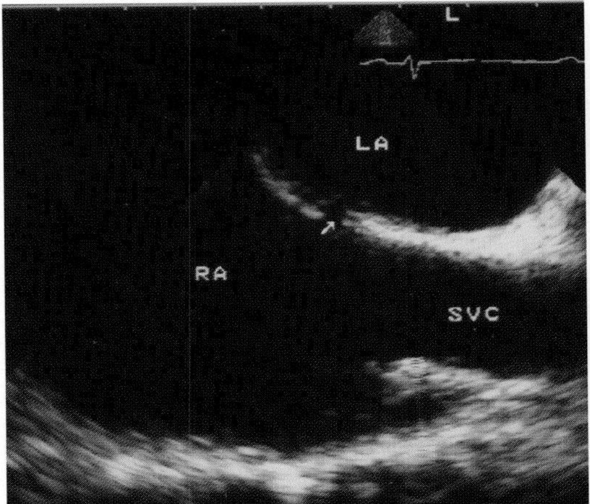

(a)

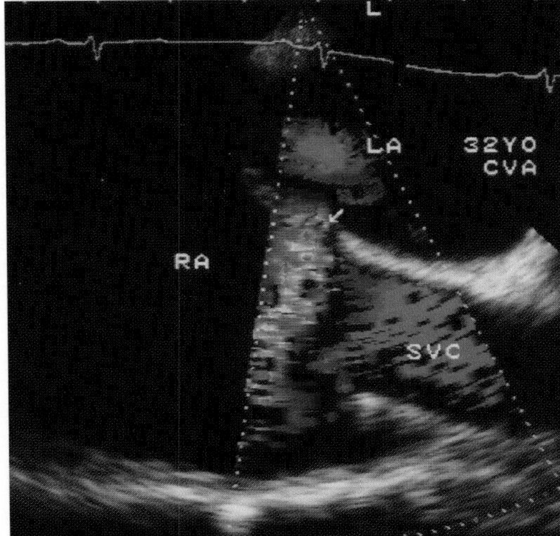

(b)

Fig. 17.29 (*above*) TEE image in the longitudinal plane of a 32-year-old-male patient with an unexplained cerebrovascular accident (CVA). The patient was found to have a small restrictive secundum-type atrial septal defect. Note the location of the defect (a) within the fossa ovalis (arrow) as compared to that of a patent formane ovale (PFO), and (b) color jet demonstrating flow from left to right.

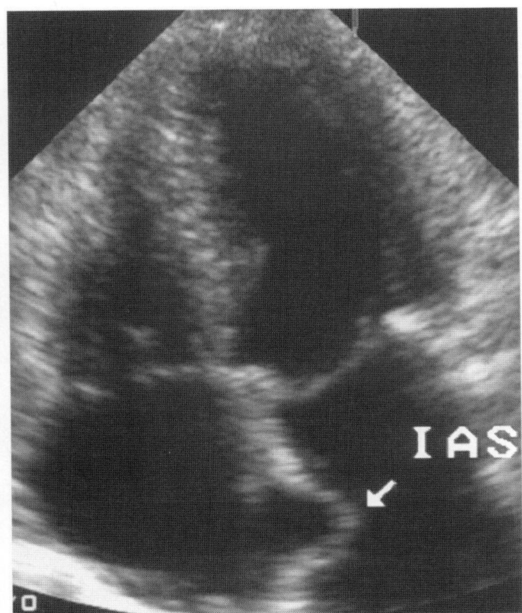

(a)

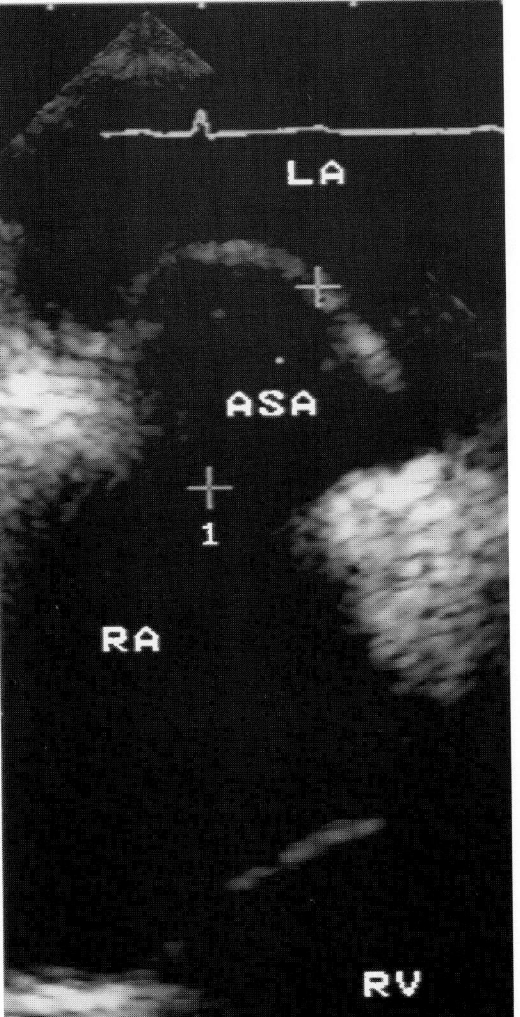

(b)

Fig. 17.30 (*right*) An atrial septal aneurysm by (a) TTE (interatrial septum (IAS)) and (b) TEE transverse image documenting a 15-mm excursion. This patient had an associated PFO visualized and documented by agitated saline venous injection.

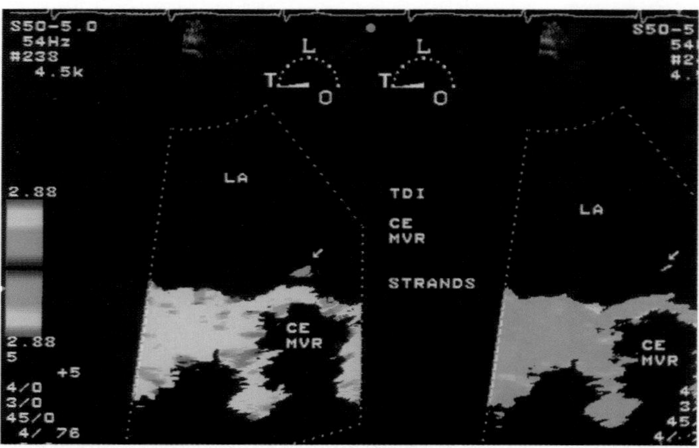

Fig. 17.31 TEE at 0° in a patient with a history of a Carpentier–Edwards mitral valve prosthesis (C-E MVR) insertion in the past. Using tissue Doppler imaging mobile valve strands were easily visualized (arrows). The color of the strands documents the "independent" motion of the strands from that of the prosthetic valve.

have been thought to be associated with unexplained neurologic events; however, others have not found an association with cardioembolism. When evaluated pathologically, fibrous strands are consistent with what has been termed Lambl's excrescence.

In summary, there exist multiple potential etiologies of cardioembolic stroke. Certain cardiac pathologies appear to have a higher association with stroke than other pathologies. Echocardiography, particularly TEE, plays a major role in detecting most of these.

18

CHAPTER 18

Endocarditis

Infective endocarditis (IE) may present in a variety of ways. It is important to diagnose IE rapidly to provide effective and prompt therapy, to improve patient outcome. Early diagnostic criteria for IE (*Beth Israel criteria* in 1981) did not include echocardiographic findings but in 1994 echocardiographic findings were added as important diagnostic criteria (the *Duke criteria*). The Duke criteria combined the Beth Israel features with echo findings and stratified patients into one of three groups: *definite* endocarditis (clinically and/or pathologically), *possible* endocarditis (not meeting definite criteria), or *rejected* endocarditis (Table 18.1). The Duke criteria gave major criteria to the following echo findings: *mobility*, *echodense masses* attached to valve leaflets or mural endocardium, *perivalvular abscesses*, and new *prosthetic valve dehiscence*. The Duke criteria were patterned after the Jones' criteria for rheumatic fever diagnosis in that "definite" IE was defined as the presence of either two major criteria or one major with three minor criteria or five minor criteria.

Transthoracic echocardiography (TTE) may detect vegetations 3 mm or less in size, whereas transesophageal echocardiography (TEE) may detect vegetations 1 mm or less in size. A vegetation usually consists of thrombus, necrotic tissue, platelet aggregates, fibrin, red blood cells, and debris. Live bacteria may also be present if the endocarditis is acute and/or antibiotic therapy is insufficient (Fig. 18.1). Vegetations are usually found on the leading edge of the involved valve and are often on the low pressure side of a regurgitant valve (i.e. left ventricular outflow tract (LVOT) side of aortic valve and atrial side of mitral or tricuspid valve). Vegetations may also form at the site where the high velocity regurgitant jet hits the myocardial wall (Fig. 18.2).

Focal valve degeneration and calcification may simulate the appearance of vegetation; however, calcification will often restrict valve mobility whereas a vegetation will not. TEE is better than TTE at detecting vegetations (especially small or prosthetic valve vegetations), allowing a more confident diagnosis and in detecting complications of endocarditis. When performing an echo in a patient with suspected IE, one should evaluate for:

- the presence, size and mobility of vegetations
- valvular involvement and destruction
- complications of IE (leaflet aneurysms/perforation, ruptured papillary structures)
- local extension (abscess and fistula)
- hemodynamic consequences (degree of regurgitation, cardiac size, and intracardiac pressures).

Frequently vegetations appear mobile and prolapsing (Figs 18.3 & 18.4). Generally, they cause some degree of valve regurgitation. They do not appear "encapsulated," but may have the appearance of having multiple appendages. *Leaflet aneurysm formation* and *leaflet perforation*, which are often best diagnosed by TEE, are very suggestive of IE (Figs 18.5–18.7).

Prosthetic valve vegetations generally are difficult to diagnose. Mechanical valves usually involve the perivalvular ring and abscess formation. Bioprosthetic valves may have evidence of infection along the valve ring, but also may involve the valve leaflets themselves. An insensitive but highly specific sign for bioprosthetic valvular endocarditis is a vegetation extending past the normal extent of a fully opened valve (see Figs 18.4 & 18.17). This helps distinguish a vegetation from a degenerated valve leaflet. Dehisced prosthetic valves may demonstrate "*rocking*" through the cardiac cycle. Often more than 40% of the circumference of the ring must be involved before this is evident.

Vegetations thought *most likely to embolize* are: (i) larger than 10 mm; (ii) attached to the mitral valve (especially anterior leaflet); and (iii) involve multiple leaflets. It has also been suggested that vegetations that are larger than 15 mm and highly mobile, irrespective of valve destruction or response to antibiotics, are at

Table 18.1 The Duke criteria for diagnosis of infective endocarditis. (Adapted with permission from: Durack DT, Lukes AS, Bright DK *et al.* New Criteria for Diagnosis of Infective Endocarditis: Utilization of Specific Echocardiographic Findings. Am J Med 1994; 96: 200–209.)

(a) Major and minor criteria

Major criteria

Positive blood culture for infective endocarditis:

- Typical microorganism for infective endocarditis from two separate blood cultures
  - Viridans streptococci,* *Streptococcus bovis*, HACEK group, *or*
  - Community-acquired *Staphylococcus aureus* or enterococci, in the absence of a primary focus, *or*
  - Persistently positive blood culture, defined as recovery of a microorganism consistent with infective endocarditis from blood cultures drawn more than 12 h apart, *or*
  - All of three, or majority of four or more separate blood cultures, with first and last drawn at least 1 h apart

Evidence of endocardial involvement:

- Positive echocardiogram for infective endocarditis
  - Oscillating intracardiac mass, on valve or supporting structures, or in the path of regurgitant jets, or on implanted material, in the absence of an alternative anatomic explanation, *or*
  - Abscess, *or*
  - New partial dehiscence of prosthetic valve, *or*
  - New valvular regurgitation (increase or change in pre-existing murmur not sufficient)

Minor criteria

Predisposition: predisposing heart condition *or* intravenous drug use

Fever ≥38.0°C (100.4°F)

Vascular phenomena: major arterial emboli, septic pulmonary infarcts, mycotic aneurysm, intracranial hemorrhage, conjunctival hemorrhages, Janeway's lesions

Immunologic phenomena: glomerulonephritis, Osler's nodes, Roth's spots, rheumatoid factor

Echocardiogram: consistent with infective endocarditis but not meeting major criterion above

Microbiologic evidence: positive blood culture but not meeting major criterion above,† *or* serologic evidence of active infection with organism consistent with infective endocarditis (e.g. Q fever serologies)

(b) Patients categorized as "Definite" (pathologically or using Duke criteria), "Possible," or "Rejected"

Definite infective endocarditis

Pathologic criteria:

- Microorganisms: demonstrated by culture or histology in a vegetation, in a vegetation that has embolized, or in an intracardiac abscess, *or*
- Pathologic lesions: vegetation or intracardiac abscess present, confirmed by histology showing active endocarditis

Clinical criteria (using specific definitions)

- Two major criteria *or*
- One major and three minor criteria *or*
- Five minor criteria

Possible infective endocarditis

Findings consistent with infective endocarditis that fall short of *definite*, but not *rejected*

Rejected

Firm alternate diagnosis explaining evidence of infective endocarditis, *or*

Resolution of endocarditis syndrome, with antibiotic therapy for 4 days or less, *or*

No pathologic evidence of infective endocarditis at surgery or autopsy, after antibiotic therapy for 4 days or less

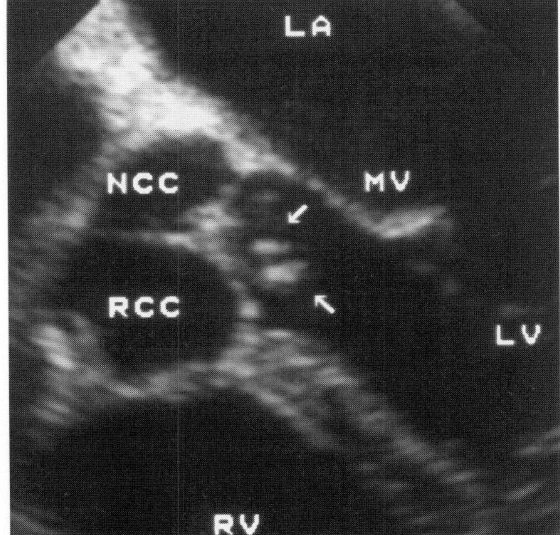

(a)

(b)

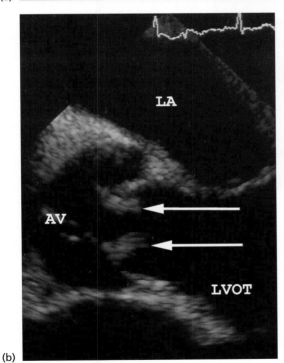

Fig. 18.1 Aortic valve endocarditis. (a) A 64-year alcoholic patient with positive blood cultures for *Streptococcus viridans* and negative (acoustically difficult) transthoracic echocardiography (TTE). By TEE, the aortic valve had two small mobile vegetations (arrows). (b) TEE horizontal plane imaging of another alcoholic patient with *S. viridans* positive blood cultures and vegetations (arrows) noted. NCC, noncoronary cusp of aortic valve; RCC, right coronary cusp of aortic valve; LVOT, left ventricular outflow tract.

significant risk of embolization, and early surgery should be considered. The relationship of vegetation size and the need for surgery, however, is somewhat controversial at this time.

A *falsely positive* TTE or TEE for IE may occur with (see Chapters 9, 10 & 17):

- flail mitral valve
- valve "strands" (Lambl's excrescences)
- papillary fibroelastoma
- prosthetic valve sutures, thrombus, or pannus
- Libman–Sacks endocarditis (antiphospholipid syndrome, systemic lupus erythematosus)
- nonbacterial thrombotic endocarditis and marantic endocarditis (Chapter 21)
- degenerative valvular changes
- acute rheumatic carditis
- rheumatoid arthritis
- ankylosing spondylitis
- nodules of Arantius
- If a flail leaflet and ruptured chordae are detected, it is often difficult to determine whether infection was the cause. Libman–Sacks endocarditis is usually sessile with leaflet thickening and no independent lesion motion
- A valve that is severely calcified may be difficult to evaluate for associated endocarditis
- The lesions of acute rheumatic carditis are usually multiple nodules 3–5 mm in size without independent mobility. There may also be focal nodular thickening of the valve tips and leaflet body with an associated clinical syndrome
- The nodular lesions of rheumatoid arthritis are usually single, less than 5 mm in size, spherical, homogeneous, and may be found on any part of the involved leaflet
- The lesion of ankylosing spondylitis is usually a subaortic valve sessile "bump" which may extend to the base of the anterior leaflet mitral valve
- If a vegetation is present, it is difficult to differentiate *old from new active vegetations*, although an old vegetation may be dense and bright, suggesting calcification.

False negative TTE or TEE studies for IE may occur with:

- prosthetic valve (also evaluate for new regurgitant lesions—see Chapter 10)
- small vegetations (<5 mm for TTE, and <3 mm for TEE)

(a)

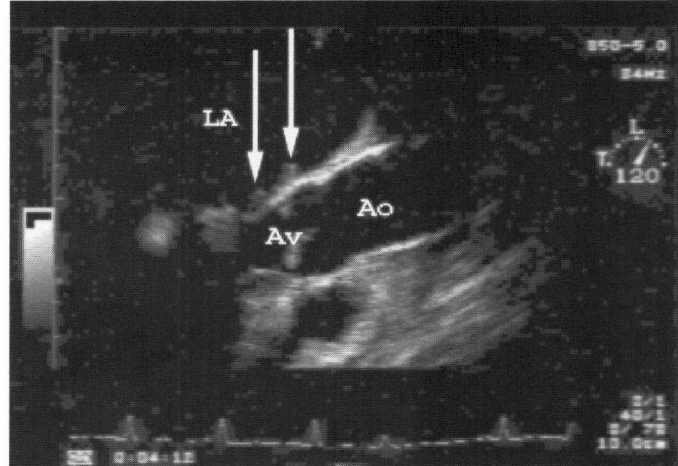

(b)

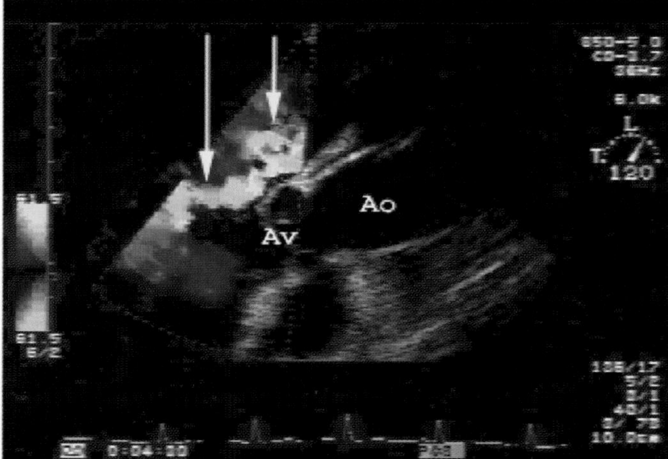

Fig. 18.2 A 57-year-old-female developed a 3-month history of subjective fevers and arthralgias after a dental visit, and grew *Streptococcus viridans* in blood cultures.
TEE imaging at 120° revealed (a) mobile small vegetations (arrows) on the LA wall, located (b) within the jet (arrows) of mitral regurgitation. Av, aortic valve; Ao, aortic root.

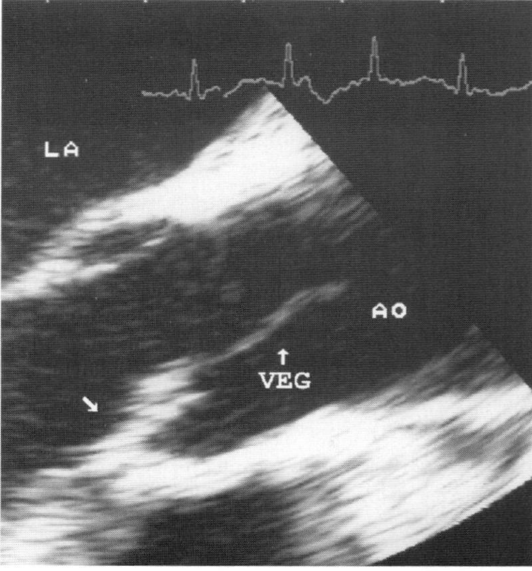

Fig. 18.3 TEE of the aortic valve and proximal aortic root in a patient with clinical evidence of endocarditis and positive blood cultures. A long mobile vegetation, seen in a systolic frame, extends into the proximal aortic root.
In diastole it prolapsed into the LVOT.

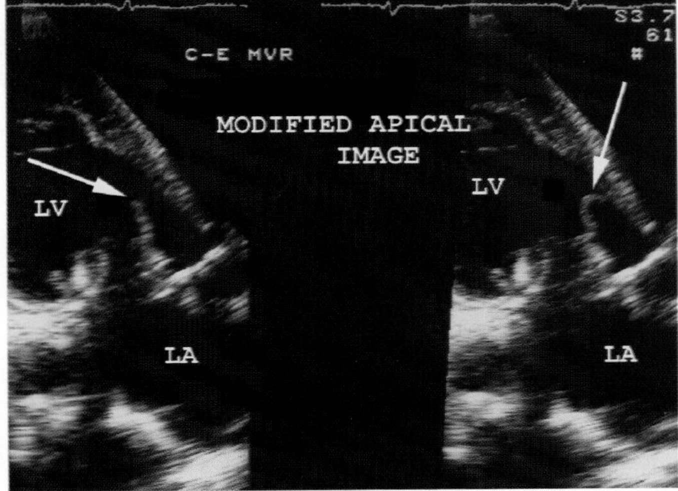

Fig. 18.4 Two sequential echo frames from a modified apical view in an elderly male with an existing bioprosthetic mitral valve. The patient grew *Enterococcus* sp. in blood cultures. A mobile vegetation is noted to "protrude" past the prosthetic valve struts. This is essentially diagnostic for bioprosthetic vegetations (see also Chapter 10).

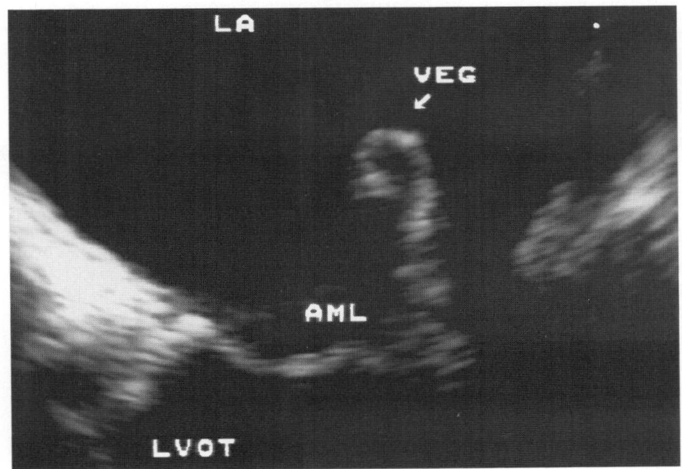

Fig. 18.5 TEE in the transverse plane of the mitral valve in a patient with positive blood cultures and severe mitral regurgitation. Leaflet perforation and a vegetation (VEG) are readily noted. AML, anterior mitral leaflet.

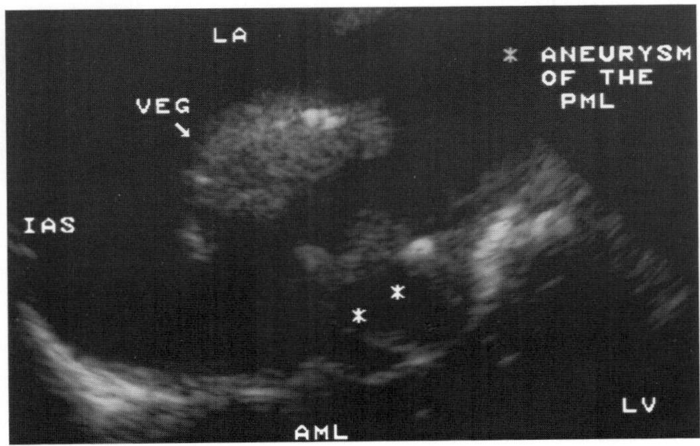

Fig. 18.6 TEE in the horizontal plane of a patient with endocarditis (VEG) involving the mitral valve. Note aneurysm formation (*) in the posterior leaflet. A large mobile vegetation is attached to the atrial surface. IAS, interatrial septum.

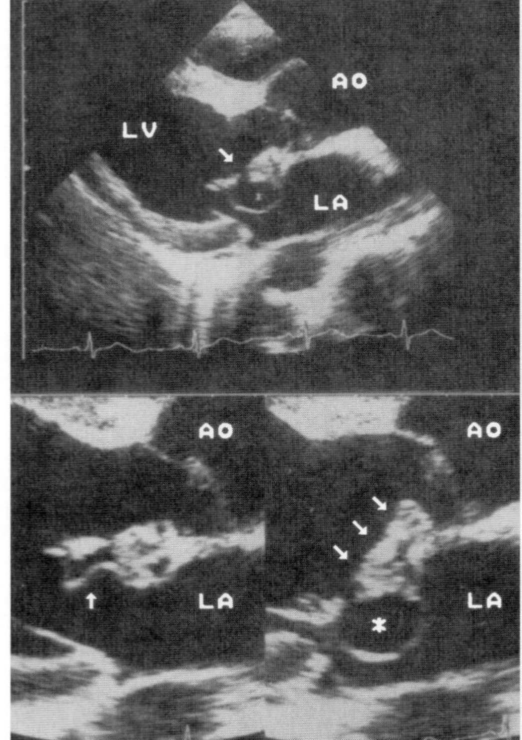

Fig. 18.7 Parasternal long axis views of a classic aneurysm of the anterior leaflet of the mitral valve with leaflet perforation. In (a) the perforation (arrow) and aneurysm (*) are well seen, in (b, left panel), the aneurysm appears collapsed (arrow) in diastole, and in (b, right panel) the aneurysm (*), perforation, and a vegetation (arrows) are seen in systole. (Reproduced with permission from: Vilacosta I, Peral V, San Roman JA, *et al.* Mitral valve aneurysm. Circulation 1997; 95: 2169.)

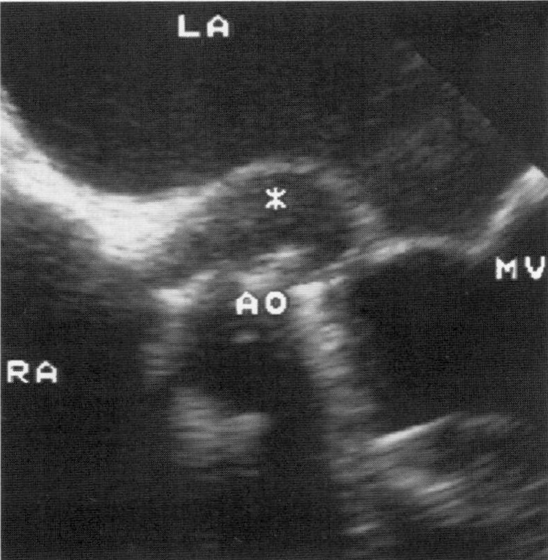

Fig. 18.8 Aortic periprosthetic valve abscess (*) in a patient with a mechanical aortic valve prosthesis. AO, prosthetic aortic valve; MV, mitral valve.

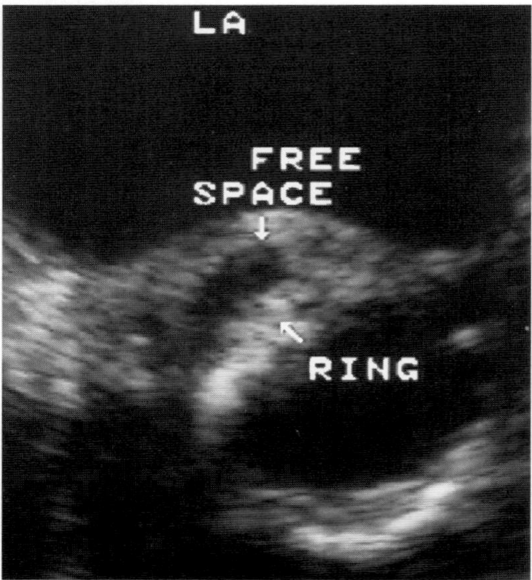

Fig. 18.9 Aortic periprosthetic valve abscess (arrows) in a patient with a bioprosthetic aortic valve. An echo-free space (FREE SPACE) defines the abscess cavity. RING, valve ring.

- poor imaging windows
- incomplete evaluation of valves, especially pulmonic valve.

When a patient has positive blood cultures, a "negative" TEE may be helpful in decreasing the odds of IE being present, but a *negative TEE does not "rule out" endocarditis!* Cases of IE may be missed, especially when the TEE is done "early" in the course of the infection, when the vegetations are small, or when they are associated with a prosthetic or heavily calcified valve. Repeat TEE or even TTE may reveal a vegetation several days later, particularly with an "aggressive" microorganism, for example *Staphylococcus* sp.

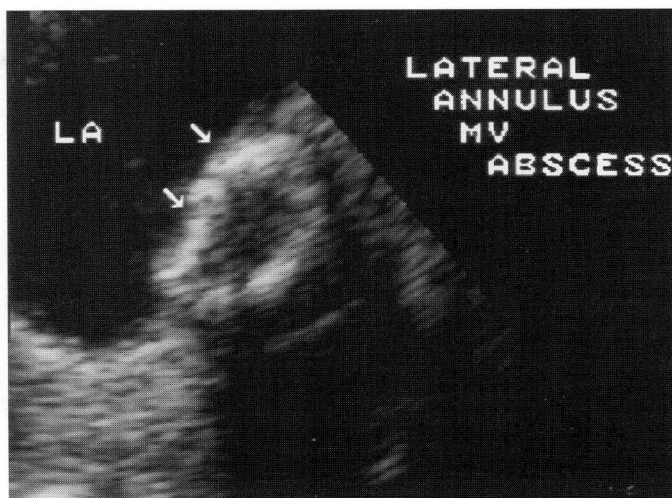

Fig. 18.10 TEE image of abscess formation (arrows) within the lateral aspect of the mitral annulus documented at surgery.

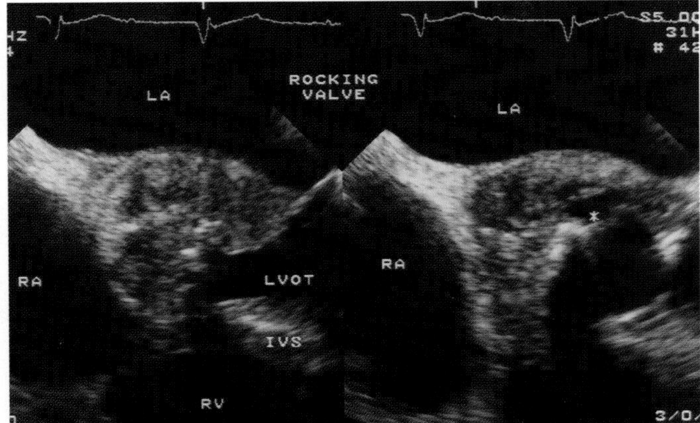

Fig. 18.11 TEE sequential images of a large abscess surrounding a large portion of a prosthetic aortic valve. The valve is partially dehisced (*).

Diagnosis of *prosthetic valve endocarditis* and its complications may be particularly difficult and TEE is clearly superior to TTE in this setting. *New* or *increasing perivalvular regurgitation* or valve dehiscence suggests IE in the proper clinical context. Comparing the TEE and/or TTE to previous studies may be extremely helpful.

In a patient with a clear diagnosis of IE, TEE should still be performed if a potential complication, such as abscess formation, is suggested. Indications for TEE in this setting include:

- persistent fever
- increasing AV conduction abnormalities on ECG
- prosthetic valve endocarditis
- recurrent embolization.

Complications of endocarditis involving the aortic or mitral valves

By definition, an *abscess* does not communicate with an intravascular space whereas a *mycotic aneurysm* does. Abscess formation often occurs within the native aortic valve annulus (usually in the region of the posterior aortic root) and occurs more frequently with aortic rather than mitral prosthetic valves. This is usually an indication for surgery (Figs 18.8–18.13). A mitral ring abscess appears as an echo-free space, most often behind the posterior mitral valve leaflet (Fig. 18.10).

Subaortic lesions in the region between the

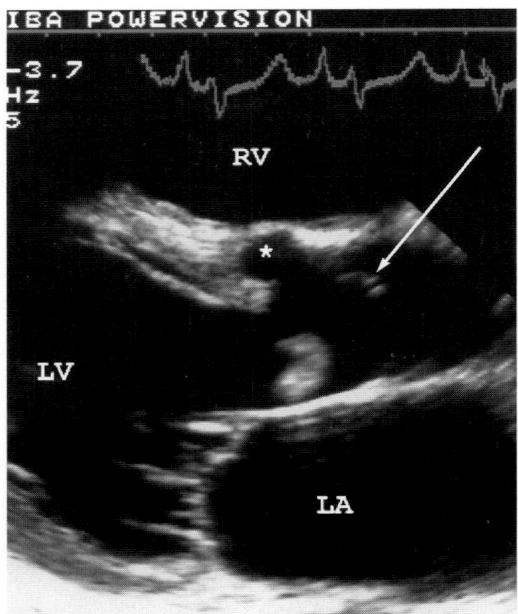

Fig. 18.12 Parasternal long axis view of a patient with a bicuspid aortic valve (arrow) and intravenous drug abuse (IVDA) history with positive blood cultures for *Staphylococcus aureus*. There is evidence of interventricular septal involvement (*).

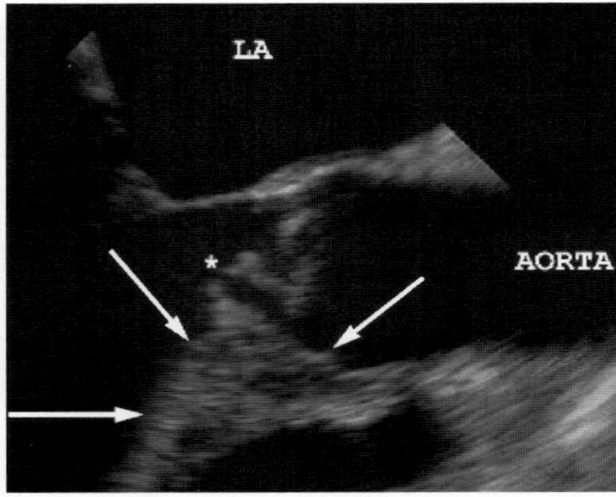

Fig. 18.13 A 42-year-old male alcohol abuser presented with fever, dyspnea, and a murmur. Blood cultures grew *Pneumococcus* organisms. By TEE at 120° there is evidence of an aortic leaflet aneurysm with perforation (*) and abscess formation (arrows) in the subaortic interventricular septum.

aortic and mitral valves (*mitral–aortic intervalvular fibrosa—MAIVF*) are best detected and delineated by TEE (Fig. 18.14). These MAIVF lesions include:

- abscess formation
- rupture of the abscess with a resultant LVOT to LA communication and shunt
- aneurysm formation of the mitral valve
- anterior mitral leaflet perforation.

TEE is helpful in differentiating severe MR due to an anterior leaflet perforation from that of an LVOT–LA shunt (Figs 18.15 & 18.16).

Right-sided endocarditis

Tricuspid valve endocarditis is often an acute rather than subacute process, often involving the *Staphylococcus* sp. organism. Intravenous drug abusers (IVDA) usually have a normal valve structure before development of infection, whereas patients who are not drug abusers who develop right-sided endocarditis often have some form of underlying heart disease, such as a left-to-right shunt or valve disease.

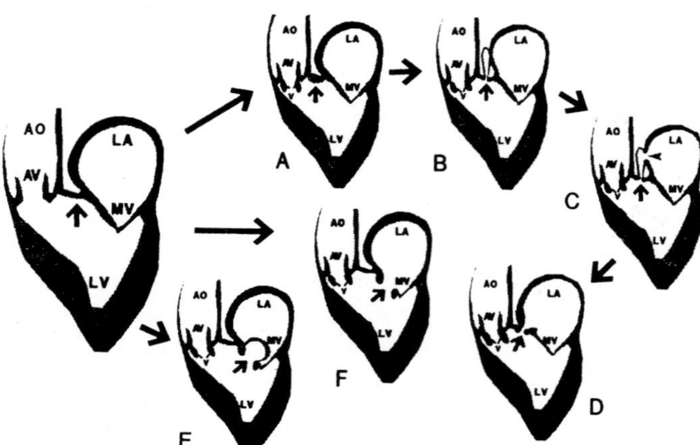

Fig. 18.14 Representation of complications of aortic valve endocarditis in relation to the mitral–aortic intervalvular fibrosa (MAIVF). (A) MAIVF abscess. (B) MAIVF aneurysm. (C) MAIVF aneurysm rupture into the left atrium. (D) MAIVF rupture into the left atrium without aneurysm formation. (E) Aneurysm of the anterior leaflet of the mitral valve. (F) Perforation of the anterior leaflet of the mitral valve. (Reproduced with permission from: Karalis GD, *et al*. Transesophageal echocardiographic recognition of subaortic complications in aortic valve endocarditis. Circulation 1992; 86: 353.)

Tricuspid vegetations are usually large (larger than those of left-sided valve lesions) and often described as "thick and shaggy" in appearance (Figs 18.17 & 18.18).

When *pulmonic valve endocarditis* occurs, it is usually in the setting of congenital heart disease (pulmonic stenosis, patent ductus arteriosus, tetralogy of Fallot, ventricular septal defect). Pulmonic valve endocarditis in the IVDA patient is much less common than with tricuspid valve involvement (Fig. 18.19).

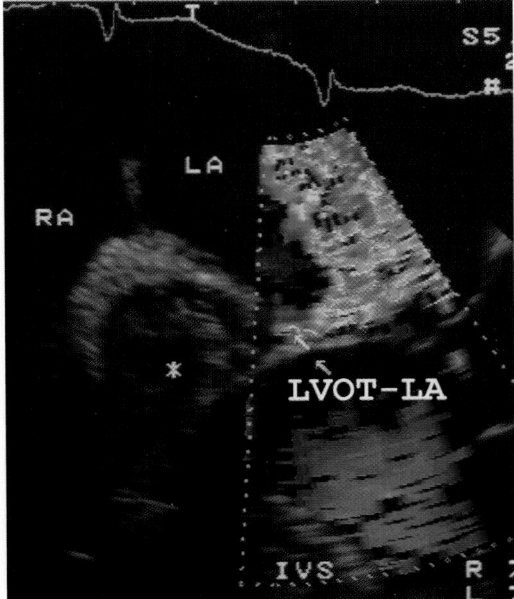

Fig. 18.15 TEE in the horizontal view of a patient with a large aortic perivalvular abscess (*) and a shunt from the LVOT into the LA (LVOT–LA). Careful evaluation of the source of the color regurgitant jet within the LA helps delineate the etiology (LVOT–LA, mitral valve regurgitation, or perforation of mitral leaflet).

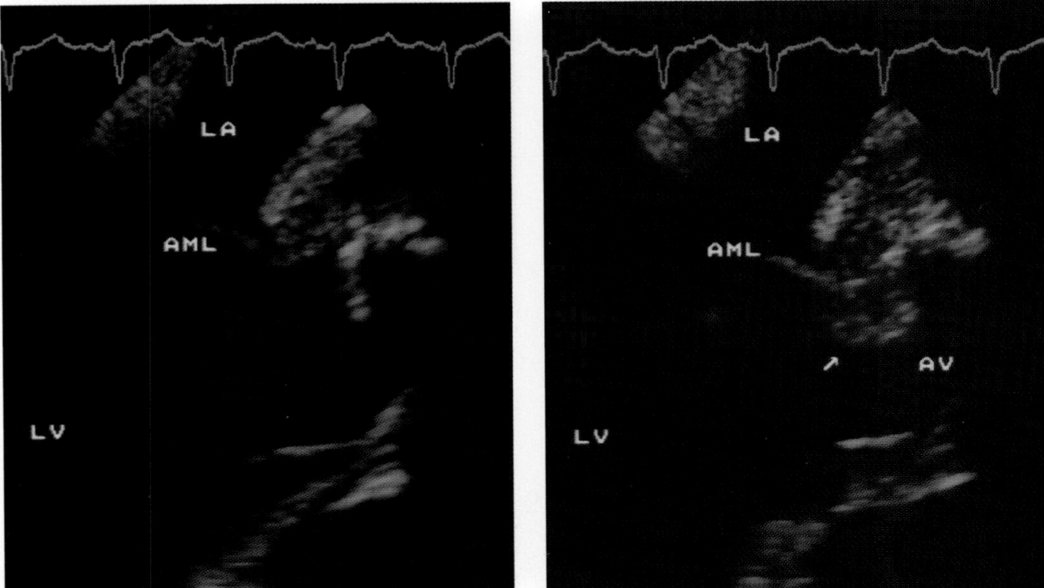

Fig. 18.16 A 46-year-old male on chronic hemodialysis with an aortic Carbomedics mechanical prosthesis, presented with fever and positive blood cultures. He underwent TEE study. (a) Systolic and (b) diastolic frames at 120°. (*Continued on p. 300.*)

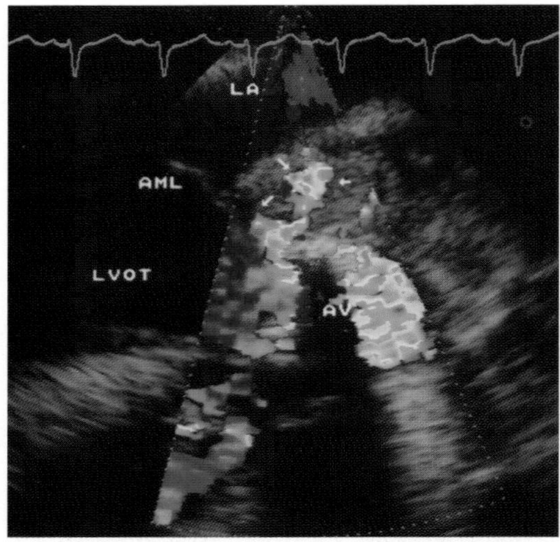

(c)

Fig. 18.16 (*cont'd*) (c) color Doppler at 135° reveal an area of systolic forward flow around the prosthesis, between the aortic prosthesis (AV) and the anterior leaflet of the mitral valve (AML). Note in this area of *valve annulus disruption* a diastolic "prolapse" into the LVOT (arrow in b). At surgery the entire aortic root was removed and replaced successfully with an aortic homograft.

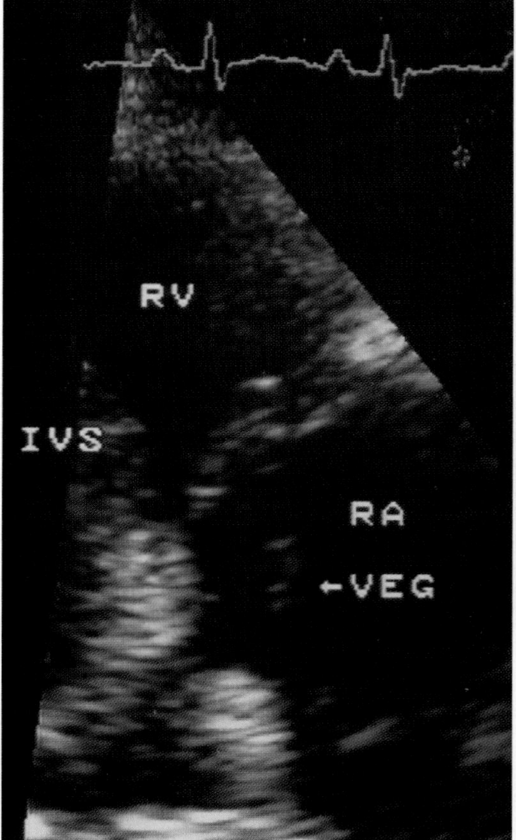

(a)

(b)

Fig. 18.17 A young man presented with spiking fevers and septic emboli on his admission chest X-ray. There was no history of intravenous drug use, but he had multiple chronic and acute abrasions on his limbs from crawling in attics of homes when he was at work servicing air-conditioning units. Blood cultures grew *Staphylococcus aureus*. (a) A systolic frame in the parasternal RV inflow view demonstrating a large tricuspid valve vegetation (VEG) prolapsing into the RA. (b) A diastolic frame demonstrating the vegetation (arrows) now in the RV. (*Cont'd.*)

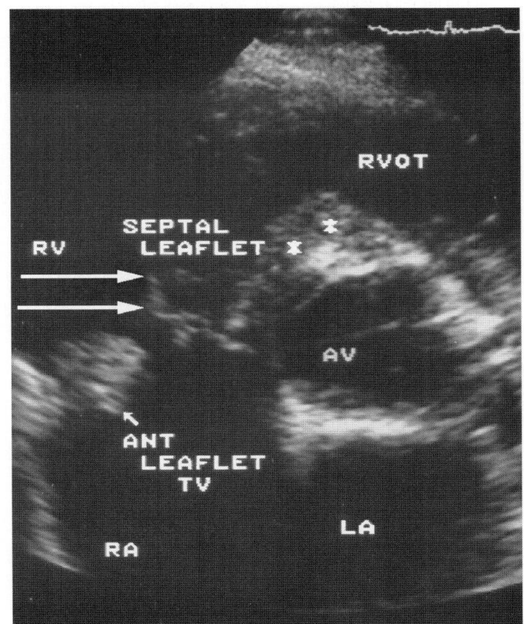

Fig. 18.17 (*cont'd*) (c) Parasternal short axis view at the aortic valve level reveals vegetations on both the septal and anterior leaflets of the tricuspid valve (TV). An abnormality (* *) noted below the tricuspid septal leaflet within the right ventricular outflow tract (RVOT) was documented to be an abscess at surgery.

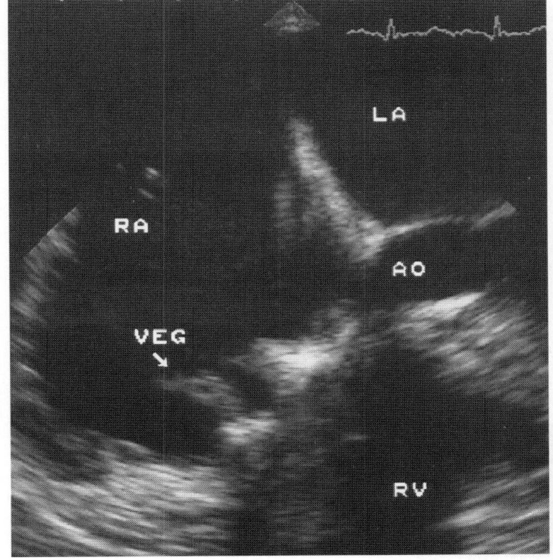

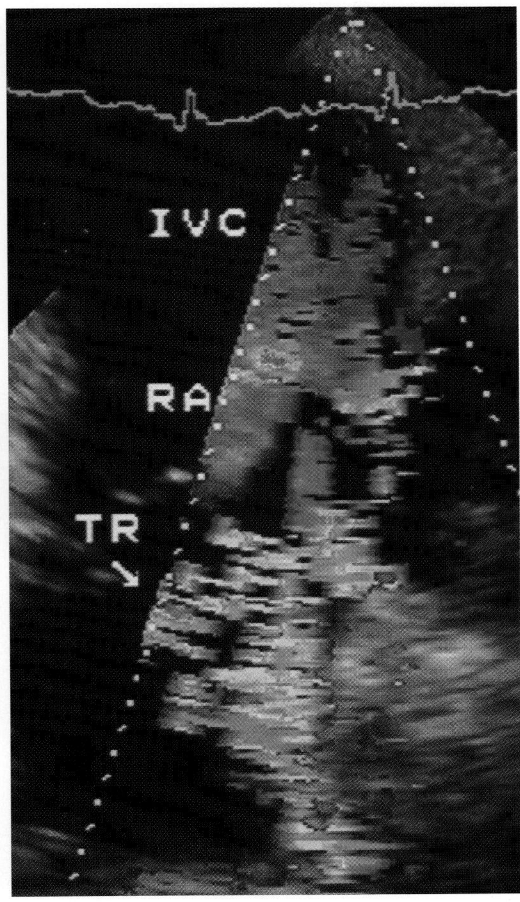

Fig. 18.18 A 32-year-old-female presented with fever and *Staphylococcus aureus* by blood culture. She had a history of IVDA, and had received a bioprosthetic tricuspid valve (TV) replacement in the past for severe tricuspid regurgitation (TR) related to drug-abuse-associated TV endocarditis. TEE in the horizontal plane demonstrates a large vegetation in (a) prolapsing into the RA in systole (VEG), and with (b) color Doppler marked valvular and peri-valvular TR was noted.

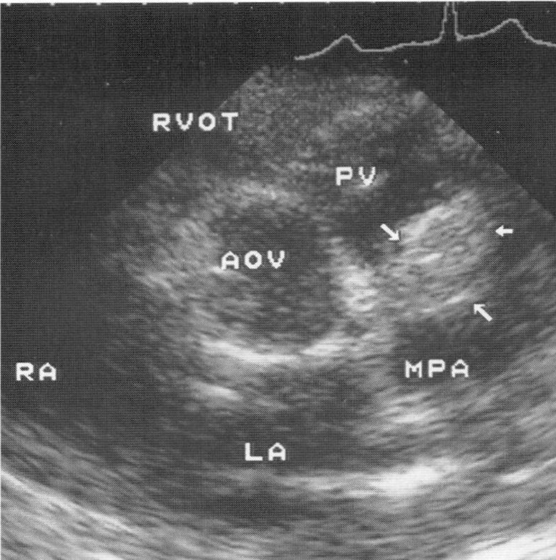

Fig. 18.19 Parasternal short axis view at the level of the aortic valve in an adult patient with a juxta-arterial doubly committed ventricular septal defect (see also Chapter 16). The patient had a history of IVDA and presented with fever and blood cultures positive for *Staphylococcus* sp. A vegetation (arrows) is noted attached to the pulmonic valve (PV). MPA, main pulmonary artery; AOV, aortic valve.

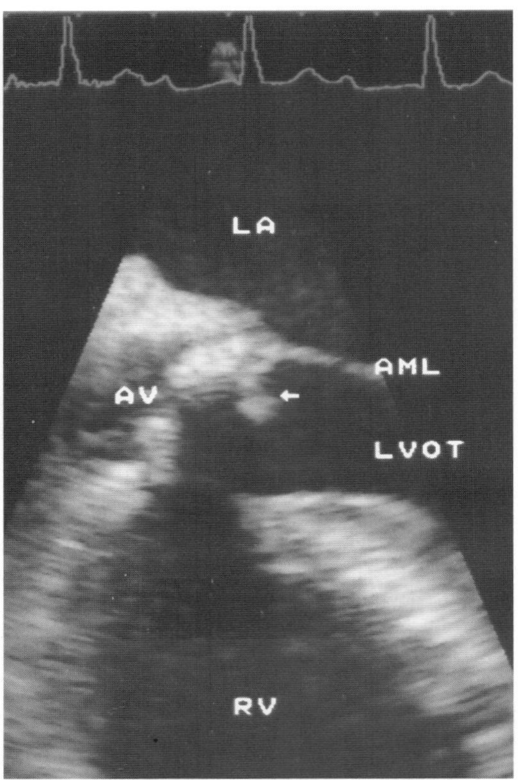

Fig. 18.21 TEE in the horizontal plane of a 72-year-old male with a chronic fistula from a ureter to the colon. He had a history of asymptomatic mild aortic stenosis, but presented with marked progressive exertional dyspnea and a noted loud murmur of aortic stenosis. Blood cultures grew *Candida tropicalis*. TTE with Doppler revealed progression of the patient's aortic stenosis over the course of 3 months, and TEE revealed a fixed mass (arrow) within the LVOT under the aortic valve. At surgery the vegetation was noted to also impede the aortic valve orifice. AV, aortic valve.

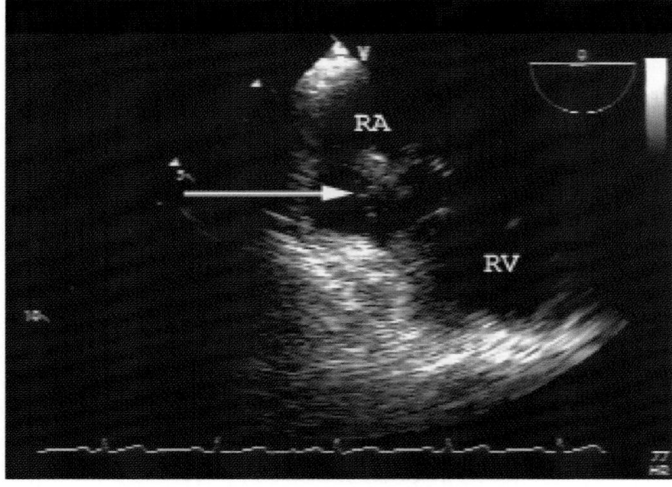

Fig. 18.20 TEE in the horizontal plane of a 43-year-old male who developed an infection after implantation of an automatic implantable cardiac defibrillator (AICD). The generator was removed, but the AICD electrode to the right ventricle could not be percutaneously removed. The patient continued with fever and a mobile friable mass, larger than 2 cm, was subsequently noted on the electrode within the right atrium.

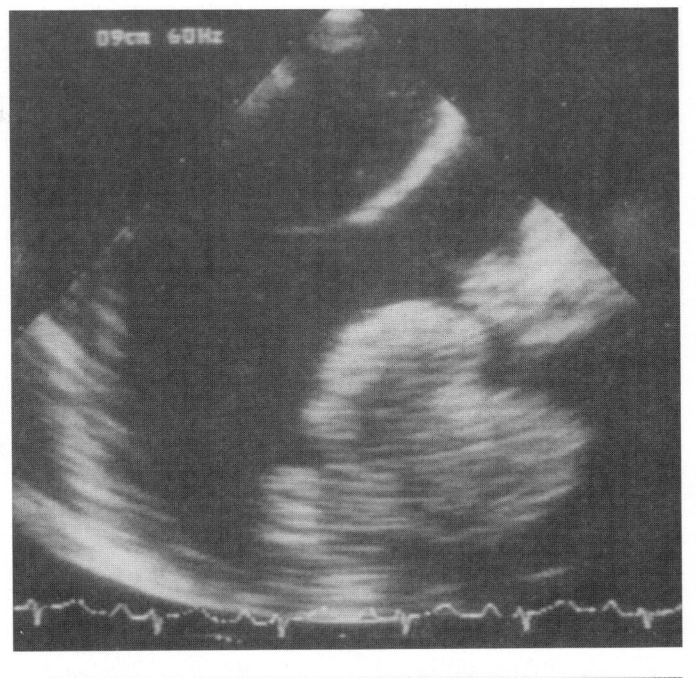

(a)

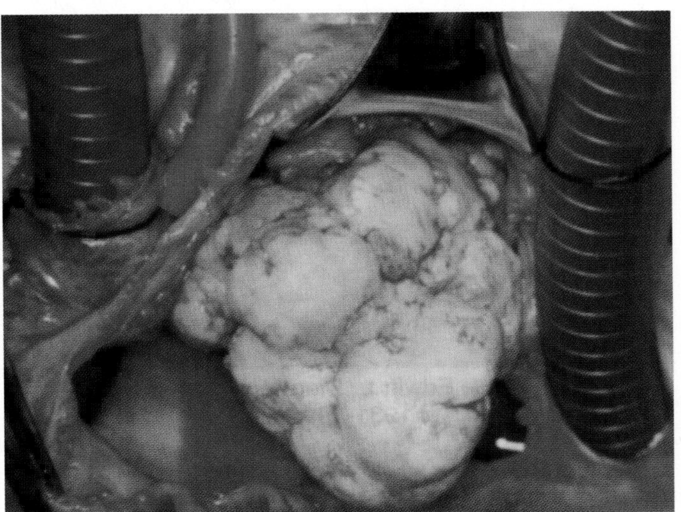

(b)

Fig. 18.22 (a) TEE in a patient with a history of intravenous drug abuse (IVDA) and blood cultures positive for *Candida albicans*. A large mass is attached to the TV. (b) Surgical image of the "cauliflower-like mass." (Reproduced with permission from: Matthew J, Gasior R, Thannoli N. Fungal mass on the tricuspid valve. Circulation 1996; 94: 2040.)

TTE is reasonably sensitive in imaging a large tricuspid vegetation but TEE appears substantially better in diagnosing pulmonic valve involvement. TEE may also be helpful in delineating the anatomy of the tricuspid valve and the etiology of tricuspid regurgitation. In addition, TEE may improve the diagnostic yield for endocarditis involving *pacemaker wires* (Fig. 18.20) or indwelling *venous catheters* (dialysis catheters).

Fungal endocarditis

Fungal endocarditis generally involves large vegetations with bulky lesions that may occasionally occlude a valve orifice. Frequently they will embolize, but generally cause less local valve leaflet destruction than do bacterial vegetations (Figs 18.21 & 18.22).

CHAPTER 19

Aorta and Aortic Dissection

Anatomy

Transesophageal echocardiography (TEE) has dramatically helped in ultrasound diagnosis of aortic pathology, especially acute dissecting aortic aneurysm. The esophagus is in close proximity to the aorta and great vessels and thus allows close evaluation (Fig. 19.1a). The aortic annulus and proximal aorta may be well visualized and measured by transthoracic echocardiography (Fig. 19.1b), but more distal segments of the thoracic aorta are difficult to image with TTE. TEE allows a more complete view of the aorta; however, the *left main stem bronchus* (LB) lies between the esophagus and upper ascending aorta limiting the ability to image that part of the aorta. The origin of the great vessels (see Fig. 4.27) may be visualized and identified by TEE. Specifically, the *left common carotid* (LC), the *left subclavian* (LS), and the *innominate artery* (IA) may be seen.

To best image the thoracic aorta with TEE, one should:

• Begin in the proximal descending aorta in the horizontal plane.
• Gradually withdraw the probe until the distal transverse aorta is visualized (the aorta will lose its circular appearance).
• Change from the horizontal plane (0°) to the vertical plane (90°). The transverse aorta will now appear "circular."
• Rotate the transducer clockwise until the IA comes into view (transducer imaging rotates toward patient's right) and then rotate the transducer counterclockwise to bring the LC and LS arteries into view.

The IA has an anterior origin from the aorta while the LC and LS arteries are posterior and smaller compared to the IA. On occasion, the branches of the IA may be visualized. Pulsed wave Doppler of IA and LS flow will reveal predominantly systolic arterial flow whereas LC Doppler will reveal systolic and diastolic flow.

The *innominate vein* (also termed *left brachiocephalic vein*) forms from the left internal jugular and left subclavian veins (Fig. 19.2). The innominate vein crosses anterior and superior to the transverse aortic arch, descending caudally into the SVC. When visualized by TEE, one should not confuse this as a localized transverse aortic dissection (see "Aortic dissection" below). Features to differentiate an innominate vein from an aortic dissection include:

• The wall of the vessel lacks the oscillating motion seen with an intimal flap.
• Pulsed and color Doppler reveal characteristic continuous venous flow in a direction from left to right (opposite of the flow direction seen within the aortic lumen).
• Sagittal imaging of the vein reveals a "tubular" structure.
• If needed, agitated saline injection into the left arm antecubital vein reveals contrast enhancement of the innominate vein.

Sinus of Valsalva aneurysm

Sinus of Valsalva aneurysm may be congenital or due to an infectious or inflammatory process. A congenital aneurysm may appear as a "wind sock" bulging into other cardiac structures. Multiple fenestrations may be present with a shunt into adjacent structures. Indistinction, patients with Marfan's syndrome have symmetric involvement of all three sinuses. A right sinus of Valsalva aneurysm is most common and a left sinus of Valsalva aneurysm is rarest, with sinus of Valsalva aneurysms. When a rupture occurs, a substantial shunt will result in left-sided volume overload.

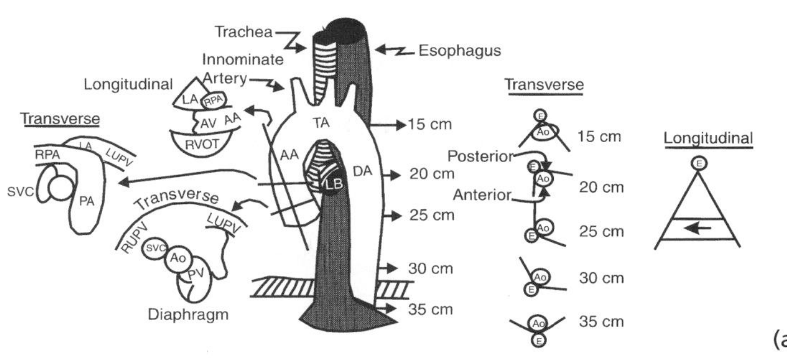

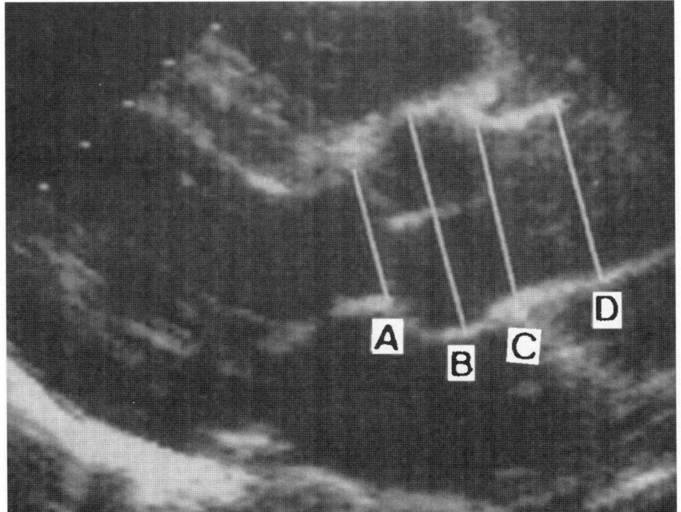

Fig. 19.1 (a) Anatomic relationship of the esophagus with the thoracic aorta. Note that the left main stem bronchus (LB) lies between the esophagus and upper ascending aorta, causing a "blind spot" in that area of the aorta. Note that the esophagus is initially posterior to the descending aorta, but becomes anterior at the level of the diaphragm. RPA, right pulmonary artery; PA, pulmonary artery; LUPV, left upper pulmonary vein; AA, ascending aorta; AV, aortic valve; RVOT, right ventricular outflow tract; RUPV, right upper pulmonary vein; SVC, superior vena cava; Ao, aorta; TA, transverse aorta; DA, descending aorta; PV, pulmonic valve. (b) Parasternal long axis of the aortic valve and proximal ascending aorta. Inner-edge to inner-edge measurements in early systole include: A, aortic annulus; B, sinus of Valsalva; C, sinotubular junction; D, ascending aorta. (Reproduced with permission from: Goldstein SA, Lindsay J. Thoracic aortic aneurysms: role of echocardiography. Echocardiography 1996; 13(2): 221.)

Rupture from the right coronary cusp results in shunting into either the RV or RA, whereas rupture from the noncoronary cusp results in shunting into the RA.

Acquired aortic aneurysms and disorders

Relatively common acquired aortic aneurysms may be divided into:

- aortic dissection and aortic intramural hematoma (AIH)
- traumatic aneurysms (see Chapter 14)
- atherosclerotic aneurysms and penetrating atherosclerotic ulcer
- pseudoaneurysm
- medial degeneration:
    - annuloaortic ectasia
    - Marfan's syndrome
    - other heritable disorders
    - associated with bicuspid aortic valve/coarctation (see Chapters 7 & 16)
- syphilis and noninfectious aortitis (giant-cell, Takayasu's) (see Chapter 21).

Aortic dissection

Transthoracic echocardiography (TTE) and TEE may be performed in the emergency room to make a rapid diagnosis (and to *rule out* dissection)). However, one must be alert to potential false positive or negative results (Figs 19.3–19.6). The most definitive finding for a dissection is an *undulating intimal aortic flap* by TEE, seen in more than one view. The flap should have

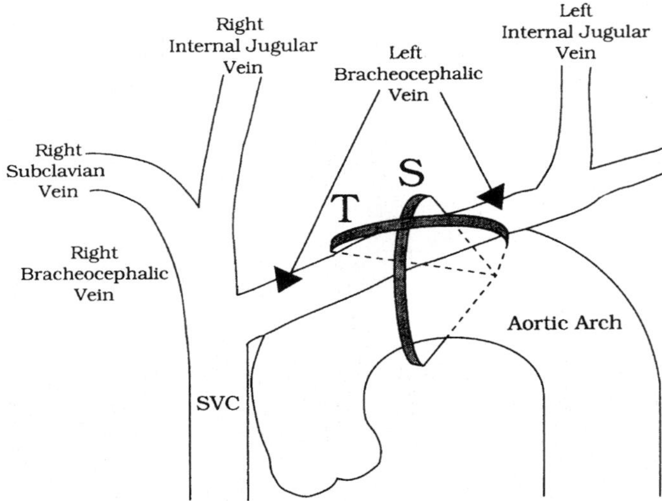

Fig. 19.2 The innominate vein (left brachiocephalic vein) crossing anterior and superior to the transverse aortic arch, descending caudally into the SVC. A TEE probe at the level of the transverse aorta images the aorta and innominate vein in its transverse plane position (T) at 0°, and in its sagittal plane (S) at 90° (see text). (Reproduced with permission from: Appelbe AF, Olson S, Biby LD, *et al.* Left brachiocephalic vein mimicking an aortic dissection on transesophageal echocardiography. Echocardiography 1993: 10(1): 67–69.)

a defined motion that is not parallel to that of any other cardiothoracic structure. With a chronic false lumen thrombosis, central displacement of intimal calcification is helpful in making a diagnosis of dissection.

Artifacts may at times simulate an intimal flap. These include *linear artifacts* in the ascending aorta (seen in up to 44% of patients) and at the level of the diaphragm, and also *mirror image artifacts* in the transverse and descending thoracic aorta (seen in >80% of patients). Linear artifacts of the ascending aorta are caused by ultrasound reflection within the left atrium, and are associated with a dilated ascending aorta. They are more frequent when the aortic diameter is greater than the left atrial diameter (Fig. 19.7). At the level of the diaphragm, an artifact from reflection of the ultrasound between the aorta and diaphragm may be seen when a left pleural effusion is present, and possibly ascites also (Fig. 19.8). Mirror image artifacts appear as a "double-barrel" aorta, and are caused by the aorta–lung interface. Other potential pitfalls in imaging include an aberrant right subclavian artery (Fig. 4.27), the innominate vein (see

(a)

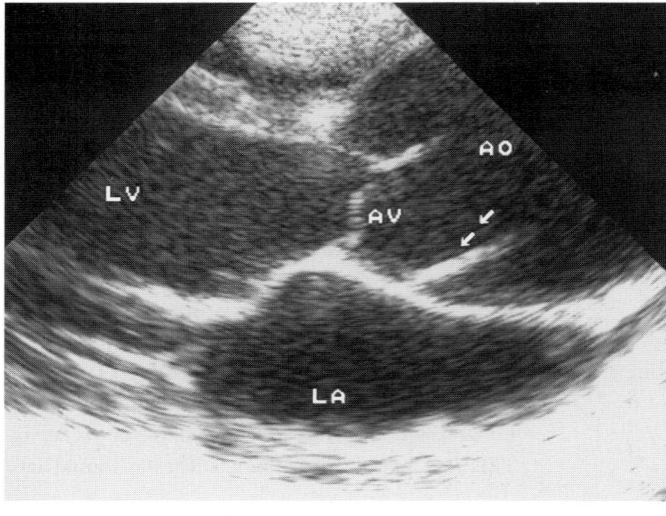

Fig. 19.3 A young adult with Marfan's syndrome who presented with severe chest pain. Transthoracic echocardiography (TTE) reveals a Type I dissection with a posterior tear in a dilated aorta. (a) Parasternal long axis of the proximal ascending aorta. (*Cont'd.*)

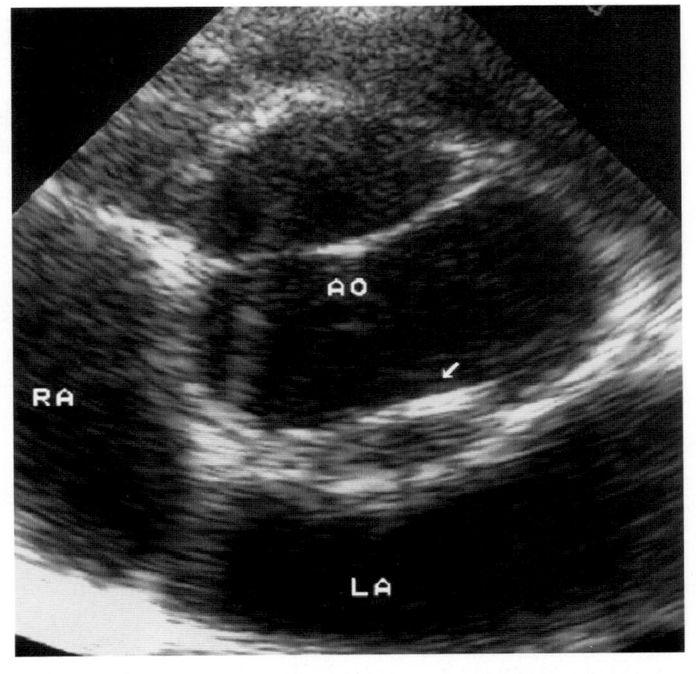

(b)

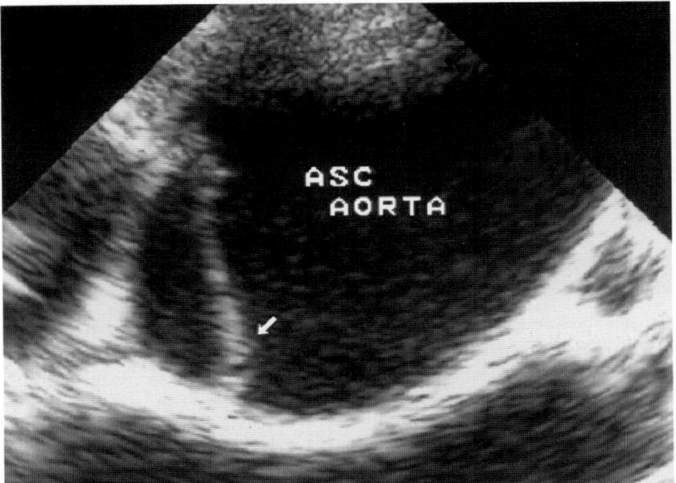

(c)

Fig. 19.3 (*cont'd*) (b) Parasternal short axis and (c) right upper parasternal image of upper ascending aorta. Arrow points to the intimal tear in all three images. AO, aorta; AV, aortic valve; ASC AORTA, ascending aorta.

discussion above), collapsed lung, hiatal hernia, the hemiazygos vein, spinal cord, and esophageal varices (Fig. 19.9).

When evaluating a patient for a potential dissection, the following information should be obtained:

- presence of dissection
- location of dissection:

  Type A

  DeBakey Type I—ascending aorta extending into descending aorta

  DeBakey Type II—ascending aorta only

  Type B

  DeBakey Type III—descending aorta
- location of entry tear

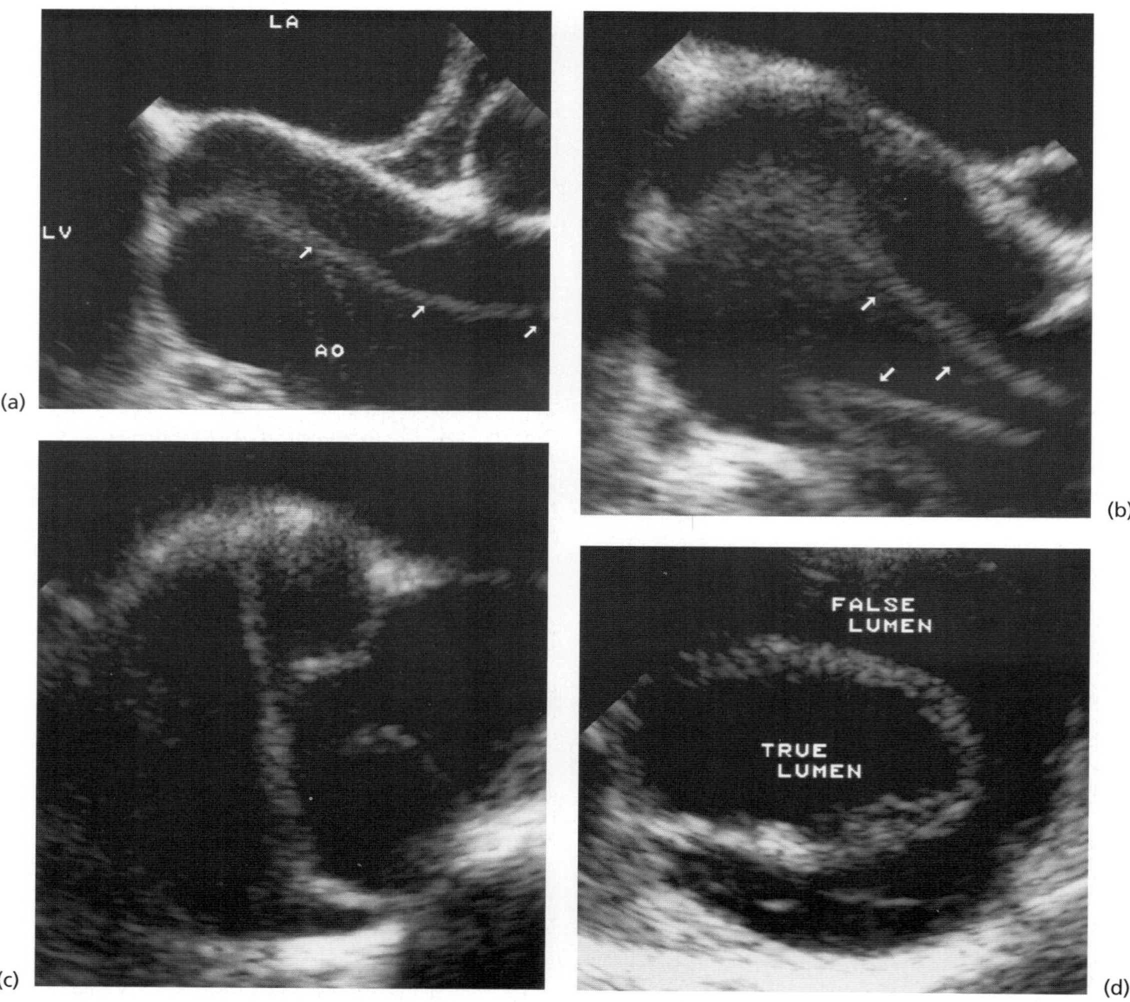

Fig. 19.4 Transesophageal echocardiography (TEE) of Type I dissection in a middle-aged hypertensive patient presenting with severe chest pain. (a,b) Sequential time-frame longitudinal images suggesting a "double lumen" with an undulating intimal flap. (c) Transverse image of the proximal aortic root tear. (d) Longitudinal image of transverse aorta demonstrating the "double lumen."

- location of re-entry tear and secondary tears
- involvement of arch and major branch vessels
- differentiation of true from false lumen
- involvement of coronary arteries (dissection frequently involves the right coronary ostium, rarely the left; coronary ostia may become obstructed by prolapse of the intimal flap in diastole or by false lumen distention impeding flow)
- presence and extent of aortic regurgitation (see discussion below)
- pericardial effusion and tamponade
- left ventricular function.

To differentiate true from false lumens, the following may be helpful:

- Using M-mode, the flap moves toward the false lumen in systole.
- Spontaneous echo contrast "smoke" and thrombus may form in the false lumen.
- Color Doppler reveals delayed systolic flow through secondary or re-entrant tears into the false lumen.

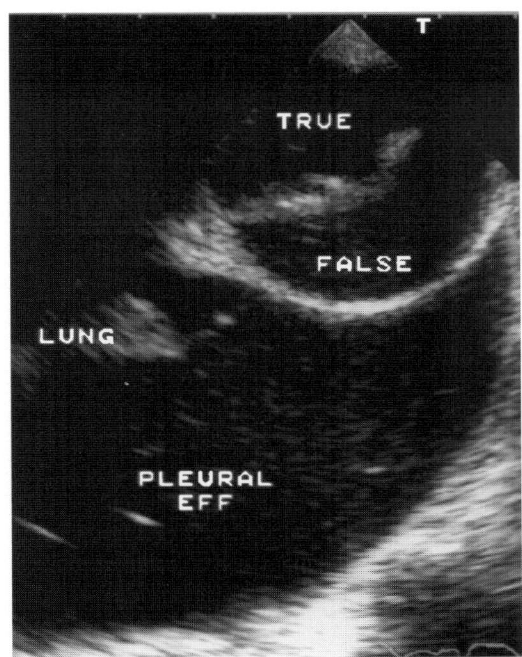

Fig. 19.5 TEE in the transverse view of the descending aorta in the same patient as the previous example. This study was performed 24 h after surgical repair of the ascending aortic tear. Spontaneous echo contrast was readily evident in the false lumen (FALSE), and flow by color flow imaging in the true lumen (TRUE). Note the left pleural effusion (PLEURAL EFF).

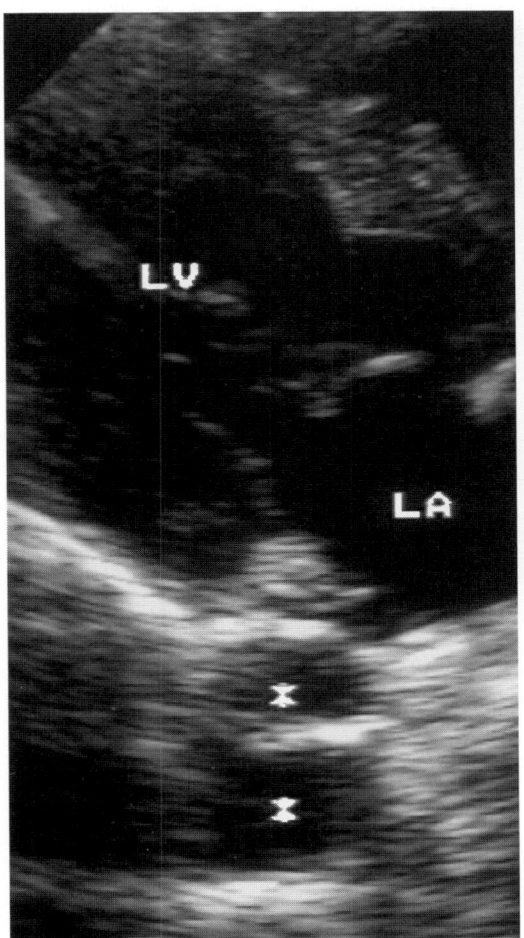

(a)

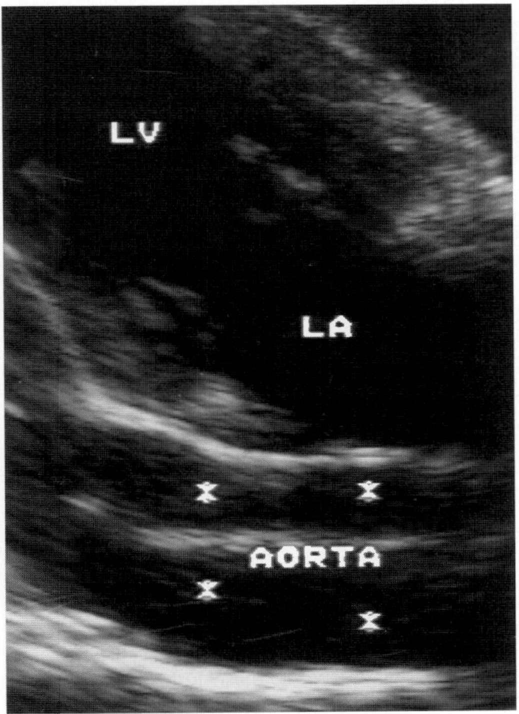

(b)

Fig. 19.6 TTE imaging in a parasternal window of a chronic dissection of the descending aorta, giving a double-lumen appearance. (a) Cross-sectional and (b) longitudinal image of the descending aorta (*).

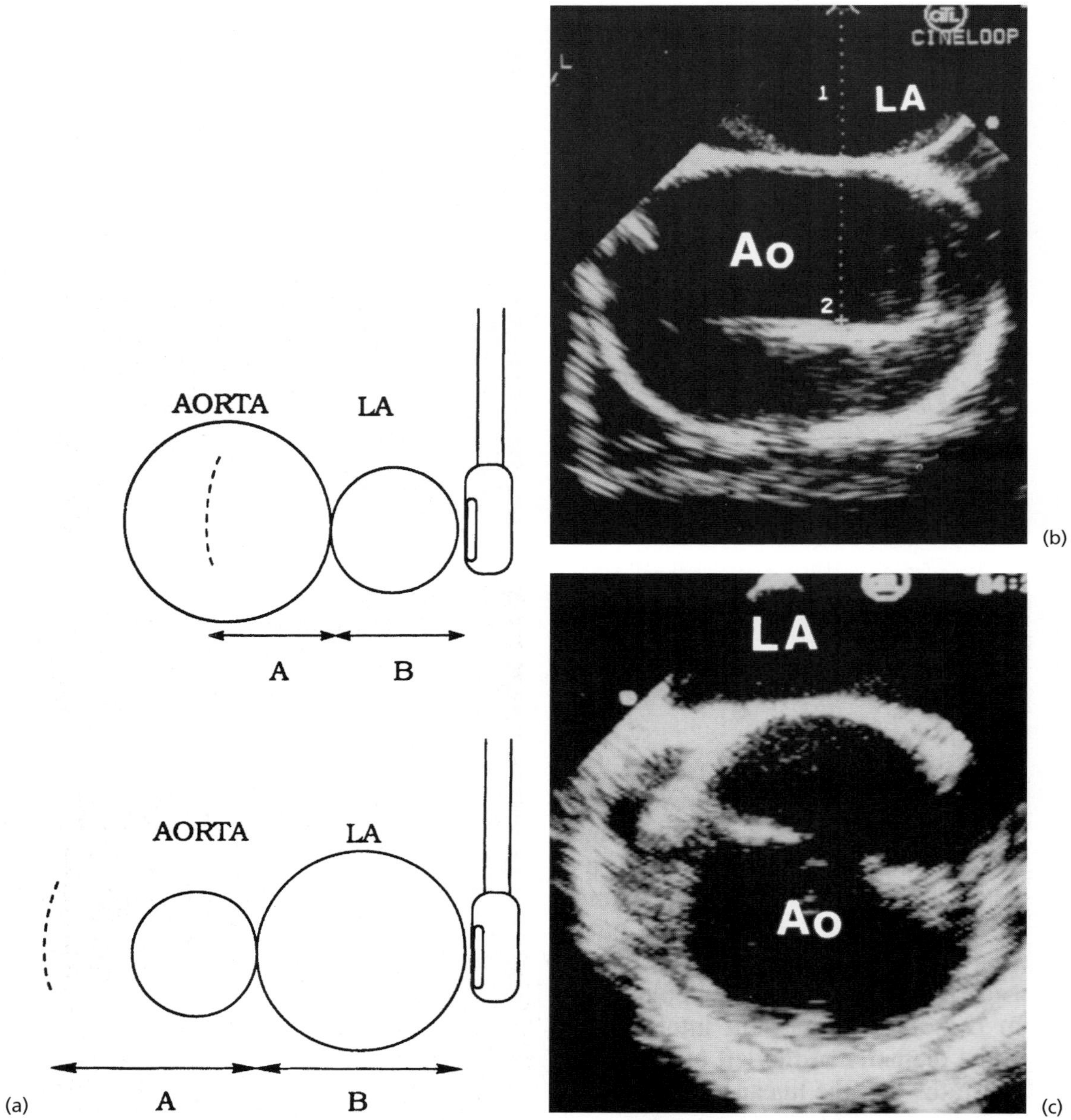

AORTA LA

A B

AORTA LA

A B

(a)

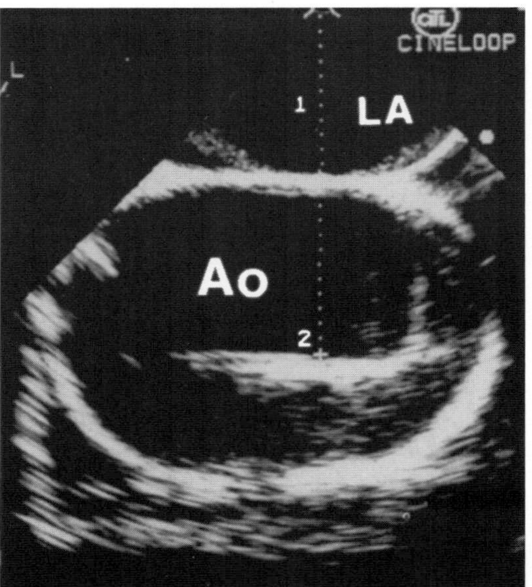

(b)

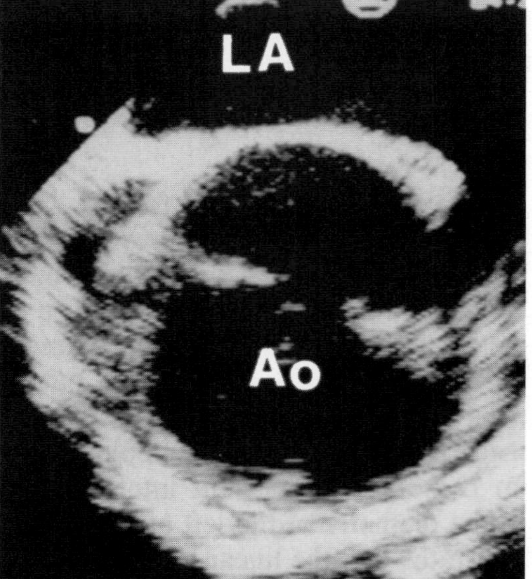

(c)

Fig. 19.7 (a) An *in vitro* model of the ascending aorta (AORTA) and left atrium (LA). An artifact (dashed curved line) will appear within the aorta (upper panel) at twice the diameter of the LA (twice the length B), and is due to ultrasound reverberation from the LA wall. If the LA is larger than the aorta (lower panel) then the artifact will appear outside the aortic lumen. (b) An example of a "balloon model" representing the LA and aorta (Ao). (c) The LA and aorta (Ao) in a patient. A linear artifact within the aortic lumen may mimic an intimal flap. (Reproduced with permission from: Appelbe AF, Walker PG, Yeoh JK, *et al.* Clinical significance and origin of artifacts in transesophageal echocardiography of the thoracic aorta. Journal of the American College of Cardiology 1993; 21: 754–760.)

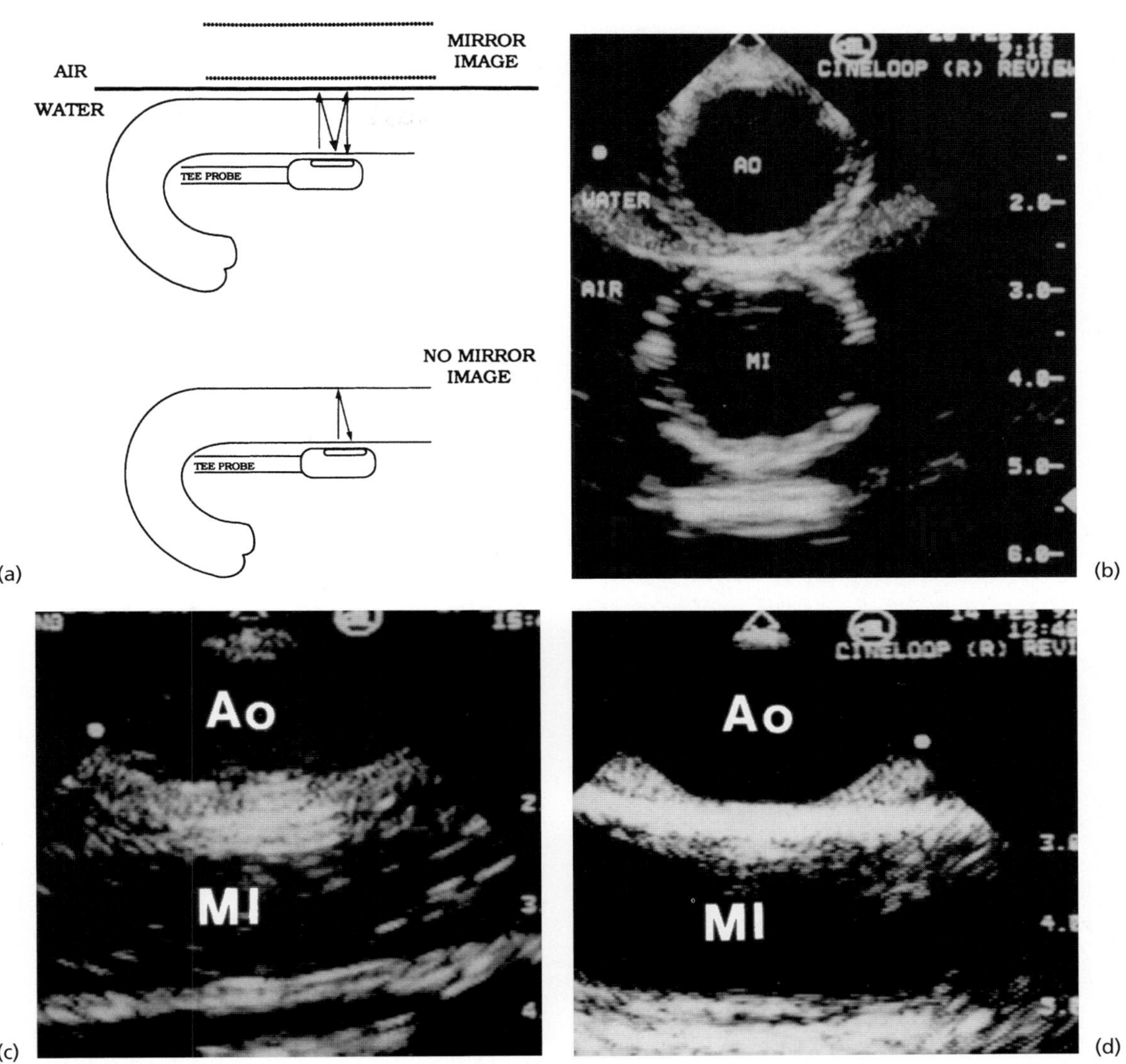

Fig. 19.8 (a) An *in vitro* model simulating the mirror image artifact of the descending aorta. When an air–water interface exists (upper panel), reverberation of the ultrasound signal will occur, and a mirror image will be generated. (b,c) A model demonstrating the mirror image (MI) phenomena. (d) The MI phenomena in a patient. Within the mirror image, Doppler color flow will appear, as in the true lumen. (Reproduced with permission from: Appelbe AF, Walker PG, Yeoh JK, *et al*. Clinical significance and origin of artifacts in transesophageal echocardiography of the thoracic aorta. Journal of the American College of Cardiology 1993; 21: 754–760.)

• False lumen (especially in chronic dissections) is usually larger than the true lumen.

If aortic regurgitation (AR) is present in a patient with dissection of the ascending aorta; one should evaluate for the mechanism of AR to determine if the aortic valve is potentially reparable. Etiologies of AR in a patient with aortic dissection are:

1 Potentially repairable valves (Fig. 19.10)

(a) Incomplete closure of an intrinsically normal leaflet due to tethering by a dilated sinotubular junction, with a resultant central regurgitant jet (Fig. 19.11).

(b) Leaflet prolapse due to leaflet attachment disruption from a dissection extending below into the aortic root.

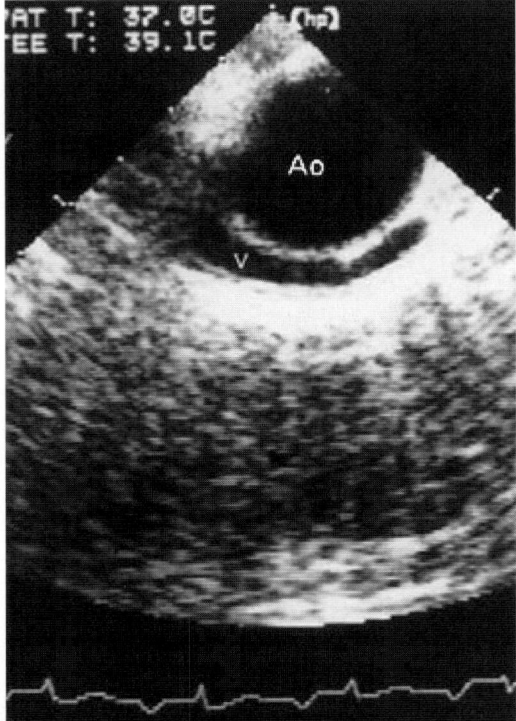

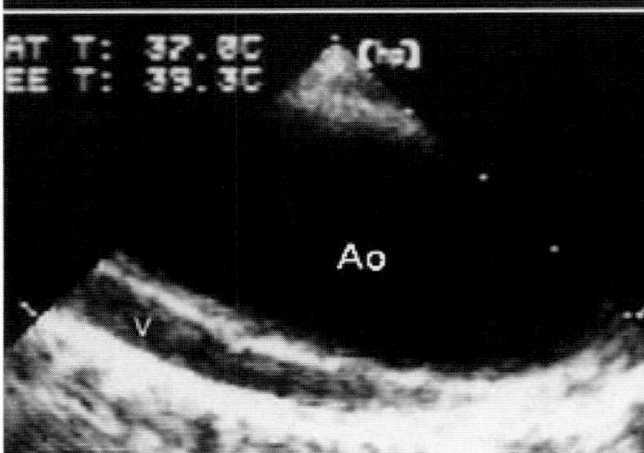

Fig. 19.9 TEE of the proximal descending aorta in both horizontal (upper panel) and vertical (lower panel) planes of a patient with previously unrecognized esophageal varices. Multiple periaortic echolucent channels were noted in the mid-distal descending aorta along the posterolateral and anterolateral aspects of the aorta. Venous flow was documented by PW Doppler. Further imaging posterior to the esophagus revealing multiple channels also confirmed varices to the authors of this case report. V, varices; AO, descending aorta. (Reproduced with permission from: Chang GL, Lynch M, Martin RP. Diagnosis of esophageal varices by transesophageal echocardiography: a mimicker of aortic disease. J Am Soc Echo 1997; 10: 231–235.)

(c) Diastolic prolapse of the dissection flap through the aortic annulus impeding leaflet coaptation (Fig. 19.12).

2 Potentially nonrepairable valves

(a) Bicuspid aortic valve with associated leaflet prolapse not related to the dissection.

(b) Degenerative leaflet thickening with abnormal leaflet coaptation.

(c) Marfan's syndrome, preexisting aortic root aneurysm, or bicuspid aortic valve with AR.

A few medical centers have performed repair of a prolapsing bicuspid valve with some success.

Aortic intramural hematoma

An *aortic intramural hematoma* (*AIH*) is thought to begin with rupture of the vasa vasorum within the aortic wall, with a circumferential hematoma developing (Fig. 19.13). AIH may be defined as:

- hemorrhage with circular or crescentic thickening of the aortic wall >0.7 cm (some use >0.5 cm as a definition of AIH)
- central displacement of intimal calcification (this is an important diagnostic clue)
- layered appearance
- longitudinal length of 1–20 cm
- absence of an intimal tear
- in some patients slight movement of aortic wall layers may be noted.

Diagnosis of AIH may be difficult. Because the intima remains intact, aortography will generally not visualize an AIH. CT or MRI may help make the diagnosis, although AIH will not enhance with contrast. AIH and *severe atherosclerotic aortic disease in conjunction with an old healing dissection* of the descending aorta may be nearly impossible to distinguish. AIH will change with time, upon repeat TEE. Also, a *descending aortic thoracic aneurysm with layered thrombus* may appear as an AIH. A *periaortic fat pad* may simulate an AIH by TEE. A subtle movement with respiration along the line between the aortic wall and adjacent fat may be seen. MRI will help diagnose a periaortic fat pad. When evaluating the ascending aorta, a periaortic fat pad or imaging the aorta with an oblique view through the aortic wall with a resultant appearance of aortic wall thickening, may mimic an AIH. Again, MRI will help in the diagnosis.

Atherosclerotic aneurysms and penetrating atherosclerotic aortic ulcer

Atherosclerosis is the most common cause of *aortic*

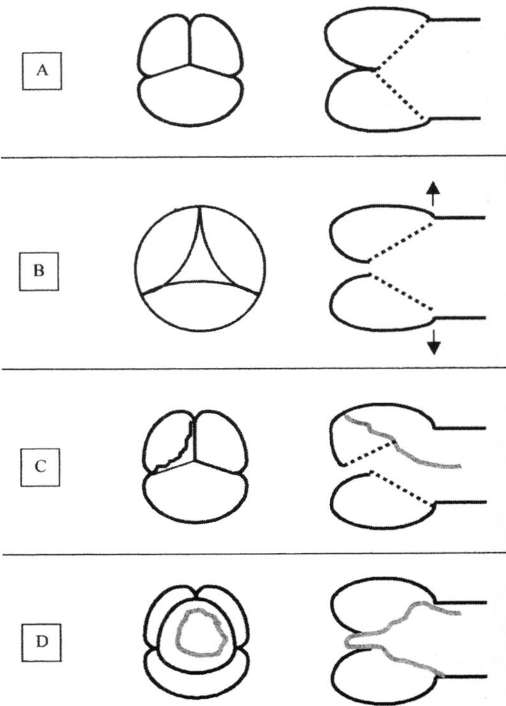

Fig. 19.10 The mechanisms of potentially repairable lesions of the aortic valve in patients with aortic dissection and aortic regurgitation (AR). Left-sided panels represent the short axis in diastole, and right-sided panels the long axis in diastole. Dotted lines in the right-sided panels represent leaflet tip attachment to the sinotubular junction. (A) Normal aortic valve anatomy in which leaflet tip coaptation is complete. Also note that the sinotubular junction diameter is similar to that of the annulus base. (B) Incomplete leaflet coaptation when the sinotubular junction dilates relative to the aortic annulus. (C) Aortic leaflet prolapse occurs when the dissection extends into the aortic root, disrupting normal leaflet attachment, with a resultant eccentric regurgitant jet. (D) Dissection flap prolapses in diastole through the aortic annulus impeding valve closure. (With permission from Mousowitz HD, Levine RA, Hilgenberg AD, Isselbacher EM. Transesophageal echocardiographic description of the mechanisms of aortic regurgitation in acute type A aortic dissection: implications for aortic valve repair. J Am Coll Cardiol 2000; 36: 884–890.)

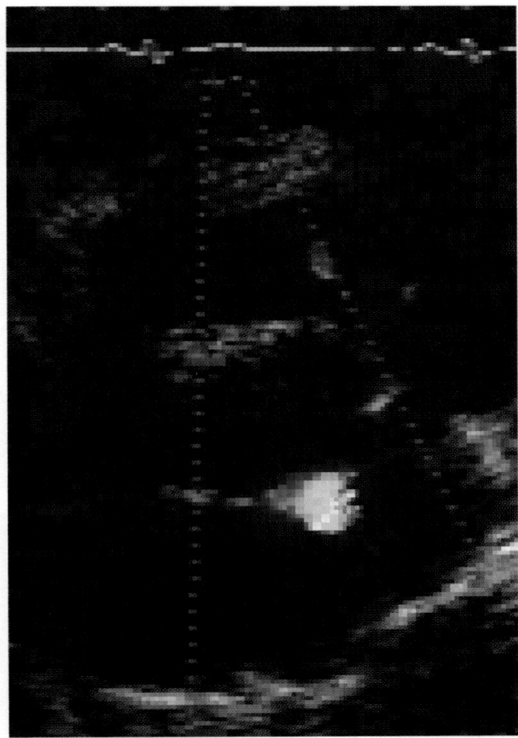

Fig. 19.11 Parasternal short axis with color flow Doppler in a patient with annuloaortic ectasia. Aortic regurgitation is due to inadequate central coaptation of the aortic leaflets, with resultant central aortic regurgitation.

aneurysm formation. Most are infrarenal in location, but up to 25% may affect the descending or occasionally the ascending thoracic aorta. These aneurysms usually are lined by irregular atherosclerotic plaque, and are best seen by TEE (see Chapter 16). Typically fusiform, they may also be saccular (Figs 19.14 & 19.15).

Penetrating atherosclerotic aortic ulcer (*PAAU*) may present with chest or back pain, especially in elderly hypertensive patients, or may be asymptomatic. Plaque erosion and ulceration penetrate into the media. A localized AIH may develop, as well as aneurysm and pseudoaneurysm formation (probably these two are most common to develop), aortic dissection, or transmural rupture. Aortography, CT or MRI, as well as TEE are helpful for diagnosis. TEE will image the ulcer as a crater or outpouching within an atherosclerotic aorta, usually in the mid or distal descending portions (Fig. 19.16).

Pseudoaneurysms of the thoracic aorta

Aortic pseudoaneurysms may occur as a result of:

- blunt chest trauma
- penetrating trauma
- infection (mycotic aneurysm)
- PAAU
- following surgical repair of aorta—coarctation of aorta, ductus arteriosus.

Rupture of the descending thoracic aorta may be contained by the adventitia and mediastinal

(a)

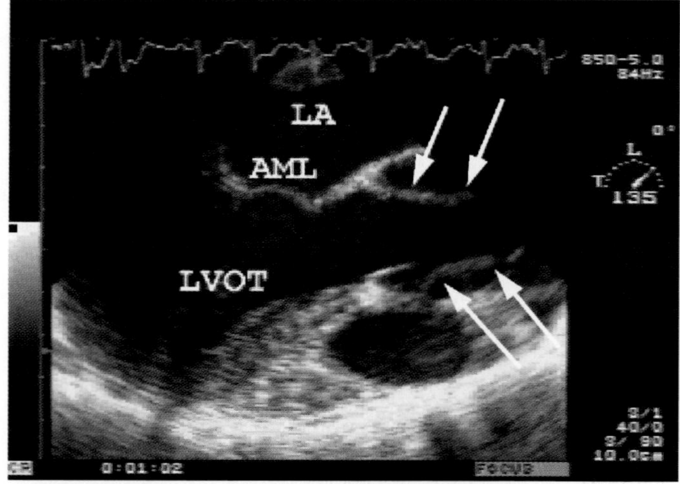

(b)

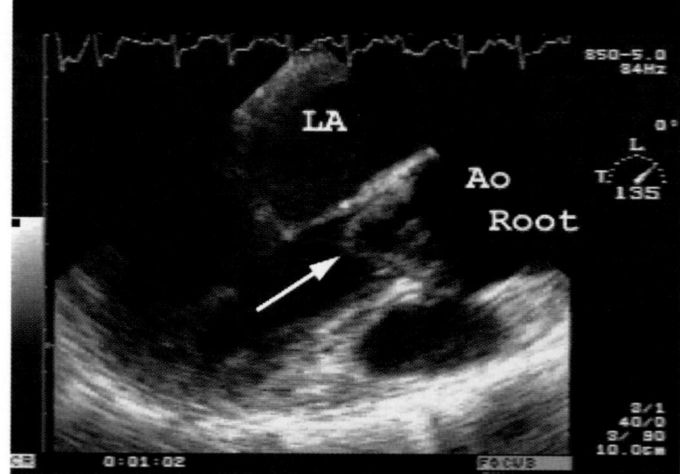

Fig. 19.12 A middle-aged female presented with acute Type I aortic dissection. Severe aortic regurgitation is due to prolapse of the intimal flap through the aortic annulus. By TEE at 135° in systole (a) the intimal tear is noted within the aortic root (arrows), and in diastole (b) the intimal tear prolapses (arrow) into the left ventricular outflow tract (LVOT). LA, left atrium; AML, anterior mitral valve leaflet; Ao Root, ascending aortic root.

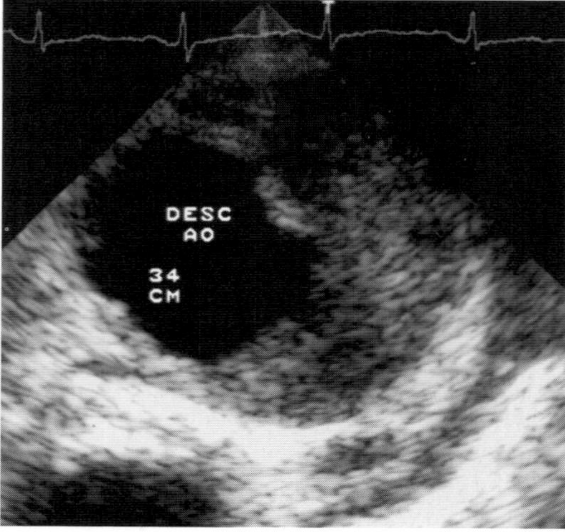

Fig. 19.13 Aortic intramural hematoma (AIH) of the descending thoracic aorta. The patient presented with severe back pain. TEE imaging revealed a hematoma extending just distal to origin of the left subclavian artery through the diaphragm level. Note the crescentic shape. The patient developed further pain and hemodynamic instability, requiring surgical correction.

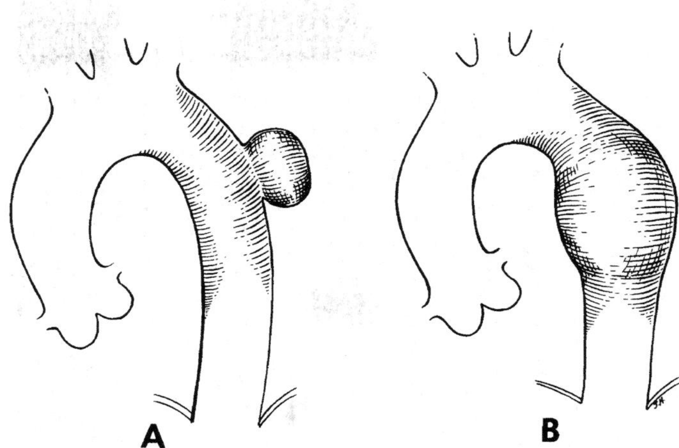

Fig. 19.14 Atherosclerotic aneurysms may be (A) saccular or (B) fusiform. Most often they are fusiform. (Reproduced with permission from: Goldstein SA, Lindsay J. Thoracic aortic aneurysms: role of echocardiography. Echocardiography 1996; 13(2): 214.)

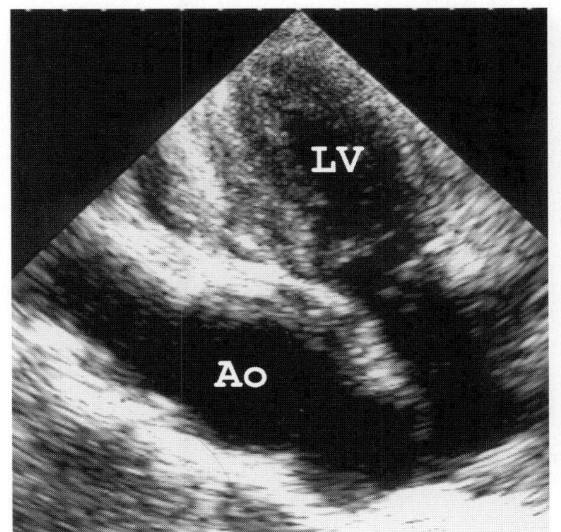

(a)

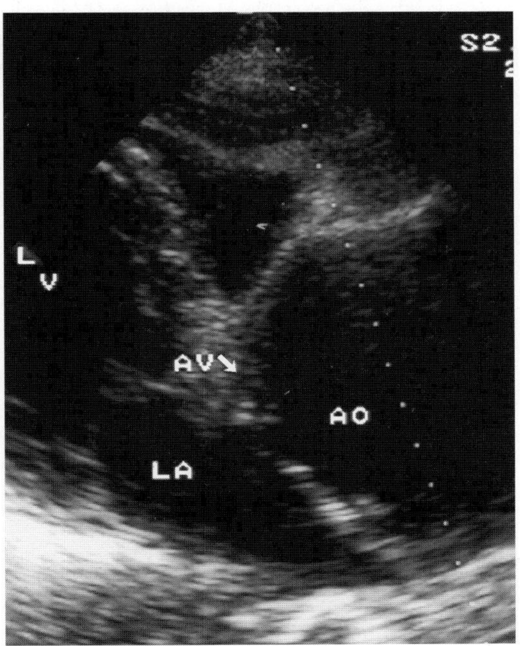

(b)

Fig. 19.15 (a) Modified transthoracic apical image of the LV and LA with a large atherosclerotic descending thoracic aneurysm compressing the left atrium. (b) Parasternal long axis image of an elderly patient with a large aneurysm of the ascending aorta, measuring more than 80 mm in diameter. Ao, aorta.

structures. Thrombus will usually line the cavity (Figs 19.17 & 19.18). As pitfalls exist for diagnosis of aortic dissection, one must be alert for pitfalls in diagnosis of aortic rupture (Fig. 19.19).

Medial degeneration (annuloaortic ectasia/Marfan's syndrome)

Annuloaortic ectasia is common in patients with *Marfan's syndrome* and probably is a result of an

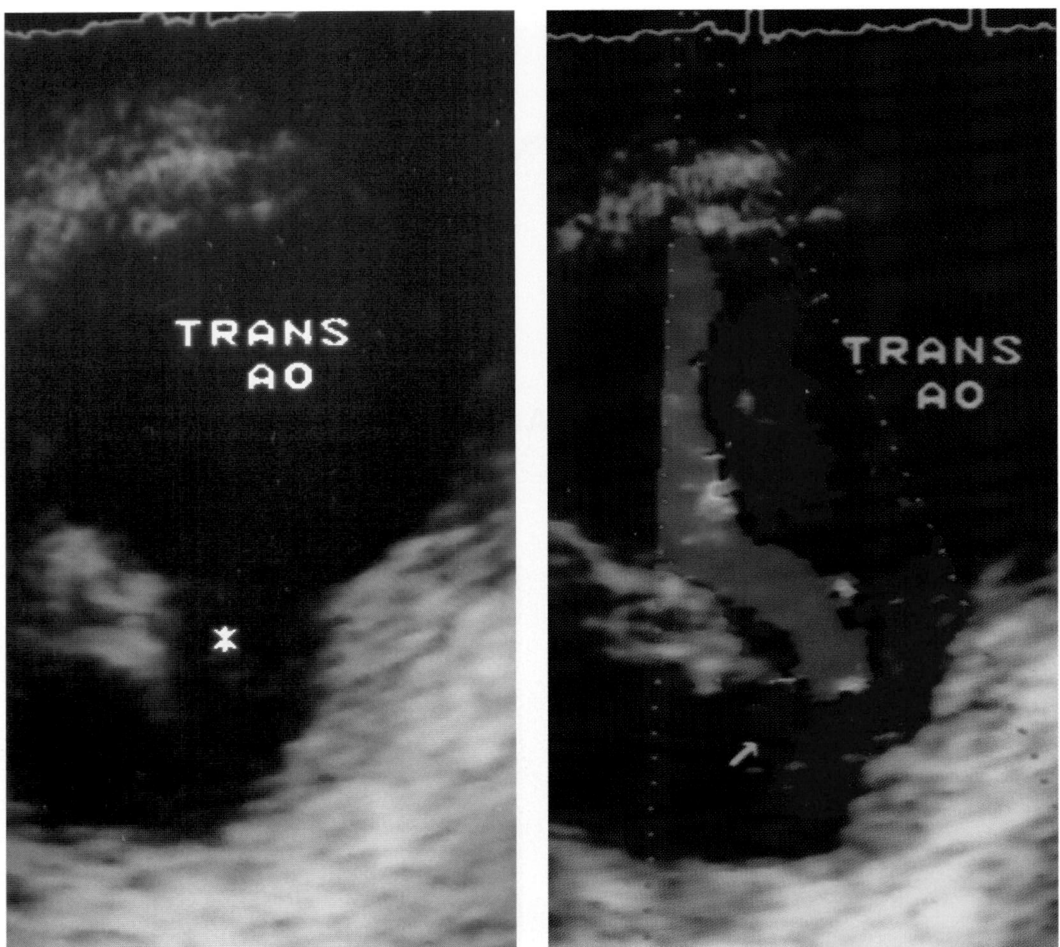

Fig. 19.16 Penetrating atherosclerotic aortic ulcer in an elderly patient, located in the distal transverse aorta. TEE (a) two-dimensional and (b) color flow Doppler image.

abnormality of the media (sometimes termed *cystic medial necrosis*). The proximal ascending aorta is symmetrically dilated, often with dilatation of the sinuses of Valsalva and aortic annulus (Figs 19.3, 19.11, 19.20–19.22). Annuloaortic ectasia may also occur with Ehlers–Danlos syndrome, osteogenesis imperfecta, and autosomal dominant polycystic kidney disease.

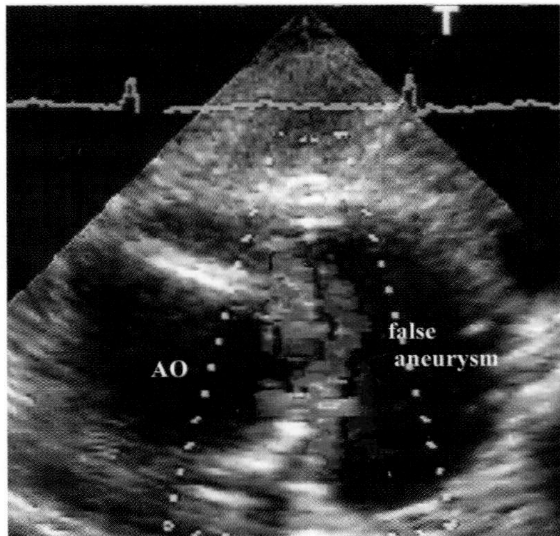

Fig. 19.17 TEE transverse view of a mycotic pseudoaneurysm (false aneurysm) of the descending thoracic aorta documented at surgery. The patient presented with fever and "tamponade" of the left heart, from the false aneurysm compressing the LA. AO, descending aorta.

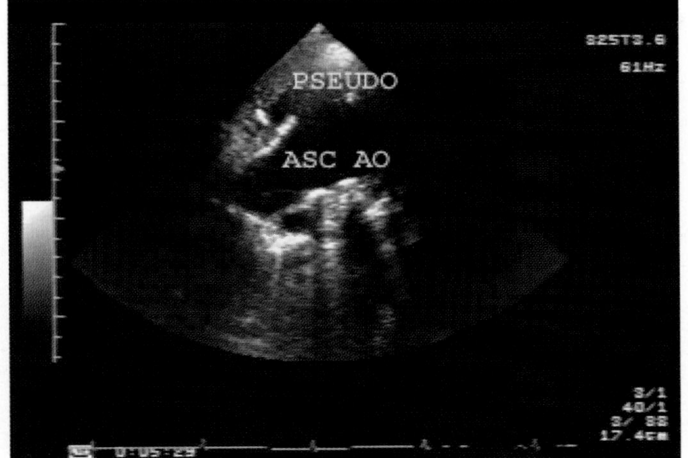

(a)

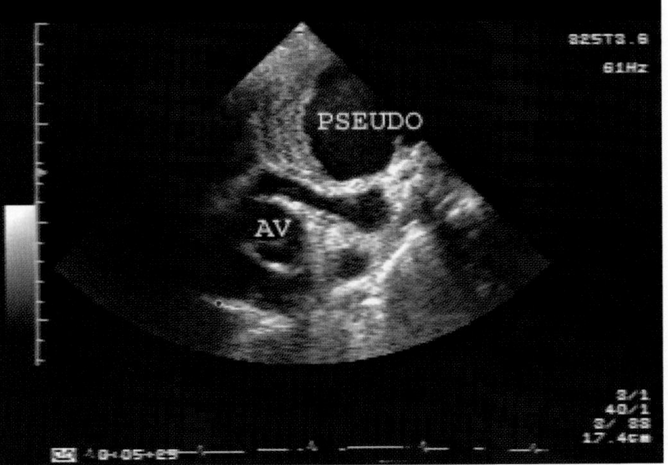

(b)

Fig. 19.18 TTE imaging from a high parasternal window in an elderly patient who presented with severe anterior upper chest pain. (a) There is a pseudoaneurysm cavity (PSEUDO) adjacent to the upper ascending aorta (ASC AO). (b) The transducer has been rotated. The aortic valve (AV) is also noted.

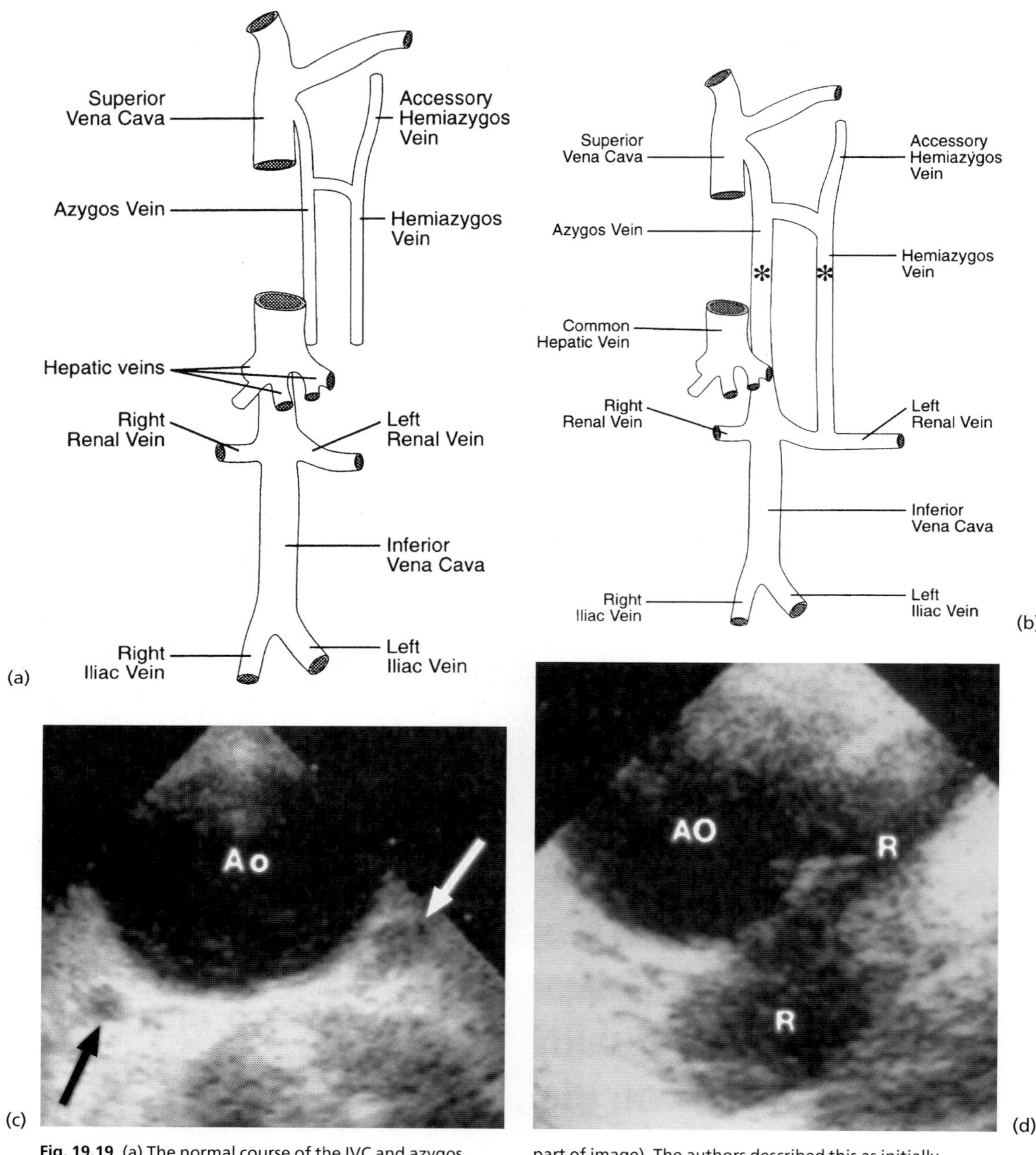

Fig. 19.19 (a) The normal course of the IVC and azygos and hemiazygos venous system. (b) With interruption of the IVC, flow continues into either the azygos or the hemiazygos system. (c) TEE in the horizontal plane of the descending aorta (AO), azygos vein (white arrow), and hemiazygos vein (black arrow). (d) TEE in the horizontal plane of the descending aorta (AO) and prominent drainage from the hepatic vein (R in lower part of image) into the azygos vein (R in upper right part of image). The authors described this as initially being misdiagnosed as a partial aortic rupture, but agitated saline injection in a foot vein documented saline enhancement of these vessels. (Reproduced with permission from: Blanchard DG, Sobel JL, Hope J, *et al.* Infrahepatic interruption of the inferior vena cava with azygos continuation: a potential mimicker of aortic pathology. Journal of the American Society of Echocardiography 1998; 11: 1079.)

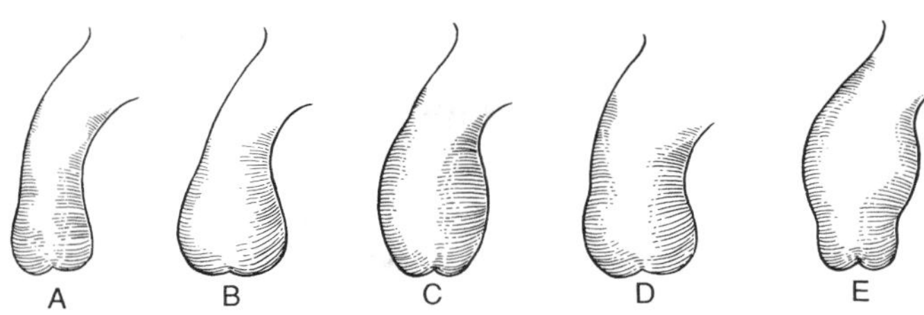

Fig. 19.20 The aortic root and ascending aorta. Normal appearance (A) and appearance of annuloaortic ectasia (B) demonstrating dilatation of the annulus and sinuses of Valsalva. (C,D) Dilatation of the aortic annulus, sinuses of Valsalva, and the ascending aorta. (E) Dilatation begins at the sinotubular junction. (Reproduced with permission from: Goldstein SA, Lindsay J. Thoracic aortic aneurysms: role of echocardiography. Echocardiography 1996; 13(2): 222.)

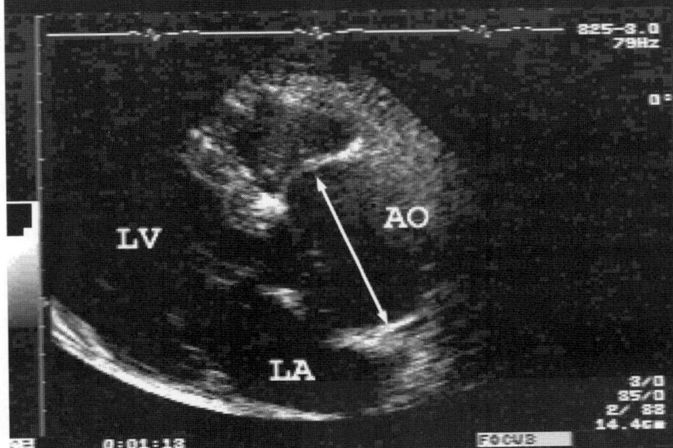

Fig. 19.21 Parasternal long axis view in a patient with annuloaortic ectasia, but not Marfan's syndrome. Arrows point to the sinuses of Valsalva.

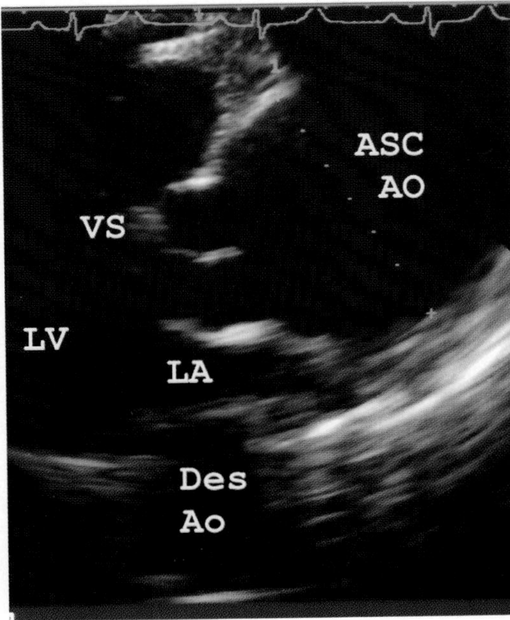

Fig. 19.22 A 67-year-old-asymptomatic female with marfanoid features has aneurysmal dilatation of the thoracic and abdominal aorta. The aorta began to dilate significantly after the sinotubular junction. The measured aortic diameter (ascending, transverse, and descending) was 66 mm. Note the dilated descending aortic compression of the LA. ASC AO, ascending aorta; Des Ao, descending aorta; VS, interventricular septum.

20

CHAPTER 20
Masses and Tumors

Evaluation of cardiac masses includes *thrombi*, *pseudomasses*, and *tumors*. Mediastinal masses may also be evaluated by TEE. (See also Chapters 13, 14 & 17.)

Foreign bodies

The most common foreign body is an intravascular catheter or pacemaker wire. Echocardiography will help determine its location and evaluate any effects it may have on the cardiac structures, such as valvular regurgitation. It will also help evaluate for thrombus or vegetations associated with the catheter or wire (Figs 20.1–20.5). The lumen of a catheter may be seen but the catheter walls may appear thicker, due to the marked difference in acoustic reflection between blood and tissue and the catheter. Catheter perforation into the pericardial space may reveal an associated pericardial effusion, and agitated saline injection through the catheter will reveal cavitations within the pericardial space.

Pseudomasses (see also Chapter 4)

Pseudomasses include papillary muscles, trabeculations, false tendons, and moderator bands among other mass-like structures. A papillary muscle may appear as a mass or thrombus but have chordae attached and a round appearance. *Hypertrophic trabeculae*, *false tendons* (Fig. 20.6), and *aberrant muscular bands* may be seen in the left ventricle and a *moderator band*, septal chordae, and the posterior papillary muscle (Fig. 20.6) may be seen in the right ventricle. Rarely an accessory papillary muscle may

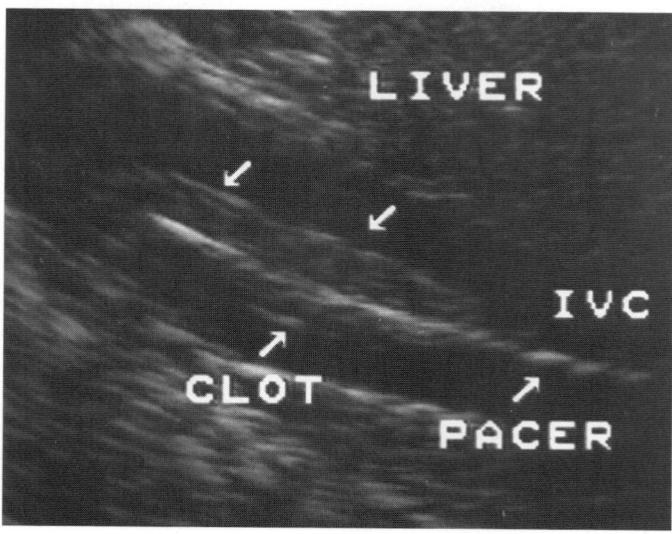

Fig. 20.1 Subcostal view of the IVC in a patient with a temporary pacing wire inserted via the right femoral vein. The wire (PACER) is noted to be encased with a fresh thrombus (arrows CLOT).

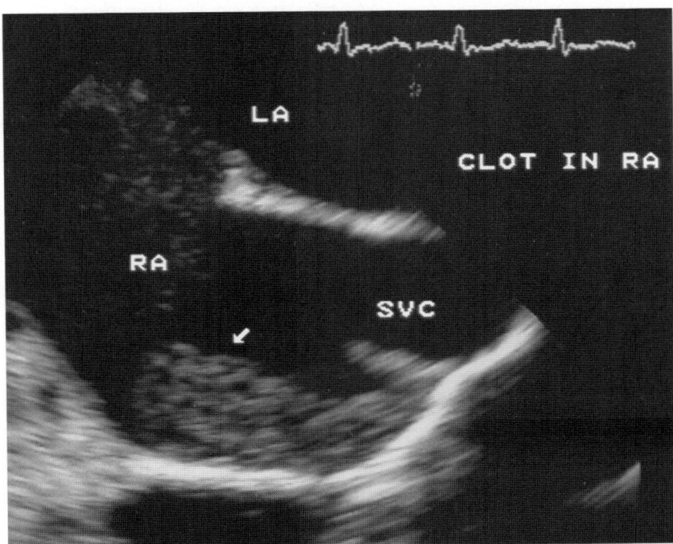

Fig. 20.2 Transesophageal echocardiography (TEE) in the longitudinal view of a patient after removal of a central venous line in which the tip had been in the right atrium. Residual thrombus is noted (arrow).

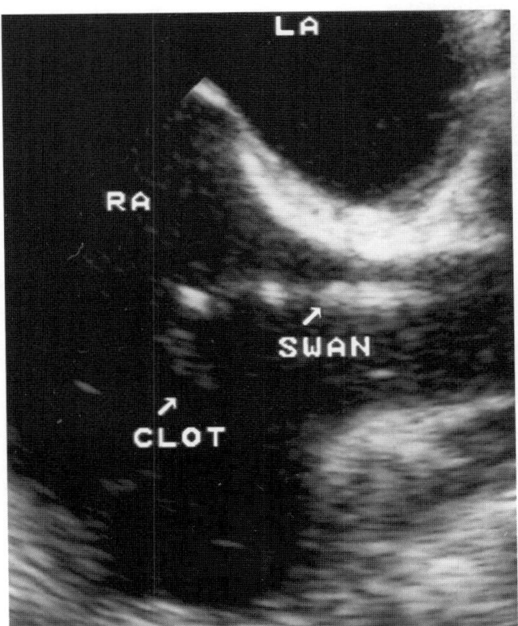

Fig. 20.3 TEE in the longitudinal plane of a Swan–Ganz catheter and a "soft" mobile clot attached within the right atrium (arrow CLOT).

be visualized in the LV but can be identified by its chordal attachment and the observation that the mitral valve has a triangular appearance. This accessory muscle is most often an extra posterior papillary muscle. Occasionally it is attached to the anterolateral wall and then termed the *papillary muscle of Moulaert.*

Apical hypertrophy of the LV, often associated with deep T wave inversions across the precordial ECG, involves obliteration of the apex of the LV cavity by hypertrophied myocardium (see Chapter 11). *Mitral annular calcification* (MAC) usually involves the posterior annulus, but may involve the entire mitral ring (Figs 17.19 & 20.7). A "mass" may appear posteriorly in the LA, behind the mitral annulus (see Chapter 17). An *atrial septal aneurysm* (ASA) is best seen in the subcostal four-chamber view or by transesophageal echocardiography (TEE), and consists of redundant tissue at the level of the foramen ovalis (Fig. 20.8; see also Fig. 17.30).

Lipomatous hypertrophy of the interatrial septum involves fat deposits within the septum (Fig. 20.9). It occurs more commonly in patients over 50 years old, particularly in those over 65 years old. There is no capsule, which distinguishes it from a lipoma, and it spares the fossa ovalis. It occurs most often in obese patients and is associated with subepicardial adipose tissue (which may be confused as a pericardial effusion). MRI will help in difficult cases. Lipomatous hypertrophy may rarely encompass and narrow the SVC, but most often is of no clinical consequence. *Tricuspid annulus fat* may appear to be a tumor, but has a typical appearance (Fig. 20.10). A bulbous infolding between the left atrial appendage and left

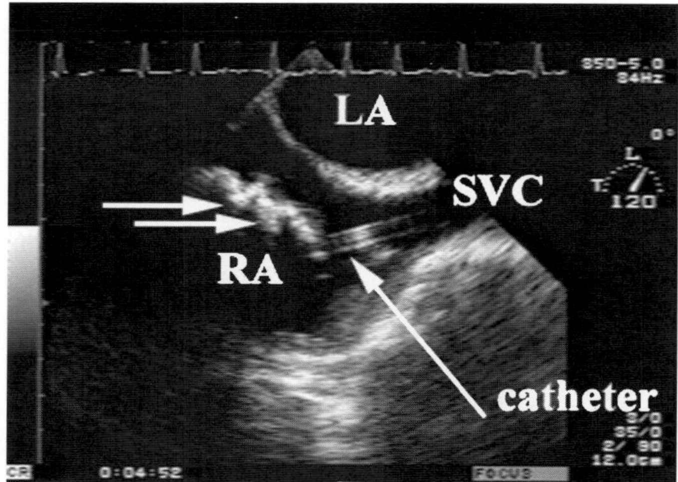

Fig. 20.4 TEE at 120° in a patient with a chronically indwelling dialysis catheter (arrow) via the SVC. Chronic thrombus/fibrosis is evident (horizontal arrows), which appeared to encase the tip of the catheter by real-time imaging. During removal of the catheter, a "tugging" on the thrombus/fibrosis was evident, remaining unchanged afterwards.

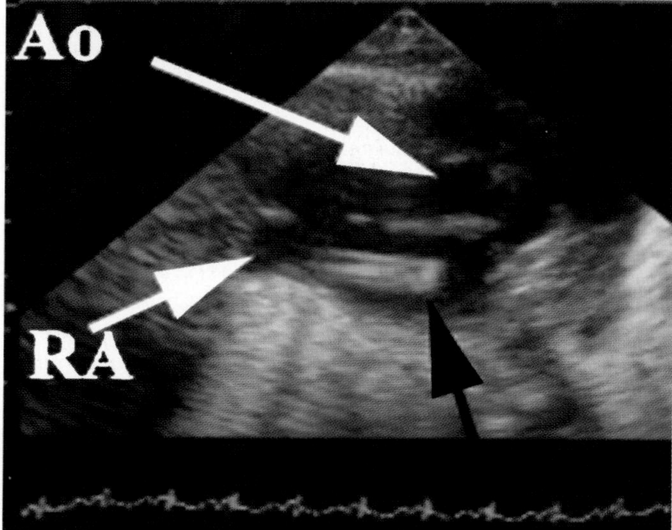

Fig. 20.5 Parasternal short axis view of a newborn infant with an umbilical venous catheter. The catheter has crossed the foramen ovale and its tip (black arrow) lies within the LA. Ao, aorta.

(a)

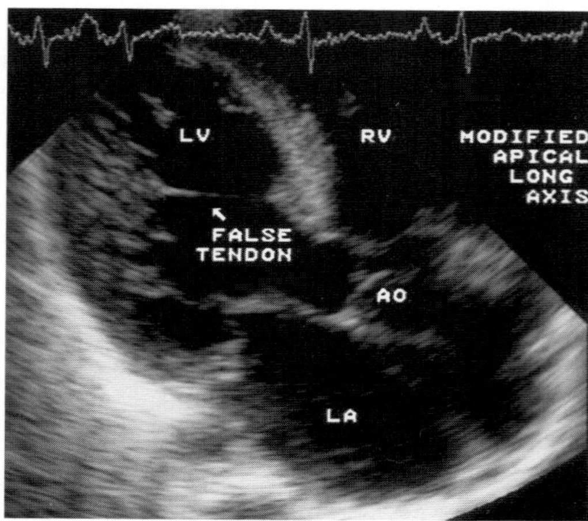

Fig. 20.6 (a) Foreshortened apical long axis view highlighting a LV false tendon. (*Cont'd.*)

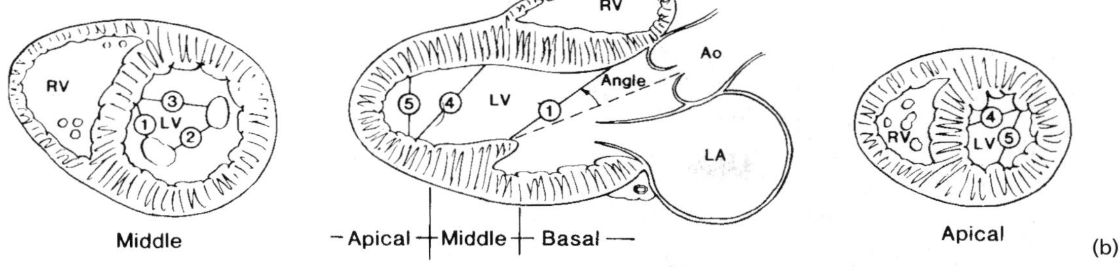

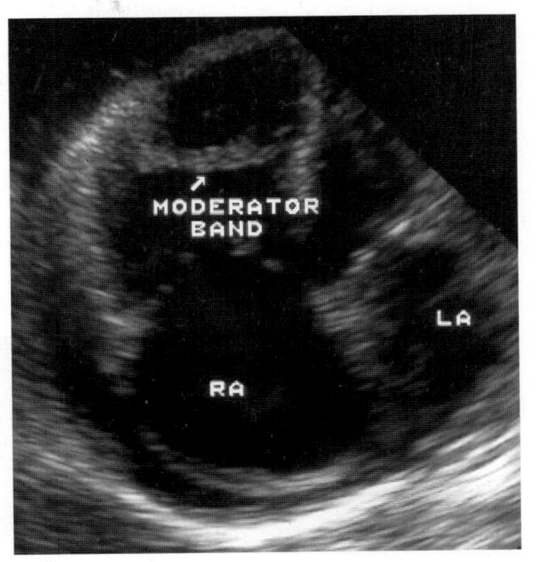

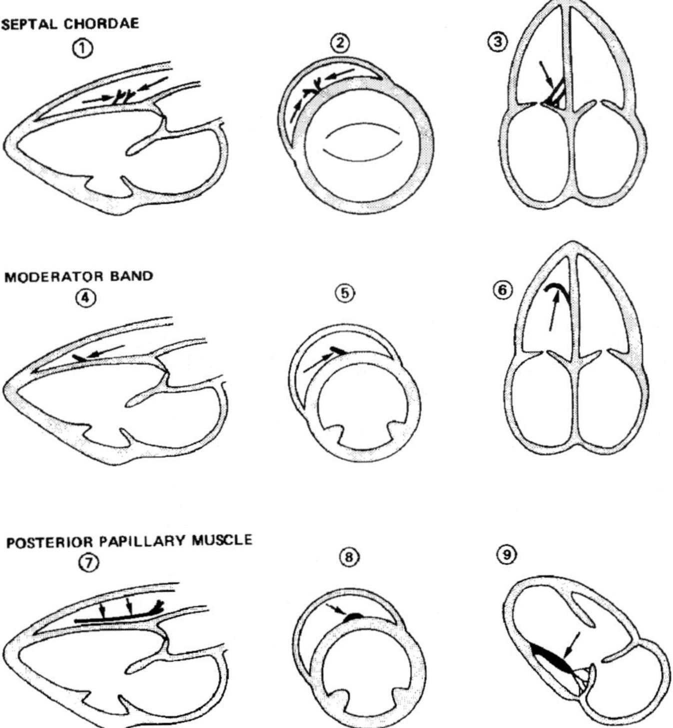

Fig. 20.6 (*cont'd*) (b) Representation of left ventricular false tendons. False tendons may occur as: (1) posterior papillary muscle (PMPM) to ventricular septum (VS); (2) anterolateral papillary muscle (ALPM) to PMPM; (3) ALPM–VS; (4) left ventricular free wall (LVFW) to VS; (5) LVFW–LVFW. (c) Apical four-chamber view demonstrates a prominent RV moderator band. (d) Representation of RV paraseptal structures ((b) Reproduced with permission from: Luetmer PH, Edwards WD, Seward JB, Tajik AJ. Incidence and distribution of left ventricular false tendons: an autopsy study of 483 normal human hearts. Journal of the American College of Cardiology 1986; 8: 179–183, figure 1. (d) Reproduced with permission from: Keren A, Billingham ME, Popp RL. Echocardiographic recognition of paraseptal structures. Journal of the American College of Cardiology 1985; 6: 913–919, figure 7.)

(a)
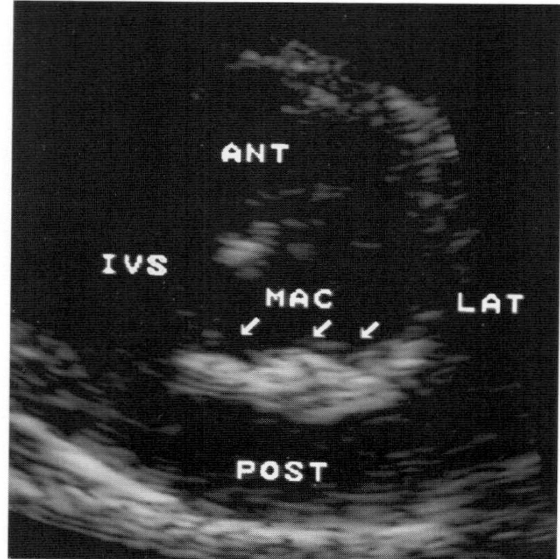

(b)
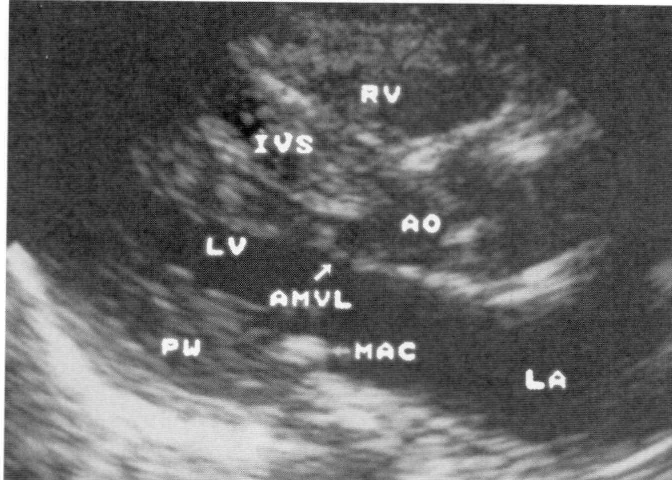

Fig. 20.7 (a) Parasternal short axis view at the mitral level illustrating mitral annular calcification (MAC). Calcification usually involves only the posterior mitral annulus. (b) Parasternal long axis view demonstrating MAC. ANT, anterior; POST, posterior; LAT, lateral; PW, left ventricular posterior wall; IVS, interventricular septum; AO, aortic valve; AMVL, anterior mitral valve leaflet; AML, anterior mitral leaflet; PML, posterior mitral leaflet.

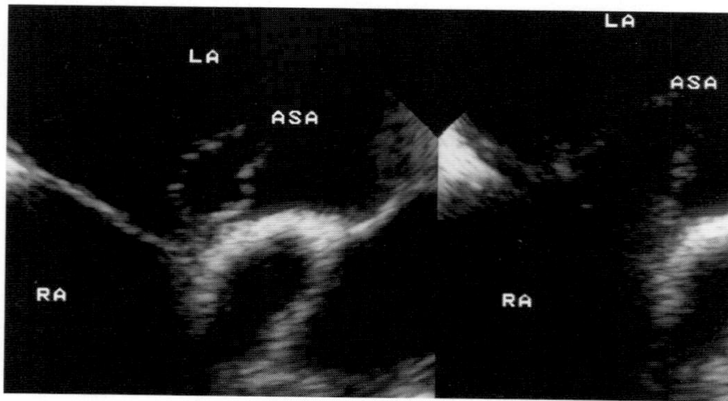

Fig. 20.8 Transverse upper esophageal sequential time-frame images of an atrial septal aneurysm (ASA). Marked redundancy may produce an image simulating a mass. Real-time imaging will readily identify this as an ASA.

upper pulmonary vein has been called the "coumadin ridge," a normal finding that has at times been misidentified as a thrombus (Fig. 20.11).

The *Chiari network* is a remnant from embryology (see Chapter 17) from the septum spurium and the right valve of the sinus venosus, resulting from incomplete resorption of these structures. These fibers have their origin from either the Eustachian or *Thebesian valve* (covers the coronary sinus) and have attachments to the upper wall of the right atrium or the interatrial septum (autopsy incidence 2–3%, TEE incidence 2%). They may be very mobile. Catheters may become caught up within the Chiari network. It is important not to confuse the Chiari network with emboli from the lower extremities (Fig. 20.12). The *Eustachian valve* is usually a small membrane that covers the IVC–RA junction. It may also be relatively mobile and fenestrated but does not attach to the upper wall of the right atrium or interatrial septum (Figs 20.13 & 20.14).

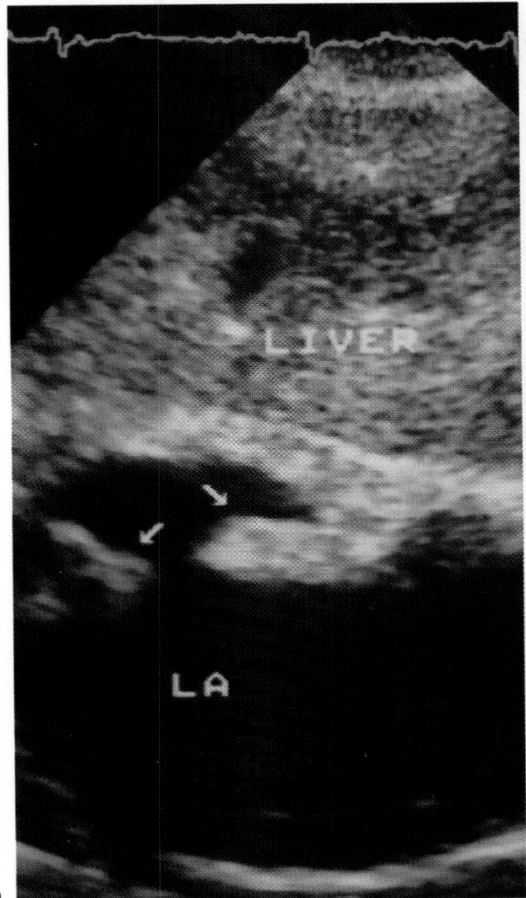

(a)

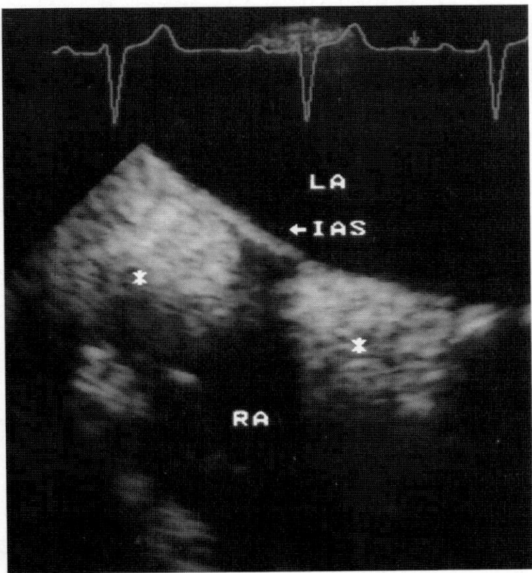

(b)

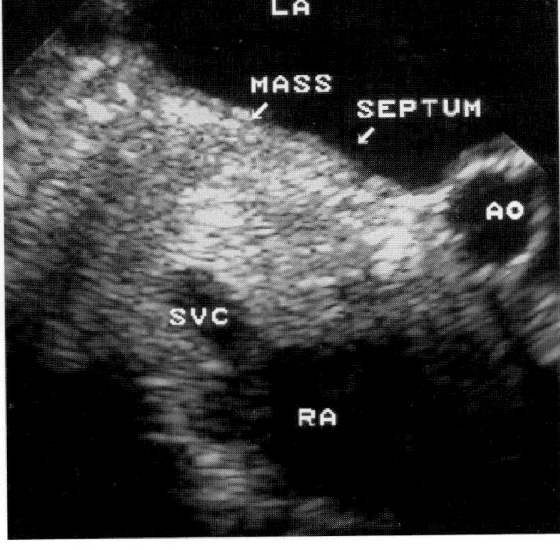

(c)

Fig. 20.9 (a) Subcostal imaging of a patient with lipomatous hypertrophy of the interatrial septum (arrows). Sparing of the fossa ovalis is readily noted. (b) TEE of lipomatous hypertrophy (*) of the interatrial septum. Note the typical appearance of sparing of the fossa ovalis. The septum may appear as a "dumbbell". (*Continued on p. 326.*)

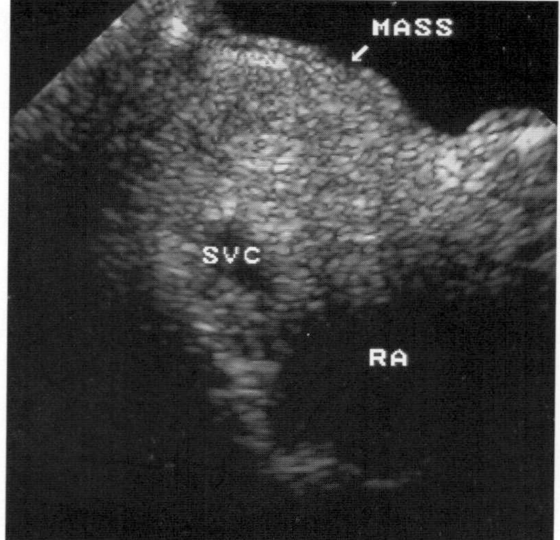

(d)

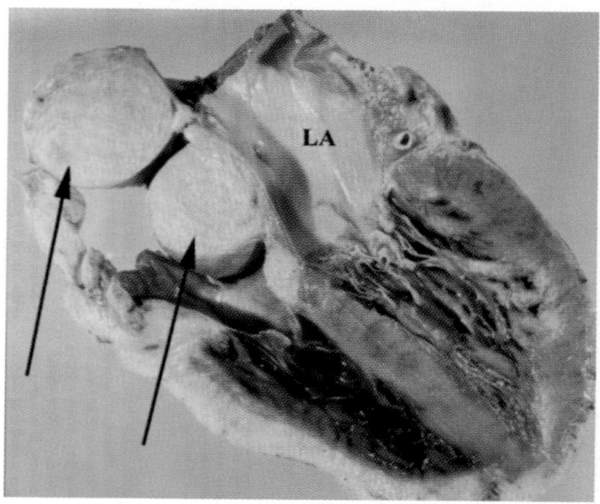

(e)

Fig. 20.9 (*cont'd*) (c,d) TEE in the horizontal plane of a patient with lipomatous hypertrophy of the interatrial septum, which has surrounded the junction of the SVC and RA. Although the SVC was narrowed, the patient did not have SVC syndrome. This patient underwent coronary artery bypass surgery. A biopsy specimen of the "mass" documented lipomatous hypertrophy. IAS, fossa ovalis of the interatrial septum; AO, aortic valve; SEPTUM, interatrial septum. (e) Pathologic specimen as would be visualized from an apical four-chamber view of impressive lipomatous hypertrophy (arrows) ((e) Reproduced with permission from: Shirani J, Roberts WC. Clinical, electrocardiographic and morphologic features of massive fatty deposits ("lipomatous hypertrophy") in the atrial septum. Journal of the American College of Cardiology 1993; 22: 226–238, figure 2.)

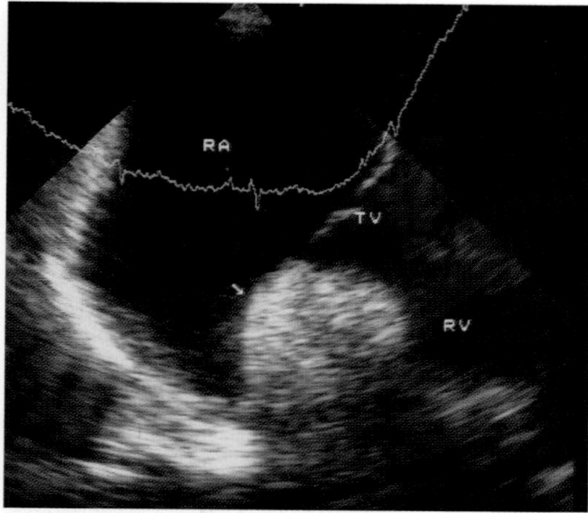

Fig. 20.10 TEE in the horizontal plane of the tricuspid valve (TV) and tricuspid annulus fat (arrow). Tricuspid annulus fat will have a typical appearance as noted.

Tumors

Valve strands (*Lambl's excrescences*), cardiac *myxomas*, and *papillary fibroelastomas* are discussed and illustrated in Chapter 17. Primary cardiac tumors are benign or malignant. Benign tumors include myxomas, rhabdomyomas, fibromas, and fibroelastomas. *Rhabdomyomas* are the most common childhood tumor, occurring in muscular parts of the heart. They are small, round, usually multiple, and have distinctive borders. A *fibroma* is usually found in the LV free wall, ventricular septum, or at the apex (may be confused with apical hypertrophy when located at the apex). It is well circumscribed, and may grow into the cavity of the LV, impairing LV filling. It is associated with ventricular arrhythmias (Fig. 20.15).

Malignant primary cardiac tumors include sarcomas and angiosarcomas. Sarcomas may affect any chamber or valve, but usually the right heart. An *angiosarcoma* usually occurs in adult males, and affects the right atrium with pericardial infiltration, hemorrhage, and resultant pericardial effusion or tamponade.

Metastatic cardiac tumors are 20–40 times more common than primary cardiac tumors (Figs 20.16 & 20.17). They may be generally classified as:

1 Myocardial involvement:
   (a) breast, lung—most common

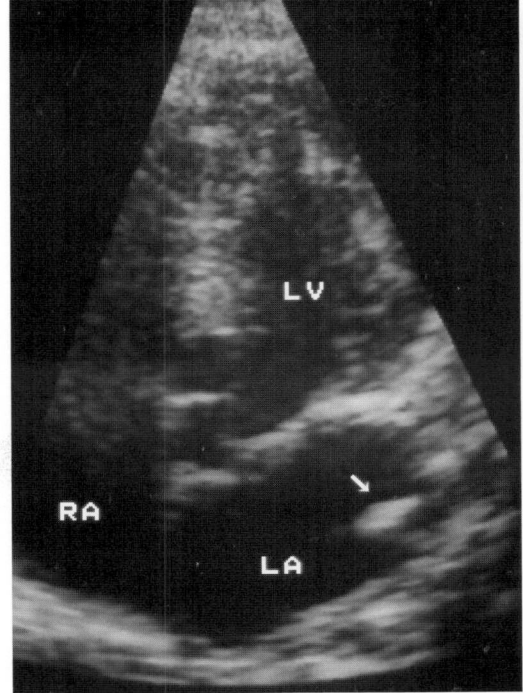

(a)

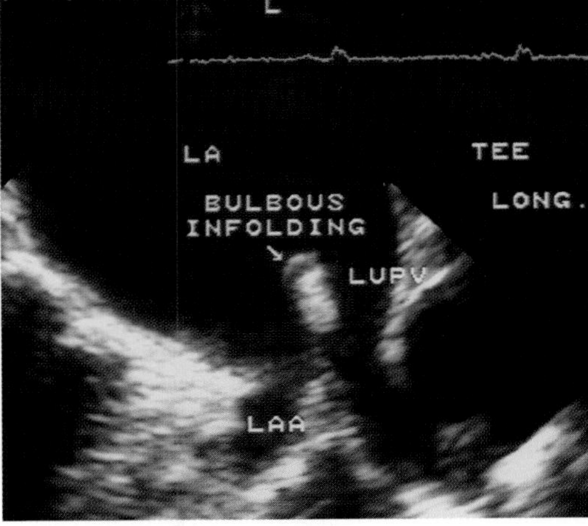

(b)

Fig. 20.11 (a) Bulbous infolding (arrow) from an apical four-chamber view, and (b) as visualized by TEE in a different patient. The bulbous infolding is seen between the left atrial appendage (LAA) and the left upper pulmonary vein (LUPV).

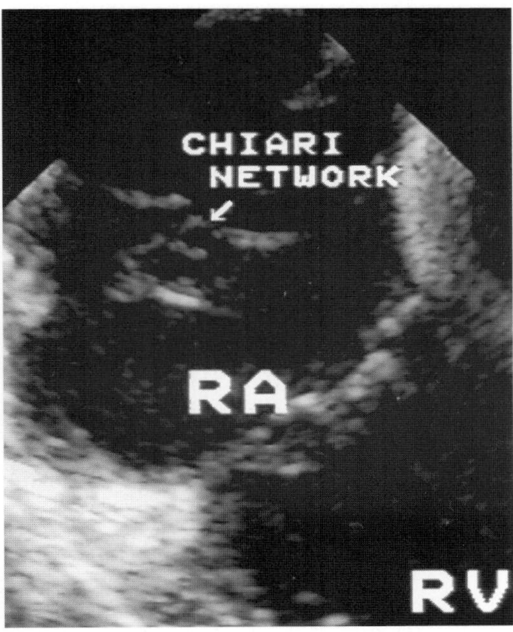

Fig. 20.12 The Chiari network as visualized by TEE in the horizontal plane. It may appear filamentous and is often very mobile.

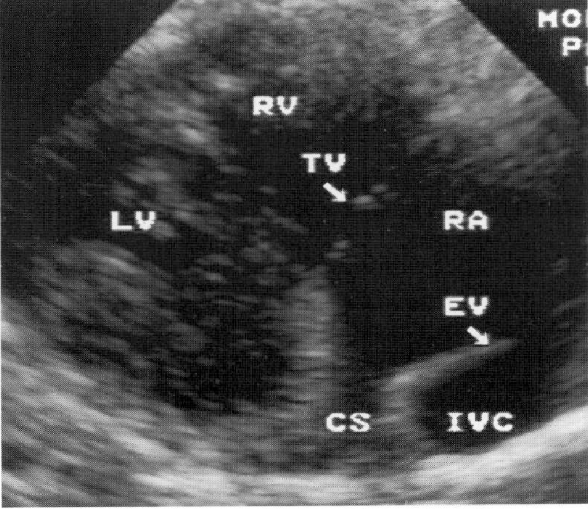

Fig. 20.13 Modified parasternal long axis (RV inflow) of the coronary sinus (CS), IVC, and the Eustachian valve (EV) covering the IVC. The posterior leaflet of the tricuspid valve (TV) is also noted.

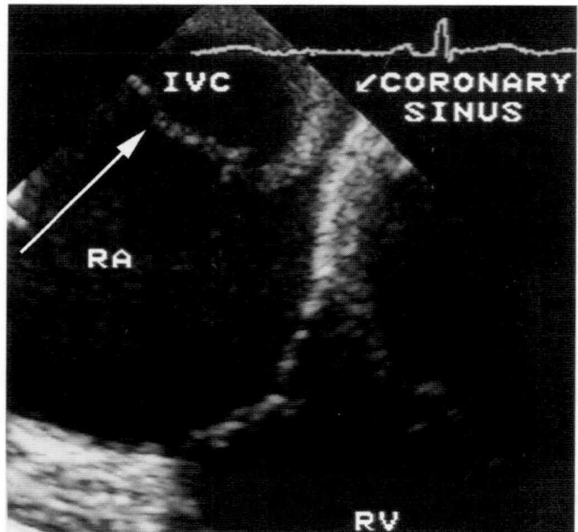

Fig. 20.14 TEE in the transverse plane from the lower esophagus demonstrates the coronary sinus, IVC, and Eustachian valve (arrow).

(b) melanoma—50% of melanomas have cardiac metastases.

2 Direct venous extension—intracavitary:

(a) SVC—often thymus

(b) IVC—hepatic carcinoma, hypernephroma.

3 Pericardial metastasis:

(a) more common than myocardial metastases

(b) often presents as a bloody effusion with tamponade.

Mediastinal masses

Thoracic echocardiography has somewhat limited applicability for evaluation of mediastinal masses. TEE may help with the following:

- identification of abnormal masses and location
- evaluation for obstruction of the cardiac chambers and great vessels
- assessment as to whether a mass is solid or cystic.

Although computed tomography (CT) and magnetic resonance imaging (MRI) are very good for identification and evaluation of mediastinal masses, TEE will on occasion be of added value (Fig. 20.18; see also Fig. 14.12). Mediastinal hematoma may be difficult to assess by TEE, but CT will help. A *hiatal hernia* may appear as a mass posterior to the LV, from a parasternal window. By having the patient drink a carbonated beverage, bubbles appearing in the field of view will document this diagnosis (Fig. 20.19). This should not be confused with an aneurysmal descending thoracic aorta. Extrinsic compression of the pulmonary artery or the SVC has also been successfully identified using TEE (Fig. 20.20).

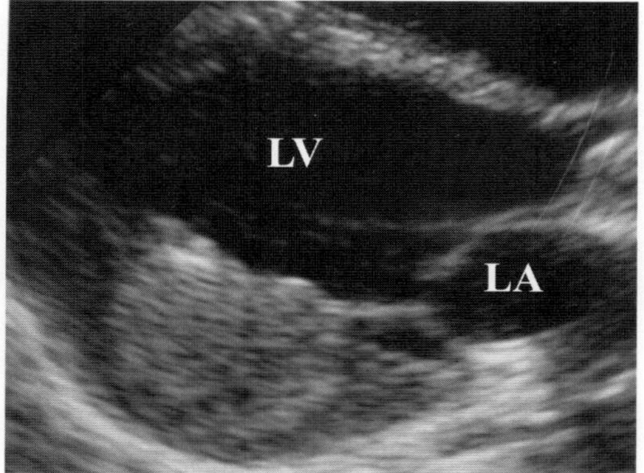

(a)

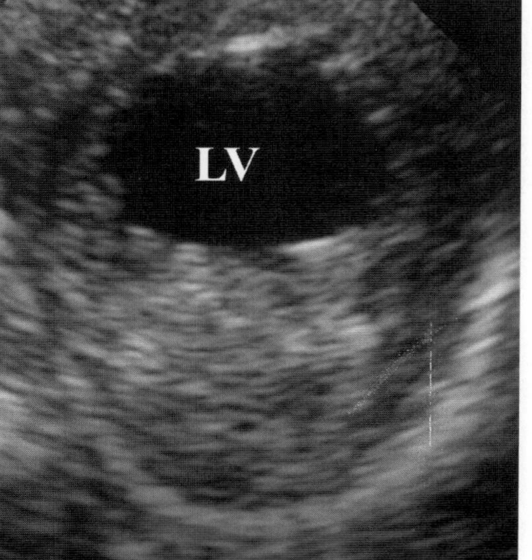

(b)

Fig. 20.15 A patient with a typical LV fibroma involving the inferior wall of the left ventricle. (a) Parasternal long axis and (b) parasternal short axis views.

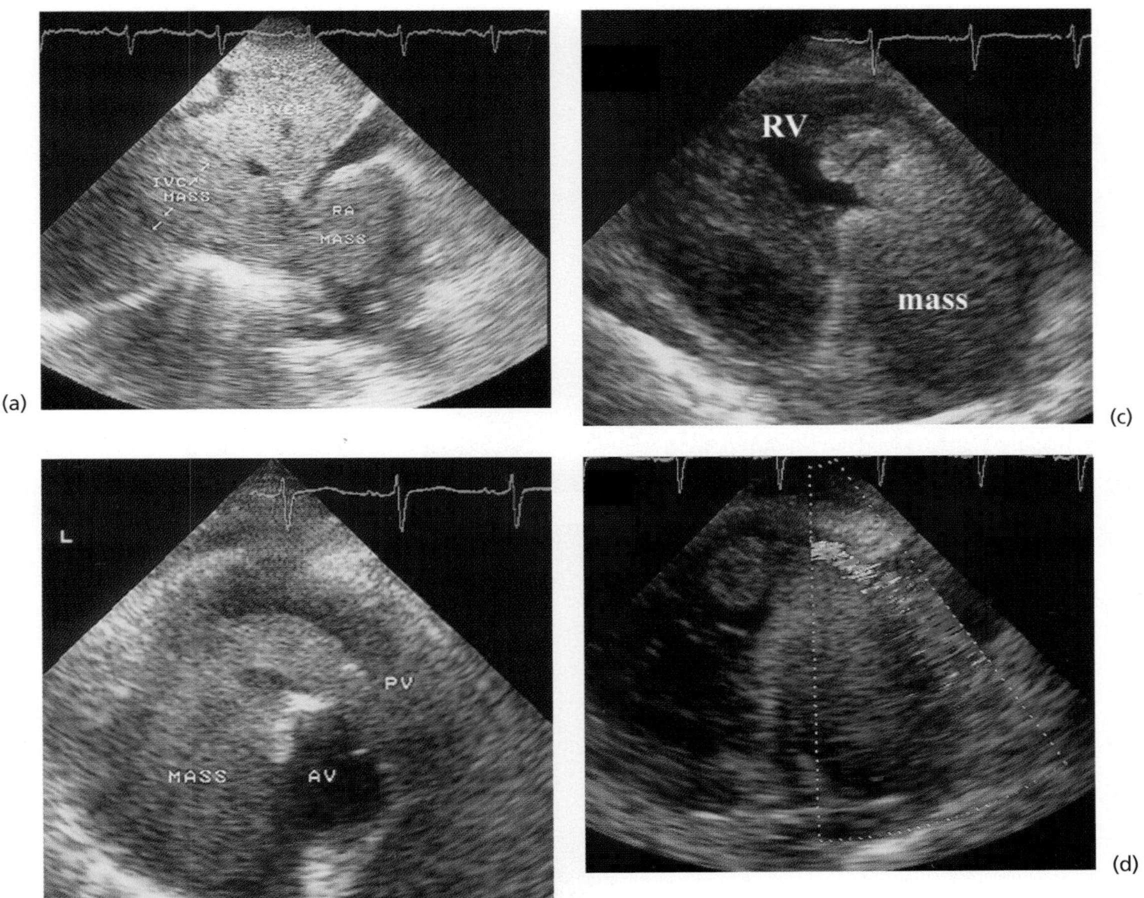

Fig. 20.16 A 50-year-old-male presented with weight loss, hematuria, abdominal discomfort, and progressive lower extremity edema. Abdominal ultrasound revealed a tumor extending from the right kidney into the IVC and up toward the heart. (a) Subcostal imaging reveals a mass essentially occluding the IVC (IVC MASS and arrows) and extending into the RA (RA MASS). (b) Parasternal short axis imaging at the aortic valve level (AV) reveals that the mass extends from the RA (MASS), into the RV and right ventricular outflow tract, towards the pulmonic valve (PV). (c,d) Parasternal RV inflow views demonstrating the RA mass (mass) extending into the right ventricle (RV). Color Doppler documents significant flow turbulence around the mass, causing obstruction to RV inflow. The working diagnosis was hypernephroma, the patient refused any further evaluation and subsequently expired.

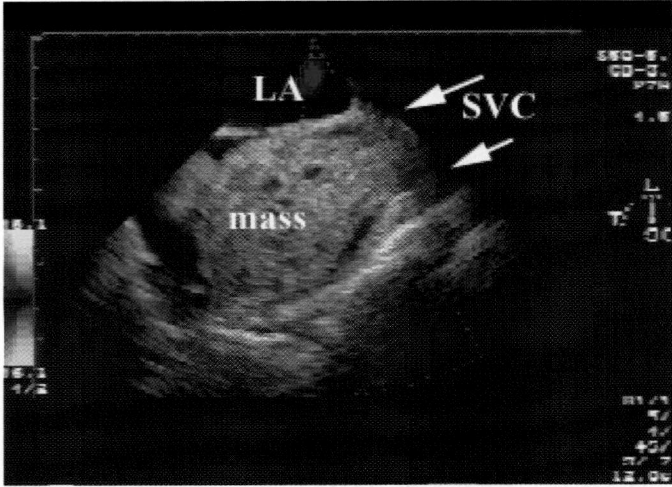

(a)

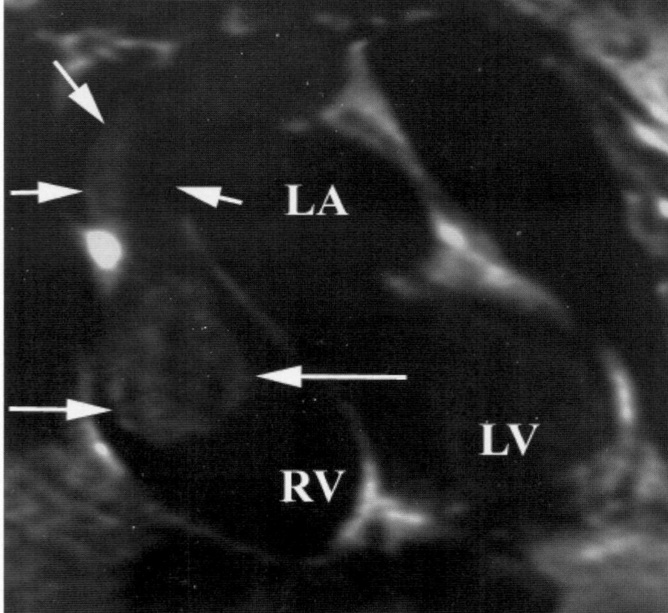

(b)

Fig. 20.17 A middle-aged female presented with hypotension, chest pain, and diffuse electrocardiographic changes across the precordium. Echocardiography revealed a mass within the right heart. (a) TEE in the longitudinal view reveals a large mass extending into the RA from the SVC. It appears to nearly completely occlude the SVC. (b) Magnetic resonance imaging (MRI) of the heart, from an anteroposterior view, shows the large mass extending intravascularly (arrows) down through the innominate vein into the SVC, and then into the right heart. The mass crossed the tricuspid annulus into the right ventricle. Pathology revealed the mass to be a Hurthle carcinoma of the thyroid.

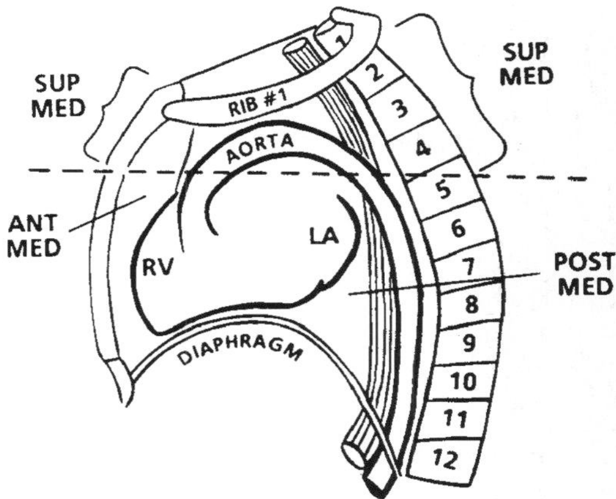

Fig. 20.18 Lateral view of the thorax demonstrates the relationship of cardiovascular structures, esophagus, and mediastinum. SUP MED, superior mediastinum; ANT MED, anterior mediastinum; POST MED, posterior mediastinum. (Reproduced with permission from: D'Cruz IA, Feghali N, Gross CM. Echocardiographic manifestations of mediastinal masses compressing or encroaching on the heart. Echocardiography 1994; 11(5): 523.)

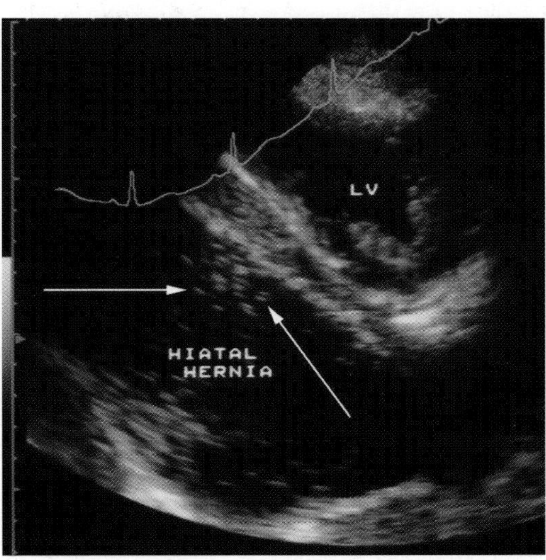

Fig. 20.19 From the left parasternal window, a patient was found to have a large mass posterior to the LV. The patient was asked to sit in a semi-upright position. While imaging, the patient slowly drank a carbonated beverage through a straw. Bubbles were noted (arrows) within the "mass," thus documenting that it was a hiatal hernia.

(a)

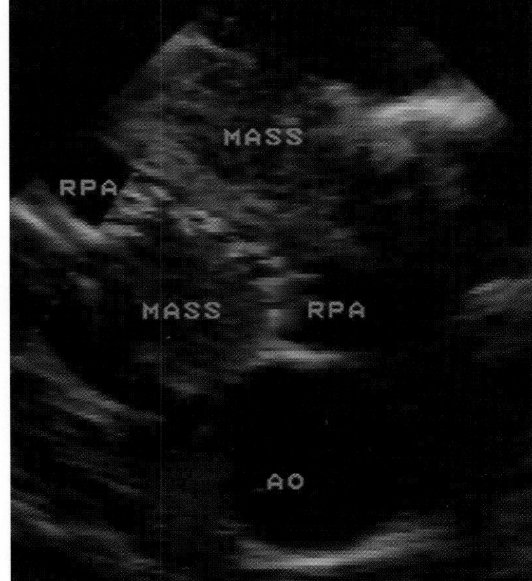

(b)

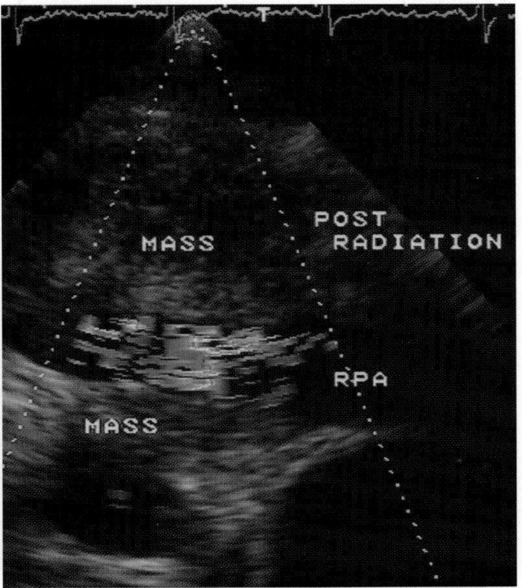

Fig. 20.20 TEE of a 50-year-old female, with a longstanding history of tobacco abuse, presented with severe SVC syndrome and hemodynamic instability. Based on TEE findings of SVC near-obstruction, radiation therapy was begun. Subsequently, the patient stabilized, and mediastinal mass biopsy identified oat cell carcinoma. (a) Transverse imaging with TEE in the mid-upper esophagus reveals extrinsic compression of the right pulmonary artery (RPA) by the lung mass, which was circumferential around the RPA. Note color flow turbulence at the level of obstruction and also distal to it. (b) TEE was performed subsequent to radiation therapy. The tumor size had regressed, and normal pulmonary artery flow restored. (*Continued on p. 332.*)

(c)

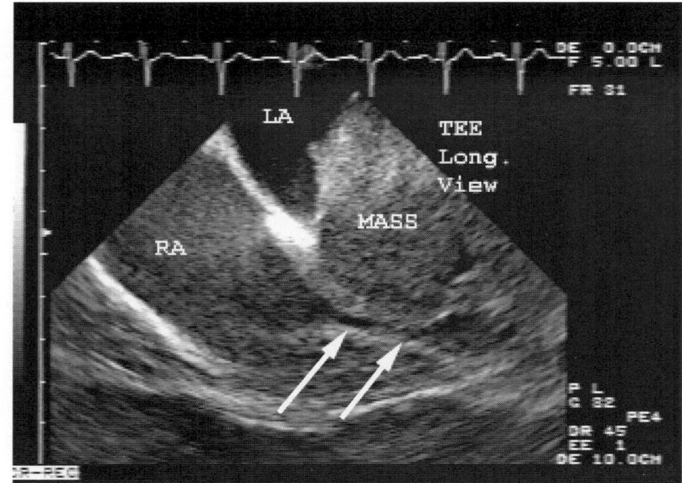

(d)

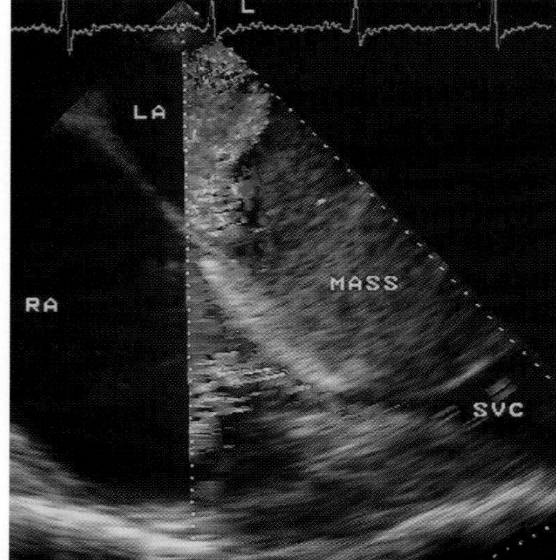

(e)

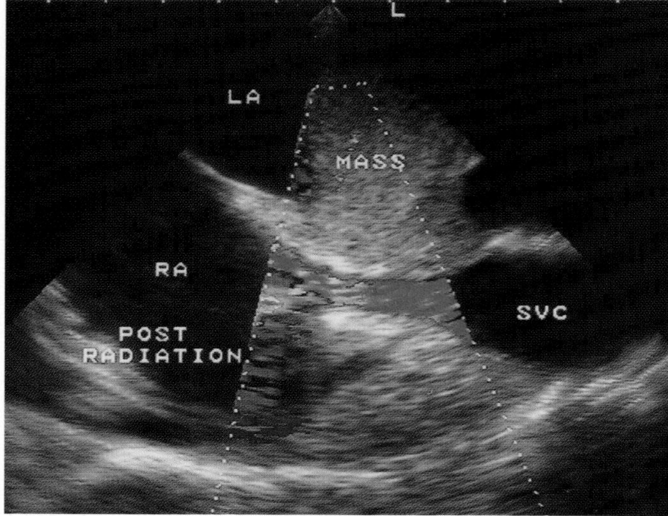

Fig. 20.20 (*cont'd*) (c) Longitudinal two-dimensional TEE and (d) two-dimensional color Doppler of the SVC and RA. Note the appearance of nearly complete obstruction of the SVC (arrows in c). (e) Repeat TEE after radiation therapy reveals tumor regression, and relief of SVC obstruction. AO, ascending aorta.

21

CHAPTER 21
Selected Topics

Nonbacterial thrombotic endocarditis and marantic endocarditis

Valvular lesions that are bacteria-free, termed *nonbacterial thrombotic endocarditis* (NBTE), are found most often in patients with autoimmune diseases and neoplasms. The reported incidence in primary antiphospholipid syndrome is 32%, in myeloproliferative disorders is 63%, and in solid malignant tumors such as adenocarcinoma is 19%. NBTE has also been described in patients with sepsis, burns, indwelling pulmonary artery catheters, disseminated intravascular coagulation (DIC), and acquired immunodeficiency syndrome (AIDS). Lesions are usually found by microscopic evaluation to be superficial and consist of fibrin and platelet thrombi, without inflammation.

Lesions involve the mitral and aortic valves with equal frequency. Right-sided involvement is uncommon. They rarely cause significant valvular disruption, but regurgitation is often found by Doppler. The appearance is most commonly a vegetation-like lesion, which is localized and mobile, attached to a normal-appearing valve. Attachment is usually on the atrial side of the mitral valve and the ventricular side of the aortic valve. The size may range from small, mobile lesions to masses over 10 mm in diameter. The differential diagnosis includes culture-negative bacterial endocarditis, fungal endocarditis, tumors, and the antiphospholipid syndrome. Another distinctive pattern is that of diffuse mitral or aortic valve thickening, or thickening and calcification of the mitral annulus or mitral chordae. As opposed to rheumatic involvement, there is no commissural fusion or valve doming with NBTE.

By definition *marantic endocarditis* involves malignant tumors that are metastatic to cardiac valves. Lesions appear similar to those of Libman–Sacks endocarditis (see section below). The most common malignancies associated with marantic endocarditis include adenocarcinoma of the lung, pancreas, stomach, and colon, and also Hodgkin's disease.

Systemic lupus erythematosus and primary antiphospholipid syndrome

The pericardium is most often involved in patients with *systemic lupus erythematosus* (SLE) and may manifest itself as pericarditis or pericardial effusion. Tamponade or constriction is uncommon. A myocardial vasculitis may cause a myocarditis, but abnormal diastolic function is not common.

The mitral valve is involved in about 50% of patients. Leaflet thickening and vegetations (termed *Libman–Sacks endocarditis*) may be noted (Fig. 21.1). Lesions are multiple, up to several millimeters in size, and occur most often on the atrial surface of the leaflets near the base (Fig. 21.2), but may extend toward the chords or papillary muscles. Lesions have irregular borders, a heterogeneous texture, and move exactly parallel with the motion of the valve leaflet (infective endocarditis lesions are usually homogeneous in appearance, are located at the line of valve closure, and often have a vibratory motion independent of the valve leaflet). Occasionally, the aortic valve may be involved with thickening and vegetations. Diffuse leaflet thickening may rarely lead to diminished mobility and stenosis.

It appears that valve lesions occur in SLE regardless of the presence or absence of antiphospholipid antibodies. In patients with *primary antiphospholipid syndrome* (PAPS), lesions appear to be the same as with Libman–Sacks endocarditis.

Spondyloarthropathies

Patients with *ankylosing spondylitis* may develop thickened aortic valve leaflets and aortic root dilatation, resulting in aortic regurgitation. Thickening

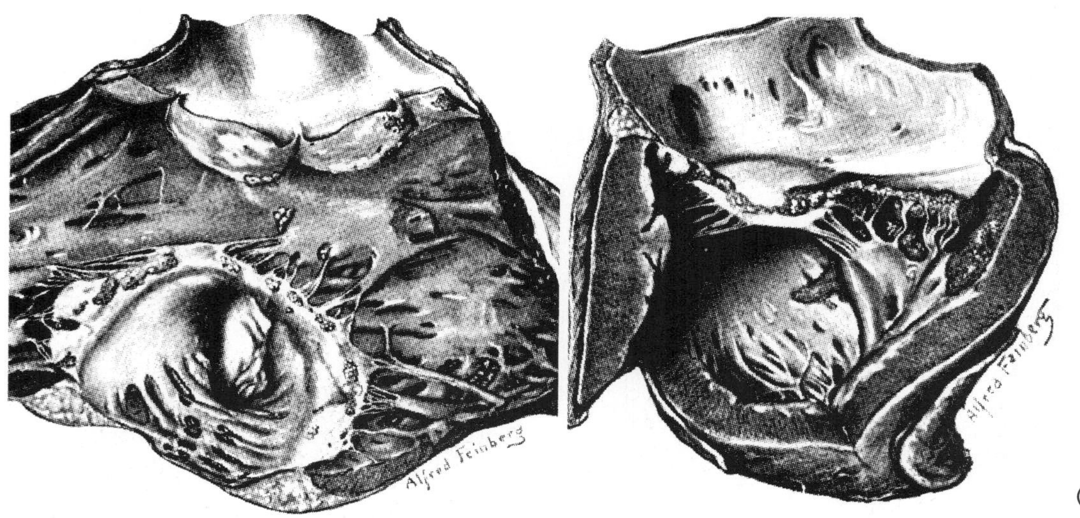

Fig. 21.1 Drawing from the original description of valvular verrucae in SLE. The right side of the heart (a) and the left side of the heart (b) are shown. Lesions on the atrial surface of the tricuspid leaflets, on the right atrial endocardium, on the RV side of the pulmonic valve cusps, and on the surface of the right ventricle are noted. Lesions are also noted on both atrial and ventricular sides of both mitral leaflets and on the endocardium in the area of the posteromedial papillary muscle. (With permission from Libman E, Sacks B. A hitherto undescribed form of valvular and mural endocarditis. Archives of Internal Medicine 1924; 33: 701–737.)

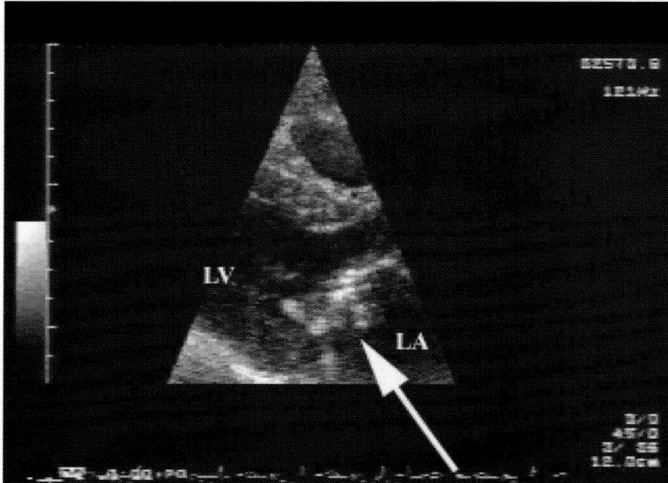

Fig. 21.2 Parasternal long axis imaging of a patient with SLE. The mitral valve is thickened and a large vegetative lesion is noted on both the anterior mitral leaflet (arrow) and posterior leaflet.

of the subaortic area near the base of the anterior leaflet of the mitral valve (posterior wall of the aortic root extending to the base of the anterior mitral leaflet) is commonly seen. A so-called *subaortic bump* results (Fig. 21.3). Patients with *Reiter's disease* have aortic valve changes similar to those of ankylosing spondylitis.

Pericarditis and pericardial effusion occur in up to 50% of patients with *rheumatoid arthritis*. Valves (most commonly mitral, followed by aortic, tricuspid, and

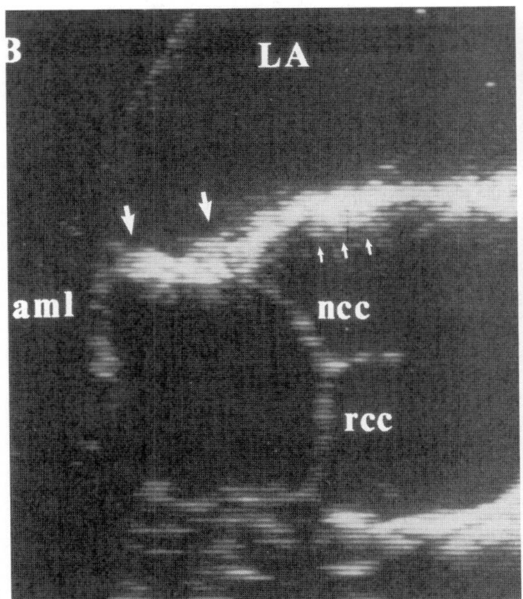

(a)

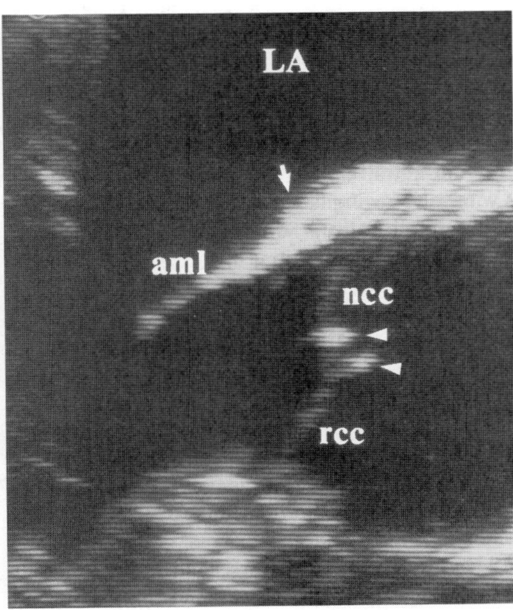

(b)

Fig. 21.3 (a) TEE from a longitudinal view of the LV outflow tract and aortic root in a patient with moderate thickening of the posterior aortic root (small upwards arrows) extending toward the base of the anterior leaflet of the mitral valve, forming a subaortic bump (downward arrows). (b) Marked thickening of the posterior aortic root and a subaortic bump (downward arrow). Anterior mitral leaflet mobility was reduced. (Reproduced with permission from: Roldan CA, Chavez J, Wiest P, *et al*. Aortic root disease and valve disease associated with ankylosing spondylitis. Journal of the American College of Cardiology 1998; 32: 1397–1404, figure 1.)

lastly pulmonic) may be involved with granulomas, and most commonly mitral regurgitation will result.

Acute rheumatic fever

Cardiac involvement is the most important part of *acute rheumatic fever*, occurring in about two thirds of patients diagnosed with acute illness. Doppler evidence of mitral regurgitation (MR) is found in more than 90% of these patients. The severity will tend to increase with recurrent bouts of acute episodes. Aortic valve involvement occurs less commonly. By echocardiography, valvular thickening with or without restriction is frequently noted. In 25% of patients with acute rheumatic carditis, focal valvular nodules have been found on the body and tips of the mitral leaflets (Fig. 21.4). These nodules tend to disappear on follow-up echocardiographic studies.

LV dilatation is more common in patients with recurrent bouts—it has been found in about one half of patients with their initial bout of acute rheumatic fever and in about two thirds of patients with recurrent bouts. Ventricular dilatation in patients with restricted leaflet mobility is the most common etiology of mitral regurgitation in patients with recurrent bouts.

Drug-related valvular disease and reproducibility/reliability of color Doppler assessment of valvular regurgitation

The Federal Drug Administration (FDA) defines *anorexigen-associated valve disease* as moderate or severe mitral regurgitation (MR) or mild or more aortic regurgitation (AR) in patients taking fenfluramine-phentermine—"fen-phen". Few patients have had surgical or pathologic confirmation, and histology in these patients has been rather nonspecific, making a definitive diagnosis and association difficult. Initially described pathology in patients on fen-phen seemed to be similar to carcinoid valve disease with

(a)

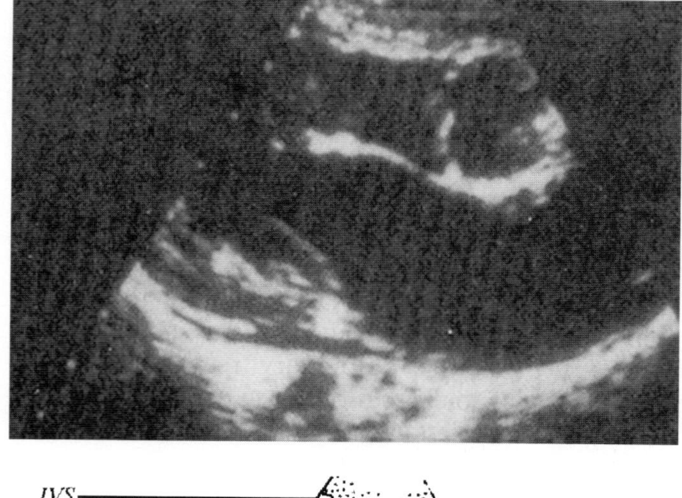

(b)

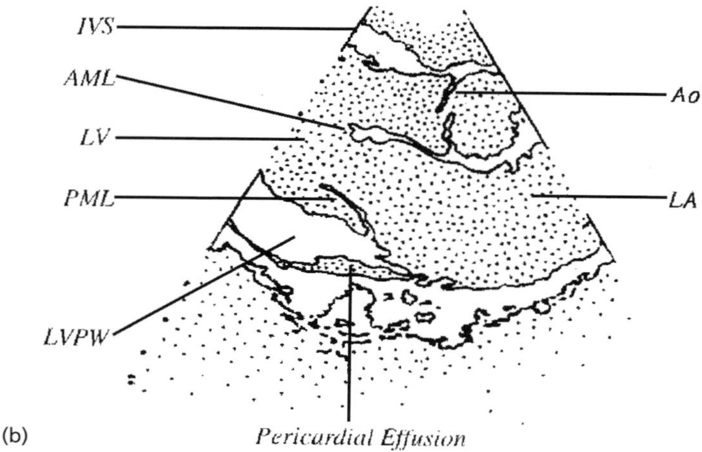

Fig. 21.4 (a) Parasternal two-dimensional echocardiogram and (b) corresponding diagram of focal nodular thickening of the tip and distal part of the anterior leaflet of the mitral valve (AML). The posterior mitral leaflet (PML) remains normal. AoV, aortic valve; LVPW, left ventricular posterior wall. (Modified with permission from: Vasan RS, Shrivastava S, Vijayakumar M, *et al.* Echocardiographic evaluation of patients with acute rheumatic fever and rheumatic carditis. Circulation 1996; 94: 73–82, figure 1.)

fibroendocardial plaque formation overlying normal valve histology. However, upwards of 90% of patients with FDA-defined "anorexigen-associated valve disease" appear to have valve morphology resembling degenerative, myxomatous, or rheumatic disease.

It is unclear exactly how many people thought to have anorexigen-associated valve disease actually have specific pathology related to anorexic drugs. Many of the patients may have other forms of valve disease. *Degenerative* valve disease is suggested by increased thickness, sclerosis and brightness at the basal portions of mitral leaflets associated with annulus calcification or involvement of the basal portion or edges of aortic leaflets associated with aortic root sclerosis. *Myxomatous* valve disease is characterized by redundant, hypermobile and thickened valve tissue. *Rheumatic* valve disease is characterized by increased leaflet thickness with or without sclerosis at the tips, commissural fusion, or subvalvular involvement with restricted motion. *Carcinoid* valve disease is characterized by a diffuse leaflet thickening of soft tissue reflectance with retraction, and decreased mobility of the entire leaflet (see next section). Anorexigen-associated valve disease may coexist (~20%) with other preexisting valvular disease. The FDA has not described a specific morphologic appearance (thickness, mobility, or brightness). There does appear to be an increased incidence of features having the appearance of chronic rheumatic disease without obstruction. True fen-phen-related valvular regurgitation seems to more commonly involve the aortic valve as opposed to the mitral valve. In addition to valvular abnormalities, pulmonary hypertension clearly appears to be related to anorexigen usage, particularly in obese individuals.

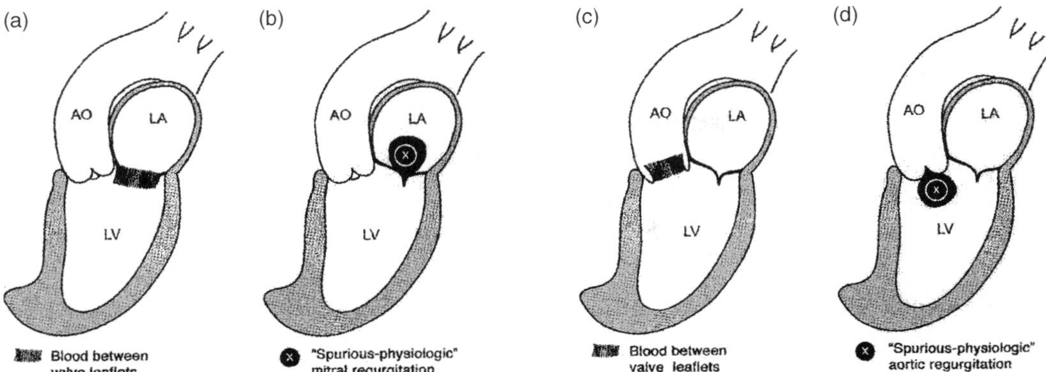

Fig. 21.5 Probable etiology of physiologic mitral regurgitation (a,b) and physiologic aortic regurgitation (c,d). (Reproduced with permission from: Rahimtoola SH. Drug-related valvular heart disease: here we go again: will we do better this time? Mayo Clinic Proceedings 2002; 77: 1275–1277, figure 1.)

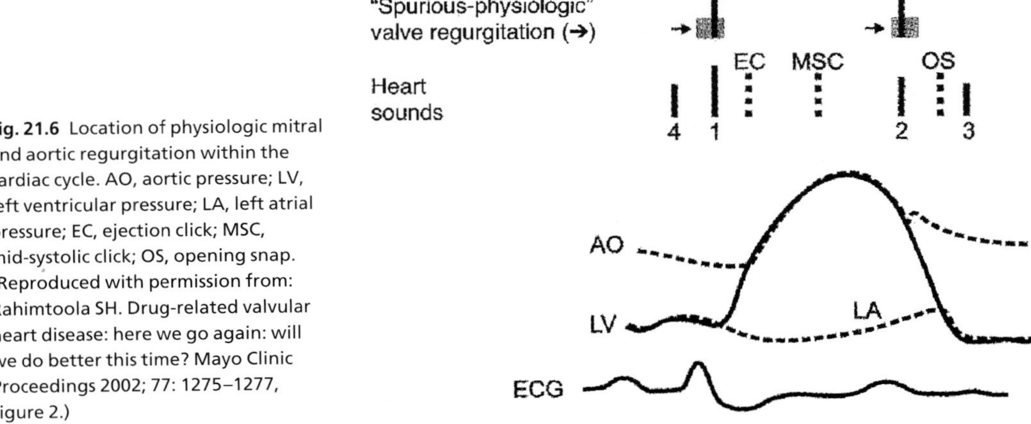

Fig. 21.6 Location of physiologic mitral and aortic regurgitation within the cardiac cycle. AO, aortic pressure; LV, left ventricular pressure; LA, left atrial pressure; EC, ejection click; MSC, mid-systolic click; OS, opening snap. (Reproduced with permission from: Rahimtoola SH. Drug-related valvular heart disease: here we go again: will we do better this time? Mayo Clinic Proceedings 2002; 77: 1275–1277, figure 2.)

Other drugs associated with valvular disease include *ergot derivatives* (*methysergide* and *ergotamine*) causing carcinoid-like lesions and *pergolide mesylate* (used for therapy of Parkinson's disease and restless legs syndrome). Pergolide mesylate has been associated with pericardial fibrosis, and may cause tricuspid valve disease with resultant severe tricuspid regurgitation. The incidence is presently not known, but is probably rare. The valve will appear as that of carcinoid heart disease. Mitral and aortic valve involvement appears to be common.

Proper interpretation of two-dimensional echocardiography and Doppler for quantification of left heart regurgitation is of paramount importance. The term physiologic (spurious or trace) is commonly seen as a small amount of closing flow (1–2 mm behind the valve) trapped between valve leaflets (Figs 21.5 & 21.6). Severity of regurgitation is variable (especially with trivial or mild regurgitation), and dependent upon blood pressure (especially diastolic blood pressure) and PR interval (mitral regurgitation severity). Variability is introduced in the recording and interpretation (~5–29%) of regurgitation. In patients with a short PR interval and hypertension, the degree of MR could be overestimated (physiologic interpreted as mild, mild as moderate, and moderate as severe). In order to minimize the amount of variability in estimation of mitral and aortic valve regurgitation, the following is recommended:

- Measure blood pressure at the time of the echo study.

• In addition to color Doppler, use other modalities to estimate valve regurgitation (most variability is noted with trace and mild regurgitation).
• Try to use the same echo machine, sonographer, and reader for serial studies.

Changes in trace and mild valve regurgitation are most likely due to a change in blood pressure and variability in interpretation.

Carcinoid heart disease

Cardiac involvement in patients with *carcinoid* almost always occurs in those with hepatic metastases. It is thought that tumor release of serotonin and bradykinin cause a fibrous deposition on endocardial surfaces of the right heart and tricuspid and pulmonic valves. The lungs apparently inactivate the substances, and therefore, in the absence of a right-to-left shunt (i.e. resting PFO) or pulmonary metastatic disease, the left side is spared. The tricuspid valve is thickened and has markedly reduced mobility. Coaptation is incomplete, resulting in severe tricuspid regurgitation. Tricuspid stenosis is usually mild. Increased thickening of the pulmonic valve results in pulmonic stenosis, usually with mild pulmonic regurgitation (Fig. 21.7).

Chemotherapeutic drugs

Several *chemotherapeutic drugs* are associated with the development of LV systolic dysfunction. Radiation therapy potentiates systolic dysfunction. With doxorubicin, dysfunction occurs with cumulative doses

(a)

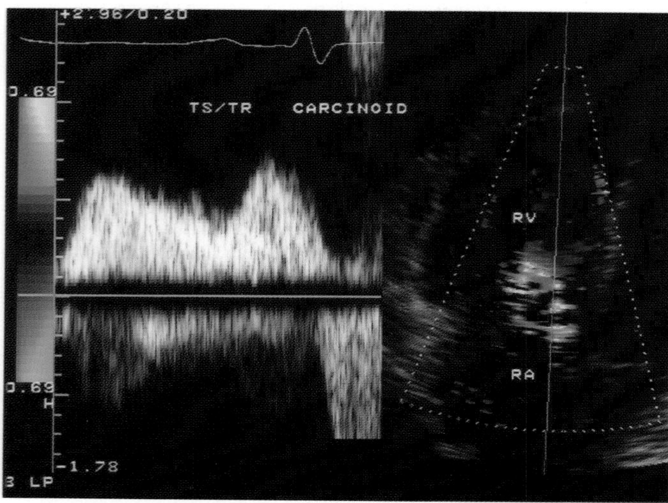

(b)

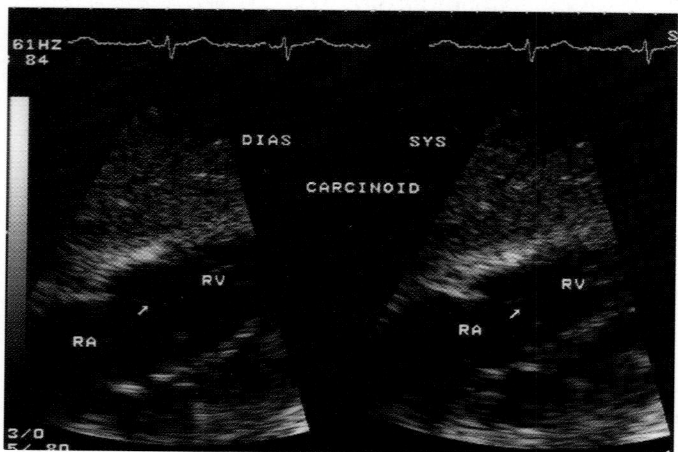

Fig. 21.7 A middle-aged male with a longstanding chronic history of diarrhea presented with progressive lower extremity oedema. (a) Apical four-chamber imaging with colour Doppler (right panel) and continuous wave Doppler (left panel) reveals mild tricuspid stenosis, as the maximum initial velocity is over 1 m/s and the deceleration time is "slow." The tricuspid regurgitant jet maximum velocity was 3 m/s and a "cut-off" sign was present. (b) Diastolic (left panel) and systolic (right panel) frames, from a subcostal window, reveal a bright tricuspid valve that appears "fixed" throughout the cardiac cycle. (*Cont'd.*)

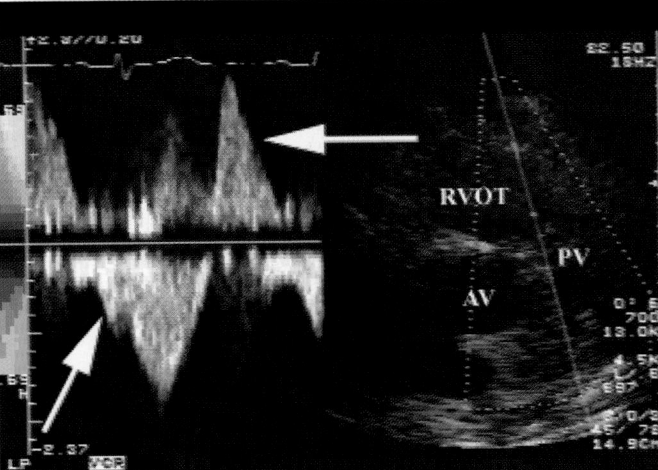

(c)

Fig. 21.7 (*cont'd*) (c) In addition, the patient had evidence of mild pulmonic stenosis with a peak velocity of 2 m/s, and pulmonic regurgitation (horizontal arrow). The PR deceleration time is short, due to rapid equilibration of pressures between the RV and pulmonary artery. Late diastolic flow (upward arrow) is present, due to the rapid rise in RV diastolic pressure.

greater than 450 g/m^2, with daunorubicin greater than 600 mg/m^2, and with cyclophosphamide greater than 6.2 g/m^2 (pericardial effusion and tamponade may be associated with cyclophosphamide).

Acquired immunodeficiency syndrome

Acquired immunodeficiency syndrome (AIDS) and the human immunodeficiency virus are associated with dilated cardiomyopathy, development of pulmonary hypertension, pericardial effusion, pericardial tamponade, and intracardiac tumors, particularly Kaposi's sarcoma and non-Hodgkin's lymphoma. (Fig. 21.8). Pericardial effusion is the most common site of cardiac involvement and is usually small. In addition, NBTE is often found at autopsy in patients with AIDS. Infective endocarditis in patients with AIDS almost always occurs in individuals who are intravenous drug users.

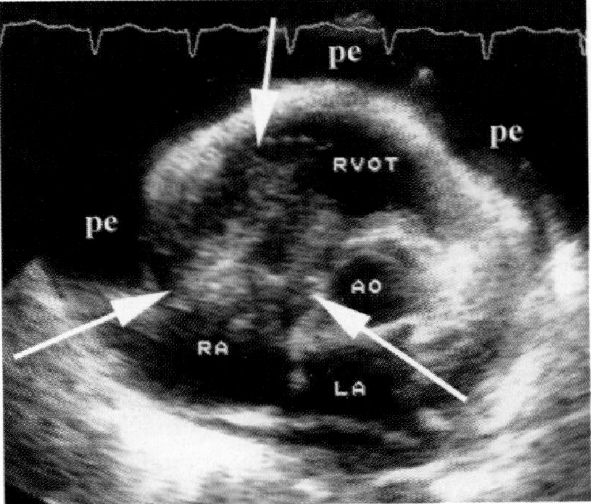

Fig. 21.8 A young adult with AIDS presented with a progressive dyspnea and oedema syndrome. Parasternal short axis imaging revealed a large pericardial effusion (pe) and a large mass within the right heart (arrows). The patient refused any further evaluation.

Syphilis

Syphilis once accounted for 5–10% of cardiovascular death, but is now uncommon. The aorta may be involved anywhere (*luetic aortitis*), but the most common site is the ascending aorta. Aneurysmal dilatation of the aorta with a described "tree-bark" appearance of the affected aorta is characteristic. In addition to aneurysm formation, aortic valvulitis with aortic regurgitation and syphilitic coronary ostial stenosis involving either one or both ostia may be seen.

Echinococcosis and hydatid cyst

Echinococcosis is a human parasitic condition caused by the larvae of *Echinococcus granulosus*. The tapeworm lives as an adult in the intestine of dogs and other canines. Hydatid infection follows closely in occurrence with its most important intermediate host, sheep. Human infection is seen in sheep-raising areas of South America, New Zealand, southern Australia, Algeria, Tanzania, and South Africa. Several cases are found each year in Canada and the United States, particularly where sheep herding is common (Southwest United States) and sled dogs are present (Alaska and northern Canada). Cardiac involvement occurs in 0.5–2% of affected patients, but most often the *Echinococcus* embryo will be found in the liver and also the lungs.

Hydatid cysts may range from 0.5 to 12 cm in dimension. Most are single, but multiple cysts may occur. Intramyocardial cysts protrude into the adjacent cardiac chamber, and pericardial and mediastinal cysts may compress the cardiac chambers or great vessels. Cysts usually appear to be cystic with well-defined edges and internal trabeculations. They may appear "solid," signifying replacement of hydatid liquid by necrotic matter with a foreign-body inflammatory reaction.

Fabry's disease

Patients with *Fabry's disease* appear to have an increased incidence of mitral valve prolapse with leaflet redundancy as the most common cardiac finding. The aortic root may be enlarged, and LV chamber dimensions and wall thickness (mass) may be increased.

Friedreich's ataxia

Friedreich's ataxia is associated with electrocardiographic and echocardiographic abnormalities. Concentric LV hypertrophy (~10%), asymmetric septal hypertrophy (~10%), and global diminished LV function (~7%) appear to be most common.

Diabetes mellitus

Diabetes mellitus is associated with LV hypertrophy and also dilatation of all four cardiac chambers, along with LV systolic dysfunction. Diastolic dysfunction (decreased E/A ratio, increased isovolumic relaxation time) is often impaired in patients with normal systolic function.

Thyroid disease

Hypothyroidism is associated with a relatively slow heart rate and depression of LV function. Diastolic abnormality is also noted. A pericardial effusion will often occur in patients with longstanding severe hypothyroidism and on occasion in patients with mild disease. Very large pericardial effusions, most often without tamponade physiology, may develop. These effusions will gradually resolve with thyroid replacement therapy.

Hyperthyroidism is associated with a relatively high heart rate and enhanced LV systolic function (increased ejection fraction and velocity of circumferential shortening). Diastolic measures will be supernormal evidenced by a decreased isovolumic relaxation time. With continued hyperthyroidism, patients may develop systolic dysfunction and evidence of congestive heart failure.

Obesity

Obesity is associated with dilatation and hypertrophy (eccentric hypertrophy) of the LV, probably in response to an increased cardiac output. Increased measures of LA dimension, aortic root, LV end-diastolic dimension, and LV septal and posterior wall thickness are found. LV mass will also increase. Equations for expected LV mass (from Gardin *et al.* 1995: see Further reading, p. 384) in an elderly population are:

$$LV_{mass}\,(\text{male}) = 16.6(Wt)^{0.51}$$

$$LV_{mass}\,(\text{female}) = 13.9(Wt)^{0.51}$$

where LV_{mass} is the expected mass of the left ventricle and Wt is patient weight in kilograms. If the measured mass to expected mass ratio is from 0.69 to 1.47, it is considered an expected value. Systolic function (ejection fraction and fractional shortening) may be reduced in morbid obesity and may improve with weight loss. In addition, diastolic abnormality (increased isovolumic relaxation time and reduced E/A ratio) may be noted in obese individuals.

Aging and the heart

LV wall thickness and mass normally increase with *aging*. LV cavity dimensions remain basically unchanged. The size of the aortic root and left atrium increase with increasing age. The aortic and mitral valves will thicken and calcify with aging, with calcium noted along the bases of the aortic cusps, at the line of closure on the atrial side of the mitral leaflets, and in the mitral annulus (*mitral annulus calcification*—more common in females). The *senile calcification syndrome* is identified as calcification of the aortic valve leaflets, mitral annulus, and coronary arteries.

Peak aortic annulus flow (pulsed wave Doppler) decreases with age, but this may in part be due to a progressive increase in aortic annulus diameter (mitral annulus diameter increases with age also), and a resultant unchanged stroke volume. As one ages, diastolic parameters change, with a pattern approaching that of abnormal relaxation. Approximately seven of eight normal persons over the age of 70 years will have a pattern of abnormal relaxation.

Optimal timing of biventricular pacemakers

Pulsed Doppler of mitral inflow helps optimize atrioventricular (AV) timing of a biventricular pacemaker. Although providing a small improvement in haemodynamics, optimizing atrioventricular delay (AVD) in a patient with LV systolic dysfunction and advanced heart failure may have significant clinical benefits. An optimal AVD is defined as the shortest AVD that allows complete ventricular filling, thereby optimizing stroke volume and minimizing presystolic mitral regurgitation. The goal of optimization is to maximally prolong LV diastolic filling without truncating the mitral A wave (Fig. 21.9).

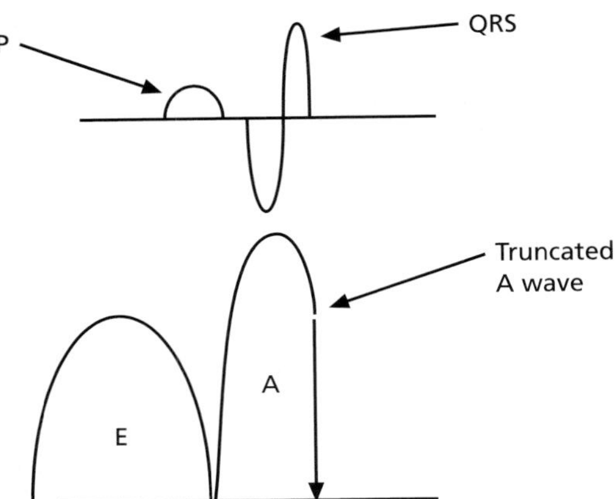

Fig. 21.9 ECG with a P wave (P) and QRS complex (QRS) with PW mitral inflow recording of an E wave and A wave. The A wave is truncated in this diagram in which the programmed AV delay is too short. (Courtesy of Medtronic, Inc, Minneapolis, MN.)

In patients with an interventricular conduction delay pattern (IVCD) with a left bundle branch block pattern (LBBB) on the ECG, there is delayed LV activation, but atrial activation is not delayed. Passive early LV filling (E wave) and the atrial component (A wave) may occur at the same time, causing fusion of the E and A waves on the pulsed wave mitral inflow pattern.

With a RA pacemaker lead, and with leads pacing both ventricles (pacer lead in the RV and pacer lead in the coronary sinus which activates the LV), the LV will finish systolic contraction and also start diastolic relaxation earlier, which will lengthen diastolic filling time. With adjustment of the pacemaker AV interval, one will find separation of the mitral E and A waves, without A-wave truncation (to make sure the A wave is not truncated follow the "outside" of the A wave and look for a mitral valve closure click to assist in timing).

Two methods for optimizing AVD using optimization of LV filling with mitral Doppler inflow patterns are the *iterative method* and the *Ritter method*. The iterative method is as described below:

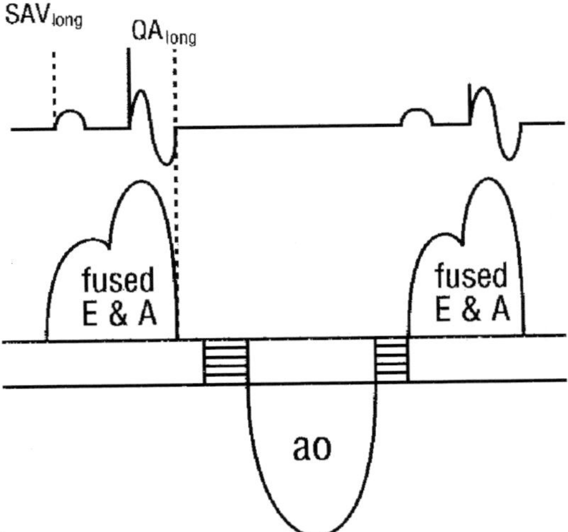

Fig. 21.10 The programmed AV delay is slightly less than the patient's own natural PR interval, causing E and A fusion, but long enough so that A wave truncation does not occur. SAV_{long}, programmed long AV delay (usually 140–160 ms); QA_{long}, time from the paced ventricular spike to the end of the A wave when the AV delay has been programmed long. (Courtesy of Medtronic, Inc., Minneapolis, MN.)

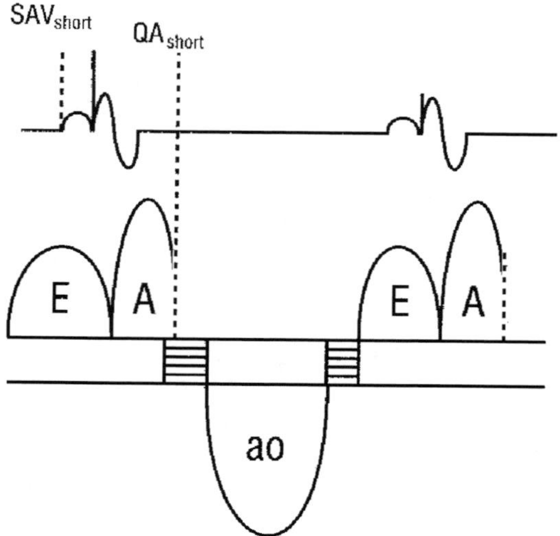

Fig. 21.11 The AV delay has been shortened until the A wave appears truncated, thus limiting the atrial contribution to LV filling. *SAV_{short}*, programmed short AV delay (around 50 ms); *QA_{short}*, time from the paced ventricular spike to the end of the A wave when the AV delay has been programmed short. (Courtesy of Medtronic, Inc., Minneapolis, MN.)

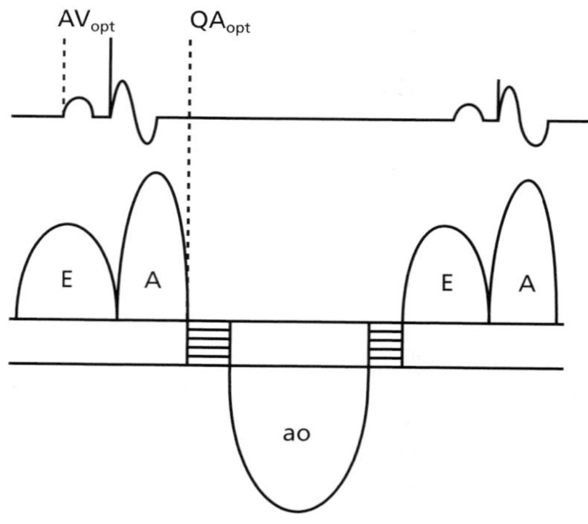

Fig. 21.12 Once truncation of the A wave is no longer evident, programmed AV delay should be optimized. Ventricular contraction occurs at the end of the completion of the A wave. *AV_{opt}*, optimized AV programmed delay; *QA_{opt}*, resultant optimized QA interval. (Courtesy of Medtronic, Inc., Minneapolis, MN.)

1 Program the pacemaker for an AVD that is slightly less than the patient's own natural PR interval. This will ensure capture of the paced ventricular beats. Fused E and A waves will probably be seen with closure of the mitral valve occurring prior to initiation of aortic forward flow, and the A wave should not be truncated (Fig. 21.10).

2 Shorten AV delay in 20-ms increments until the A wave begins to truncate, thus limiting the atrial contribution to LV filling (Fig. 21.11).

3 Once truncation of the A wave is noted, begin to lengthen the AV delay in 10-ms increments until truncation is no longer evident. This should be the optimized AV delay, whereby ventricular contraction is occurring at the end of the A wave (Fig. 21.12).

The Ritter method uses the following equation:

$$AV_{opt} = AV_{short} + [(AV_{long} + QA_{long}) - (AV_{short} + QA_{short})]$$

where AV_{opt} is the optimal programmed AV delay. The other parameters are defined in Figs 21.10 and 21.11. One programs the AV delay at ~150 ms for AV_{long} and then measures the QA_{long} from the Doppler recording (Fig. 21.10). Similarly, one then programs the AVD at ~50 ms for AV_{short} and measures the QA_{short} from the Doppler recording (Fig. 21.11).

Appendices

Appendix 1

With permission: Zabalgoitia M. Echocardiography of Prosthetic Heart Valves, RG Landes Co., Austin, Texas 1994, p 52 – 55.

Normal Doppler Values for Mechanical Aortic Prostheses

Prosthesis	*Peak Velocity (M/sec)*	*Mean Gradient (mmHg)*
Starr Edwards	3.1 ± 0.5	24 ± 4
Bjork-Shiley	1.9 ± 0.2 to 2.8 ± 0.9	14 ± 3 to 31 ± 2
19 mm	—	21.0 ± 7.00
21 mm	2.76 ± 0.90	16.0
23 mm	2.59 ± 0.42	14.0 ± 5.00
25 mm	2.14 ± 0.31	13.3 ± 2.53
27 mm	1.91 ± 0.20	9.7 ± 2.53
29 mm	1.87 ± 0.20	7.0 ± 6.00
St. Jude Medical	2.2 ± 0.5 to 3.0 ± 0.8	22 ± 11 to 11 ± 6
19 mm	3.00 ± 0.77	22.2 ± 11.0
21 mm	2.70 ± 0.26	14.4 ± 5.0
23 mm	2.32 ± 0.60	10.8 ± 6.3
25 mm	2.20 ± 0.46	11.0 ± 6.0
Medtronic-Hall	2.6 ± 0.3	12 ± 3
Omniscience	2.8 ± 0.4	14 ± 3

Appendix 2

With permission: Zabalgoitia M. Echocardiography of Prosthetic Heart Valves, RG Landes Co., Austin, Texas 1994, p 52 – 55.

Normal Doppler Values for Mechanical Mitral Prostheses

Prosthesis	*Peak Velocity (M/sec)*	*Mean Gradient (mmHg)*	*Pressure Half-time (ms)*	*Valve Area*	
				Mean (cm^2)	*Range (cm^2)*
Starr Edwards	1.8 ± 0.4	4.6 ± 2.4	110 ± 27	2.1	1.2–2.5
Bjork-Shiley	1.6 ± 0.3	2.9 ± 1.6	90 ± 22	2.4	1.6–3.7
St. Jude Medical	1.5 ± 0.3	3.5 ± 1.3	77 ± 17	2.91–4.4	
27 mm	1.54 ± 0.20	5.00 ± 2.00	137.5	1.60	
29 mm	1.59 ± 0.27	2.71 ± 1.36	78.0 ± 16.0	2.93 ± 0.60	
31 mm	1.54 ± 0.36	5.00 ± 3.00	57.9 ± 6.10	3.80 ± 0.40	
Medtronic-Hall	1.7 ± 0.3	3.1 ± 0.9	89 ± 19	2.41–3.9	
Omniscience	1.8 ± 0.3	3.3 ± 0.9	125 ± 29	1.9	1.6–3.1

Appendix 3

With permission: Zabalgoitia M. Echocardiography of Prosthetic Heart Valves, RG Landes Co., Austin, Texas 1994, p 52 – 55.

Normal Doppler Values for Biologic Aortic Prosthesis

Prosthesis	Peak Velocity (M/sec)	Mean Gradient (mmHg)	Valve Area	
			Mean (cm^2)	Range (cm^2)
Aortic Homograft	0.8 ± 0.4	7.1 ± 3	2.2	1.7–3.1
Hancock	2.4 ± 0.4	11 ± 2	1.8	1.4–2.3
Carpentier-Edwards	2.4 ± 0.5	14 ± 6	1.8	1.2–3.1

Appendix 4

With permission: Zabalgoitia M. Echocardiography of Prosthetic Heart Valves, RG Landes Co., Austin, Texas 1994, p 52 – 55.

Normal Doppler Values for Biological Mitral Prostheses

Prosthesis	Peak Velocity (M/sec)	Mass Gradient (mmHg)	Valve Area	
			Mean (cm^2)	Range (cm^2)
Hancock	1.5 ± 0.3	4.3 ± 2.1	129 ± 31	1.3–2.7
Carpentier-Edwards	1.8 ± 0.2	6.5 ± 2.1	90 ± 25	1.6–3.5

Appendix 5

With permission: Zabalgoitia M. Echocardiography of Prosthetic Heart Valves, RG Landes Co., Austin, Texas 1994, p 52 – 55.

Normal Doppler Values for Mitral Annular Rings

Ring	Peak Velocity (M/sec)	Mean Gradient (mmHg)	Pressure Half-time (ms)	Valve Area	
				Mean (cm^2)	Range (cm^2)
Carpentier-Edwards	1.4 ± 0.3	3.8 ± 0.4	98 ± 16	2.6	1.8–3.8
Duran	1.3 ± 1.1	3.8 ± 1.1	89 ± 19	2.8	1.9–3.9

Appendix 6

With permission: Zabalgoitia M. Echocardiography of Prosthetic Heart Valves, RG Landes Co., Austin, Texas 1994, p 52 – 55.

Aortic Valve Hemodynamics at Rest and Exercise Using Doppler

Prosthesis	*Valve Size (mm)*	*Peak Gradient (mmHg)*			*Mean Gradient (mmHg)*		
		Rest	*Exercise*	*Increase*	*Rest*	*Exercise*	*Increase*
St. Jude Medical	21–31	24	41	71%	11	18	64%
		21	39	86%	9	17	89%
		23	63	74%	—	—	—
Medtronic-Hall	21–31	21	35	67%	9	15	67%
		21	35	67%	9	15	67%
	20	33	48	—	18	26	72%
	21	30	46	—	15	24	80%
Carpentier-Edwards	21	27	36	—	15	24	70%

Appendix 7

With permission: Zabalgoitia M. Echocardiography of Prosthetic Heart Valves, RG Landes Co., Austin, Texas 1994, p 52 – 55.

Mitral Valve Hemodynamics at Rest and Exercise Using Doppler

Prosthesis	*Valve Size (mm)*	*Peak Gradient (mmHg)*			*Valve Area (cm^2)*		
		Rest	*Exercise*	*Increase*	*Rest*	*Exercise*	*Increase*
Starr-Edwards	28–32	4.6	12.6	174%	1.8		
St. Jude Medical	25–33	2.5	5.1	104%	3.4		
		2.3	4.6	100%	3.7	3.2	14%
		4.8	9.5	98%			
Medtronic-Hall	25–33	3.0	7.0	133%	3.4		
		2.9	7.1	145%	2.9	2.9	0

Appendix 8a

Normal Cross-Sectional Values for Echocardiography, as obtained from the Cardiac Ultasound Laboratory at Massachusetts General Hospital. All measurements are in cm (linear) and cm^2 (area). (With permission: Triulzi M, *et al.* Normal Adult Cross-Sectional Echocardiographic values: Linear dimensions and Chamber Areas. Echocardiography 1984; 1: 403).

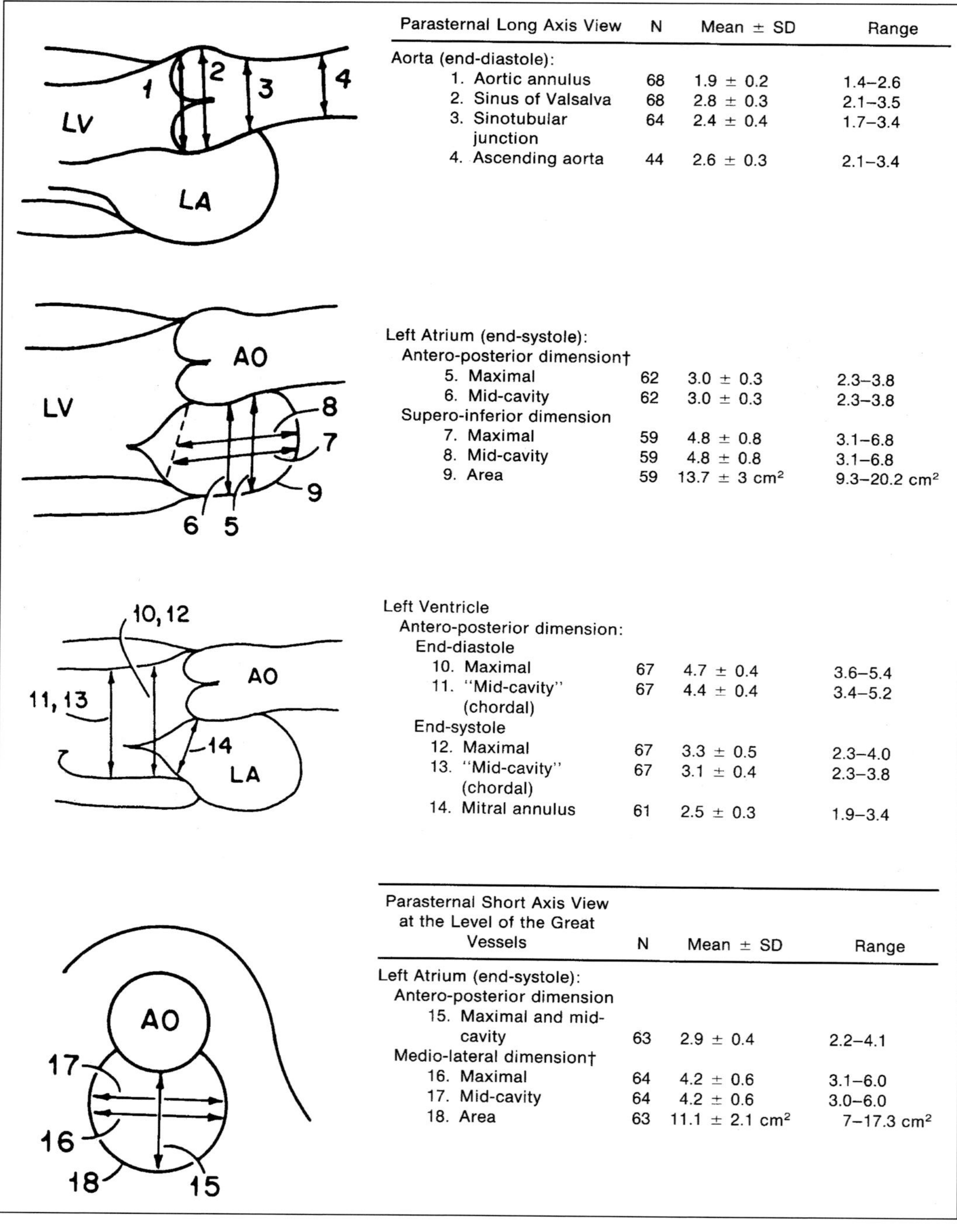

Parasternal Long Axis View	N	Mean ± SD	Range
Aorta (end-diastole):			
1. Aortic annulus	68	1.9 ± 0.2	1.4–2.6
2. Sinus of Valsalva	68	2.8 ± 0.3	2.1–3.5
3. Sinotubular junction	64	2.4 ± 0.4	1.7–3.4
4. Ascending aorta	44	2.6 ± 0.3	2.1–3.4
Left Atrium (end-systole):			
Antero-posterior dimension†			
5. Maximal	62	3.0 ± 0.3	2.3–3.8
6. Mid-cavity	62	3.0 ± 0.3	2.3–3.8
Supero-inferior dimension			
7. Maximal	59	4.8 ± 0.8	3.1–6.8
8. Mid-cavity	59	4.8 ± 0.8	3.1–6.8
9. Area	59	13.7 ± 3 cm^2	9.3–20.2 cm^2
Left Ventricle			
Antero-posterior dimension:			
End-diastole			
10. Maximal	67	4.7 ± 0.4	3.6–5.4
11. "Mid-cavity" (chordal)	67	4.4 ± 0.4	3.4–5.2
End-systole			
12. Maximal	67	3.3 ± 0.5	2.3–4.0
13. "Mid-cavity" (chordal)	67	3.1 ± 0.4	2.3–3.8
14. Mitral annulus	61	2.5 ± 0.3	1.9–3.4

Parasternal Short Axis View at the Level of the Great Vessels	N	Mean ± SD	Range
Left Atrium (end-systole):			
Antero-posterior dimension			
15. Maximal and mid-cavity	63	2.9 ± 0.4	2.2–4.1
Medio-lateral dimension†			
16. Maximal	64	4.2 ± 0.6	3.1–6.0
17. Mid-cavity	64	4.2 ± 0.6	3.0–6.0
18. Area	63	11.1 ± 2.1 cm^2	7–17.3 cm^2

Appendix 8b

Parasternal Short Axis View at the Level of the Great Vessels	N	Mean ± SD	Range
Pulmonary Artery (end-diastole):†			
19. Right ventricular outflow tract (subvalvular)	53	2.5 ± 0.4	1.8–3.4
20. Pulmonary valve	51	1.5 ± 0.3	1.0–2.2
21. Supravalvular	48	1.8 ± 0.3	0.9–2.9
22. Right pulmonary artery	39	1.2 ± 0.2	0.7–1.7
23. Left pulmonary artery	11	1.1 ± 0.2	0.6–1.4

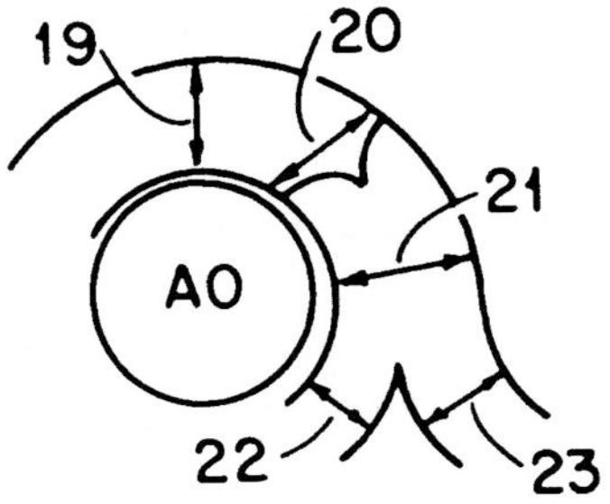

Parasternal Short Axis View at the Ventricular Level	N	Mean ± SD	Range
Right Ventricle (tricuspid valve level):			
Septal-free wall maximal dimension			
24. Diastole	36	3.0 ± 0.4	2.5–3.8
25. Systole	36	2.6 ± 0.3	2.0–3.4

Parasternal Short Axis View at the Ventricular Level	N	Mean ± SD	Range
Left Ventricle (mitral valve level):			
Antero-posterior diameter			
26. Diastole	57	5.1 ± 0.5	3.4–5.8
27. Systole	57	3.6 ± 0.3	2.8–4.3
Medio-lateral diameter			
28. Diastole	57	5.0 ± 0.5	3.6–5.8
29. Systole	57	3.8 ± 0.5	2.6–4.8
Area			
30. Diastole	57	24.7 ± 5.1 cm^2	16.3–38.4 cm^2
31. Systole	57	12.3 ± 2.8 cm^2	6–20.2 cm^2
32. Fractional change	57	50.5 ± 6.8%	33.8–69.9%

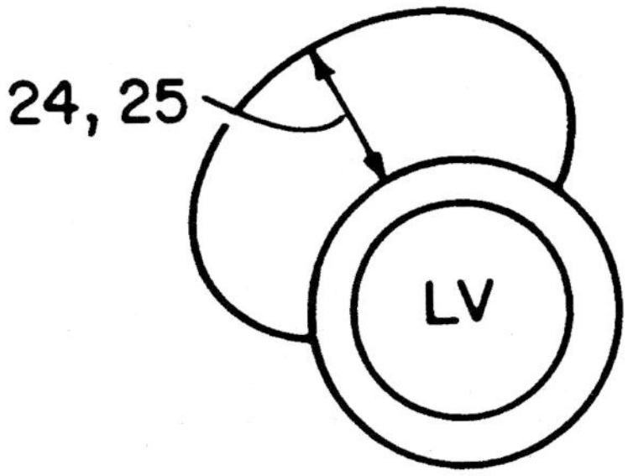

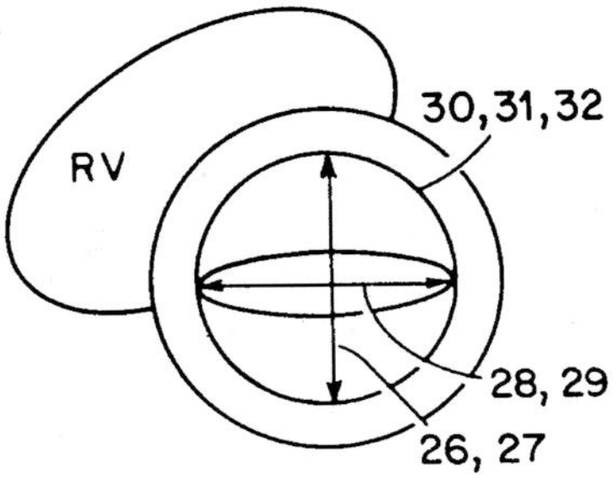

Appendix 8c

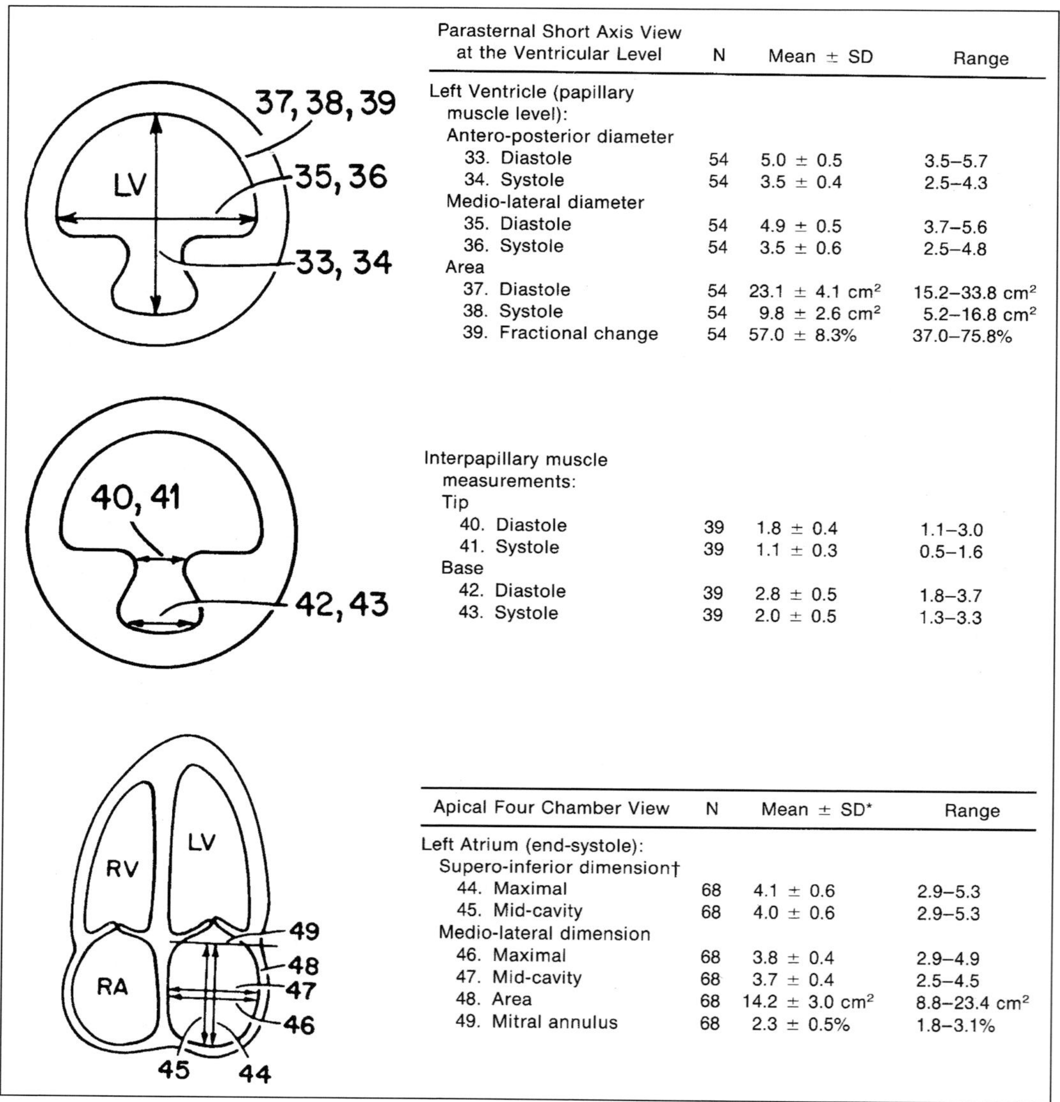

Parasternal Short Axis View at the Ventricular Level	N	Mean ± SD	Range
Left Ventricle (papillary muscle level):			
Antero-posterior diameter			
33. Diastole	54	5.0 ± 0.5	3.5–5.7
34. Systole	54	3.5 ± 0.4	2.5–4.3
Medio-lateral diameter			
35. Diastole	54	4.9 ± 0.5	3.7–5.6
36. Systole	54	3.5 ± 0.6	2.5–4.8
Area			
37. Diastole	54	23.1 ± 4.1 cm^2	15.2–33.8 cm^2
38. Systole	54	9.8 ± 2.6 cm^2	5.2–16.8 cm^2
39. Fractional change	54	57.0 ± 8.3%	37.0–75.8%
Interpapillary muscle measurements:			
Tip			
40. Diastole	39	1.8 ± 0.4	1.1–3.0
41. Systole	39	1.1 ± 0.3	0.5–1.6
Base			
42. Diastole	39	2.8 ± 0.5	1.8–3.7
43. Systole	39	2.0 ± 0.5	1.3–3.3

Apical Four Chamber View	N	Mean ± SD*	Range
Left Atrium (end-systole):			
Supero-inferior dimension†			
44. Maximal	68	4.1 ± 0.6	2.9–5.3
45. Mid-cavity	68	4.0 ± 0.6	2.9–5.3
Medio-lateral dimension			
46. Maximal	68	3.8 ± 0.4	2.9–4.9
47. Mid-cavity	68	3.7 ± 0.4	2.5–4.5
48. Area	68	14.2 ± 3.0 cm^2	8.8–23.4 cm^2
49. Mitral annulus	68	2.3 ± 0.5%	1.8–3.1%

Appendix 8d

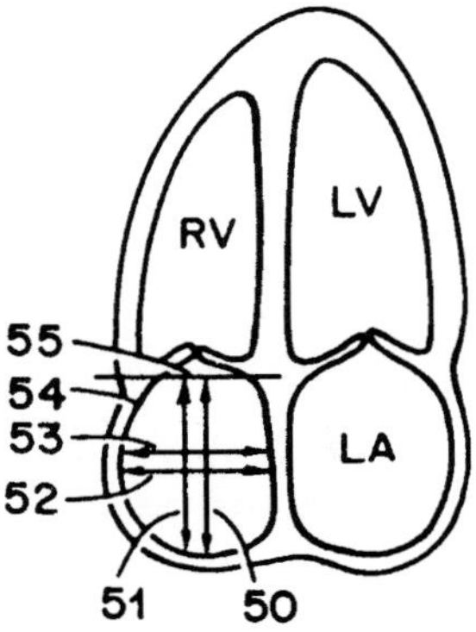

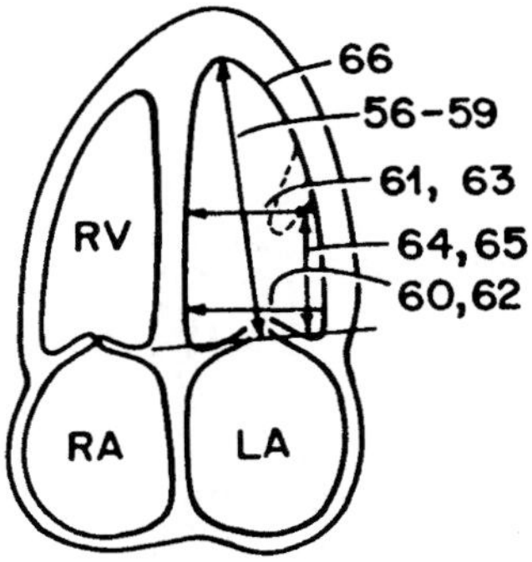

Apical Four Chamber View	N	Mean ± SD	Range
Right Atrium (end-systole):			
Supero-inferior dimension			
50. Maximal	67	4.2 ± 0.4	3.4–4.9
51. Mid-cavity	67	4.2 ± 0.4	3.4–4.9
Medio-lateral dimension			
52. Maximal	67	3.7 ± 0.4	3.0–4.6
53. Mid-cavity	67	3.7 ± 0.4	2.9–4.6
54. Area	67	13.5 ± 2 cm^2	8.3–19.5 cm^2
55. Tricuspid annulus	53	2.2 ± 0.3	1.3–2.8
Left Ventricle			
Length (diastole)			
56. Maximal	67	7.8 ± 0.7	6.3–9.5
57. Mid-cavity	67	7.8 ± 0.7	6.2–9.5
Length (systole)			
58. Maximal	67	6.1 ± 0.8	4.6–8.5
59. Mid-cavity	67	6.1 ± 0.8	4.6–8.4
Medio-lateral dimension			
Diastole			
60. Maximal	67	4.7 ± 0.4	3.7–5.8
61. Mid-cavity	67	4.2 ± 0.5	3.3–5.2
Systole			
62. Maximal	67	3.7 ± 0.4	2.8–4.7
63. Mid-cavity	67	3.1 ± 0.4	2.4–4.2
Papillary muscle to mitral annulus			
64. Diastole	9	3.0 ± 0.4	2.2–3.6
65. Systole	9	2.2 ± 0.3	1.6–2.6
Area			
66. Diastole	62	33.2 ± 7.7 cm^2	17.7–47.3 cm^2
67. Systole	62	17.6 ± 5.2 cm^2	7.9–31.5 cm^2
68. Fractional change	63	47.2 ± 8.8%	31–67.9%
Right Ventricle:			
Length (diastole)			
69. Maximal	61	7.1 ± 0.8	5.5–9.1
70. Mid-cavity	61	7.1 ± 0.9	5.5–9.1
Length (systole)			
71. Maximal	61	5.5 ± 0.8	4.2–8.1
72. Mid-cavity	61	5.5 ± 0.8	4.2–8.1
Medio-lateral dimensions			
Diastole			
73. Maximal	61	3.5 ± 0.4	2.6–4.3
74. Mid-cavity	61	3.0 ± 0.5	2.1–4.2
Systole			
75. Maximal	61	2.9 ± 0.4	2.2–3.6
76. Mid-cavity	61	2.4 ± 0.3	1.9–3.1
Area			
77. Systole	41	20.1 ± 4.0 cm^2	10.7–35.5 cm^2
78. Diastole	41	10.9 ± 2.9 cm^2	4.5–20 cm^2
79. Fractional change	41	45.9 ± 7.3%	30–59.5%

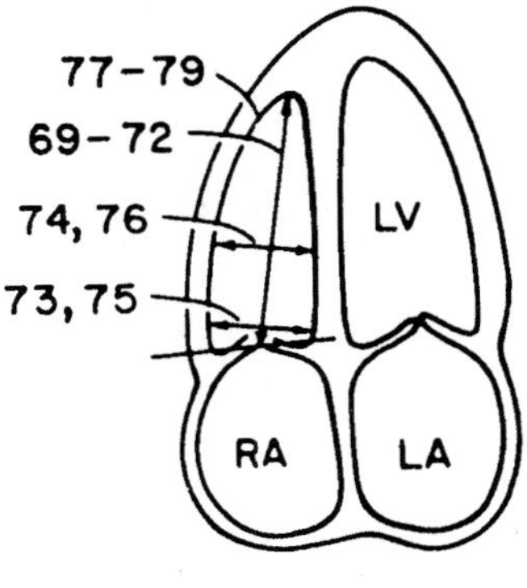

Appendix 8e

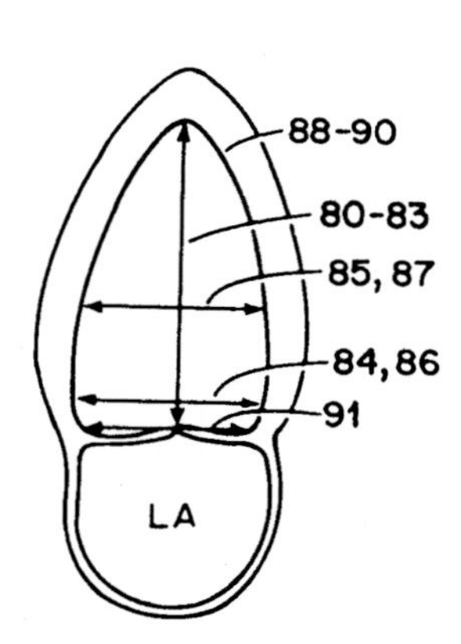

Apical Two Chamber View	N	Mean ± SD	Range
Left Ventricle:			
Length (diastole)			
80. Maximal	54	8.0 ± 0.7	6.8–9.5
81. Mid-cavity	54	8.0 ± 0.7	6.8–9.5
Length (systole)			
82. Maximal	54	6.3 ± 0.9	4.4–7.8
83. Mid-cavity	54	6.2 ± 0.9	4.4–7.8
Transverse dimension			
Diastole			
84. Maximal	52	4.7 ± 0.6	3.8–5.8
85. Mid-cavity	52	4.2 ± 0.6	2.6–5.5
Systole			
86. Maximal	52	3.6 ± 0.6	2.6–4.8
87. Mid-cavity	52	3.2 ± 0.6	2.1–4.5
Area			
88. Diastole	42	34.2 ± 7.4 cm^2	19.3–48.8 cm^2
89. Systole	42	17.3 ± 5.2 cm^2	8.9–28.1 cm^2
90. Fractional change	42	49.8 ± 8.2%	33.7–69.0%
91. Mitral annulus	46	2.3 ± 0.3	1.8–2.8

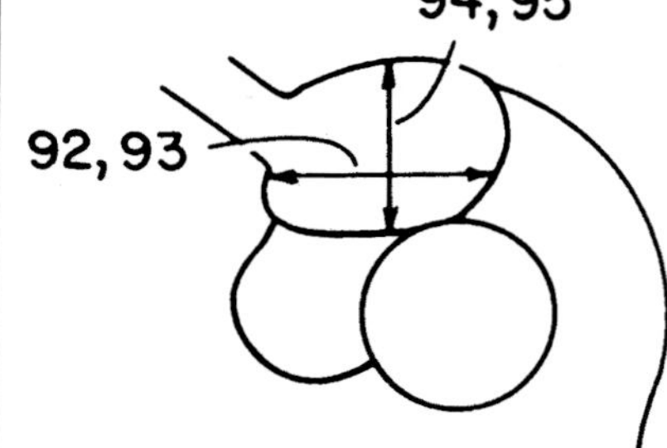

Subcostal View	N	Mean ± SD	Range
Right Atrium (end-systole):			
Antero-posterior diameter			
92. Maximal	22	4.5 ± 0.5	3.7–5.7
93. Mid-cavity	22	4.5 ± 0.5	3.7–5.7
Medio-lateral diameter			
94. Maximal	31	4.0 ± 0.5	3.3–5.7
95. Mid-cavity	31	4.0 ± 0.4	3.3–4.9

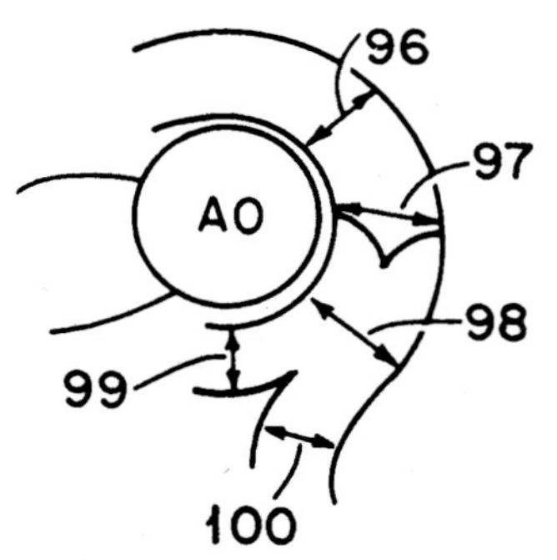

	N	Mean ± SD	Range
Pulmonary Artery (end-diastole)§			
96. Right ventricular outflow tract (subvalvular)	18	2.0 ± 0.4	1.4–2.9
97. Pulmonary valve	19	1.4 ± 0.2	1.1–1.7
98. Supravalvular	19	1.6 ± 0.3	1.2–2.3
99. Right pulmonary artery	7	1.2 ± 0.2	0.9–1.3
100. Left pulmonary artery	5	1.1 ± 0.4	0.8–1.6

Appendix 8f

Subcostal View	N	Mean ± SD	Range
Inferior Vena Cava			
101. Proximal	52	1.6 ± 0.2	1.2–2.3
102. Distal	49	1.6 ± 0.3	1.1–2.5
103. Hepatic vein	12	0.8 ± 0.2	0.5–1.1

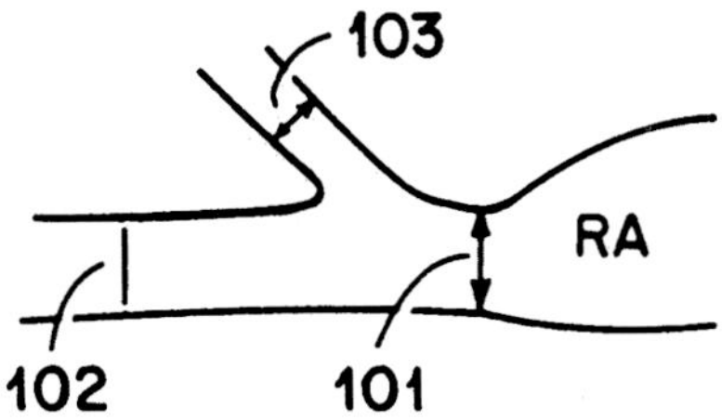

Suprasternal Notch View	N	Mean ± SD	Range
End-diastole			
104. Aortic arch	42	2.7 ± 0.3	2.0–3.6
105. Right pulmonary artery	37	1.8 ± 0.3	1.4–2.7

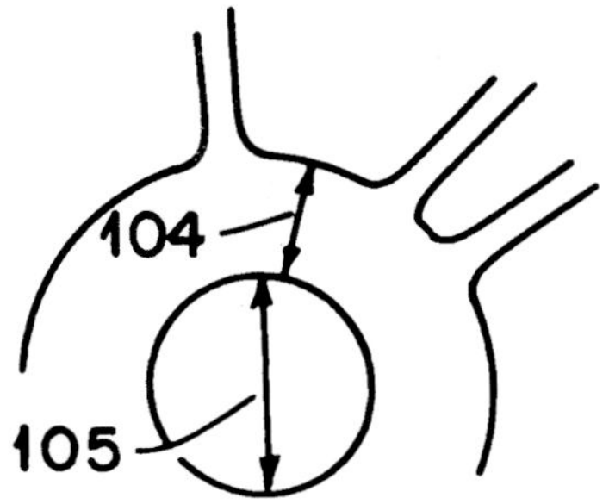

Appendix 9

Measures of left ventricular mass using the truncated ellipsoid method in 44 normal males, and 40 normal females. From Helak JW, Reichek N. Quantitation of Human Left Ventricular Mass and Volume By Two-Dimensional Echocardiography: In Vitro Anatomic Validation. Circulation 1981; 63: 1398–1407.

Normal Left Ventricular Mass
(Truncated Ellipse Methodology)

	Mean ± SD	
Mass	Males	Females
Grams	148 ± 26	108 ± 21
Index (Gm/m^2)	76 ± 13	66 ± 11

Appendix 10

Suggested algorithm for evaluation and therapy for suspected methemoglobinemia. (With permission: Novaro GM, Aronow HD, Militello MA, *et al.* Benzocaine-Induced Methemoglobinemia: Experience From a High-Volume Transesophageal Echocardiogarphy Laboratory. JASE 2003; 16: 170–175, fig. 1, page 173.)

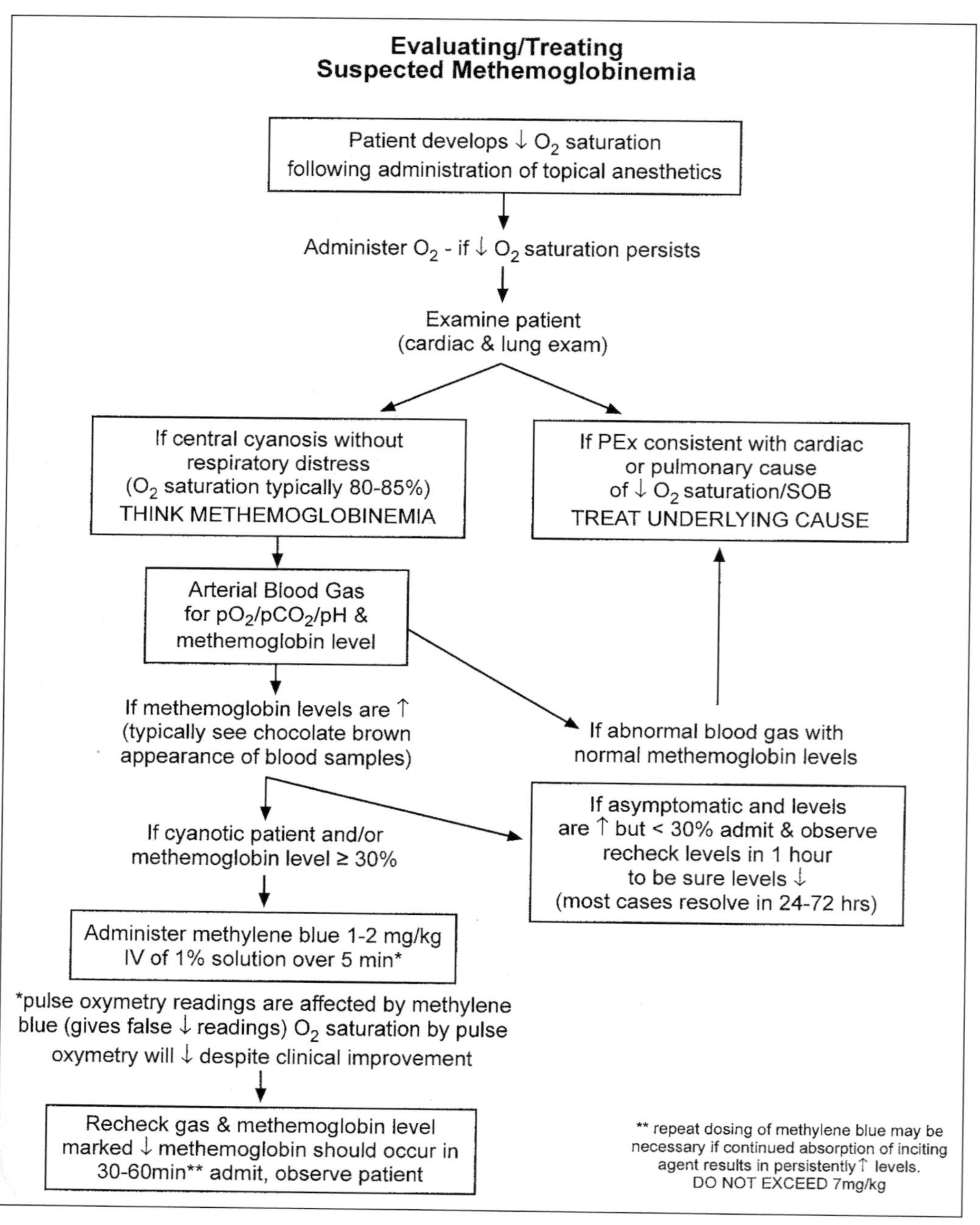

Further Reading

General

Cheitlin MD, Armstrong WF, Aurigemma GP, *et al.* ACC/AHA/ASE 2003 Guidelines Update for the Clinical Application of Echocardiography: a report of the American College of Cardiology/American Heart Association Task Force on Practice Guidelines (ACC/AHA/ASE Committee to Update the 1997 Guidelines for the Clinical Application of Echocardiography). 2003.

This 96 page document is available at www.acc.org/clinical/guidelines/echo/index.pdf.

Quinones MA, Douglas PS, Foster EF, *et al.* American College of Cardiology/American Heart Association Clinical Competence Statement on Echocardiography. Circulation 2003; 107: 1068–1089.

This is a revision of the 1990 guidelines, written in conjunction with the American College of Cardiology, American Heart Association, American College of Physicians, American Society of Echocardiography, Society of Pediatric Echocardiography, and the Society of Cardiovascular Anesthesiologists. These guidelines discuss training requirements and competence in transthoracic echocardiography, Transesophageal echocardiography, perioperative echocardiography, stress echocardiography, coronary heart disease, fetal, and emerging technologies—hand-carried devices, contrast, intracoronary and intracardiac ultrasound, and echo-directed pericardiocentesis.

Books

Feigenbaum H. Echocardiography, 5th edn. Philadelphia: Lea & Febiger, 1994.

This textbook should be available to echo laboratories and persons involved in echocardiography.

Fung YC. A First Course in Continuum Mechanics, 3rd edn. Englewood Cliffs, NJ: Prentice Hall, 1994.

Fung YC. Biodynamics: circulation. New York: Springer Verlag, 1984.

Fung YC. Biomechanics: motion, flow, stress, and growth. New York: Springer Verlag, 1990.

Fung YC. Biomechanics: mechanical properties of living tissues, 2nd Edn. New York: Springer Verlag, 1993.

These four texts provide material for those interested in more in-depth coverage of principles related to bioengineering.

Oh JK, Seward JB, Tajik AJ. The Echo Manual, 2nd edn. Philadelphia: Lippincott Williams & Wilkins, 1999.

This is a clinically useful text written by cardiologists from the Mayo Clinic. The illustrations and photographs are instructive.

Otto CM. Textbook of Clinical Echocardiography, 2nd edn. Philadelphia: Saunders, 2000.

A concise and practical text covering echocardiography and an echo perspective of specific clinical problems.

Otto CM. The Practice of Clinical Echocardiography, 2nd edn. Philadelphia: Saunders, 2002.

Aspects of clinical echocardiography and significant investigational areas are covered.

Snider AR, Serwer GA, Ritter SB. Echocardiography in Pediatric Heart Disease, 2nd edn. St Louis: Mosby, 1997.

This text covers echocardiographic aspects of pediatric cardiology along with a presentation of echo hemodynamics and quantitative methods.

Weyman AE. Principles and Practice of Echocardiography, 2nd edn. Philadelphia: Lea & Febiger, 1994.

This textbook discusses technical aspects of ultrasound machines and physics, along with quantitative methods.

Video and CD-ROM media

Kerut EK, McIlwain EF, Plotnick, Giles TD. Video Case Studies of Echocardiography: An interactive CD-ROM. New York: Futura Publishing, 2000.
Collection of over 100 short case presentations of adult disorders with video clips of echocardiography and TEE cases.

Shirali GS, Lombano F, Dyar D, *et al.* Congenital Heart Disease Visualized. New York: Futura Publishing, 1997.
Pathology and echo correlates in a large number of congenital cases.

Journals

Echocardiography: A Journal of Cardiovascular Ultrasound and Allied Techniques. Editor—Dr Navin C Nanda. Futura Publishing Co., Armonk, NY.
Original investigations, the "Image Section," "Echo Rounds," case reports, and timely reviews of specific echo topics are presented by investigators from around the world.

European Journal of Echocardiography. Editor—JRTC Roelandt. Elsevier Science, 32 Jamestown Road, London NWI 7BY, UK.
The journal of the Working Group on Echocardiography of the European Society of Cardiology. Original investigations, case reports, and review articles on all aspects of echocardiography.

Journal of the American Society of Echocardiography. Editor—Dr Harvey Feigenbaum. Mosby, Orlando, FL.
The official journal of the American Society of Echocardiography (ASE) with original investigations and case reports.

Ultrasound in Medicine and Biology. Editor—Professor PNT Wells. Elsevier Science Publishing Co. New York, NY.
A technical journal with articles at the forefront of ultrasound.

Chapters 1 and 2

AIUM Bioeffects Committee: Bioeffects and Safety of Diagnostic Ultrasound, Laurel, MD: American Institute of Ultrasound in Medicine, 1992.
Statement summarizing bioeffects of ultrasound exposure based on animal studies performed.

Edelman SK. Understanding Ultrasound Physics, 2nd edn. Houston: Armstrong Inc., 1994.
Fundamentals of ultrasound physics with sample questions make this a tool in preparation for ultrasound certifying examinations.

Erbel R, Nesser HJ, Drozdz J. Atlas of Tissue Doppler Echocardiography. New York: Springer Verlag, 1995.
Presentation of the basics of color tissue Doppler and its applications.

Kremkau FW. Diagnostic Ultrasound, 4th edn. Philadelphia: Saunders, 1993.
Covers basic ultrasound principles and physics. Good questions are at the end of each chapter to help prepare for examinations.

Medical Ultrasound Safety. Part 1: bioeffects and biophysics, Part 2: prudent use, Part 3: implementing ALARA. Laurel, MD: American Institute of Ultrasound in Medicine, 1994.
Written particularly for the sonographer.

O'Brien WD. Biological effects of ultrasound: rationale for measurement of selected ultrasonic output quantities. Echocardiography 1986; 3: 165.
Ultrasound energy parameters and why they are used are discussed.

Skorton DJ, Collins SM, Greenleaf JF, *et al.* Ultrasound bioeffects and regulatory issues: an introduction for the echocardiographer. J Am Soc Echocardiogr 1988; 1: 240–251.
Discussion of ultrasound bioeffects, basic concepts, and review of safety standard documents.

Zagzebski JA. Essentials of Ultrasound Physics. St Louis: Mosby, 1996.
An introduction to the physics of ultrasound, and how it affects clinical ultrasonography.

Chapter 3

Cape EG, Yoganathan AP, Weyman AE, Levine RA. Adjacent solid boundaries alter the size of regur-

gitant Doppler color flow maps. J Am Coll Cardiol 1991; 17: 1094–1102.
Theoretical and experimental demonstration of the Coanda effect.

Deng YB, *et al.* Estimation of mitral valve area in patients with mitral stenosis by the flow convergence region method: selection of aliasing velocity. J Am Coll Cardiol 1994; 24: 683–689.
Discussion of practical use of PISA for calculation of the mitral valve area in mitral stenosis.

Levine RA, Jimoh A, Cape EG, McMillan S, Yoganathan AP, Weyman AE. Pressure recovery distal to a stenosis: potential cause of gradient "overestimation" by Doppler echocardiography. J Am Coll Cardiol 1989; 13: 706–715.
Definition of pressure recovery and explanation of its manifestation in clinical echocardiography.

Popp RL, Teplitsky I. Lessons from in vitro models of small, irregular, multiple and tunnel-like stenoses relevant to clinical stenoses of valves and small vessels. J Am Coll Cardiol 1998; 13: 716–722.
Discussion of when the simplified Bernoulli equation may not be valid.

Richards KL. Assessment of aortic and pulmonic stenosis by echocardiography. Circulation 1991; 84(suppl I): I182–I187.
Theory behind the Doppler calculations for quantitation of valvular stenosis.

Simpson IA, Sahn DJ. Quantification of valvular regurgitation by Doppler echocardiography. Circulation 1991; 84(suppl I): I188–I192.
Theory and application of color Doppler for quantitation of valvular regurgitation.

Sitges M, Jones M, Shiota T, *et al.* Interaliasing distance of the flow convergence surface for determining mitral regurgitant volume: a validation study in a chronic animal model. J Am Coll Cardiol 2001; 38: 1195–1202.
Background calculations and description of methodology for using the PISA method and two color aliasing "shells" for determination of mitral regurgitant volume. This is a well-illustrated paper. See also the accompanying editorial by R Hoffmann and P Hanrath, pp 1203–1206.

Stamm RB, Martin RP. Quantification of pressure gradients across stenotic valves by Doppler ultrasound. J Am Coll Cardiol 1983; 2: 707–718.
An early paper describing the method of measurement of pressure gradients across a stenotic aortic or mitral valve.

Thomas JD, Liu CM, Flachskampf FA, *et al.* Quantification of jet flow by momentum analysis: an in vitro color Doppler flow study. Circulation 1990; 81: 247–259.
Mathematics, computer simulation, and in vitro analysis of color jet flow by momentum analysis.

Utsunomiya T, Ogawa T, Doshi R, *et al.* Doppler color flow "proximal isovelocity surface area" method for estimating volume flow rate: effects of orifice shape and machine factors. J Am Coll Cardiol 1991; 17: 1103–1111.
Definition of PISA discussion of its utility through various shaped orifices. Influence of machine settings is also discussed.

Vandervoort PM, Greenberg NL, Pu M, Powell KA, Cosgrove DM, Thomas JD. Pressure recovery in bileaflet heart valve prostheses. Circulation 1995; 92: 3464–3472.
A discussion of pressure recovery and its relationship to single and double disc mechanical prostheses.

Yoganathan AP, Cape EG, Sung HW, *et al.* Review of hydrodynamic principles for the cardiologist: applications to the study of blood flow and jets by imaging techniques. J Am Coll Cardiol 1988; 12: 1344–1353.
This technical article reviews concepts of the physics of blood-flow and derivation of equations (Bernoulli and Continuity equations) used in clinical practice.

Chapter 4

Aepfelbacher FC, Breen P, Manning WJ. Methemoglobinemia and topical pharyngeal anesthesia [correspondence]. N Engl J Med 2003; 348: 85–86.
Two cases of patients developing methemoglobinemia after topical anesthesia in preparation for the TEE procedure. Typical presentation and therapy is discussed.

Agrawal G, LaMotte LC, Nanda NC, Parekh HH. Identification of the aortic arch branches using

transesophageal echocardiography. Echocardiography 1997; 14: 461–466.
This article describes how to find and identify the great vessels as they arise from the aortic arch.

ASE/SCA Guidelines for Performing a Comprehensive Intraoperative Multiplane Transesophageal Echocardiography Examination. Recommendations of the American Society of Echocardiography Council for Intraoperative Echocardiography and the Society of Cardiovascular Anesthesiologists Task Force for Certification in Perioperative Transesophageal Echocardiography. J Am Soc Echocardiogr 1999; 12: 884–900.
Each physician performing TEEs, especially in the OR, should read this manuscript, and have it accessible for reference.

Feigenbaum H. Current status of M-mode echocardiography. ACC Curr J Rev 1994; Jan/Feb: 58–59.
A brief description of the added utility of M-mode echocardiography in light of continuously developing echo imaging and Doppler modalities.

Foster E (guest ed). Transesophageal echocardiography. Cardiol Clin 2000; Nov.
This issue of the Cardiology clinics covers indications and use of TEE.

Gardin JM, Adams DB, Douglas PS, *et al.* Recommendations for a standardized report for adult transthoracic echocardiography: A Report from the American Society of Echocardiography's Nomenclature and Standards Committee and Task Force for a Standardized Echocardiography Report. J Am Soc Echocardiogr 2002; 15: 275–290.
A guideline as to what measurements and what items should be included in an echo report. The entire document may be accessed at the web site of the ASE at www.asecho.org.

Marcella CP, Johnson LE. Right parasternal imaging: an underutilized echocardiographic technique. J Am Soc Echocardiogr 1993; 6: 453.
An illustrated review of use of the right parasternal window.

Novaro GM, Aronow HD, Militello MA, Garcia MJ, Sabik EM. Benzocaine-induced methemoglobinemia: experience from a high-volume transesophageal echocardiography laboratory. J Am Soc Echocardiogr 2003; 16: 170–175.
A review of this potentially life-threatening complication of benzocaine spray. A good flowchart of diagnosis and management is provided on p. 173 of this paper.

Pandian NG, *et al.* Multiplane transesophageal echocardiography: imaging planes, echocardiographic anatomy, and clinical experience with a prototype phased array omniplane probe. Echocardiography 1992; 9: 649.
Images and description of multiplane TEE anatomy.

Report of the American Society of Echocardiography Committee on Nomenclature and Standards in Two-Dimensional Echocardiography. Raleigh, NC: American Society of Echocardiography (ASE).
This publication of the ASE sets the standard for transthoracic imaging.

Reynolds T, Santos T, Weidemann J, Langenfeld K, Warner MG. The evaluation of the abdominal aorta: a "how-to" for cardiac sonographers. J Am Soc Echocardiogr 1990; 3: 336–346.
This is a practical review for the sonographer describing normal and abnormal anatomy, and how to perform an ultrasound examination of the abdominal aorta.

Sahn DJ, DeMaria A, Kisslo J, Weyman A. Recommendations regarding quantitation in M-mode echocardiography: results of a survey of echocardiographic measurements. Circulation 1978; 58: 1072–1083.
This sets the standard for M-mode measurements.

Saphir JR, Cooper JA, Kerbavez RJ, *et al.* Upper airway obstruction after transesophageal echocardiography. J Am Soc Echocardiogr 1997; 10: 977–978.
A rare case of retropharyngeal hematoma development 24 hours after TEE, in a patient on aspirin and therapeutic intravenous heparin.

Tajik AJ, *et al.* Two-dimensional real-time ultrasonic imaging of the heart and great vessels. Mayo Clinic Proc 1978; 53: 271.
A historical description of two-dimensional echocardiography.

Waller BF, Taliercio CP, Slack JD, *et al.* Tomographic views of normal and abnormal hearts: the anatomic basis for various cardiac imaging techniques. Part I. Clin Cardiol 1990; 13: 804–812.

Waller BF, Taliercio CP, Slack JD, *et al.* Tomographic views of normal and abnormal hearts: the anatomic basis for various cardiac imaging techniques. Part II. Clin Cardiol 1990; 13: 877–884.

These two papers present cardiac anatomy in terms of standard imaging planes.

Chapter 5

Alam M, Rosenhamer G. Atrioventricular plane displacement and left ventricular function. J Am Soc Echocardiogr 1992; 5: 427–433.

Displacement of the atrioventricular plane as measured using M-mode echo through the AV plane from an apical window helps characterize systolic function. Although not used in many echo labs, the method of recording and its utility is described.

Aurigemma GP, Gaasch WH, Villegas B, Meyer TE. Noninvasive assessment of left ventricular mass, chamber volume, and contractile function. Curr Prob Cardiol 1995; 20: 361–440.

Coverage of echo-Doppler methods (and nuclear) for quantitation of ventricular systolic function along with volume and mass.

Devereux RB, Wallerson DC, de Simone G, *et al.* Evaluation of left ventricular hypertrophy by m-mode echocardiography in patients and experimental animals. Am J Card Imaging 1994; 8: 291–304.

Methodology for M-mode measurements, including mass, stress, and fractional shortening in humans and animals.

D'hooge J, Heimdal A, Jamal F, *et al.* Regional strain and strain rate measurements by cardiac ultrasound: principles, implementation and limitations. Eur J Echo 2000; 1: 154–170.

A discussion of strain and strain rate measurements in ultrasound.

Heimdal A, Stoylen A, Torp H, Skjaerpe T. Real-time strain rate imaging of the left ventricle by ultrasound. J Am Soc Echocardiogr 1998; 11: 1013–1019.

Description of the strain rate concept and its clinical significance.

King DL, Coffin LEK, Maurer MS. Myocardial contraction fraction: a volumetric index of myocardial shortening by freehand three-dimensional echocardiography. J Am Coll Cardiol 2002; 40: 325–329.

A volumetric (3-dimensional) method of calculating mid-wall shortening, analogous to mid-wall shortening fraction (2-D) is presented. This may be a useful way to assess differences in myocardial performance in patients with hypertrophy of different etiologies (hypertensive hypertrophy vs. physiologic hypertrophy).

Park SH, Shub C, Nobrega TP, Bailey KR, Seward JB. Two-dimensional echocardiographic calculation of left ventricular mass as recommended by the American Society of Echocardiography: correlation with autopsy and M-mode echocardiography. J Am Soc Echocardiogr 1996; 9: 119–128.

Compares methodologies recommended by the ASE and autopsy findings.

Schiller NB. Considerations in the standardization of measurement of left ventricular myocardial mass by two-dimensional echocardiography. Hypertension 1987; 9(suppl II): II33–II35.

The discussion particularly in the image acquisition section provide guidelines for making precise recordings for careful echo measurements.

Schiller NB. Two-dimensional echocardiographic determination of left ventricular volume, systolic function, and mass: summary and discussion of the 1989 recommendations of the American Society of Echocardiography. Circulation 1991; 84(suppl I): I280–I287.

Review of recommendations and practical advice on performance of quantitative studies.

Schiller NB, Shah PM, Crawford M, *et al.* Recommendations for quantitation of the left ventricle by two-dimensional echocardiography. American Society of Echocardiography Committee on Standards, Subcommittee on Quantitation of Two-Dimensional Echocardiograms. J Am Soc Echocardiogr 1989; 2: 358–367.

Establishes guidelines and sets the standard for LV quantitation by two-dimensional imaging methods.

Schiller NB, Skiolkebrand CG, Schiller EJ, *et al.* Canine left ventricular mass estimation by

two-dimensional echocardiography. Circulation 1983; 68: 210–216.
This work helped determine the equations used for mass calculations.

Tavel ME. Clinical Phonocardiography and External Pulse Recording, 4th edn. Chicago: Year Book Medical Publishers, 1985.
This text describes phonocardiography, carotid and jugular pulse tracings, apex cardiography, and M-mode measurement of time intervals in normal and abnormal states.

Tei C, Dujardin KS, Hodge DO, *et al.* Doppler echocardiographic index for assessment of global right ventricular function. J Am Soc Echocardiogr 1996; 9: 838–847.
This paper describes the utility of the Index of Myocardial Performance (IMP) as the best index to categorize patients with normal pulmonary artery pressure and those with primary pulmonary hypertension.

Tei C, Ling LH, Hodge DO, *et al.* New index of combined systolic and diastolic myocardial performance: a simple and reproducible measure of cardiac function—a study in normals and dilated cardiomyopathy. J Cardiol 1995; 26: 357–366.
Description of the IMP to evaluate global ventricular performance.

Tortoledo FA, Quinones MA, Fernandez G, *et al.* Quantitation of left ventricular volumes by two-dimensional echocardiography: a simplified and accurate approach. Circulation 1983; 67: 579–584.
This article describes a method for LV volume determination that is easier to perform in the clinical laboratory.

Chapter 6

Appleton CP, Firstenberg MS, Garcia MJ, Thomas JD. The echo-Doppler evaluation of left ventricular diastolic function: a current perspective. Cardiol Clin 2000; 18: 513–546.
A review of echo-Doppler techniques for practical clinical evaluation of diastolic properties.

Appleton CP, Jensen JL, Hatle LK, Oh JK. Doppler evaluation of left and right ventricular diastolic function: a technical guide for obtaining optimal flow velocity recordings. J Am Soc Echocardiogr 1997; 10: 271–291.
This article describes practical aspects of diastolic evaluation.

Chirillo F, Brunazzi MC, Barbiero M, *et al.* Estimating mean pulmonary wedge pressure in patients with chronic atrial fibrillation from transthoracic Doppler indexes of mitral and pulmonary venous flow velocity. J Am Coll Cardiol 1997; 30: 19–26.
Describes estimation of pulmonary capillary wedge pressure from pulmonary vein recordings.

Cohen GI, Pietrolungo JF, Thomas JD, Klein AL. A practical guide to assessment of ventricular diastolic function using Doppler echocardiography. J Am Coll Cardiol 1996; 27: 1753–1760.
Discussion of mitral/pulmonary vein flow, color M-mode Doppler, and tissue Doppler imaging.

D'Cruz IA, Kleinman D, Aboulata H, Orander P, Hand RC. A reappraisal of the mitral B-bump (B-inflection): its relationship to left ventricular dysfunction. Echocardiography 1990; 7: 69–75.
This study and review describes the M-mode B-bump in detail, along with its clinical utility.

Firstenberg MS, Levine BD, Garcia MJ, *et al.* Relationship of echocardiographic indices to pulmonary capillary wedge pressures in healthy volunteers. J Am Coll Cardiol 2000; 36: 1664–1669.
In patients with normal hearts the E, septal E′, and E divided by the wave propagation velocity correlate with PCWP.

Firstenberg MS, Vandervoort PM, Greenberg NL, *et al.* Noninvasive estimation of transmitral pressure drop across the normal mitral valve in humans: importance of convective and inertial forces during left ventricular filling. J Am Coll Cardiol 2000; 36: 1942–1949. Editorial: Isaaz K. Expanding the frontiers of Doppler echocardiography for the noninvasive assessment of diastolic hemodynamics. J Am Coll Cardiol 2000; 36: 1950–1951.
Color M-mode was used to quantitate inertial forces across the normal mitral valve. These measurements may improve understanding of diastolic filling.

Gaasch WH, LeWinter MM. Left Ventricular Diastolic Dysfunction and Heart Failure. Philadelphia: Lea & Febiger, 1994.

This text provides a discussion of diastole including theory, research, and clinical application.

Garcia MJ, Thomas JD, Klein AL. New Doppler echocardiographic applications for the study of diastolic function. J Am Coll Cardiol 1998; 32: 865–875.

Describes method and practical implementation of tissue Doppler echocardiography and also color M-mode Doppler of LV flow propagation to assess diastolic function.

Hurrell DG, Nishimura RA, Ilstrup DM, Appleton CP. Utility of preload alteration in assessment of left ventricular filling pressure by Doppler echocardiography: a simultaneous catheterization and Doppler echocardiographic study. J Am Coll Cardiol 1997; 30: 459–467.

Changes in preload help with assessment of LV filling pressures.

Nagueh SF, Middleton KJ, Kopelen HA, *et al.* Doppler tissue imaging: a noninvasive technique for evaluation of left ventricular relaxation and estimation of filling pressures. J Am Coll Cardiol 1997; 30: 1527–1533.

Description of the method of tissue Doppler imaging of the mitral annulus to estimate LV filling pressures.

Nishimura RA, *et al.* Assessment of diastolic function of the heart: background and current applications of Doppler echocardiography. Part I. Physiologic and pathophysiologic features. Mayo Clin Proc 1989; 64: 71.

Nishimura RA, *et al.* Assessment of diastolic function of the heart: background and current applications of Doppler echocardiography, Part II. Physiologic and pathophysiologic features. Mayo Clin Proc 1989; 64: 71.

These two reviews by Dr Nishimura provide a concise introduction and give examples of practical application.

Oh JK, Appleton CP, Hatle LK, Nishimura RA, Seward JB, Tajik AJ. The noninvasive assessment of left ventricular diastolic function with two-dimensional and Doppler echocardiography. J Am Soc Echocardiogr 1997; 10: 246–270.

This article along with the Appleton et al article from J Am Soc Echocardiogr 1997 discuss diastolic assessment using mitral and pulmonary vein flow patterns.

Pritchett AM, Jacobsen SJ, Mahoney DW, *et al.* Left atrial volume as an index of left atrial size: a population-based study. J Am Coll Cardiol 2003; 41: 1036–1043.

A simplified method to calculate LA volume is presented. Values for normal and cardiovascular disease are presented. LA volume is most sensitive when normalized to body surface area.

Rakowski H, Appleton C, Chan KL, *et al.* Canadian Consensus Recommendations for the measurement and reporting of diastolic dysfunction by echocardiography. J Am Soc Echocardiogr 1996; 9: 736–760.

Routine assessment of mitral pulmonary vein flow patterns along with integration of this information with the clinical scenario and other echo features are discussed.

Scalia GM, Greenberg NL, McCarthy PM, Thomas JD, Vandervoort PM. Noninvasive assessment of the ventricular relaxation time constant (τ) in humans by Doppler echocardiography. Circulation 1997; 95: 151–155.

Discussion of Doppler methods for estimation of τ.

Sohn DW, Chai IH, Lee DJ, *et al.* Assessment of mitral annulus velocity by Doppler tissue imaging in the evaluation of left ventricular diastolic function. J Am Coll Cardiol 1997; 30: 474–480.

A description of mitral annulus velocity determination with Doppler tissue echocardiography, and its application.

Tenenbaum A, *et al.* Shortened Doppler-derived mitral a wave deceleration time: an important predictor of elevated left ventricular filling pressure. J Am Coll Cardiol 1996; 27: 700–705.

This paper describes use of the mitral A wave deceleration time to help evaluate for an elevated LVEDP.

Thomas JD, Weyman AE. Echocardiographic Doppler evaluation of left ventricular diastolic function: physics and physiology. Circulation 1991; 84: 977–990.

Discussion of factors that affect mitral filling, and computer modeling of such.

Thomas L, Levett K, Boyd A, *et al.* Compensatory changes in atrial volumes with normal aging: is atrial enlargement inevitable? J Am Coll Cardiol 2002; 40: 1630–1635.

Left atrial volume does not change in the normal aging process.

Tsang TSM, Barnes ME, Gersh BJ, *et al.* Left atrial volume as a morphophysiologic expression of left ventricular diastolic dysfunction and relation to cardiovascular risk burden. Am J Cardiol 2002; 90: 1284–1289.

Left atrial volume is indicative of diastolic dysfunction and is reflective of cardiovascular risk.

Tsang TSM, Gersh BJ, Appleton CP, *et al.* Left ventricular diastolic dysfunction as a predictor of the first diagnosed nonvalvular atrial fibrillation in 840 elderly men and women. J Am Coll Cardiol 2002; 40: 1636–1644.

Left atrial volume is predictive of risk for development of atrial fibrillation.

Waggoner AD, Bierig SM. Tissue Doppler imaging: a useful echocardiographic method for the cardiac sonographer to assess systolic and diastolic ventricular function. J Am Soc Echocardiogr 2001; 14: 1143–1152.

A review of how to perform a pulsed wave tissue Doppler examination for assessment of systolic and diastolic function.

Chapter 7

Cannon JD, Zile MR, Crawford FA, Carabello BA. Aortic valve resistance as an adjunct to the Gorlin formula in assessing the severity of aortic stenosis in symptomatic patients. J Am Coll Cardiol 1992; 20: 1517–1523.

Some patients with relatively mild AS may have severe AS by the Continuity equation. Aortic valve resistance with the Gorlin formula helps to differentiate truly severe AS from milder disease.

Fedak PWM, Verma S, David TE, *et al.* Clinical and pathophysiological implications of a bicuspid aortic valve. Circulation 2002; 106: 900–904.

A discussion of the histology, manifestations, complications and therapy of bicuspid aortic valve.

Garcia D, Pibarot P, *et al.* Assessment of aortic valve stenosis severity: a new index based on the energy loss concept. Circulation 2000; 101: 765–771.

For aortic stenosis, presentation of an index to calculate energy loss as potentially better than calculation of the aortic valve area by the Continuity equation.

Hoffmann R, Flachskampf FA, Hanrath P. Planimetry of orifice area in aortic stenosis using multiplane transesophageal echocardiography. J Am Coll Cardiol 1993; 22: 529–534.

TEE is useful and accurate for planimetry of stenotic aortic valves.

Levine RA, Jimoh A, Cape E, McMillan S, Yoganathan A, Weyman A. Pressure recovery distal to a stenosis: potential cause of gradient "overestimation" by Doppler echocardiography. J Am Coll Cardiol 1989; 13: 706.

Discussion of pressure recovery with aortic stenosis and prosthetic aortic valves.

Monin JL, Monchi M, Gest V, *et al.* Aortic stenosis with severe left ventricular dysfunction and low transvalvular pressure gradients. J Am Coll Cardiol 2001; 37: 2101–2107.

In patients with severe aortic stenosis, left ventricular dysfunction and a low transvalvular gradient, contractile reserve (average increase in ejection fraction of ~12%) with dobutamine infusion is associated with a relatively low operative risk. Operative mortality is high in the absence of contractile reserve. The maximal dose used was 20 μg/kg/min or when heart rate acceleration greater than 10 beats/min was reached.

Oh JK, Taliercia CP, Holmes DR, *et al.* Prediction of the severity of aortic stenosis by Doppler aortic valve area determination: prospective Doppler–catheterization correlation in 100 patients. J Am Coll Cardiol 1988; 11: 1227.

Comparison of catheterization and Doppler results for evaluation of aortic stenosis.

Otto CM, *et al.* Determination of the stenotic aortic valve area in adults using Doppler echocardiography. J Am Coll Cardiol 1986; 7: 509.

Utilization of the Continuity equation and Dimensionless Index to calculate the severity of aortic stenosis.

Perry GJ, Helmcke F, Nanda NC, *et al.* Evaluation of aortic insufficiency by color flow mapping. J Am Coll Cardiol 1987; 9: 95.
Original description of color flow Doppler in quantitating aortic regurgitation.

Plotnick GD, White SJ. Shortness of breath and hypotension (echocardiographic quiz). Choices Cardiol 1993; 7: 64.
A clinical example of severe aortic regurgitation.

Shively BK. Transesophageal echocardiographic (TEE) evaluation of the aortic valve, left ventricular outflow tract, and pulmonic valve, in transesophageal echocardiography. Cardiol Clin 2000; 18: 711–729.
Discussion of the role of TEE in evaluation of aortic stenosis and aortic regurgitation.

Timperley J, Milner R, Marshall AJ, Gilbert TJ. Quadricuspid aortic valves. Clin Cardiol 2002; 25: 548–552.
Discussion and illustration of quadricuspid aortic valve.

Chapter 8

Block PC. Who is suitable for percutaneous balloon mitral valvotomy. Int J Cardiol 1988; 20: 9.
Echo clues for successful balloon mitral valvotomy.

Carabello BA. Mitral valve regurgitation. Curr Probl Cardiol 1998; 23: 202–241.
A discussion of mitral regurgitation with a discussion on timing of valve surgery.

Fenster MS, Feldman MD. Mitral regurgitation: an overview. Curr Probl Cardiol 1995; 20: 193–280.
A discussion of the etiology, diagnosis and therapy of MR.

Fontana ME, *et al.* Mitral valve prolapse and the mitral valve prolapse syndrome. Curr Probl Cardiol 1991; 16(5).
A review of the MVP syndrome.

Foster GP, Isselbacher EM, Rose GA, *et al.* Accurate localization of mitral regurgitant defects using multiplane transesophageal echocardiography. Ann Thorac Surg 1998; 65: 1025–1031.
TEE helps to localize mitral regurgitant lesions and helps preoperatively to assess in anticipation of repair.

Grayburn PA, Smith MD, Gurley JC, *et al.* Effect of aortic regurgitation on the assessment of mitral valve orifice area by Doppler pressure half-time in mitral stenosis. Am J Cardiol 1987; 60: 322.
The problem of aortic regurgitation is discussed if one intends to use the pressure half-time method in mitral stenosis.

Hatle L, Brubakk A, Tromsdal A, *et al.* Non-invasive assessment of pressure drop in mitral stenosis by Doppler ultrasound. Br Heart J 1978; 40: 131.
An original paper describing Doppler evaluation of mitral stenosis.

Helmcke F, Nanda NC, Hsiung MC, *et al.* Color Doppler assessment of mitral regurgitation with orthogonal planes. Circulation 1987; 75: 175.
Use of color Doppler for assessment of mitral regurgitation.

Hurst JW. Memories of patients with a giant left atrium. Circulation 2001; 104: 2630–2631.
Discussion of giant left atrium. Dr Hurst's definition of giant left atrium is one that touches the right lateral side of the chest wall by chest X-ray. He noted that the condition is caused by rheumatic mitral valve disease with mitral regurgitation more prominent than mitral stenosis. The chest X-ray often is thought to show right pleural fluid.

Klein AL, *et al.* Effects of mitral regurgitation on pulmonary venous flow and left atrial pressure: an intraoperative transesophageal echocardiographic study. J Am Coll Cardiol 1992; 20: 1345.
The effect of mitral regurgitation on mitral and pulmonary vein Doppler flow patterns.

Kwan J, Shiota T, Agler DA, *et al.* Geometric differences of the mitral apparatus between ischemic and dilated cardiomyopathy with significant mitral regurgitation. Circulation 2003; 107: 1135–1140.
With real-time three-dimensional echocardiography several geometrical differences are noted in patients with functional mitral regurgitation and ischemic vs. dilated cardiomyopathy. With an ischemic cardiomyopathy, tethering of both leaflets on the medial aspect of the mitral valve, but only significant posterior leaflet tethering on the lateral aspect of the mitral valve, is seen. With

a dilated cardiomyopathy significant tethering of both mitral leaflets medially and laterally is noted.

Levine RA, Handschumaacher MD, Sanfilippo AJ, *et al.* Three-dimensional echocardiographic reconstruction of the mitral valve, with implications for the diagnosis of mitral valve prolapse. Circulation 1989; 80: 589.
This article explains that based upon mitral annulus geometry, mitral valve prolapse has been previously overdiagnosed.

Levine RA, *et al.* The relationship of mitral annular shape to the diagnosis of mitral valve prolapse. Circulation 1987; 75: 756–767.
This paper explains how mitral annular geometry has led to overdiagnosis of mitral vale prolapse.

MacIsaac AI, *et al.* Quantification of mitral regurgitation by integrated Doppler backscatter power. J Am Coll Cardiol 1994; 24: 690–695.
Description of a method to use CW Doppler of aortic and mitral flow to estimate mitral regurgitant fraction. The method is difficult and has not been routinely used.

Madu EC, D'Cruz IA. The vital role of papillary muscles in mitral and ventricular function: echocardiographic insights. Clin Cardiol 1997; 20: 93–98.
Illustrated with diagrams, this paper discusses the role of the papillary muscles normally and in various disorders. A review of papillary muscle anatomy and pathologic abnormalities.

Minagoe S, *et al.* Obstruction of inferior vena caval orifice by giant left atrium in patients with mitral stenosis: a Doppler echocardiographic study from the right parasternal approach. Circulation 1992; 86: 214.
A potential cause of right heart failure.

Nakatani S, Masuyama T, Kodama K, *et al.* Value and limitations of Doppler echocardiography in the quantification of stenotic mitral valve area: comparison of the pressure half-time and continuity equation methods. Circulation 1987; 77: 78.
Discussion of both of these methods for calculation of mitral valve area.

Oh JK. Echocardiographic evaluation of morphological and hemodynamic significance of giant left atrium. Circulation 1992; 86: 328–330.
An excellent short editorial about previous descriptions and the definition of giant left atrium.

Pai RG, Bansal RC, Shah PM. Doppler-derived rate of left ventricular pressure rise: its correlation with the postoperative left ventricular function in mitral regurgitation. Circulation 1990; 82: 514–520.
The Doppler derived value of the rate of rise of left ventricular pressure (dp/dt), obtained from the mitral regurgitation profile, along with LV end-systolic dimension are good predictors of postoperative ejection fraction, after mitral valve replacement for chronic, severe mitral regurgitation.

Pearlman AS. Role of echocardiography in the diagnosis and evaluation of severity of mitral and tricuspid stenosis. Circulation 1991; 84(suppl I): I193–I197.
Doppler evaluation of mitral and tricuspid stenosis.

Pearlman AS, Otto CM. Quantification of valvular regurgitation. Echocardiography 1987; 4: 271.
Review of Doppler techniques used to detect and quantify severity of valvular regurgitation.

Plotnick GD. A candidate for mitral balloon valvuloplasty (echocardiographic quiz). Choices Cardiol 1991; 5: 61.
An example of the use of transthoracic and transesophageal echocardiography in a patient with mitral stenosis.

Rifkin RD, Harper K, Tighe D. Comparison of proximal isovelocity surface area method with pressure half-time and planimetry in evaluation of mitral stenosis. J Am Coll Cardiol 1995; 26:458–465.
Explanation of the PISA method for evaluation of mitral stenosis.

Shah PM. Echocardiographic diagnosis of mitral valve prolapse. J Am Soc Echocardiogr 1994; 7: 286.
An excellent discussion of mitral valve prolapse, evaluating both structure and function.

Stewart WJ, Currie PJ, Salcedo EE, *et al.* Evaluation of mitral leaflet motion by echocardiography and jet direction by Doppler color flow mapping to

determine the mechanisms of mitral regurgitation. J Am Coll Cardiol 1992; 15: 1353.
Explains with excellent illustrations how regurgitant jet direction helps determine the etiology of mitral regurgitation.

Vilacosta I, *et al.* Clinical, anatomic, and echocardiographic characteristics of aneurysms of the mitral valve. Am J Cardiol 1999; 84: 110–113.
An illustrated discussion of mitral valve aneurysms.

Wilkens GT, Weyman AE, Abascal VM, *et al.* Percutaneous mitral valvotomy: an analysis of echocardiographic variables related to outcome and the mechanism of dilatation. Br Heart J 1988; 60: 299.
Discussion of percutaneous mitral valvuloplasty and echo features that predict results.

Chapter 9

Appleton CP, Hatle LK, Popp RL. Superior vena cava and hepatic vein Doppler echocardiography in healthy adults. J Am Coll Cardiol 1987; 10: 1032–1039.
Normal PW Doppler flow patterns in the SVC and the hepatic vein.

Bajzer CT, Stewart WJ, Cosgrove DM, *et al.* Tricuspid valve surgery and intraoperative echocardiography: factors affecting survival, clinical outcome, and echocardiographic success. J Am Coll Cardiol 1998; 32: 1023–1031.
The Cleveland Clinic experience with tricuspid valve repair is discussed.

Berger M, Haimowitz A, Van Tosh A, *et al.* Quantitative assessment of pulmonary hypertension in patients with tricuspid regurgitation using continuous wave Doppler ultrasound. J Am Coll Cardiol 1985; 6: 359.
Use of the modified Bernoulli Equation in patients with pulmonary hypertension, especially when greater than 50 mmHg is very accurate.

Daniels SJ, Mintz GS, Kotler MN. Rheumatic tricuspid valve disease: two-dimensional echocardiographic, hemodynamic, and angiographic correlations. Am J Cardiol 1983; 51: 492–496.
A discussion of the echo findings in tricuspid stenosis with several two-dimensional images.

Eichhorn P, Ritter M, Suetsch G, *et al.* Congenital cleft of the anterior tricuspid leaflet with severe tricuspid regurgitation in adults. J Am Coll Cardiol 1992; 20: 1175–1179.
Echocardiographic findings in patients with this disorder and surgical results are discussed.

Kircher BJ, *et al.* Noninvasive estimation of right atrial pressure from the inspiratory collapse of the inferior vena cava. Am J Cardiol 1990; 66: 493.
Discussion of evaluation of the IVC to estimate RA pressure.

McQuillan BM. Picard MH, Leavitt M, Weyman AE. Clinical correlates and reference intervals for pulmonary artery systolic pressure among echocardiographically normal subjects. Circulation 2001; 104: 2797–2802.
Pulmonary artery systolic pressure may be "normal" up to 40 mmHg in older or obese individuals. Use of age and body mass index may be needed to evaluate the patient and determine if the pulmonary artery systolic pressure is "normal."

Nanna M, *et al.* Value of two-dimensional echocardiography in detecting tricuspid stenosis. Circulation 1983; 67: 221.
M-mode and two-dimensional echo findings in four cases of tricuspid stenosis out of 100 patients with rheumatic heart disease.

Parris TM, Panidis IP, Ross J, Mintz GS. Doppler echocardiographic findings in rheumatic tricuspid stenosis. Am J Cardiol 1987; 60: 1414–1416.
Echo and Doppler findings in tricuspid stenosis.

Pearlman AS. Role of echocardiography in the diagnosis and evaluation of severity of mitral and tricuspid stenosis. Circulation 1991; 84(suppl I): I193–I197.
A review of evaluation of mitral and tricuspid stenosis.

Perez JE, Ludbrook PA, Ahumada GG. Usefulness of Doppler echocardiography in detecting tricuspid valve stenosis. Am J Cardiol 1985; 55: 601–603.
One of the earliest examples of the utility of Doppler to characterize tricuspid stenosis.

Raman SV, Sparks EA, Boudoulas H, Wooley CF. Tricuspid valve disease: tricuspid valve complex perspective. Curr Probl Cardiol 2002; 27: 103–142.
The tricuspid valve and classification of its disorders.

Raymond RJ, Hinderliter AL, Willis PW, *et al.* Echocardiographic predictors of adverse outcomes in primary pulmonary hypertension. J Am Coll Cardiol 2002; 39: 1214–1219.
Pericardial effusion, right atrial enlargement and ventricular septal displacement are associated with right heart failure and are predictive of a poor outcome in patients with severe primary pulmonary hypertension (PPH).

Reynolds T, Appleton CP. Doppler flow velocity patterns of the superior vena cava, inferior vena cava, hepatic vein, coronary sinus, and atrial septal defect: a guide for the echocardiographer. J Am Soc Echocardiogr, 1991; 4: 503–512.
Discussion and images of PW Doppler patterns of the SVC, IVC, hepatic vein, coronary sinus, and ASD.

Reynolds T, Szymanski K, Langenfeld K, Appleton CP. Visualization of the hepatic veins: new approaches for the echocardiographer. J Am Soc Echocardiogr 1991; 4: 93–96.
Discussion and illustrations of hepatic vein flow patterns.

Scapellato F, Temporelli PL, Eleuteri E, *et al.* Accurate noninvasive estimation of pulmonary vascular resistance by Doppler echocardiography in patients with chronic heart failure. J Am Coll Cardiol 2001; 37: 1813–1819.
A method to estimate pulmonary vascular resistance is presented.

Stevenson JG. Comparison of several noninvasive methods for estimation of pulmonary artery pressure. J Am Soc Echocardiogr 1989; 2: 157.
A study of several methods used for estimation of pulmonary artery pressures.

Chapter 10

Alan M, Rosman HS, Lakier JB, *et al.* Doppler and echocardiographic features of normal and dysfunctioning bioprosthetic valves. J Am Coll Cardiol 1987; 10: 851–858.
One of the early discussions of normal and abnormal bioprosthetic valves. This paper is well illustrated with echo and Doppler features.

Alton ME, Pasierski TJ, Orsinelli DA, *et al.* Comparison of transthoracic and transesophageal echocardiography in evaluation of 47 Starr–Edwards prosthetic valves. J Am Coll Cardiol 1992; 20: 1503–1511.
TEE is helpful in diagnosis of Starr–Edwards dysfunction.

Back DS. Echocardiographic assessment of stentless aortic bioprosthetic valves. J Am Soc Echocardiogr 2000; 13: 941–948.
Echocardiographic features of stentless aortic bioprostheses.

Barbetseas J, Nagueh SF, Pitsavos C, Toutouzas PK, Quinones MA, Zoghbi WA. Differentiating thrombus from pannus formation in obstructed mechanical prosthetic valves: an evaluation of clinical transthoracic and transesophageal echocardiographic parameters. J Am Coll Cardiol 1998; 32: 1410–1417.
Patient history on presentation along with ultrasound intensity of the obstructing mass may help differentiate pannus from thrombus. Mass size and shape could not differentiate pannus from thrombus.

Connolly HM, *et al.* Doppler hemodynamic profiles of 82 clinically and echocardiographically normal tricuspid valve prostheses. Circulation 1993; 88: 2722.
Review of prosthetic valves in the tricuspid position. Normal ranges for Doppler hemodynamics and emphasis of recording throughout the respiratory cycle is presented.

Kerut EK, Hanawalt C, Everson CT, Frank RA, Giles TD. Left ventricular apex to descending aorta valved conduit: description of transthoracic and transesophageal echocardiographic findings in four cases. Echocardiography 2001; 18: 463–468.
Description of the echocardiographic findings in patients with an LV apex to descending aorta valved conduit. All patients had critical aortic valvular stenosis with a "porcelain" aorta.

Flachskampf FA, O'Shea JP, Griffin BP, *et al.* Patterns of normal transvalvular regurgitation in mechan-

ical valve prostheses. J Am Coll Cardiol 1991; 18: 1493–1498.
Normal Doppler flow patterns in mechanical valves.

Freedberg RS, Kronzon I, Gindea AJ, Culliford AT, Tunick PA. Noninvasive diagnosis of left ventricular outflow tract obstruction caused by a porcine mitral prosthesis. J Am Coll Cardiol 1987; 9: 698–700.
Obstruction of the left ventricular outflow tract may occur as a consequence of a mitral bioprosthesis with a strut obstructing the LVOT.

Gelsomino S, Morocutti G, Frassani R, *et al.* Usefulness of the Cryolife O'Brien stentless suprannular aortic valve to prevent prosthesis-patient mismatch in the small aortic root. J Am Coll Cardiol 2002; 39: 1845.
This stentless aortic valve is placed above the aortic annulus, allowing a larger effective valve to be inserted.

Girard SE, Miller FA, Montgomery S, *et al.* Outcome of reoperation for aortic valve prosthesis-patient mismatch. Am J Cardiol 2001; 87: 111–114.
Discussion of prosthesis–patient mismatch and risk of reoperation.

Glancy DL, O'Brien KP, Reis RL, Epstein SE, Morrow AG. Hemodynamic studies in patients with 2M and 3M Starr–Edwards prostheses: evidence of obstruction to left atrial emptying. Circulation 1969; 14,15(suppl 1): I113–I118.
Relative obstruction in a structurally normal prosthesis has long been recognized as a problem with prosthetic heart valves.

Grigg L, Fulop J, Daniel L, *et al.* Doppler echocardiography assessment of prosthetic heart valves. Echocardiography 1990; 7: 97–114.
Discussion of the value and limitations of transthoracic echocardiography for assessment of prosthetic valves.

Gueret P, Vignon P, Fournier P, *et al.* Transesophageal echocardiography for the diagnosis and management of nonobstructive thrombosis of mechanical mitral valve prosthesis. Circulation 1995; 91: 103–110.
TEE helps identify thrombi on a mitral mechanical prosthesis, and may be helpful in formulating a therapeutic plan.

Harpaz D, Shah P, Bezante G, *et al.* Transthoracic and transesophageal echocardiographic sizing of the aortic annulus to determine prosthesis size. Am J Cardiol 1993; 72: 1411–1417.
Measurement of aortic annulus size appears to be more accurate when measured at end-diastole, as compared to end-systole. Inner-edge to inner-edge measurements were made from the transthoracic (TTE) parasternal long-axis and TEE transverse plane from the lower esophagus by anteflexion of the probe, obtaining a four-chamber view, revealing the left ventricular outflow tract and the aortic valve. Measurements were made at the insertion point of the anterior right coronary cusp on the anterior root to the insertion point of the posterior noncoronary cusp on the posterior root. TTE may be more accurate than TEE when measurements are performed at end-diastole.

Hurrell DG, Schaff HV, Tajik AJ. Thrombolytic therapy for obstruction of mechanical prosthetic valves. Mayo Clin Proc 1996; 71: 605–613.
Review of the literature on use of thrombolysis for obstructed mechanical prosthetic valves. Recommendations for thrombolysis in clinical practice are given.

Lengyel M, Fuster V, Keltai M, *et al.* Guidelines for management of left-sided prosthetic valve thrombosis: a role for thrombolytic therapy. Consensus Conference on Prosthetic Valve Thrombosis. J Am Coll Cardiol 1997; 30: 1521–1526.
TEE helps to visualize abnormal mechanical leaflet motion and characterize thrombus. Recommendations and risks of thrombolysis are discussed.

Mann DL, Gillam LD, Marshall JE, King ME, Weyman AE. Doppler and two-dimensional echocardiographic diagnosis of Bjork–Shiley prosthetic valve malfunction: importance of interventricular septal motion and the timing of onset of valve flow. J Am Coll Cardiol 1986; 8: 971–974.
Description with echo and Doppler features of an intermittently "sticking" single-disc prosthetic valve in the mitral position.

Mehlman DJ. A Pictorial and radiographic guide for identification of prosthetic heart valve devices. Prog Cardiovasc Dis 1988; 6: 441–464.
Appearance and radiographic appearance of prosthetic heart valves.

Montorsi P, Caroretto D, Parolari A, *et al.* Diagnosing prosthetic mitral valve thrombosis and the effect of the type of prosthesis. Am J Cardiol 2002; 90: 73–76.

Prosthetic mechanical valve thrombosis is often associated with normal Doppler gradients, most often occurring with bileaflet (as opposed to single leaflet) valves. Cinefluoroscopy helps to diagnosis a dysfunctional leaflet, demonstrating reduced motion. Although all patients in this study underwent TEE along with surface echocardiography/Doppler, TEE findings were not discussed.

Nihoyannopoulos P, Kambouroglou D, Athanassopoulos G, *et al.* Doppler hemodynamic profiles of clinically and echocardiographically normal mitral and aortic valve prosthesis. Eur Heart J 1992; 13: 348.

Doppler parameters of normally functioning prosthetic valves.

Pibarot P, Dumesnil JG. Hemodynamic and clinical impact of prosthesis–patient mismatch in the aortic valve position and its prevention. J Am Coll Cardiol 2000; 36: 1131–1141.

An explanation of prosthetic valve mismatch and how it occurs in the clinical setting. Suggestions are given to prevent this prior to valve surgery.

Rao V, Jamieson WRE, Ivanov J, *et al.* Prosthesis–patient mismatch affects survival after aortic valve replacement. Circulation 2000; 102(suppl III): III5–III9.

Prosthesis–patient mismatch results in an increased post-operative (early and late) mortality. An effective orifice area/body surface area (EOA/BSA) ratio of $>0.75\ cm^2/m^2$ *may avoid this problem.*

Reisner SA, Meltzer RS. Normal values of prosthetic valve Doppler echocardiographic parameters: a review. J Am Soc Echocardiogr 1988; 1: 201.

A review of 18 prior studies of normally functioning prosthetic valves with tables and figures that can be used for reference.

Rothbart RM, *et al.* Determination of aortic valve area by two-dimensional and Doppler echocardiography in patients with normal and stenotic bioprosthetic valves. J Am Coll Cardiol 1990; 15: 817.

Demonstration that calculation of the effective valve area in stenosed prosthetic aortic valves is accurate.

Sakai K, Nakamura K, Ishizuka N, *et al.* Echocardiographic findings and clinical features of left ventricular pseudoaneurysm after mitral valve replacement. Am Heart J 1992; 124: 975–982.

Echo and Doppler features of LV pseudoaneurysm post mitral valve surgery are discussed.

Shahid M, Sutherland G, Hatle L. Diagnosis of intermittent obstruction of mechanical mitral valve prostheses by Doppler echocardiography. Am J Cardiol 1995; 76: 1305–1309.

Discussion and illustrations of intermittent prosthetic valve obstruction.

Smith MD, Harrison MR, Pinton R, *et al.* Regurgitant jet size by transesophageal compared with transthoracic Doppler color flow imaging. Circulation 1991; 83: 79–86.

The backflow jet area will appear larger by TEE than by TTE imaging.

Staab ME, Nishimura RA, Dearani JA, Orszulak TA. Aortic valve homografts in adults: a clinical perspective. Mayo Clin Proc 1998; 73: 231–238.

A review of indications for use, and complications.

Vongpatanasin W, Hillis LD, Lange RA. Prosthetic heart valves. N Engl J Med 1996; 335: 407–415.

A review of prosthetic heart valves.

Zabalgoitia M, Garcia M. Pitfalls in the echo-Doppler diagnosis of prosthetic valve disorders. Echocardiography 1993; 10: 203.

Emphasis on potential problems encountered when evaluating prosthetic valves for abnormalities.

Chapter 11

Acquatella H, Schiller NB, Puigbo JJ, *et al.* Value of two-dimensional echocardiography in endomyocardial disease with and without eosinophilia. Circulation 1983; 67: 1219–1226.

Description of the two-dimensional echo features of endomyocardial fibrosis.

Bax JJ, Lamb HJ, Poldermans D, *et al.* Noncompaction cardiomyopathy—echocardiographic diagnosis. Eur J Echocardiogr 1992; 3; 301–302.

Case presentation and discussion of noncompaction of the left ventricle.

Burke AP, Farb A, Taashko G, Virmani R. Arrhythmogenic right ventricular cardiomyopathy and fatty replacement of the right ventricular myocardium: are they different diseases? Circulation 1998; 97: 1571–1580.
Iillustrated with pathologic specimens, this paper discusses the histologic findings and differentiation of both arrhythmogenic RV cardiomyopathy and fatty replacement of the RV myocardium.

Claessens PJM, Claessens CWF, Claessens MMM, *et al.* Supernormal left ventricular diastolic function in triathletes. Texas Heart Inst J 2001; 28: 102–110.
Findings of LV mass and dimensions with comparison of diastolic features in elite triathletes.

D'Cruz IA, Rouse CC. The hypertrophied ventricular septum: anatomic variants and their echocardiographic diagnosis. J Noninvasive Cardiol 1997; Summer: 9–15.
Ventricular septum anatomy, its appearance with "benign" variations and variations of hypertrophic cardiomyopathy, are illustrated and discussed.

Fontaine G, Fontaliran F, Frank R. Arrhythmogenic right ventricular cardiomyopathies: clinical forms and main differential diagnoses. Circulation 1998; 97: 1532–1535.
An editorial discussing the differential diagnosis of this disorder compared to other diagnoses that may be confused with it.

Flores-Ramirez R, Lakkis NM, Middleton KJ, *et al.* Echocardiographic insights into the mechanisms of relief of left ventricular outflow tract obstruction after nonsurgical septal reduction therapy in patients with hypertrophic obstructive cardiomyopathy. J Am Coll Cardiol 2001; 37: 208–214.
Altered LV ejection dynamics and basal septal function cause acute changes in the LVOT gradient after nonsurgical septal reduction therapy (alcohol injection into the first major septal coronary artery). Long-term improvement occurs secondary to LVOT remodeling and a change in LV ejection.

Gemayel C, Pelliccia A, Thompson PD. Arrhythmogenic right ventricular cardiomyopathy. J Am Coll Cardiol 2001; 38: 1773–1781.
A review of the etiology, clinical presentation, diagnosis, and management of arrhythmogenic RV dysplasia. Echo features of diagnosis are discussed.

Giannuzzi P, Temporelli PL, Bosimini E, *et al.* Independent and incremental prognostic value of Doppler-derived mitral deceleration time of early filling in both symptomatic and asymptomatic patients with left ventricular dysfunction. J Am Coll Cardiol 1996; 28: 383–390.
In patients with an LV EF ≤35%, whether or not having a history of heart failure, a shortened mitral E deceleration time (≤125 ms) is predictive of hospitalization for heart failure and mortality.

Giles TD, Kerut EK. Restrictive and obliterative cardiomyopathy. In: Parmley WW, Chatterjee K, eds. Cardiology. New York: Lippincott-Raven, ch 49.
This book chapter reviews restrictive and obliterative cardiomyopathy and discusses echo and pulsed wave Doppler findings.

Gottdiener JS, Maron BJ, Schooley RT, *et al.* Two dimensional echocardiographic assessment of the idiopathic hypereosinophilia syndrome. Circulation 1983; 67: 572.
Echo features of hypereosinophilia syndrome are discussed.

Hansen A, Haass M, Zugck C, *et al.* Prognostic value of Doppler echocardiographic mitral inflow patterns: implications for risk stratification in patients with chronic congestive heart failure. J Am Coll Cardiol 2001; 37: 1049–1055.
Mitral Doppler inflow patterns help determine prognosis in patients with heart failure and LV systolic dysfunction.

Harrison MR, Grigsby CG, Souther Sk, Smith MD, DeMaria AN. Midventricular obstruction associated with chronic systemic hypertension and severe left ventricular hypertrophy. Am J Cardiol 1991; 68: 761–765.
Description of imaging, color, pulsed wave and continuous wave Doppler features of LV cavity obliteration.

Henry WL, Clark CE, Epstein SE. Asymmetric septal hypertrophy (ASH): echocardiographic

identification of the pathognomonic anatomic abnormality of IHSS. Circulation 1973; 47: 225.
A historical paper by the NIH group.

Kaul S, Pearlman JD, Touchstone DA, Esquival L. Prevalence and mechanisms of mitral regurgitaiton in the absence of intrinsic abnormalities of the mitral leaflets. Am Heart J 1989; 118: 963–972.
One of the first descriptions of functional mitral regurgitation in patients with heart failure.

Keren G, Belhassen B, Sherez J, *et al.* Apical hypertrophic cardiomyopathy: evaluation by noninvasive and invasive techniques in 23 patients. Circulation 1985; 71: 45–56.
Catheterization, EKG, and echo findings of apical hypertrophy.

Klein AL, Hatle LK, Taliercio CP, *et al.* Prognostic significance of Doppler measures of diastolic function in cardiac amyloidosis: a Doppler echocardiography study. Circulation 1991; 83: 808–816.
Comparison of LV wall thickness and diastolic filling parameters with its prognostic value.

Klein AL, *et al.* Two-dimensional and Doppler echocardiographic assessment of infiltrative cardiomyopathy. J Am Soc Echocardiogr 1988; 1: 48.
Discussion and illustration of amyloid, hemochromatosis, sarcoid and glycogen storage disease.

Klues HG, Roberts WC, Maron BJ. Anomalous insertion of papillary muscle directly into anterior mitral leaflet in hypertrophic cardiomyopathy. Circulation 1991; 84: 1188–1197.
Approximately 10–15% of patients with hypertrophic cardiomyopathy have anomalous insertion of one or both left ventricular papillary muscles directly into the anterior mitral leaflet. By echo, a direct continuity between the papillary muscle and mitral leaflet, resulting in a long rigid area of midcavity narrowing, appeared to be responsible for outflow obstruction.

Klues HG, Schiffers A, Maron BJ. Phenotypic spectrum and patterns of left ventricular hypertrophy in hypertrophic cardiomyopathy: morphologic observations and significance as assessed by two-dimensional echocardiography in 600 patients. J Am Coll Cardiol 1995; 26: 1699–1708.
A discussion of the heterogeneity of hypertrophic cardiomyopathy.

Kullo IJ, Edwards WD, Seward JB. Right ventricular dysplasia: the Mayo Clinic Experience. Mayo Clin Proc 1995; 70: 541–548.
Discussion of the clinical presentation of RV dysplasia and also several echo images.

Lapu-Bula R, Robert A, Craeynest DV, *et al.* Contribution of exercise-induced mitral regurgitation to exercise stroke volume and exercise capacity in patients with left ventricular systolic dysfunction. Circulation 2002; 106: 1342–1348.
MR associated with a dilated cardiomyopathy is secondary to relative apical displacement of papillary muscles, and apical displacement of mitral leaflet coaptation, reducing the contact between the two leaflets and compromising valvular competence. Exercise bicycle stress testing with color Doppler identifies patients with marked increases in MR with exercise. Exercise tolerance seems to be related to the degree of exercise-associated MR.

Lebrun F, Lancellotti P, Pierard LA. Quantitation of functional mitral regurgitation during bicycle exercise in patients with heart failure. J Am Coll Cardiol 2001; 38: 1685–1692.
An exercise associated increase in MR appears to be associated with exercise-limiting dyspnea, and also an exercise-associated elevation in pulmonary artery pressure.

Lewis JF, Maron BJ. Elderly patients with hypertrophic cardiomyopathy: a subset with distinctive left ventricular morphology and progressive clinical course late in life. J Am Coll Cardiol 1989; 13: 36–45.
Elderly patients with obstructive hypertrophic cardiomyopathy are described as having relatively small hearts with only modest hypertrophy. LV geometry is distorted with exaggerated anterior displacement of the mitral valve. Heavy calcium is also described between the posterior mitral leaflet and LV free wall endocardium.

Louie EK, Maron BJ. Apical hypertrophic cardiomyopathy: clinical and two-dimensional echocardiographic assessment. Ann Intern Med 1987; 196: 663–670.
ECG and echo findings in apical LV hypertrophy.

McKenna WJ, Thiene G, Nava A, *et al.* Diagnosis of arrhythmogenic right ventricular dysplasia/cardiomyopathy: Task Force of the Working Group Myocardial and Pericardial Disease of the European Society of Cardiology and of the Scientific Council on Cardiomyopathies of the International Society and Federation of Cardiology. Br Heart J 1994; 71: 215–218.
Criteria for diagnosis of right ventricular dysplasia modeled after the "Jones criteria" are presented.

Maron BJ (guest ed). The athlete's heart. Cardiol Clin 1992; May.
Most aspects of athlete's heart are covered in detail.

Maron BJ, Spirito P. Implications of left ventricular remodeling in hypertrophic cardiomyopathy. Am J Cardiol 1998; 81: 1339–1344.
LV remodeling in hypertrophic cardiomyopathy appears to be different at different phases of life. In childhood, marked wall thickening with a small increase in cavity size and clinical stability is typical. In the adult, marked LV wall thinning with a large increase in cavity size and systolic dysfunction with clinical deterioration occurs. Throughout life it appears that mild/gradual wall thinning with a small change in LV cavity size is found.

Maron BJ, Gottdiener JS, Arce J, *et al.* Dynamic sybaortic obstruction in hypertrophic cardiomyopathy: analysis by pulsed Doppler echocardiography. J Am Coll Cardiol 1985; 6: 1–15.
Hemodynamic findings in obstructive and nonobstructive hypertrophic cardiomyopathy.

Maron BJ, Pelliccia A, Spirito P. Cardiac disease in young trained athletes. Circulation 1995; 91: 1596–1601.
Differentiation of athlete heart from that of hypertrophic cardiomyopathy is presented.

Maron BJ, Spirito P, *et al.* Unusual distribution of left ventricular hypertrophy in obstructive hypertrophic cardiomyopathy: localized posterobasal free wall thickening in two patients. J Am Coll Cardiol 1985; 5: 1474–1477.
Illustrations and discussion of two patients with LV wall thickening confined to the posterobasal LV segment with dynamic LVOT obstruction.

Menapace FJ, Hammer WJ, Ritzer TF, *et al.* Left ventricular size in competitive weight lifters: an echocardiographic study. Med Sci Sports Exerc 1983; 14: 72–75.
The diastolic septal to end-systolic LV internal dimension ratio helps to differentiate HCM from athlete heart.

Movsowitz HD, *et al.* Pitfalls in the echo-Doppler diagnosis of hypertrophic cardiomyopathy. Echocardiography 1993; 10: 167.
Doppler findings along with other conditions that may mimic hypertrophic cardiomyopathy.

Oechslin EN, *et al.* Long-term follow-up of 34 adults with isolated left ventricular noncompaction: a distinct cardiomyopathy with poor prognosis. J Am Coll Cardiol 2000; 36: 493–500.
This uncommon disorder is presented in detail.

Ommen SR, Seward JB, Tajik AJ. Clinical and echocardiographic features of hypereosinophilic syndromes. Am J Cardiol 2000; 86: 110–113.
Idiopathic hypereosinophilic syndrome is a heterogeneous group of disorders characterized by eosinophil overproduction., Approximately 40–50% have cardiac involvement.

Passen EL, Rodriguez ER, Neumann A, *et al.* Cardiac hemochromatosis. Circulation 1996; 94: 2302–2303.
Discussion and echo images of a patient with cardiac hemochromatosis.

Pelliccia A, Maron BJ, Spataro A, Proschan MA, Spirito P. The upper limit of physiologic cardiac hypertrophy in highly trained elite athletes. N Engl J Med 1991; 324: 295–301.
A comparison of patterns of LV hypertrophy in various types of athletes and those with a primary hypertrophic cardiomyopathy.

Rakowski H, *et al.* Echocardiographic and Doppler assessment of hypertrophic cardiomyopathy. J Am Soc Echocardiogr 1988; 1: 31.
Discussion and illustrations of hypertrophic cardiomyopathy.

Sakamoto T, Tei C, Murayama M, *et al.* Giant T wave inversion as a manifestation of asymmetrical apical hypertrophy (AAH) of the left ventricle. Echocardiographic and ultrasonocardiotomographic study. Jap Heart J 1976; 17: 611.

The original description of LV apical hypertrophy was found in a Japanese cohort.

Sasson Z, Yock PG, Hatle LK, Alderman EL, Popp RL. Doppler echocardiographic determination of the pressure gradient in hypertrophic cardiomyopathy. J Am Coll Cardiol 1988; 11: 752–756.

Dynamic LV outflow obstruction characterized by continuous wave Doppler.

Schwengel RH, Hawke MW, Gottlieb SS, Fisher ML, Plotnick GD. Abnormal Valsalva blood pressure response in dilated cardiomyopathy—association with pseudonormalized Doppler transmitral filling velocity pattern. Am Heart J 1993; 126: 1182.

Clinical and Doppler tools to risk stratify patients with dilated cardiomyopathy.

Sheikhzadeh A, Eslami B, Stierle U, *et al.* Midventricular obstruction—a form of hypertrophic obstructive cardiomyopathy—and systolic anterior motion of the mitral valve. Clin Cardiol 1986; 9: 607–613.

Description of midventricular hypertrophy and dynamic obstruction in nine patients. Only one manifested SAM.

Shindo T, Kurihara H, Ohishi N, *et al.* Cardiac sarcoidosis. Circulation 1998; 97: 1306–1307.

Discussion and echocardiographic images of a patient with cardiac sarcoidosis.

Symposium: dilated and amyloid cardiomyopathy. Echocardiography 1991; 8: 137.

A collection of papers covering many facets of dilated and restrictive cardiomyopathy.

Temporelli PL, Corra U, Imparato A, *et al.* Reversible restrictive left ventricular diastolic filling with optimized oral therapy predicts a more favorable prognosis in patients with chronic heart failure. J Am Coll Cardiol 1998; 31: 1591–1597.

In patients with a history of heart failure and EF <35%, prolongation of a short mitral E deceleration time (DT) with optimal oral therapies is associated with an improved prognosis compared to those patients whose DT remains shortened.

Waller BF. Pathology of the cardiomyopathies. J Am Soc Echocardiogr 1988; 1: 1.

The first paper in the first issue of the Journal of the American Society of Echocardiography (J Am Soc Echocardiogr). It is an illustrated discussion of the pathology of the cardiomyopathies.

Webb JG, Sasson Z, Rakowski H, *et al.* Apical hypertrophic cardiomyopathy: clinical follow-up and diagnostic correlates. J Am Coll Cardiol 1990; 15: 83.

The 7-year clinical course of 26 patients with apical hypertrophic cardiomyopathy.

Whalley GA, Doughty RN, Gamble GD, *et al.* Pseudonormal mitral filling pattern predicts hospital re-admission in patients with congestive heart failure. J Am Coll Cardiol 2002; 39: 1787–1795.

Patients with clinical heart failure were evaluated. Over 90% had an EF <50%. A pseudonormal mitral pattern prior to discharge was predictive of readmission within 1 year.

Wigle ED, Rakowski H, Kimball BP, Williams WG. Hypertrophic cardiomyopathy: clinical spectrum and treatment. Circulation 1995; 92: 1680–1692.

Definition, pathology, clinical spectrum, and therapy of hypertrophic cardiomyopathy are discussed.

World Health Organization/International Society and Federation of Cardiology. Report of the 1995 World Health Organization/International Society and Federation of Cardiology Task Force on the Definition and Classification of Cardiomyopathies. Circulation 1996; 93: 841.

Classification of cardiomyopathy by the World Health Organization.

Xie G, Smith MD. Pseudonormal or intermediate pattern? J Am Coll Cardiol 2002; 39: 1796–1798.

An editorial describing how Doppler patterns may help therapy and be predictive in patients with LV dysfunction and heart failure.

Xie G, Berk MR, Smith MD. Prognostic value of Doppler transmitral flow patterns in patients with congestive heart failure. J Am Coll Cardiol 1994; 24: 132–139.

A mitral restrictive pattern in patients with heart failure and LV EF <40% is associated with an increased mortality.

Chapter 12

Appleton CP, Hatle LK, Popp RL. Cardiac tamponade and pericardial effusion: respiratory variation in transvalvular flow velocities studied by Doppler echocardiography. J Am Coll Cardiol 1988; 11: 1020.
Doppler clues to pericardial tamponade.

Bansal RC, Chandrasekaran K. Role of echocardiography and Doppler techniques in the evaluation of pericardial diseases. Echocardiogrpahy 1989; 6: 293.
The differential diagnosis of various pericardial disorders, with discussion of hepatic vein hemodynamics.

Chuttani K, Pandian NG, Mohanty PK, *et al.* Left ventricular diastolic collapse: an echocardiographic sign of regional cardiac tamponade. Circulation 1991; 83: 1991.
An important clue in those with loculated postoperative effusions is presented.

D'Cruz IA, Constantine A. Problems and pitfalls in the echocardiographic assessment of pericardial effusion. Echocardiography 1993; 10: 151.
A review covering the differential of pericardial and pleural effusions, along with echo signs of tamponade.

D'Cruz IA, Kanuru N. Echocardiography of serous effusions adjacent to the heart. Echocardiography 2001; 18: 445–456.
Discussion and photos of pericardial (circumferential and localized) effusions, pleural effusions, and ascites

Di Segni E, Feinberg MS, Sheinowitz M, *et al.* Left ventricular pseudohypertrophy in cardiac tamponade: an echocardiographic study in a canine model. J Am Coll Cardiol 1993; 21: 1286–1294.
Pseudohypertrophy of the LV is often noted in cardiac tamponade.

Engel PJ, Fowler NO, Tei C, *et al.* M-mode echocardiography in constrictive pericarditis. J Am Coll Cardiol 1985; 6: 471–474.
One of the early descriptions of multiple M-mode findings in constrictive pericarditis.

Garcia MJ, Rodriguez L, Ares M, *et al.* Differentiation of constrictive pericarditis from restrictive cardiomyopathy: assessment of left ventricular diastolic velocities in longitudinal axis by dopler tissue imaging. J Am Coll Cardiol 1996; 27: 108–114.
Doppler tissue imaging from the apex of the lateral mitral annulus revealed that the early diastolic velocity was higher in normal volunteers and constriction ~14.5 +4.5 cm/s than those with restriction 5.1 +1.4 cm/s.

Gillam LD, Guyer DE, Gibson TC, *et al.* Hydrodynamic compression of the right atrium: a new echocardiographic sign of cardiac tamponade. Circulation 1983; 68: 294–301.
Description of RA collapse as a sign of cardiac tamponade.

Ha JW, Oh JK, Ommen SR, Ling LH, Tajik AJ. Diagnostic value of mitral annular velocity for constrictive pericarditis in the absence of respiratory variation in mitral inflow velocity. J Am Soc Echocardiogr 2002; 15: 1468–1471.
Discussion of tissue Doppler imaging of the mitral annulus to help identify patients with constrictive pericarditis, even if there is no identifiable mitral inflow respiratory variation.

Himelman RB, Kircher B, Rockey DC, Schiller NB. Inferior vena cava plethora with blunted respiratory response: a sensitive echocardiographic sign of cardiac tamponade. J Am Coll Cardiol 1988; 12: 1470–1477.
Original description of IVC plethora as a useful sign of cardiac tamponade.

Hoit B, Sahn DJ, Shabetai R. Doppler-detected paradoxus of mitral and tricuspid valve flows in chronic lung disease. J Am Coll Cardiol 1986; 8: 706–709.
Respiratory variation in mitral and tricuspid Doppler flow secondary to lung disease is described.

Klodas E, Nishimura RA, Appleton CP, Redfield MM, Oh JK. Doppler evaluation of patients with constrictive pericarditis: use of tricuspid regurgitation velocity curves to determine enhanced ventricular interaction. J Am Coll Cardiol 1996; 28: 652–657.
Respiratory changes in the CW tricuspid regurgitant jet in constrictive pericarditis is presented.

Ling LH, *et al.* Pericardial thickness measured with transesophageal echocardiography: feasibility and potential clinical usefulness. J Am Coll Cardiol 1997; 29: 1317.

Describes and illustrates accurate measurement of pericardial thickness using TEE.

Oh JK, *et al.* Preload reduction to unmask the characteristic Doppler features of constrictive pericarditis: a new observation. Circulation 1997; 95: 796.

Reducing preload with head-up tilt or sitting unmasked respiratory variation in patients with markedly elevated LV preload and little respiratory variation.

Oh JK, Hatle LK, Seward JB, *et al.* Diagnostic role of Doppler echocardiography in constrictive pericarditis. J Am Coll Cardiol 1994; 23: 154–162.

Doppler features of pericardial constriction, along with a comparison with restrictive cardiomyopathy.

Sharma S, Maron BJ, Whyte G, *et al.* Physiologic limits of left ventricular hypertrophy in elite junior athletes: relevance to differential diagnosis of athlete's heart and hypertrophic cardiomyopathy. J Am Coll Cardiol 2002; 40: 1431–1436.

Trained adolescent athletes rarely will have a left ventricular wall thickness (LVWT) >12 mm, and then always with chamber enlargement. Hypertrophic cardiomyopathy should be considered in a trained adolescent male athlete with an LVWT >12 mm (females >11 mm) and a nondilated LV.

Tsang TSM, Enriquez-Sarano M, Freeman WK, *et al.* Consecutive 1127 therapeutic echocardiographically guided pericardiocenteses: clinical profile, practice patterns, and outcomes spanning 21 years. Mayo Clin Proc 2002; 77: 429–436.

Echo-guided pericardiocentesis has been performed routinely for years at the Mayo Clinics. Cardiothoracic surgery has replaced malignancy as the leading cause of pericardial effusion requiring pericardiocentesis. This along with malignancy and perforation from catheter-based procedures accounted for ~70% of all pericardiocenteses. The success rate was 97% with 1.2% major (14 total—death (1), chamber lacerations requiring surgery (5), intercostals vessel injury (1), pneumothorax requiring a chest tube (5), ventricular tachycardia (1), bacteremia (1) possibly related to pericardial catheter placement) and 3.5% minor complications noted. Presently, 75% of cases require a pericardial drainage catheter left in place for a period of time.

Chapter 13

Buda AJ. The role of echocardiography in the evaluation of mechanical complications of acute myocardial infarction. Circulation 1991; 84(suppl I): I109–I121.

Mechanical complications of myocardial infarction (papillary muscle rupture, myocardial rupture, ventricular septal defect) are illustrated and discussed.

Cerqueira MD, Weissman NJ, Dilsizian V, *et al.* Standardized myocardial segmentation and nomenclature for tomographic imaging of the heart. Circulation 2002; 105: 539–549.

Standardized description of myocardial segments for imaging . . . MRI, CT, PET, coronary arteriography, nuclear cardiology, and echocardiography.

Gaither NS, Roagan KM Stajduhar K, *et al.* Anomalous origin and course of coronary arteries in adults: identification and improved imaging utilizing transesophageal echocardiography. Am Heart J 1991; 122: 69–75.

TEE is a good tool to help identify anomalous proximal coronary arteries.

Gibson RS, Bishop HL, Stamm RB, *et al.* Value of early two dimensional echocardiography in patients with acute myocardial infarction. Am J Cardiol 1982; 1: 49: 1110–1118.

It has been long recognized that echocardiography not only helps in prognostication in acute myocardial infarction, but also in patient management.

Hoffmann R, Altiok E, Nowak B, *et al.* Strain rate measurement by Doppler echocardiography allows improved assessment of myocardial viability in patients with depressed left ventricular function. J Am Coll Cardiol 2002; 39: 443–449.

Strain rate imaging with low dose dobutamine appears to be better than two-dimensional dobutamine stress echocardiography and also tissue Doppler imaging with dobutamine.

Moore CA, Nygaard TW, Kaiser DL, *et al.* Postinfarction ventricular septal rupture: the importance of

location of infarction and right ventricular function in determining survival. Circulation 1986; 74: 45.
In patients with ventricular septal rupture and RV dysfunction, survival is diminished.

Moursi MH, Bhatnagar SK, Vilacosta I, *et al.* Transesophageal echocardiographic assessment of papillary muscle rupture. Circulation 1996; 94: 1003–1009.
Discussion and images of TEE evaluation of ruptured papillary muscle.

Oh JK, Miller FA, Shub C, *et al.* Evaluation of acute chest pain syndromes by two-dimensional echocardiography: its potential application in the selection of patients for acute reperfusion therapy. Mayo Clin Proc 1987; 62: 59–66.
Echocardiography has long been known to be helpful in evaluation of patients with acute chest pain syndromes.

Raisinghani A, Mahmud E, Sadeghi M, *et al.* Paradoxical inferior-posterior wall systolic expansion in patients with end-stage liver disease. Am J Cardiol 2002; 89: 626–629.
An observation of abnormal LV inferior wall motion secondary to external compression of those segments from an elevated diaphragm in patients with increased intra-abdominal pressures.

Raitt MH, Kraft CD, Gardner CJ, Pearlman AS, Otto CM. Subacute ventricular free wall rupture complicating myocardial infarction. Am Heart J 1993; 126: 946–955.
Four case reports of subacute LV free wall rupture, and review of the literature with discussion.

Roelandt JRTC, Sutherland GR, Yoshida K, Yoshikawa J. Improved diagnosis and characterization of left ventricular pseudoaneurysm by Doppler color flow imaging. J Am Coll Cardiol 1988; 12: 807–811.
Doppler features of pseudoaneurysm are illustrated.

Samdarshi TE, Nanda NC, Gatewood RP, *et al.* Usefulness and limitations of transesophageal echocardiography in the assessment of proximal coronary artery stenosis. J Am Coll Cardiol 1992; 19: 572–580.
Visualization of the proximal coronary arteries and identification of proximal stenosis.

Shiina A, Tajik Aj, Smith HC, *et al.* Prognostic significance of regional wall motion abnormality in patients with prior myocardial infarction: a prospective correlative study of two-dimensional echocardiography and angiography. Mayo Clin Proc 1986; 61: 254–262.
The wall motion score index (WMSI) is a good prognosticator after myocardial infarction.

Smyllie JH, Sutherland GR, Geuskens R, *et al.* Doppler color flow mapping in the diagnosis of ventricular septal rupture and acute mitral regurgitation after myocardial infarction. J Am Coll Cardiol 1990; 15: 1449–1455.
Echocardiography and color Doppler are excellent to differentiate and diagnose ventricular septal rupture and acute mitral regurgitation in the postinfarction patient with a new systolic murmur.

Waller BF. Anatomy, histology, and pathology of the major epicardial coronary arteries relevant to echocardiographic imaging techniques. J Am Soc Echocardiogr 1989; 2: 232–252.
Illustrated discussion of coronary anatomy relevant to the echocardiographer.

Waller BF, Orr CM, Slack JD, *et al.* Anatomy, histology, and pathology of coronary arteries: a review relevant to new interventional and imaging techniques—Part I. Clin Cardiol 1992; 15: 451–457.
Anatomic diagrams of coronary anatomy as it relates to imaging tools available.

Weyman AE, Peskoe SM, Williams ES, *et al.* Detection of left ventricular aneurysm by cross-sectional echocardiography. Circulation 1976; 54: 936.
An original description of echocardiographic diagnosis of LV aneurysm.

Chapter 14

Berenfield A, Barraud P, Lusson JR, *et al.* Traumatic aortic ruptures diagnosed by transesophageal echocardiography. J Am Soc Echocardiogr 1996; 9: 657–662.
TEE is helpful for rapid diagnosis of aortic trauma. Periaortic hematoma diagnosis may be difficult. Part of the ascending aorta, the innominate artery, proximal left carotid artery, and the abdominal aorta are not visualized by TEE, a potential site of trauma.

Bortolotti U, Scioti G, Milano A, *et al.* Post-traumatic tricuspid valve insufficiency. Texas Heart Inst J 1997; 24: 223–225.

Illustrations and discussion of tricuspid valve abnormalities after blunt trauma.

Brooks SW, Young JC, Cmolik B, *et al.* The use of transesophageal echocardiography in the evaluation of chest trauma. J Trauma 1992; 32: 761–766.

TEE is helpful in identifying aortic trauma in patients with blunt chest trauma.

Heidenreich PA. Transesophageal echocardiography (TEE) in the critical care patient, in transesophageal echocardiography (Elyse Foster, guest editor). Cardiol Clin 2000; 18: 789–805.

Indications for TEE and findings in the critical care setting.

Heidenreich PA, Stainback RF, Redberg RF, *et al.* Transesophageal echocardiography predicts mortality in critically ill patients with unexplained hypotension. J Am Coll Cardiol 1995; 26: 152–158.

TEE contributes to diagnosis and management of unexplained hypotension and is predictive of prognosis in the critically ill patient.

Herregods MC, Timmermans C, Frans E, *et al.* Diagnostic value of transesophageal echocardiography in platypnea. J Am Soc Echocardiogr 1993; 6: 624–627.

Case presentation of use of TEE to diagnose this syndrome.

Konstantinides S, Geibel A, Kasper W, *et al.* Patent foramen ovale is an important predictor of adverse outcome in patients with major pulmonary embolism. Circulation 1998; 97: 1946–1951.

With major pulmonary embolism, echo detection of a patent foramen ovale is associated with a high risk of death and paradoxical arterial embolism.

Le Bret F, Ruel P, Rosier H, *et al.* Diagnosis of traumatic mediastinal hematoma with transesophageal echocardiography. Chest 1994; 105: 373–376.

TEE is useful for identification of mediastinal hematoma, but CT appears to be a noninvasive "gold standard."

Pearson AC, Castello R, Labovitz AJ. Safety and utility of transesophageal echocardiography in the critically ill patient. Am Heart J. 1990; 119: 1083.

TEE is safe in the critically ill patient.

Plotnick GD, Hamilton S, Lee YC. The cardiologist and the trauma patient: non-invasive testing. Sem Thorac Cardiovas Surg 1992; 4: 168.

Use and limitations of laboratory and imaging modalities in patients with possible cardiac trauma.

Pretre R, Chilcott M. Blunt trauma to the heart and great vessels. N Engl J Med 1997; 336: 626–632.

A review of mechanism of injury, diagnosis, and management.

Seward JB, Hayes DL, Smith HC, *et al.* Platypnea-orthodeoxia: clinical profile, diagnostic workup, management, and report of seven cases. Mayo Clin Proc 1984; 59: 221–231.

Discussion of etiology and diagnosis of this disorder.

Sohn DW, Shin GJ, Oh JK, *et al.* Role of transesophageal echocardiography in hemodynamically unstable patients. Mayo Clinic Proc 1995; 70: 925–931.

TEE is safe in hemodynamically unstable patients, and provides a high diagnostic yield with information that affects therapy.

Vignon P, Land RM. Use of transesophageal echocardiography for the assessment of traumatic aortic injuries. Echocardiography 1999; 16: 207–219.

TEE is a useful tool for initial assessment of patients at high risk for trauma of the thoracic aorta or its branches. Echocardiographic features and findings are discussed in detail.

Vignon P, Gueret P, Vedrinne JM, *et al.* Role of transesophageal echocardiography in the diagnosis and management of traumatic aortic disruption. Circulation 1995; 92: 2959–2968.

TEE is very helpful in evaluation of the trauma patient with suspected injury of the thoracic aorta.

Chapter 15

Agricola E, Oppizzi M, De Bonis M, *et al.* Multiplane transesophageal echocardiography performed according to the guidelines of the American Society of Echocardiography in patients with mitral valve prolapse, flail, and endocarditis: diagnostic accuracy in the identification of mitral regurgitant defects by correlation with surgical findings. J Am Soc Echocardiogr 2003; 16: 61–66.

By following ASE guidelines for TEE imaging of the mitral valve, using four midesophageal and two transgastric views, the correct section of the anterior mitral leaflet, and correct posterior scallop was identified over 96% of the time.

Chopdra HK, Nanda NC, Fan P, *et al.* Can two-dimensional echocardiography and Doppler color flow mapping identify the need for tricuspid valve repair? J Am Coll Cardiol 1989; 14: 1266–1274.

These techniques help identify patients who will need tricuspid valve repair during mitral or aortic valve surgery.

Foster GP, Isselbacher EM, Rose GA, *et al.* Accurate localization of mitral regurgitant defects using multiplane transesophageal echocardiography. Ann Thorac Surg 1998; 65: 1025–1031.

TEE helps to localize mitral regurgitant lesions and helps preoperatively to assess in anticipation of repair.

Gewertz BL, Dremser PC, Zarins CK, *et al.* Transesophageal echocardiographic monitoring of myocardial ischemia during vascular surgery. J Vasc Surgery 1987; 5: 607.

TEE was quickly noted to help in monitoring during vascular surgical procedures.

Jebara VA, *et al.* Left ventricular outflow tract obstruction after mitral valve repair: results of the sliding leaflet technique. Circulation 1993; 88(part 2): 30–34.

Risks for dynamic LV outflow obstruction and prevention are discussed by Dr Carpentier's group in this well-illustrated paper.

Kochar GS, Jacobs LE, Kotler MN. Right atrial compression in postoperative cardiac patients: detection by transesophageal echocardiography. J Am Coll Cardiol 1990; 16: 511–516.

Description and illustrations of postcardiac surgery localized tamponade from a clot within the pericardium, adjacent to the right atrium.

Lee KS, *et al.* Mechanism of outflow tract obstruction causing failed mitral valve repair: anterior displacement of leaflet coaptation. Circulation 1993; 88(part 2): 24–29.

Discussion and diagrams of post mitral valve repair dynamic LV outflow tract obstruction, from the group at the Cleveland Clinics.

Maslow AD, Regan MM, Haering JM, Johnson RG, Levine RA. Echocardiographic predictors of left ventricular outflow tract obstruction and systolic anterior motion of the mitral valve after mitral valve reconstruction for myxomatous valve disease. J Am Coll Cardiol 1999; 34: 2096–2104.

TEE analysis of the mitral apparatus can identify patients at risk for postoperative SAM and LVOT obstruction. The lengths of the coapted anterior and posterior leaflets and the distance from the coaptation point to the ventricular septum appear to be useful measures.

Recommendations of the American Society of Echocardiography Council for Intraoperative Echocardiography and the Society of Cardiovascular Anesthesiologists Task Force for Certification in Perioperative Transesophageal Echocardiography. ASE/SCA guidelines for performing a comprehensive intraoperative multiplane transesophageal echocardiography examination. J Am Soc Echocardiogr 1999; 12: 884–900.

Each physician performing TEEs, especially in the OR, should read this manuscript, and have it accessible for reference.

Stewart WJ, Currie PJ, Salcedo EE, *et al.* Evaluation of mitral leaflet motion by echocardiography and jet direction by Doppler color flow mapping to determine the mechanism of mitral regurgitation. J Am Coll Cardiol 1992; 20: 1353–1361.

Discussion of the mechanisms of mitral regurgitation and echo findings prior to surgical repair.

Uva MS, *et al.* Transposition of chordae in mitral valve repair. Circulation 1993; 88(part 2): 35–38.

Dr Carpentier's group discusses and illustrates the technique of chordal transfer for repair of anterior mitral leaflet prolapse.

Yeo TC, Freeman WK, Schaff HV, Orszulak TA. Mechanisms of hemolysis after mitral valve repair: assessment by serial echocardiography. J Am Coll Cardiol 1998; 32: 717–723.

Color Doppler identified high shear stress in patients with significant hemolysis post mitral valve repair. The majority (92%) were not detected during intraoperative postbypass TEE after the initial mitral repair, but developed in the early postoperative period.

Chapter 16

Ammash N, Seward JB, Warnes CA, *et al.* Partial anomalous pulmonary venous connection: diagnosis by transesophageal echocardiogaphy. J Am Coll Cardiol 1997; 29: 1351–1358.
Discussion of various forms of anomalous pulmonary venous return, with drawings and echo images.

Child JS. Echocardiographic assessment of adults with tetralogy of Fallot. Echocardiography 1993; 10: 629.
Echocardiographic evaluation before and after surgical repair.

Cooke JC, Gelman JS, Harper RW. Echocardiologists' role in the deployment of the Amplatzer atrial septal occluder device in adults. J Am Soc Echocardiogr 2001; 14: 588–594.
Description and illustrations of the echocardiographer's role in deployment of the Amplatzer device for closure of atrial septal defects.

Cyran SE. Coarctation of the aorta in the adolescent and adult: echocardiographic evaluation prior to and following surgical repair. Echocardiography 1993; 10: 553.
A discussion of the evaluation both pre- and postoperatively, and long-term followup of patients with coarctation of the aorta.

Hijazi ZM, Cao QL, Heitschmidt M, Lang R. Residual inferior atrial septal defect after surgical repair: closure under intracardiac echocardiographic guidance. J Invasive Cardiol 2001; 13: 810–811. Comment by P Syamasundar Rao: 812.
A case of a residual inferior ASD that was diagnosed by intracardiac echocardiography (ICE) and missed by TEE twice is presented. Excellent TEE and ICE images are shown.

Humes RA, Hagler DJ, Julsrud PR, *et al.* Aortico-left ventricular tunnel: diagnosis based on two-dimensional echocardiography, color flow Doppler imaging, and magnetic resonance imaging. Mayo Clin Proc 1986; 61: 901–907.
Echocardiographic and MRI aspects of this disorder is presented in a 10-month-old infant.

King TD, Mills NL. Nonoperative closure of atrial septal defects. Surgery 1974; 75: 383–388.
First report of percutaneous closure of an ASD.

Mulhern KM, Skorton DJ. Echocardiographic evaluation of isolated pulmonary valve disease in adolescents and adults. Echocardiography 1993; 10: 533.
The echo evaluation of the right ventricular outflow tract and pulmonic valve before and after surgical correction.

O'Murchu B, Seward JB. Adult congenital heart disease: obstructive and nonobstructive cor triatriatum. Circulation (Images Cardiovasc Med) 1995; 92: 3574.
TEE images of cor triatriatum.

Pascoe RD, Oh JK, Warnes CA, *et al.* Diagnosis of sinus venosus atrial septal defect with transesophageal echocardiography. Circulation 1996; 94: 1049–1055.
TEE images of superior sinus venosus ASD.

Rahko PS. Doppler echocardiographic evaluation of ventricular septal defects in adults. Echocardiography 1993; 10: 517.
The echocardiographic findings and classification of VSDs are discussed.

Reller MD, McDonald RW, Gerlis LM, Thornburg KL. Cardiac embryology: basic review and clinical correlations. J Am Soc Echocardiogr 1991; 4: 519–532.
Illustrations and text present cardiac embryology. This is helpful in understanding congenital heart defects.

Salaymeh KJ, Taeed R, Michelfelder EC, *et al.* Unique echocardiographic features associated with deployment of the Amplatzer atrial septal defect device. J Am Soc Echocardiogr 2001; 14: 128–137.
Discussion and illustrations of deployment of the Amplatzer device. Complications and inadequate anatomy for device deployment are also discussed.

Seward JB. Ebstein's anomaly: ultrasound imaging and hemodynamic evaluation. Echocardiography 1993; 10: 641.

A discussion of the various anatomic abnormalities, and discussion of intra- and post-operative evaluation.

Staffen RN, Davidson WR. Echocardiographic assessment of atrial septal defects. Echocardiography 1993; 10: 545.
The echocardiographic evaluation of a patient with a known or suspected atrial septal defect.

Chapter 17

Agmon Y, Khandheria BK, Gentile F, Seward JB. Echocardiographic assessment of the left atrial appendage. J Am Coll Cardiol 1999; 34: 1867–1877.
Illustrations and discussion of LAA anatomy and LAA flow patterns.

Bakris N, Tighe DA, Rousou JA, *et al.* Nonobstructive membranes of the left atrial appendage cavity: report of three cases. J Am Soc Echocardiogr 2002; 15: 267–270.
Membranes may rarely traverse the LAA, and may be obstructive or nonobstructive.

Chen C, Koschyk D, Hamm C, *et al.* Usefulness of transesophageal echocardiography in identifying small left ventricular apical thrombus. J Am Coll Cardiol 1993; 21: 208–215.
TEE may be of benefit to evaluate for LV thrombus in TTE studies that reveal unclear structures or are acoustically difficult.

Cohen A, Tzourio C, Bertrand B, *et al.* Aortic plaque morphology and vascular events: a follow-up study in patients with ischemic stroke. Circulation 1997; 96: 3838–3841.
Patients with stroke were studied by TEE. Those with aortic atheroma >4 mm or without plaque calcification were at highest risk of further arterial events.

Davila-Roman V, Phillips KJ, Daily BB, *et al.* Intraoperative transesophageal echocardiography and epiaortic ultrasound for assessment of atherosclerosis of the thoracic aorta. J Am Coll Cardiol 1996; 28: 942–947.
Epiaortic ultrasound appears to be superior to TEE for identification of ascending aortic atherosclerosis, but both techniques are superior to direct palpation. Both ultrasound techniques provide complementary information.

Di Salvo, G, Habib G, Pergola V, *et al.* Echocardiography predicts embolic events in infective endocarditis. J Am Coll Cardiol 2001; 37: 1069–1076.
Staphyloccus organism, right-sided infection, vegetations >15 mm and those that were mobile were associated with a high incidence of embolism.

Falk RH. Medical progress: atrial fibrillation. N Engl J Med 2001; 344: 1067–1078.
A review of atrial fibrillation and its management.

Fatkin D, Kelly RP, Feneley MP. Relations between left atrial appendage blood flow velocity, spontaneous echocardiographic contrast and thromboembolic risk in vivo. J Am Coll Cardiol 1994; 23: 961–969.
Categorizes types of LAA flow in normal sinus rhythm and atrial fibrillation, and identifies SEC as strongly associated with LAA thrombus.

Fatkin D, Kuchar DL, Thorburn CW, Feneley MP. Transesophageal echocardiography before and during direct current cardioversion of atrial fibrillation: evidence for "atrial stunning" as a mechanism of thromboembolic complications. J Am Coll Cardiol 1994; 23: 307–316.
Describes and illustrates SEC formation and clot formation within the LA and left atrial appendage after electrical cardioversion.

Ferrari E, Vidal R, Chevallier T, Baudouy M. Atherosclerosis of the thoracic aorta and aortic debris as a marker of poor prognosis: benefit of oral anticoagulants. J Am Coll Cardiol 1999; 33: 1317–1322.
Patients with protruding aortic atheroma (>4 mm) are at increased risk of embolization, and those treated with coumadin have a better outcome than those treated with antiplatelet agents.

Foale RA, Gibson TC, Guyer DE, *et al.* Congenital aneurysms of the left atrium: recognition by cross-sectional echocardiography. Circulation 1982; 66: 1065–1069.
Echocardiograms with drawings of various LA aneurysms are presented. They may arise as aneuryms of the LA or the left atrial appendage.

Ha JW, Kang WC, Chung N, *et al.* Echocardiographic and morphologic characteristics of left atrial myxoma and their relation to systemic embolism. Am J Cardiol 1999; 83: 1579–1582.

This paper identifies polypoid, prolapsing myxomas as the type most associated with embolization.

Katz ES, Tsiamtsiouris T, Applebaum RM, *et al.* Surgical left atrial appendage ligation is frequently incomplete: a transesophageal echocardiographic study. J Am Coll Cardiol 2000; 36: 468–471.

Description with illustrations and discussion of possible risk of embolic events.

Katz ES, Tunick PA, Rusinek H, *et al.* Protruding aortic atheromas predict stroke in elderly patients undergoing cardiopulmonary bypass: experience with intraoperative transesophageal echocardiography. J Am Coll Cardiol 1992; 20: 70–77.

Description of aortic atheroma and a grading scale for embolic risk.

Kerut EK, Norfleet WT, Plotnick GD, Giles TD. Patent foramen ovale: a review of associated conditions and the impact of physiological Size. J Am Coll Cardiol 2001; 38: 613–623.

Anatomical and functional size of a PFO probably is important in evaluating patients in the context of platypnea-orthodeoxia, stroke, and decompression sickness in underwater divers and aviators/astronauts.

Klarich KW, Enriquez-Sarano M, Gura GM, *et al.* Papillary fibroelastoma: echocardiographic characteristics for diagnosis and pathologic correlation. J Am Coll Cardiol 1997; 30: 784–790.

Discussion of echocardiographic characteristics and clinical correlates.

Klein AL, Grimm RA, Murray RD, *et al.* Use of transesophageal echocardiography to guide cardioversion in patients with atrial fibrillation. N Engl J Med 2001; 344: 1411–1420. Accompanying editorial by Silverman DI and Manning WJ, pp. 1469–1470.

Report of the ACUTE trial and recommendations from that study.

Lanzarotti CJ, Olshansky B. Thromboembolism in chronic atrial flutter: is the risk underestimated? J Am Coll Cardiol 1997; 30: 1506–1511.

Chronic atrial flutter is associated with thromboembolism, both during flutter and after cardioversion.

Lund GK, Schroder S, Koschyk DH, Nienaber CA. Echocardiographic diagnosis of papillary fibroelastoma of the mitral and tricuspid valve apparatus. Clin Cardiol 1997; 20: 175–177.

Two case reports and a discussion of papillary fibroelastomas.

Mas JL, Arquizan C, Lamy C, *et al.* Recurrent cerebrovascular events associated with patent foramen ovale, atrial septal aneurysm, or both. N Engl J Med 2001; 345: 1740–1746.

Patients with a patent foramen ovale and an atrial septal aneurysm who have had a stroke are at markedly increased risk of another event. Those patients with patent foramen ovale but without an atrial septal aneurysm appear to be at a much lower risk of a recurrent event.

Movsowitz C, Podolsky LA, Meyerowitz CB, *et al.* Patent foramen ovale: a nonfunctional embryological remnant or a potential cause of significant pathology? J Am Soc Echocardiogr 1992; 5: 259–270.

A review of embryology and associated pathologies with patent foramen ovale.

Mugge A, Daniel WG, Angermann C, *et al.* Atrial septal aneurysm in adult patients: a multicenter study using transthoracic and transesophageal echocardiography. Circulation 1995; 91: 2785–2792.

TEE is best for ASA diagnosis. ASA is associated with PFO and embolic events.

Roldan CA, Shively BK, Crawford MH. Valve excrescences: prevalence, evolution and risk for cardioembolism. J Am Coll Cardiol 1997; 30: 1308–1314. Accompanying editorial: Armstrong WF, pp. 1315–1316.

In this study excrescences were frequent findings and did not appear to be a primary source of cardioembolism.

Rubin DC, Burch C, Plotnick GD, Hawke MW. The relationship between complex intraaortic debris and extrcranial carotid artery disease in patients with stroke. Am Heart J 1993; 126: 233.

The relationship found between carotid disease and aortic atheroma points out the possibility of the aorta as a source of embolic events.

Rubin DC, Hawke MW, Plotnick GD. Relationship between mitral annular calcification and complex intraaortic debris. Am J Cardiol 1993; 71: 1251.

Demonstration of the relationship of MAC with aortic atheroma.

Schneider B, Hofmann, Justen MH, Meinertz T. Chiari's network: normal anatomic variant or risk factor for arterial embolic events? J Am Coll Cardiol 1995; 26: 203–210.
Defines the Chiari network and its association with patent foramen ovale and an increased embolic risk.

Shirani J, Zafari AM, Roberts WC. Morphologic features of fossa ovalis membrane aneurysm in the adult and its clinical significance. J Am Coll Cardiol 1995; 26: 466–471.
Aneurysm of the fossa ovalis is not associated with thrombus or fibrin. Associated is mitral valve prolapse, dilated atria, intracardiac thrombi, and patent foramen ovale, which may explain the increased frequency of embolic stroke in patients with these aneurysms.

Song JM, Kang DH, Song JK, *et al.* Clinical significance of echo-free space detected by transesophageal echocardiography in patients with type b aortic intramural hematoma. Am J Cardiol 2002; 89: 548–551.
An echo free space (EFS) is often found within the wall of a aortic intramural hematoma (AIH). Often these will enhance when evaluated by contrast-enhanced computed tomography. An EFS does not appear to affect the prognosis of type B AIH, in that it appears that a similar number will progress to aortic dissection and a similar number resorb, as compared to patients with type B AIH without an EFS. This paper is well illustrated.

Stollberger C, Slany J, Schuster I, *et al.* The prevalence of deep venous thrombosis in patients with suspected paradoxical embolism. Ann Intern Med 1993; 119: 461–465.
In patients with patent foramen ovale and embolic events, occult leg venous thrombosis is relatively common (24 of 42 cases).

Thamilarasan M, Klein AL. Transesophageal echocardiography (TEE) in atrial fibrillation. Cardiol Clin 2000; 18: 819–831.
Atrial fibrillation and the role of TEE in its management.

Tunick PA, Nayar AC, Goodkin GM, *et al.* Effect of treatment on the incidence of stroke and other emboli in 519 patients with severe thoracic aortic plaque. Am J Cardiol 2002; 90: 1320–1325.
A retrospective evaluation of patients with severe thoracic plaque (>4 mm thickness) found that coumadin and also aspirin had no effect on the incidence of recurrent stroke and other embolic events, but statin therapy provided significant protection from recurrent events.

Vaduganathan P, Ewton A, Nagueh SF, *et al.* Pathologic correlates of aortic plaques, thrombi and mobile "aortic debris" imaged in vivo with transesophageal echocardiography. J Am Coll Cardiol 1997; 30: 357–363.
Pathologic description of atheroma, which were found to be thrombi.

Vargas-Barron J, Espinola-Zavaleta N, Roldan FJ, *et al.* Transesophageal echocardiographic diagnosis of thrombus in accessory lobes of the left atrial appendage. Echocardiography 2000; 17: 689–691.
Several cases presented demonstrate the need to carefully evaluate the LAA for thrombus.

Chapter 18

Afridi I, Apostolidou MA, Saad RM, Zoghbi WA. Pseudoaneurysms of the mitral-aortic intervalvular fibrosa: dynamic characterization using transesophageal echocardiographic and Doppler techniques. J Am Coll Cardiol 1995; 25: 137–145.
Pseudoaneurysm of the mitral-aortic intervalvular fibrosa (MAIVF) are more often diagnosed by TEE than by TTE or aortography. Typical Doppler features are discussed.

Bansal RC, Graham BM, Jutzy KR, *et al.* Left ventricular outflow tract to left atrial communication secondary to rupture of mitral-aortic intervalvular fibrosa in infective endocarditis: diagnosis by transesophageal echocardiography and color flow imaging. J Am Coll Cardiol 1990; 15: 499–504.
Description and illustrations of MAIVF communication to the LA, and also ruptured mitral leaflet aneurysm.

Bayer AS, Bolger AF, Tauber KA, *et al.* Diagnosis and management of infective endocarditis and its complications. Circulation 1998; 98: 2936–2948.
Description of the Duke criteria and outline of TTE and TEE indications.

De Castro S, Magni G, Beni S. Role of transthoracic and transesophageal echocardiography in predicting embolic events in patients with active infective endocarditis involving native cardiac valves. Am J Cardiol 1997; 80: 1030–1034.
This group failed to find any feature of a vegetation that would predict an embolic event.

Di Salvo G, Habib, G, Pergola V. Echocardiography predicts embolic events in infective endocarditis. J Am Coll Cardiol 2001; 37: 1069–1076.
From this study, early surgery may be indicated for patients with vegetations >15 mm and that are highly mobile.

Durack DT, Lukes AS, Bright DK, *et al.* New criteria for diagnosis of infective endocarditis: utilization of specific echocardiographic findings. Am J Med 1994; 96: 200–209.
Presentation of the Duke criteria for diagnosis of infective endocarditis.

Ferrieri P, Gewitz MH, Gerber MA, *et al.* Unique features of infective endocarditis in childhood. Pediatrics 2002; 109: 931–943.
A discussion of infective endocarditis with particular emphasis on unique aspects in the pediatric population.

Graupner C, Vilacosta I, San Roman JA, *et al.* Periannular extension of infective endocarditis. J Am Coll Cardiol 2002; 39: 1204–1211.
Risk factors for periannular complications include aortic infection, prosthetic endocarditis, new atrio-ventricular (AV) block, and coagulase-negative staphylococci. There appears to be no difference in vegetation size or embolism frequency in those with or without periannular complications.

Habib G, Derumeaux G, Avierinos JF, *et al.* Value and limitations of the Duke criteria for the diagnosis of infective endocarditis. J Am Coll Cardiol 1999; 33: 2023–2039.
Adding value to echo criteria in patients with prior antibiotic therapies and typical echo findings with serologic diagnosis of Q fever would improve the Duke classification for diagnosis of IE.

Joffe II, Jacobs LE, Owen AN, *et al.* Noninfective valvular masses: review of the literature with emphasis on imaging techniques and management. Am Heart J 1996; 131: 1175–1183.
A review of lesions that may be confused with infective endocarditis, including systemic lupus erythematosus, primary antiphospholipid syndrome, nonbacterial thrombotic endocarditis, and tumors.

Karalis DG, Bansal RC, Hauck AJ, *et al.* Transesophageal echocardiographic recognition of subaortic complications in aortic valve endocarditis: clinical and surgical implications. Circulation 1992; 86: 353–362.
Subaortic involvement in patients with aortic valve endocarditis may be more common than previously thought. Recognition of these complications by TEE affects the surgical management of these patients.

Mathew J, Gasior R, Thannoli N. Fungal mass on the tricuspid valve. Circulation (Images Cardiovasc Med) 1996; 94: 2040.
A TEE and pathologic image of a large fungal vegetation involving the tricuspid valve.

Reisner SA, Brenner B, Haim N, *et al.* Echocardiography in nonbacterial thrombotic endocarditis: from autopsy to clinical entity. J Am Soc Echocardiogr 2000; 13: 876–881.
The prevalence and echocardiographic findings of nonbacterial thrombotic endocarditis (bacteria-free verrucae) are discussed.

Ryan EW, Bolger AF. Transesophageal echocardiography (TEE) in the evaluation of infective endocarditis, in transesophageal echocardiography (Foster E, guest ed). Cardiol Clin 2000; 18: 773–787.
TEE and its use in IE.

Sanfilippo AJ, Picard MH, Newell JB, *et al.* Echocardiographic assessment of patients with infectious endocarditis: prediction of risk for complications. J Am Coll Cardiol 1991; 18: 1191–1199.
With native left-sided endocarditis, size extent, mobility, and consistency appear to be independent predictors of complications.

San Roman JA, Vilacosta I, Zamorano JL, *et al.* Transesophageal echocardiography in right-sided endocarditis. J Am Coll Cardiol 1993; 21: 1226–1230.

TEE does not appear to improve the diagnostic yield of TTE in the detection of vegetations associated with right-sided endocarditis in intravenous drug abusers.

Shively BK, Gurule FT, Roldan CA, *et al.* Diagnostic value of transesophageal compared with transthoracic echocardiography in infective endocarditis. J Am Coll Cardiol 1991; 18: 391–397.
TEE is sensitive and specific for diagnosis of IE, and more sensitive than TTE.

Vilacosta I, Sarria C, San Roman JA, *et al.* Usefulness of transesophageal echocardiography for diagnosis of infected transvenous permanent pacemakers. Circulation 1994; 89: 2684–2687.
TEE appears to be superior to TTE for detection of pacemaker lead vegetations.

Chapter 19

Agrawal G, LaMotte LC, Nanda NC, Parekh HH. Identification of the aortic arch branches using transesophageal echocardiography. Echocardiography 1997; 14: 461–466.

Appelbe AF, Walker PG, Yeoh JK, *et al.* Clinical significance and origin of artifacts in transesophageal echocardiography of the thoracic aorta. J Am Coll Cardiol 1993; 21: 754–760.
Artifacts are a frequent occurrence during TEE when imaging the aorta. This is a excellent well-illustrated discussion of how to recognize them.

Avegliano G, Evangelista A, Elorz C, *et al.* Acute peripheral arterial ischemia and suspected aortic dissection: usefulness of transesophageal echocardiography in differential diagnosis with aortic thrombosis. Am J Cardiol 2002; 90; 674–677.
Aortic thrombosis may appear as an aortic dissection by CT, but be correctly identified by TEE. TEE may be necessary for a correct diagnosis when a patient presents with acute peripheral ischemia, even if CT suggests dissection.

Bansal RC, Chandrasekaran K, Ayala K, Smith DC. Frequency and explanation of false negative diagnosis of aortic dissection by aortography and transesophageal echocardiography. J Am Coll Cardiol 1995; 25: 1393–1401.
Discussion of dissection and intramural hematoma (IMH). Aortography will miss IMH, and TEE may miss localized type II dissections in the upper ascending aorta because the trachea-left main stem bronchus lies between the esophagus and aorta at that level.

Blanchard DG, Sobel JL, Hope J, *et al.* Infrahepatic interruption of the inferior vena cava with azygos continuation: a potential mimicker of aortic pathology. J Am Soc Echocardiogr 1998; 11: 1078–1083.
A case presentation demonstrating how a prominent azygos system may mimic aortic rupture.

Bluth EI, LoCascio L. Ultrasonic evaluation of the abdominal aorta. Echocardiography 1996; 13: 197–205.
Review of the technique of scanning the abdominal aorta, and diagnosis of abdominal aortic aneurysms.

Chan KL. Usefulness of transesophageal echocardiography in the diagnosis of conditions mimicking aortic dissection. Am Heart J 1991; 122: 495–504.
Aortic disease is relatively common in patients suspected of having aortic dissection in whom it has been excluded.

Elefteriades JA (guest ed). Diseases of the aorta. Cardiol Clin 1999; 17(4).
This issue of the Cardiology Clinics covers many aspects of the thoracic aorta, including penetrating ulcers and intramural hematoma.

Flachskampf FA, Daniel WG. Aortic dissection, in Transesophageal echocardiography (Foster E, guest ed). Cardiol Clin 2000; 18: 807–817.
Illustrations and discussion of the role of TEE in diagnosis of aortic dissection with its complications.

Flachskampf FA, Banbury M, Smedira N, Thomas JD, Garcia M. Transesophageal echocardiography diagnosis of intramural hematoma of the ascending aorta: a word of caution. J Am Soc Echocardiogr 1999; 12: 866–870.
Two cases of IMH of the ascending aorta that were difficult to diagnose by TEE. CT or MRI may help the diagnostic accuracy.

Goldstein SA, Mintz GS, Lindsay J. Aorta: comprehensive evaluation by echocardiography and transesophageal echocardiography. J Am Soc Echocardiogr 1993; 6: 634–659.

Evaluation of the aorta in a systematic fashion and discussion of dissection, thoracic aneurysms, IMH, and traumatic blunt injury.

Ionescu AA, Vinereanu D, Wood A, Fraser AG. Periaortic fat pad mimicking an intramural hematoma of the thoracic aorta: lessons for transesophageal echocardiography. J Am Soc Echocardiogr 1998; 11: 487–490.
Case report of what appeared to be an IMH by TEE, but MRI helped make the diagnosis of a periaortic fat pad.

Janssen M, Breburda CS, van Geuns RJM, *et al.* Aberrant right subclavian artery mimics aortic dissection. Circulation (Images Cardiovasc Med) 2000; 101: 459–460.
Illustration of an aberrant right subclavian artery originating from the descending aorta that mimicked a localized aortic dissection of the transverse aorta. Discussion of how to avoid this potential pitfall.

Januzzi JL, Sabatine MS, Eagle KA, *et al.* Iatrogenic aortic dissection. Am J Cardiol 2002; 89: 623–626.
One should consider iatrogenic aortic dissection especially in patients with unexplained hemodynamic instability or myocardial ischemia following an invasive vascular procedure or coronary artery bypass surgery (CABG).

Keren A, Kim CB, Hu BS, *et al.* Accuracy of biplane and multiplane transesophageal echocardiography in diagnosis of typical acute aortic dissection and intramural hematoma. J Am Coll Cardiol 1996; 28: 627–636.
A presentation of the difficulty at times when evaluating a patient for acute aortic pathology. TEE sensitivity and specificity for acute aortic dissection is 98% and 95%, sensitivity and specificity for IMH was 90% and 99%. A discussion and illustrations of two false-positive TEEs for type A are presented.

Kronzon I (guest ed). Imaging of the aorta. Echocardiography 1996; 13: 165–256.
A collection of review papers covering aspects of imaging the thoracic and abdominal aorta, along with aortic atherosclerosis, aortic trauma, dissection, and thoracic aortic aneurysms.

Mohr-Kahaly S, Erbel R, Kearney P, Puth M, Meyer J. Aortic intramural hemorrhage visualized by transesophageal echocardiography: findings and prognostic implications. J Am Coll Cardiol 1994; 23: 658–664.
IMH and its diagnosis by TEE

Montgomery DH, Ververis JJ, McGorisk G, *et al.* Natural history of severe atheromatous disease of the thoracic aorta: a transesophageal echocardiographic study. J Am Coll Cardiol 1996; 27: 95–101.
Severe atherosclerosis of the aorta is associated with a high mortality rate. Over 1 year, lesions appeared to resolve and new ones form.

Movsowitz HD, Levine RA, Hilgenberg AD, Isselbacher EM. Transesophageal echocardiographic description of the mechanisms of aortic regurgitation in acute type A aortic dissection: implications for aortic valve repair. J Am Coll Cardiol 2000; 36: 884–890.
Discussion and TEE images of the aortic valve and various mechanisms for aortic regurgitation in dissection.

Nienaber CA, von Kodolitsch Y, Petersen B, *et al.* Intramural hemorrhage of the thoracic aorta. Diagnostic and therapeutic implications. Circulation 1995; 92: 1465–1472.
Comprehensive discussion and CT images are presented.

Robbins RC, McManus RP, Mitchell RS, *et al.* Management of patients with intramural hematoma of the thoracic aorta. Circulation 1993; 88 (part 2): 1–10.
MRI images of IMH and discussion of management.

Song JK, Kim HS, Kang DH, *et al.* Different clinical features of aortic intramural hematoma versus dissection involving the ascending aorta. J Am Coll Cardiol 2001; 37: 1604–1610.
Aortic intramural hematoma was associated with an older patient and female gender as compared to aortic dissection. Mediastinal hemorrhage and pericardial and pleural effusions were more frequent in AIH than AD, but in those that received medical therapy only, the AIH patient had a better prognosis that AD (6% vs. 58% mortality rate).

Svensson LG, Labib SB, Eisenhauer AC, Butterly JR. Intimal tear without hematoma: an important variant of aortic dissection that can elude current imaging techniques. Circulation 1999; 99: 1331–1336.
More than one imaging modality may be needed to help diagnose small localized dissections, especially of the ascending aorta.

Tacy TA, Silverman NH. Systemic venous abnormalities: embryologic and echocardiographic considerations. Echocardiography 2001; 18: 401–413.
Embryology and echo correlation of the SVC, IVC, CS, and innominate vein

Vilacosta I, San Roman JA, Aragoncillo P, *et al.* Penetrating atherosclerotic aortic ulcer: documentation by transesophageal echocardiography. J Am Coll Cardiol 1998; 32: 83–89.
Discussion and illustrations of penetrating atherosclerotic aortic ulcer.

Chapter 20

Adam M. Pitfalls in the echocardiographic diagnosis of intracardiac and extracardiac masses. Echocardiography 1993; 10: 181.
Masses and their differential diagnosis including normal variants.

Atilgan D, Kudat H, Tukek T, *et al.* Role of transesophageal echocardiography in diagnosis and management of cardiac hydatid cyst: report of three cases and review of the literature. J Am Soc Echocardiogr 2002; 15: 271–274.
A illustrated paper with a discussion of hydatid cyst of the heart.

Chen YT, Kan MN, Chen JS, *et al.* Transesophageal two-dimensional echocardiography for detection of left atrial masses. Am J Noninvas Cardiol 1989; 3: 337.
Discussion and illustrations of masses noted within the left atrium.

D'Cruz IA, Hancock HL. Echocardiographic characteristics of diaphragmatic hiatus hernia. Am J Cardiol 1995; 75: 308.
Images and discussion of diagnostic features of hiatal hernia.

D'Cruz IA, *et al.* Echocardiographic manifestations of mediastinal masses compressing or encroaching on the heart. Echocardiography 1994; 11: 523.
A review of how TEE helps in evaluation of mediastinal masses.

Keren A, Billingham ME, Popp RL. Echocardiographic recognition and implications of ventricular hypertrophic trabeculations and aberrant bands. Circulation 1984; 70: 836–842.
Echocardiographic and pathologic correlates of ventricular bands and trabeculations.

Keren A, Billingham ME, Popp RL. Echocardiographic recognition of paraseptal structures. J Am Coll Cardiol 1985; 6: 913–919.
Echocardiographic illustrations with pathologic specimens describing right paraseptal structures.

Kmetzo J, Peters RW, Plotnick GD, *et al.* Left atrial mass: thrombus mimicking myxoma. Chest 1985; 88: 906.
An unusual case detected by transthoracic echocardiography.

Luetmer PH, Edwards WD, Seward JB, Tajik AJ. Incidence and distribution of left ventricular false tendons: an autopsy study of 483 normal human hearts. J Am Coll Cardiol 1986; 8: 179–183
Autopsy description and illustrations of LV false tendons.

Nishimura RA, Tajik AJ, Schattenberg TT, Seward JB. Diaphragmatic hernia mimicking an atrial mass: a two-dimensional echocardiographic pitfall. J Am Coll Cardiol 1985; 5: 992–995.
Echo features of diaphragmatic hernia are presented.

Normeir AM, Watts LE, Seagle R, *et al.* Intracardiac myxomas: twenty-year echocardiographic experience with review of the literature. J Am Soc Echocardiogr 1989; 2: 139.
A concise discussion of myxomas.

Plotnick GD. A mass in the apex (echocardiographic quiz). Choices Cardiol 1994; 8: 41.
An example of a left ventricular apical thrombus with a good discussion of the differential diagnosis.

Roberts WC. Primary and secondary neoplasms of the heart. Am J Cardiol 1997; 80: 671–682.
Pathologic discussion and illustrations of cardiac tumors.

Rubin DC, Ziskind AA, Hawke MW, Plotnick GD. TEE guided percutaneous biopsy of a right atrial cardiac mass. Am Heart J 1994; 127: 935.
Discussion and illustration of use of TEE to help guide percutaneous biopsy of a right atrial mass.

Schnittger I. Cardiac and extracardiac masses: echocardiographic evaluation. In: Marcus ML, Schelbert HR, Skorton DJ, *et al.* Cardiac Imaging: a companion to Braunwald's Heart Disease. Philadelphia: WB Saunders, 1991: 511.
A discussion of both cardiac and extracardiac masses.

Shirani J, Roberts WC. Clinical electrocardiographic, and morphologic features of massive fatty deposits, "lipomatous hypertrophy", in the atrial septum. J Am Coll Cardiol 1993; 22: 226.
This is an excellent anatomic study with many photographs of specimens.

Straus R, Merliss R. Primary tumors of the heart. Arch Pathol 1945; 39: 74.
This historical paper discusses the pathology of cardiac primary tumors.

Voros S, Nanda NC, Thakur AC, Winokur TS, Samal AD. Lambl's excrescences (valvular strands). Echocardiography 1999; 16: 399–414.
A review with illustrations describing the echocardiographic and histologic features of Lambl's excrescences. The differential diagnosis is well discussed, followed by clinical implications.

Chapter 21

Ansari A, Maron BJ. Cardiovascular disease in ankylosing (Marie–Strumpell) spondylitis. Circulation (Images Cardiovasc Med) 1997; 96: 2585–2586.
X-ray, EKG, and echo features of ankylosing spondylitis are presented in this case.

Aupetit JF, Ritz B, Ferrini M, *et al.* Hydatid cyst of the interventricular septum. Circulation (Images Cardiovasc Med) 1997; 95: 2325–2326.
Presentation of a case and illustrations of a cystic-appearing hydatid cyst involving the interventricular septum.

Burstow DJ, Tajik AJ, Bailey KR, *et al.* Two-dimensional echocardiographic findings in systemic sarcoidosis. Am J Cardiol 1989; 63: 478–482.
Approximately 14% of patients had echo evidence of LV systolic dysfunction, with two-thirds having segmental hypokinesis, and the other third global hypokinesis.

Child JS, Perloff JK, Bach PM, *et al.* Cardiac involvement in Friedreich's ataxia: a clinical study of 75 patients. J Am Coll Cardiol 1986; 7: 1370–1378.
Description of electrocardiographic and echo features of this disorder. A pathologic specimen is also illustrated.

Connolly HM, Crary JL, *et al.* Valvular heart disease associated with fenfluramine-phentermine. N Engl J Med 1997; 337: 581–588.
The original description of valvular disease associated with fenfluramine-phentermine.

Dominguez FJ, Lopez de Sa E, Calvo L, *et al.* Two-dimensional echocardiographic features of echinococcosis of the heart and great blood vessels. Circulation 1988; 78: 327–337.
Description and illustrations of hydatid cysts affecting the heart or great vessels.

Frank MW, Mehlman DJ, Tsai F, *et al.* Syphilitic aortitis. Circulation (Images Cardiovasc Med) 1999; 100: 1582–1583.
TEE image of the ascending aorta along with CT scan and histologic findings in a patient with syphilitic aortitis.

Gardin JM, Siscovick D, Anton-Colver H. Sex, age and disease affect echocardiographic left ventricular mass and systolic function in the free living elderly: the Cardiovascular Health Study. Circulation 1995; 91: 1739–1748.
Expected LV mass as a function of sex and weight in the elderly.

Gerstenblith G, Frederiksen J, Yin FCP. Echocardiographic assessment of a normal adult aging population. Circulation 1977; 56: 273–277.
An M-mode evaluation of measurements of LV dimensions as normal individuals age.

Goldman ME, Cantor R, Schwartz MF, *et al.* Echocardiographic abnormalities and disease severity in Fabry's disease. J Am Coll Cardiol 1986; 7: 1157–1161.
Echocardiographic features are discussed.

Gottdiener JS, Panza JA, St John Sutton M, *et al.* Testing the test: the reliability of echocardiography in the sequential assessment of valvular regurgitation. Am Heart J 2002; 144: 115–121.
Variability exists in color interpretation of mitral and aortic regurgitation. A significant predictor of change was the initial grade, change in diastolic blood pressure, and variability in recording from day to day.

Henry WL, Gardin JM, Ware JH. Echocardiographic measurement in normal subjects from infancy to old age. Circulation 1980; 62: 1054–1061.
Left atrial and aortic root size increases normally with increasing age.

Joffe II, Jacobs LE, Owen AN, *et al.* Noninfective valvular masses: review of the literature with emphasis on imaging techniques and management. Am Heart J 1996; 131: 1175–1183.
Discussion and the contrasting features of Lambl's excrescences, systemic lupus erythematosus, primary antiphospholipid syndrome, nonbacterial thrombotic endocarditis, and several tumors are presented.

Katz AS, Sadaniantz A. Echocardiography in HIV cardiac disease. Prog Cardiovasc Dis 2003; 45: 285–292.
Review of echocardiographic findings in HIV infection, including pericardial effusion, myocarditis, dilated cardiomyopathy, endocarditis, pulmonary hypertension, tumors, and drug-related toxicity.

Markides V, Nihoyannopoulos P. Non-bacterial thrombotic endocarditis. Eur J Echocardiogr 2000; 1: 291–294.
Discussion of etiology and illustrations of NBTE, along with therapy.

Pandya UH, Pellikka PA, Enriquez-Sarano M, *et al.* Metastatic carcinoid tumor to the heart: echocardiographic–pathologic study of 11 patients. J Am Coll Cardiol 2002; 40: 1328–1332.
Although rare, metastatic lesions to the heart may be the only manifestation of carcinoid heart disease. These tumors appear intramyocardial and are well-circumscribed, noninfiltrating, and homogeneous in appearance.

Pearson AC, Grudipath CV, Labovitz AJ. Effects of aging left ventricular structure and function. Am Heart J 1991; 121: 871–873.
Increasing age is normally associated with increasing LV mass.

Pellikka PA, *et al.* Carcinoid heart disease: clinical and echocardiographic spectrum in 74 patients. Circulation 1993; 87: 1188.
A review of carcinoid involving not only the tricuspid and pulmonic valves, but the left heart and pericardium

Pritchett AM, Morrison JF, Edwards WD, *et al.* Valvular heart disease in patients taking pergolide. Mayo Clin Proc 2002; 77: 1280–1286.
Description of pergolide-associated valvular disease, along with echo and histologic images.

Reisner SA, Brenner B, Haim N, *et al.* Echocardiography in nonbacterial thrombotic endocarditis: from autopsy to clinical entity. J Am Soc Echocardiogr 2000; 13: 876–881.
This is a review with illustrations of NBTE.

Roberts WC. A unique heart disease associated with a unique cancer: carcinoid heart disease. Am Heart J 1997; 80: 251–256.
Discussion of the pathology and echocardiographic features of carcinoid.

Roldan CA, Chavez J, Wiest PW, *et al.* Aortic root disease and valve disease associated with ankylosing spondylitis. J Am Coll Cardiol 1998; 32: 1397–1404.
Echocardiographic features of aortic root and aortic valve involvement in this disorder.

Roldan CA, Gelgand EA, *et al.* Morphology of anorexigen-associated valve disease by transthoracic and transesophageal echocardiography. Am J Cardiol 2002; 90: 1269–1273.
Discussion with several illustrations of anorexigen-associated valvular disease.

Roldan CA, Shively BK, Crawford MH. An echocardiographic study of valvular heart disease associated with systemic lupus erythematosus. N Engl J Med 1996; 335: 1424–1430.

Valvular heart disease is commonly found in patients with SLE, and often changes over the course of time.

Roldan CA, Shively BK, Lau CC, *et al.* Systemic lupus erythematosus valve disease by transesophageal echocardiography and the role of antiphospholipid antibodies. J Am Coll Cardiol 1992; 20: 1127–1134.

Characterization of mitral and aortic valve lesions found in patients with SLE, both with and without antiphospholipid antibodies. This paper is well illustrated.

Schiller NB. Color me variable: the irreproducible nature of color flow Doppler in mitral and aortic regurgitation. Am Heart J 2002; 144: 5–7.

An editorial discussing the difficulty in reproducibility of left-sided valve regurgitation, measured using color Doppler.

Vasan RS, Shrivastava S, Vijayakumar M, *et al.* Echocardiographic evaluation of patients with acute rheumatic fever and rheumatic carditis. Circulation 1996; 94: 73–82.

A large cohort of patients (108) with acute rheumatic fever were evaluated by echocardiography. A description of cardiac and valvular function is provided.

Index

Note: Abbreviations used in subentries are the same as those listed on pages vii to x.